Medical Care of Refugees

Medical Care of Refugees

Edited by

Richard H. Sandler, M.D.
Division of Pediatric Gastroenterology and Nutrition
The Children's Hospital, and
The Massachusetts General Hospital
Harvard Medical School

Thomas C. Jones, M.D.
Division of International Medicine
Cornell University Medical College

New York Oxford
OXFORD UNIVERSITY PRESS
1987

Oxford University Press

Oxford New York Toronto
Delhi Bombay Calcutta Madras Karachi
Petaling Jaya Singapore Hong Kong Tokyo
Nairobi Dar es Salaam Cape Town
Melbourne Auckland

and associated companies in
Beirut Berlin Ibadan Nicosia

Published by Oxford University Press, Inc.,
200 Madison Avenue, New York, New York 10016

Oxford is a registered trademark of Oxford University Press

Library of Congress Cataloging-in-Publication Data

Medical care of refugees.

Includes bibliographies and index.
1. Refugees—Medical care—Developing countries—Handbooks, manuals, etc. 2. Communicable diseases—Developing countries—Prevention—Handbooks, manuals, etc. I. Sandler, Richard H., 1949- . II. Jones, Thomas C. (Thomas Clifford), 1937- . [DNLM: 1. Communicable Disease Control—handbooks. 2. Developing Countries—handbooks. 3. Refugees—handbooks. WA 39 M489]
RA564.9.R43M43 1987 616.9'09172'4 86-18274
ISBN 0-19-504181-X

9 8 7 6 5 4 3 2 1

Printed in the United States of America
on acid-free paper

Preface

"Scratch any headline," observed a former UN High Commissioner on Refugees, "and you will find refugees." With such ongoing problems as famines, political upheavals, earthquakes and wars, dislocation of large groups of people will remain a reality. Their medical needs are often great and *Medical Care of Refugees* should help by serving as a practical guide.

Although focused specifically on refugee medicine, this book should also be useful more generally for health care efforts in less developed nations. Written for those trained in "Western" countries, this book assumes that the reader has a limited background in tropical diseases or refugee medical care but is familiar with basic medical vocabulary and concepts at the level of a third or fourth year medical student.

For easy reference this book is divided into three parts: General considerations, medical specialty issues, and management of infectious diseases. Depending on the reader's background, some sections should be studied before going abroad. Other sections may be most useful as a practical guide in a clinical setting, or in helping plan or set up such services as a dental clinic, a rehabilitation facility, a minor surgery clinic, a tuberculosis surveillence system, or a small laboratory. It is important to note that although every effort has been made to ensure the accuracy of the drug dosage information provided here, the clinician should check other sources for possible errors or recent changes.

In preparing for refugee health care, one may first want to obtain the kind of overview that is presented in Chapters 1–3, 8–11, and 22; then scan specialty considerations as in the chapters on pediatrics, dental care, surgery, obstetrics, and ophthalmology; and finally direct attention to diagnosis and management of malnutrition, dehydration, and infectious diseases important in the area to be served. Review of the references before departure may point to special texts for use in specific situations. Some texts we consider particularly helpful are listed in Appendix A and as suggested reading at the end of Chapter 1.

We have observed and experienced the conflicts that arise among health workers in many refugee situations over how best to set the level of care. In acute refugee settings, abundant resources may be available initially, enabling delivery of a fairly intensive level of medical care. However, as discussed in Chapter 9, there are numerous factors weighing against that goal, such as the wishes of the host government, the likelihood of future shortages of resources, or a more pressing need for public health expenditures. We hope that those who find themselves confronting these obstacles will always press for the highest possible level of care.

Many of the medical problems of refugees are caused by poor nutrition, contaminated water, improper sanitation, poor organization of health care delivery, and other public health factors that must be addressed. Although public health issues are not the main focus of this book, the time, effort, and money spent to combat public health problems, as discussed here in Chapters 2, 3, and 9, can be very effective in reducing morbidity and mortality of refugees.

There is a definite need for training health care workers for their service abroad. The importance of prior training has been well stated by Jelliffe and Jelliffe: "The brutal fact is that a well-trained American or European physician or nurse, without past experience in developing countries, [or] without prior orientation, can have only a limited effect and may even prove a liability in refugee camps . . . These health workers are likely to be lost without the support of laboratories. Clinical approaches they have learned are often inappropriate for community health work . . . Common clinical problems such as chloroquine-resistant malaria, protein-energy malnutrition in young children, cholera, intestinal parasites, etc., are virtually unknown to them."* This book can

*Jelliffe DB, Jelliffe EF: Education for refugee health workers: The UCLA experience. Disasters 1983;7:8.

be useful as a training manual for health workers before they serve abroad, as a basic text in the refugee setting, or as a companion to a public health volume.

Implicit in the preparation of this book was the conviction that a body of knowledge concerning the particulars of refugee medical care could be summarized and used to help prepare others. This has been referred to as "institutional memory"—a resource too often neglected in the medical care of refugees. Those working with refugees sometimes reject "academic preparation" as being of limited value, but we believe that study and reassessment that combine an accurate information base with a clear focus on anticipated challenges are essential to providing optimal health care for refugees and others in less developed nations. We hope this book will contribute to that end.

Boston, Massachusetts R.H.S.
Basle, Switzerland T.C.J.
April 1987

Acknowledgments

A heartfelt thanks to all of the people whose efforts were required to make this book possible. We particularly appreciate the efforts of the 45 contributing authors who overcame formidable distances, postal barriers, and busy schedules to make their special contributions. Much gratitude is due the Cornell University Medical College, especially the Division of International Medicine and the Departments of Medicine and Public Health. Sincere appreciation goes to Betsy M. Chalfin, a contributor as well as our principal copyeditor and manuscript coordinator. Special thanks to Irene Doyle Sandler for her thoughtful and critical review of the manuscript; to the International Rescue Committee, Inc.; to Dr. Marie Cole, Richard Fritzler, and Pauline Thomas, our medical illustrators; to Corinne Naden for her copyediting; to Bill Bower, Barry Bunting, Carolyn Kleinmann, Dr. Lee Andersen, Dr. Richard Steketee, and the Bay Medical Center of Bay City, Michigan. Finally, we want to express our deepest appreciation to our finest teachers, the refugees with whom we have been privileged to work.

Contents

Contributors[a]

[a]Supplied for identification purposes only. Institutional endorsement of this book is not expressed or implied.

Abdi-Kamal Ali-Salad, M.D.
Director, Refugee Health Unit
Ministry of Health
Mogidishu, Somalia

Ravi Balasubramanyan, M.D.
United Family Practice
St. Paul, MN

Angela Berry, M.Sc.
London School of Hygiene and Tropical Medicine
London, UK

Rudolf H. Bock, M.D.
Clinical Professor of Ophthalmology
Stanford University Medical School
Palo Alto, CA

Roy E. Brown, M.D.
Health Advisor, CARE USA
Chairman of Community Medicine
St. Joseph Hospital
Paterson, NJ

Wolfe Bulle, M.D.
Visiting Scientist
International Health Program Office
Centers for Disease Control
Atlanta, GA

Betsy M. Chalfin, M.Ed.
Words & Type Unlimited
New York City, NY

L. Mason Cobb, M.D.
Assistant Professor of Pediatric Surgery
College of Human Medicine
Michigan State University
East Lansing, MI

James C. Cobey, M.D., M.P.H.
Clinical Instructor of Orthopedic Surgery
Georgetown University Medical Center
Washington, DC

Kyle L. Coble, D.D.S., M.P.H.
New York City, NY

Timothy J. Dondero, M.D.
International Health Program Office
Centers for Disease Control
Atlanta, GA

John Dyke, Ph.D.
Clinical Professor of Microbiology
Michigan State University
Director of Microbiology
E.W. Sparrow Hospital
Lansing, MI

Paul J. Edelson, M.D.
Professor of Pediatrics
New York Hospital
Cornell Medical Center
New York City, NY

Margaret Edwards, M.D.
Assistant Professor of Pediatrics
New York Medical College
Bronx, NY

Robert H. Gelber, M.D.
Director, Hansen's Disease Program
Seton Medical Center
Daly City, GA

Miriam Gilday, M.S.N., P.N.P.
Osborn Family Health Center
Camden, NJ

Stephen Gloyd, M.D., M.P.H.
Director, International Health Programs
University of Washington Schools of Public Health and Family Medicine
Seattle, WA

Jonathan W. M. Gold, M.D.
Associate Professor of Medicine
Division of Infectious Diseases
Sloan Kettering Memorial Hospital
New York City, NY

Fred Gordin, M.D.
Division of Infectious Diseases
Veterans Administration Medical Center
Washington, DC

Sandra Gove, M.D., M.P.H.
Assistant Clinical Professor of Medicine, Epidemiology, and International Health
University of California in San Francisco
San Francisco, CA

William Hawks, M.D.
Medical Director of the Seva Foundation
Chelsea, MI

Warren D. Johnson, Jr., M.D.
Professor of Medicine
Division of International Medicine
Cornell University Medical College
New York City, NY

Thomas C. Jones, M.D.
Professor of Medicine
Chief, Division of International Medicine
Cornell University Medical College
New York City, NY

Joan Kreiss, M.D., M.P.H.
Division of Infectious Diseases
University of Washington School of Medicine
Seattle, WA

Gifford S. Leoung, M.D.
Division of Infectious Diseases
San Francisco General Hospital
San Francisco, CA

Theodore C. M. Li, M.D.
Assistant Professor of Medicine
Georgetown Medical Center
Washington, DC

William C. MacLean, Jr., M.D.
Clinical Professor of Pediatrics
Medical Director, Pediatric Nutrition
Ross Laboratories
Columbus, OH

Phillip Nieburg, M.D., M.P.H.
Nutrition Division
Centers for Disease Control
Atlanta, GA

Karen Olness, M.D.
Associate Professor of Pediatrics
University of Minnesota
Minneapolis, MN

Etienne Ott, M.D.
Geneva, Switzerland

Jean W. Pape, M.D.
Assistant Professor of Medicine
Cornell University Medical College and State University of Haiti
Petionville, Haiti

Stanley E. Read, M.D., Ph.D.
Associate Professor of Pediatrics and Microbiology
Hospital for Sick Children
Toronto, Ontario, Canada

Jean Baptiste Richardier, M.D.
Program Co-Director
Operation Handicapp Internationale
Lyon, France

Jon E. Rohde, M.D.
Adjunct Professor of Medicine
Cornell University Medical College
Representative, Management Sciences for Health
Port-au-Prince, Haiti

Richard H. Sandler, M.D.
Fellow
Division of Pediatric Gastroenterology and Nutritio
Childrens Hospital, and
Massachusetts General Hospital
Harvard Medical School
Boston, MA

William P. Schecter, M.D.
Associate Professor of Surgery
University of California San Francisco
San Francisco, CA

Edwin J. Schodorf, Jr., M.P.A.
Public Health International of Oregon
Roseburg, OR

Ira K. Schwartz, M.D.
Division of Infectious Diseases
University of Chicago Hospitals & Clinics
Chicago, IL

Gary Slutkin, M.D.
Assistant Clinical Professor of Medicine, International Health, and Epidemiology
University of California San Francisco
Advisor, National Primary Health Care Programme
Ministry of Health, Mogadishu, Somalia

Barry N. Stein, Ph.D.
Professor of Social Sciences
Michigan State University
E. Lansing, MI

Richard H. Swenson, R.S.
Director
Public Health International of Oregon
Roseburg, OR

Cynthia S. Weikel, M.D.
Assistant Professor of Medicine
University of Virginia School of Medicine
Charlottesville, VA

David Werner
Director
Hesperian Foundation
Palo Alto, CA

Joseph Westermeyer, M.D., Ph.D.
Professor of Psychiatry
University of Minnesota
Minneapolis, MN

Joe Wray, M.D.
Associate Director
Center for Population and Health
Columbia University Medical Center
New York City, NY

Abbreviations

ac	Before meals
AFB	Acid fast bacillus
bid	Twice a day
°C	Degrees Celsius
cc	Cubic centimeter
CDC	Centers for Disease Control
cm	Centimeter
CSF	Cerebral spinal fluid
°F	Degrees Fahrenheit
g	Gram
h	Hour
hs	Bedtime
IM	Intramuscular route of injecting medication
IV	Intravenous route of injecting medication
KW	Kwashiorkor
l	Liter
MCH	Maternal Child Health center
μg	Microgram, one millionth of a gram
mEq	Milli-Equivalent (number of grams of a solute contained in one milliliter of normal solution)
mg	Milligram, one thousandth of a gram
ml	Milliliter, one thousandth of a liter
mm	Millimeter, one thousandth of a meter
#	Number
OPD	Out-patient department
ORS	Oral rehydration salts
ORT	Oral rehydration therapy
pc	After meals
PEM	Protein energy malnutrition
PO	Oral route of drug administering medication, food or fluids
PRN	As needed
q	Each, every
qid	Four times a day
RBC	Red blood cell
rpm	Revolutions per minute
SQ	Subcutaneous route of drug administration
STAT	Immediately
tab	Tablet
tid	Three times a day
WBC	White blood cell
WHO	World Health Organization

BASIC CONSIDERATIONS

1
Basic Considerations in Refugee Medicine

JAMES C. COBEY
RICHARD H. SANDLER
THOMAS C. JONES
BETSY M. CHALFIN

"Health" defines the condition of individuals when they are free of disease. Numerous factors are compounded to deny many refugees this status. These include carrying diseases from the refugees' home country into a crowded area and being exposed to infectious agents in the host country. Both conditions are magnified by the type and degree of contributing factors present, such as malnutrition, trauma, and severe psychological stress. Dick and Simmonds (1983) have reviewed the studies that describe the spectrum and incidence of pathology among refugees (Glass et al 1980; Seaman 1981; Gardiner et al 1972). They point out that the major causes of morbidity and mortality among refugees are diarrheal and infectious diseases, malnutrition, pneumonia, upper respiratory tract infections, and skin diseases.

Medical training in developed nations is usually directed toward technology-intensive diagnosis and treatment of individual patients with acute or chronic disease, while the most pressing health problems in underdeveloped nations often require a focus on preventive public health measures and basic low-technology treatment. Physicians and nurses in the refugee setting will be called to play an important role in initiating cost-effective medical interventions rather than technology-intensive therapies that drain precious resources but benefit few individuals.

One example of a low-technology focus that can aid millions of children was provided by the United Nations Children's Fund (UNICEF), which documented that each day more than 40,000 children die from malnutrition and infection (Grant 1985). UNICEF estimated that if four simple measures were instituted, more than 20,000 children could be saved daily. These measures, which cost no more than a few dollars per child, are as follows:

- Use of oral rehydration therapy (Chapter 15). Diarrhea kills over 5 million children each year and is by far the leading cause of pediatric mortality in underdeveloped nations. Oral rehydration therapy provides effective treatment when the parent or health worker gives a solution of salt, sugar, and water in the proper proportions.
- Universal childhood immunization (Chapter 6). Measles, diphtheria, tetanus, whooping cough, poliomyelitis, and tuberculosis kill an estimated 5 million children each year. More than 1 million die annually from tetanus alone.
- Promotion of breastfeeding. Diarrhea and malnutrition result from use of improperly sterilized bottles and overdiluted formula. UNICEF estimates that a change from bottle to breastfeeding could save 1 million infants each year.
- Use of growth charts. Morley (1973) and others have documented the value of maintaining growth charts for each child. This facilitates early recognition of undernutrition, chronic infection, or other factors that result in a failure to thrive.

Important tasks of health care workers in the refugee setting are to assess the problem areas rapidly, to assist in integrating the goals and balancing the pressures of different groups, and to make maximum use of their own skills.

ENTRY INTO THE SYSTEM

A few basic considerations for being an "effective donor" are summarized in Table 1-1. A well-meaning medical professional reads of a disaster or refugee crisis in the newspaper and wants to drop everything and help. He or she excitedly calls a relief organization to offer medical expertise and cannot understand why

Table 1–1. Basic Considerations on Being an Effective Donor in Emergency Relief Operations

For Individuals Wishing to Assist:
- Consult national health authorities, the Red Cross, or the WHO office in your country.
- Do not travel to the disaster site unless you are certain you can be useful and welcome. It is better to offer services and stand by.
- Do not collect food, clothing, or medical supplies unless you are certain they are needed and someone is willing to pay for transportation and distribution.
- Consider giving cash, as this is the most flexible and versatile type of assistance. Many reputable agencies can assist in channeling donations (see Appendix B).

For Governments, Private Organizations, and Nongovernmental Organizations (NGOs)
- Consult with your own national health sector disaster preparedness and relief experts, the Ministry of Health of the disaster-stricken country, and WHO before sending supplies or health personnel.
- Avoid donations of:
  1. Food and used clothing.
  2. Medicines close to or past their expiration date.
  3. Blood, plasma, water purification tablets, and vaccines, as these are often not needed.
  4. Field hospitals and medical teams. These often arrive in time for good public relations but too late for good emergency relief.
- If consultation cannot take place, provide:
  1. Drugs from the WHO list of essential drugs with a long shelf life.
  2. Funds for, or assistance with, rehabilitation and restoration of basic health services.
  3. Small equipment for primary health care, environmental health, and water supply.

Adapted from the Pan American Health Organization: International assistance: The delicate balance between donor and recipient. Disaster Preparedness in the Americas 1986;26:7.

the offer to volunteer for a month in some distant locale is not immediately accepted.

The desire among health professionals to help is certainly commendable. But for the relief agency, which provides medical relief both before and after the fanfare of prime-time news, the mechanics of placing medical teams in stressful and remote situations can be a Herculean task. The need is great for medical professionals with more than good intentions and a "free" month. Relief medicine, from the viewpoint of a relief agency administrator or program coordinator, is quite different from the adventurous "MASH" stereotype often conjured up in the minds of medical personnel not yet acquainted with its reality.

What, then, can one do to provide the combination of skills and attitude that will be most attractive to a relief agency recruiter and enable the health professional to make a real contribution to the relief setting?

Scheduling

The potential volunteer should realize that a month of his or her time is not of great value to a relief agency. Assessing credentials and verifying references is costly to the agency, and transportation and orientation to a new geographic and cultural environment consumes at least one week. Depending on the cohesiveness and efficiency of the medical team already present, a newcomer can be either flexible and quickly productive or troublesome, slow to adapt, and counterproductive. A month of service from an individual inexperienced with relief work usually is not worth the agency's investment of time and money. The shortest commitment one can usually expect is three months, if arranged through the rare medical school program, or six months if arranged directly with a relief agency.

Assessment of Professional Experience and Personality Traits

After reconciling time considerations, several professional and personal aspects should be considered. Recruiters for voluntary relief agencies (VOLAGs) are eager to find medical staff who are stable and well-adjusted, with a supportive family, a history of steady employment in the medical setting, and a self-assured temperament. A willingness to be adaptable, not only professionally but personally, is crucial because team members often live in communal settings that lack the amenities most are accustomed to. Other important attributes are an interest in being part of a team rather than an individual crusader; a good sense of humor and the capacity to accept the montage of cultures, languages, and attitudes that exist in a relief setting; and the ability to compromise and benefit from the experience of those already in the field. On the other hand, a need to "run the show," to be catered to, or to have special arrangements made are red flags to wary recruiters who have had the occasional unpleasant experience of dealing with finicky staff more interested in devising a fulfilling tourist experience than in focusing on the relief situation at hand.

A commitment to work in the field for a VOLAG also implies acceptance of the potential risks and political realities in the area where one has decided to work. An agency recruiter assumes that adult professionals have done their homework and are aware of the complicated and sometimes tense political or military situations that create refugee settings. Most VOLAGs are candid with their applicants and outline the existing situation. They are not anxious to send volunteers into areas of heated combat; however, military lines of demarkation can change unexpectedly and there is often a possibility of exposure to military intrusion and the need for treatment of wounded villagers or combat personnel. Those who know they would be very uneasy in a politically unstable setting should look for some other way to offer humanitarian assistance.

Health professionals who served in the Peace Corps are welcome applicants to almost any VOLAG. Peace Corps training and field work are invaluable in teaching self-reliance, flexibility, and the art of improvisation, which are often crucial in a relief setting. A second language, particularly French or Spanish, is a plus. Special medical training emphases on pediatrics, infectious diseases, tropical medicine, and public health are helpful in the long-term relief setting; critical care and trauma experience are helpful in catastrophic disaster situations. Nurses with pediatric or emergency room experience are often sought, as are midwives and nurse practitioners capable of organizing and running maternal-child health programs. A major component of any relief program is the training of local health workers (Chapter 4). Therefore, an interest or experience in teaching and sharing skills is helpful.

Assuming recruits have the previously discussed characteristics, VOLAG recruiters want individuals who are flexible in regard to scheduling. Most people like to volunteer for the fall through early spring, so those available in late spring and summer are more easily placed. Those who present an iron-clad schedule will be more difficult to place than those who offer alternative time periods. Because medical personnel often use "stand-by" status or travel on off peak days on airlines for lower rates, exact departure times are often unknown until several days before. The uncertainty of flight schedules and ticketing arrangements is the first hurdle a health worker faces. Ability to cope with this mild aggravation can be an indication of how well the health worker will be able to cope with major difficulties in the field.

WHOM TO CALL WHEN A CRISIS OCCURS

The component pieces have been analyzed, the time is available, a crisis is at hand. How does one sign up as a volunteer?

Often, newspaper or television accounts of an international refugee crisis or disaster will include the names of relief organizations directly involved in providing medical assistance. Appendix B also provides a comprehensive list of international relief agencies to which direct inquiries can be made.

Relief organizations provide a broad spectrum of activities and services including resettlement of refugees, feeding centers, emergency medical intervention, health clinics, public health and sanitation programs, and education programs. Some organizations emphasize development through long-term educational programs, agriculture, and irrigation and water projects. Organizations may be backed by churches, government agencies, and private foundations, each with its own political approach and geographic interests. Some of the church-supported organizations are interested in promoting their religious concepts; others are not. It is up to the individual to investigate which VOLAG best suits his or her needs and interests.

When calling or writing to a relief agency to volunteer, be prepared to provide complete information on educational and professional background and experience. You should have an up-to-date curriculum vita or resume prepared and several recent letters of recommendation available. If you have an interest in providing long-term services overseas, the same agencies can make future assignment as well as immediate disaster relief. This is best done six months to one year before the desired time of departure.

Following are summaries of two organizations often referred to in the context of refugee relief, disaster assistance, and refugee resettlement. This information provides only a brief overview of representative organizations.

International Rescue Committee

The International Rescue Committee, Inc. (IRC) was founded in 1933. IRC's initial purpose was to assist refugees fleeing from Germany, but soon it was assisting refugees from a number of countries. Today, IRC provides resettlement services throughout the world, as well as public health and medical services, sanitation, and education programs in a number of refugee settings including Thailand, Hong Kong, the Sudan, Pakistan, and Central America.

IRC's medical programs vary according to on-site needs but include adult and pediatric out-patient clinics, tuberculosis prevention and treatment, immunization programs, well-baby clinics, trauma units, laboratory facilities, and mobile field units. An important part of IRC's activities includes the recruitment and training of local nationals and refugees.

IRC prefers to recruit individuals who can make a one-year commitment to a particular location, though shorter stints are possible, in some instances. Having previous field experience or an appropriate medical subspecialty such as infectious diseases, pediatrics, tropical medicine, or public health is helpful when applying for a position. IRC is a voluntary agency in that they provide their services at no cost to the country in which they operate, but staff members are provided with transportation, a modest stipend, and, in some locations, housing. IRC is among those organizations that hire a relatively large number of medical personnel; their expatriate field personnel number anywhere from 50 to 300 at any given time.

Catholic Relief Services

One of the largest international humanitarian organizations involved in relief and development is Catholic Relief Services (CRS). CRS addresses health needs created by lack of food, contaminated water, and poor sanitation.

Generally, CRS operates feeding and nutrition programs, mother-child health centers, sanitation and water projects, leprosy patient services, psychiatric services, physical rehabilitation programs and prosthetic workshops, and public health projects including preventive medicine and the training of village health providers. Projects are located in 50 countries throughout the world.

CRS recruits a small number of physicians and nurses with appropriate experience who are able to make a commitment of one year. Because of their interest in development projects, CRS has positions for technical advisers with experience in agriculture, water systems, and sanitation. Volunteers are provided with transportation, housing, and a small stipend.

The work of VOLAGs has been successful in some areas, including immunization programs, emergency feeding, and crisis intervention, but they suffer from an overall lack of institutional memory and long-term organizational planning. Every crisis requires starting projects from scratch and recruiting new personnel.

Although the relief experience is challenging and satisfying for the small number of medical professionals who have found their way into the system, one basic consideration we seek to explore is how the medical community can provide a greater number of skilled, experienced staff members on short notice.

It is apparent that the activities of health professionals are best used within the organized structure of a known VOLAG rather than independently. VOLAGs offer an established administrative structure to ensure that volunteers are placed in areas of need and transported and oriented in an orderly fashion. In addition, VOLAGs establish the vital field and government contacts needed to ensure that volunteers will be admitted to the refugee setting and allowed to work.

One option in blending the experience of VOLAGs and the interests of health professionals is a program administered by a VOLAG in conjunction with a recognized university-based medical program. This setting can provide a plentiful source of trained health professionals from fourth-year medical students and nurses to senior residents and faculty. The short rotation (two to six months) is incumbent in this setting; this makes orientation to a distant site easier and eliminates the mental and physical burnout syndrome often seen in those who have served abroad for longer periods.

The potential problems of Western-trained health professionals include adapting their medical background and expertise to the needs and available technology of the field setting, making the mental and physical adjustments required for work in an underdeveloped setting, and ensuring program continuity with a short rotation system, but these challenges can and have been met (Li et al 1981).

There is no question that humanitarian concern exists throughout the medical community. In the university setting, however, that concern is more easily channelled if an established program of education, service, and training is an accepted part of the curriculum. A major task of organizers of such a program is to study and promote the educational merit of relief activities and to convince academic colleagues and administrators of their value. To compete for limited funding within the academic institution, the educational as well as humanitarian aspects of medical programs within the refugee setting must be clearly defined.

After completing a long-term assignment or several shorter-term assignments, one may consider a more permanent role in relief work. The opportunities are few but may be found in development projects rather than disaster relief. Jobs of a more permanent nature can be sought through the United Nations Development Program (UNDP), Save the Children Fund, or the World Health Organization (WHO). However, for the most effective use of experienced personnel, and perhaps of greater personal and professional benefit to the individual, a goal is to create a pool of medical personnel from which VOLAGs can draw at a time of crisis.

ASSESSMENT OF PROBLEM AREAS

It is important for health workers to define their roles in relation to problem assessment. Some of the skill required to do this are taught in clinical medicine. Clinicians are skilled at gathering data on medical problems of individual patients, weighing therapeutic options, and assessing the results of intervention. Similar skills are needed in refugee health care, but often with different parameters.

The first thing that refugees need is usually not medical care but food, water, and shelter. Although this is obvious, it may not immediately come to the minds of many clinicians. Doctors and nurses are often the first to volunteer for emergency relief efforts when what might be more needed are technical advisers to design and build latrines, civil engineers to provide a water supply and shelter, and food distribution organizers. In the absence of trained professionals and technicians to provide these essential services, the clinician can assess the size and distribution of the present population, calculate the food, water, and shelter needs, and help in procuring the necessary technical and material resources.

An adequate and clean water supply is essential. It is disheartening to see health care workers diagnose and treat diarrheal and parasitic diseases when the contaminated water at the source of the problem remains uncorrected.

Food should be considered an important medicine. Passing out vitamins is, in part, an admission that the available diet is inadequate. Distributing large quantities of powdered skimmed milk or high-protein soybean foods provides temporary relief but does not solve the problem. Once acute hunger has abated, people will not continue proper nourishment unless the foods agree with the local customs and palate. Food that does not meet local tastes, no matter how nutritious, will not be eaten.

If others are already performing the initial essential tasks, then the health worker is free to focus directly on health care needs. Health care efforts can be more appropriately expended if health needs are surveyed first. This involves assessing the distribution, magnitude, and type of health care needs present, and then planning for the most efficient use of available time, money, personnel, and supplies. All health workers, especially those arriving early in the evolution of a refugee camp, should have a basic knowledge of epidemiology to perform these tasks (Chapter 2).

It is essential to train health care workers from the refugee population. To sweep in, briefly "do one's thing," and depart is of marginal value. The elements of refugee training programs are presented in Chapter 4.

Acute medical care serves two main functions in the refugee setting. First is the obvious benefit to individual patients. Also important are the goodwill and trust engendered in the refugee population, which will later facilitate cooperation for public health projects.

The level of acute medical care should be appropriate for the refugee setting. Highly sophisticated diagnostic and therapeutic interventions should usually be avoided as they are not cost-effective and might create long-term expectations that cannot be fulfilled. Occasionally, certain usually treatable diseases might have to be left untreated. For example, in the Kampuchean refugee border camps, a very high rate of treatment failure for tuberculosis was found because patients failed to comply in completing a proper course of therapy. Initiating treatment under this condition is of little value to the individual patient and it allows resistant organisms to spread throughout the community. (For a general discussion of setting the level of care, see Chapter 9. For further discussion of the important issues of tuberculosis program management, see Chapter 33.)

The tendency for health care workers to want to do something, only to pass out vitamin pills, is overwhelming. This behavior, however, does little more than create dependence in the refugee population. It is more helpful to teach that all medical problems cannot be solved with a pill.

INTEGRATING VARIED GOALS

To carry out meaningful public health efforts, one must work with the entire community. To do this effectively, one needs to appreciate the political leaders and the dynamics between competing power groups. Each component group and subgroup has its own power structure and set of goals. Most of the refugees may be concerned with food, water, shelter, and security, but the top priority of powerful community leaders may be to return home and regain political control. The host country has its own goals, which vary depending, in part, on its historical relationship with the refugees' home country. Finally, health workers have their own set of explicit and implicit goals as to treating patients and feeling important. The health workers' goal of building a latrine system may be thwarted by refugees who use the supplies to build trenches and fortifications. Clean water might be procured to help children avoid diarrheal diseases, only to find the water given to water buffaloes because of their great value.

The population of host countries often suffers from malnutrition, water shortages, and poor medical care and sometimes becomes envious of the assistance provided to the refugees. This is fertile ground for anger and resentment, especially when the refugees come from a country that has traditionally been regarded with hostility. It is not surprising, then, that host-country government representatives sometimes obstruct refugee relief efforts. Patience, understanding, and creativity are required to overcome these conflicts as in 1980, when the International Rescue Committee and other groups formed mobile health care teams to serve Thai villages surrounding the Kampuchean refugee camps.

The conflicting goals of health workers may be manifest in a number of ways. They wish to return home with a sense of accomplishment, yet have only a short time in which to fulfill this goal. Often, health workers have little or no previous experience in international relief work and feel a great need to define their roles. Frequent complaining, lack of cooperation, and poor morale may result. To help prevent these problems, it is important to set realistic goals. Apart from direct service and teaching, goals should include learning as much as possible while in the refugee setting. This learning might include the language, culture, and history of the people involved, and learning about the diseases encountered.

FLEXIBILITY

The ability to be flexible involves recognizing and doing what is required, even if it does not meet one's job description. For example, everyone may prefer to be on the front line treating patients, but if no one stays behind to sort out the drugs in the pharmacy, the work of an entire ward or clinic can come to a halt.

Flexibility also includes accepting, with patience and humor, a multitude of daily frustrations. Murphy's laws apply to refugee medicine: "Anything that can go wrong, will," and "in general, things tend to go from bad to worse." Supplies are often unavailable when most needed, and host country administrators and health workers do not always share the same priorities or sense of urgency.

Cross-cultural communication can be difficult, especially since most volunteers lack knowledge of refugee or host country languages and customs. Developing a sensitivity to cultural differences is particularly important (see Chapter 11). As Jelliffe and Jelliffe (1983) have commented, "Some of the more important, underappreciated cross-cultural issues in the

Table 1-2. Estimate of World Refugee Populations

Africa	
Algeria[a]	54,000
W. Sahara[b]	50,000
Chile	1,000
Others	3,000
Angola	93,000
Namibia	70,000
Zaire	18,000
S. Africa	5,000
Botswana	1,300
Angola, Namibia, S. Africa, Lesotho	
Burundi	55,000
Rwanda	50,000
Others	5,000
Cameroon	1,000
Chad	
Central Af. Rep.	5,600
Chad	
Djibouti	31,500
Ethiopia	
Egypt	1,200
Ethiopia, Armenia, Chad, Afghanistan	
Ethiopia	5,400
Sudan	
Kenya	3,800
Ethiopia	1,500
Rwanda	1,200
Other	1,100
Lesotho	1,100
South Africa	
Niger	5,500
Chad	
Nigeria	400
Chad	
Rwanda	60,000
Uganda	45,000
Burundi	15,000
Senegal	5,200
Guinea-Bissaur and others	
Somalia	500,000
Ethiopia	
Sudan	513,000
Ethiopia	350,000
Uganda	150,000
Chad	5,000
Zaire	8,000
Swaziland	6,300
S. Africa	6,000
Other	300
Tanzania	155,000
Burundi	124,700
Zaire	23,000
S. Africa	3,000
Rwanda	2,300
Malawi	2,000
Uganda	102,900
Rwanda	69,900
Zaire	32,000
Ethiopia	1,000
Zaire	270,000
Angola	200,000
Uganda	35,000
Rwanda	22,000
Burundi	11,000
Zambia	2,000
Zambia	49,800
Angola	37,000
Zaire	5,800
Namibia	4,800
S. Africa	2,200
TOTAL AFRICA	1,921,000
East Asia and the Pacific	
Burma	1,000
China, Malaysia, Other Asia	
China	1,500
Vietnam	
Hong Kong	12,000
Vietnam	
Indonesia	12,800
Vietnam	7,000
*Processing Center	5,800
Japan	1,800
Vietnam	
Laos	3,500
Cambodia	
Macau	1,000
Vietnam	
Malaysia	8,400
Vietnam	
Philippines	14,900
Vietnam	3,900
*Processing Center	11,000
Singapore	500
Vietnam	
Thailand	**169,000
Cambodia	84,000
Laos	76,000
Vietnam	9,000
**(does not include border camps)	
Vietnam	30,000
Cambodia	
TOTAL E. ASIA/PACIFIC	256,400

*In transit to third country.

Table 1-2. Estimate of World Refugee Populations (*Continued*)

Europe	
Austria	17,700
Poland	14,600
Other E. Eur.	3,100
Greece	3,400
Iraq, Iran	
Italy	6,500
E. Eur., Ethiopia, Iraq	
Turkey	300
E. Eur., Afghanistan, Iran	
Yugoslavia	2,800
E. Eur.	
TOTAL EUROPE	30,700
Latin America and the Caribbean	
Argentina	12,300
Europe, Latin Amer., S.E. Asia	
Belize	5,000
El Salvador	
Brazil	5,400
Europe, Latin Amer.	
Chile	1,500
Europe	
Costa Rica	15,000
El Salvador	10,000
Other Latin Amer.	5,000
Dominican Rep.	5,000
Haiti	
Guatemala	70,000
El Salvador	
Honduras	33,300
El Salvador	20,000
Nicaragua	12,000
Other	1,300
Mexico	140,000
El Salvador	120,000
Guatemala	20,000
Nicaragua	22,500
El Salvador	22,000
Guatemala	500
Panama	1,500
El Salvador	1,000
Other	500
Peru	500
Europe, Latin Amer.	
Venezuela	500
Europe, Latin Amer.	
TOTAL LATIN AMERICA AND THE CARIBBEAN	312,500
Middle East/South Asia	
Gaza Strip	377,000
Palestinians	
India	4,700
Afghanistan	4,000
Iran	700
Iran	560,000
Afghanistan	500,000
Iraq	60,000
Jordan	749,000
Palestinians	
Lebanon	242,100
Palestinians	239,000
Other	3,100
Pakistan	2,800,800
Afghanistan	2,800,000
Iran	800
Syria	221,000
Palestinians	
West Bank	341,000
Palestinians	
TOTAL MIDDLE EAST/ S. ASIA	5,295,600
TOTAL	7,816,200

From The World Refugee Survey. New York, US Committee for Refugees, 1983.
[a]Country or area of refugee asylum.
[b]Source country or area.

development of refugee health services may include [certain limitations on] the roles of female health workers, special beliefs and customs related to food, and reliance on indigenous forms of medical treatment. The surprise, irritation, and misunderstanding often experienced by health workers can be minimized if they are prepared for such cultural differences."

While health workers may leave the refugee camp recounting the number of people treated or the number of latrines built, perhaps a greater benefit will be the education provided to facilitate the refugees' self-sufficiency. If the health worker can assess problems correctly, integrate conflicting goals, and maintain a high level of personal skills, he or she may realize that an even greater service has been provided by engaging in this activity with concern, gentleness, and humility. This might also be contagious.

REFERENCES AND SUGGESTED READING

Allegra DT, Nieburg P, Grabe M: Emergency Refugee Health Care—A Chronicle of the Khmer Refugee Assistance Operation. Washington, DC, US Department of Health and Human Services, 1984.
Braham M: Refugee Abstracts. Geneva, International Refugee Integration Resource Centre, 1982.
Cambodian Refugee Relief: Lessons Learned and Future Directions. Workshop Report. Washington, DC, National Council for International Health, 1980.
Caritas Internationalis: Emergency Manual: Disaster Relief and Rehabilitation. Rome, Caritas International, 1979.
Cobey JC: A Guide for Short-Term Volunteer Medical Workers in Developing Countries. Washington, DC, Orthopaedics Overseas, 1985.
Council of Europe, Division for Higher Education and Research: European Workshop on Educational Aspects of Health in Disasters. Strasbourg, Council of Europe, 1982.
Cuny FC: Disasters and Development. New York, Oxford University Press, 1983.
Cuny FC: Refugee camps and camp planning: The state of the art. Disasters 1977;1:125–44.
De Ville de Goyet C, Lechat MF: Health aspects in natural disasters. Tropical Doctor 1976;6:152–57.
Dick B: Diseases of refugees: Causes, effects and control. Trans R Soc Trop Med Hyg 1984; 78:734–41.
Dick B, Simmonds SP: Refugee health care: Similar but different? Disasters 1983;7:291–303.
Disaster assessment: The weak link in international relief efforts. Bull Pan Am Health Organ 1985;19:97–99.
The health of refugees. Lancet 1985;1:673–74.
Djukanovic V, Mach EP: Alternative Approaches to Meeting Basic Health Needs in Developing Countries. Geneva, World Health Organization, 1975.
Durham TW, McCammon SL, Allison EJ Jr: The psychological impact of disaster on rescue personnel. Ann Emerg Med 1985;14:664–68.
Feldstein B, Frelick G, Frye E: Training international refugee relief health workers. Disasters 1983;7:26–29.
Fisher R, Ury W: Getting to Yes: Negotiating Agreement Without Giving In. New York, Penguin Books, 1981.
Gardiner P, Rohde JE, Majumdar MB: Health priorities among Bangladesh refugees. Lancet 1972;1:834–36.
Glass RI, Cates WJr, Nieburg P et al: Rapid assessment of health status and preventive medicine needs of newly arrived Kampuchean refugees in SaKaeo, Thailand. Lancet 1980;1:868–72.
Grant JP: The State of the World's Children 1985. New York, United Nations Children's Fund, 1985.
Hamilton VL, Silk J, Papanicolas K, et al (eds): World Refugee Survey. 1985 in Review. New York, US Committee for Refugees and the American Council of Nationalities Service, 1986.
The health of refugees. Lancet 1985;1:673—74.
INTERTECT: Relief Operations Guidebook: Administration and Resource Management. Dallas, INTERTECT, 1979.
Jelliffe DB, Jelliffe EF: Education for refugee health workers: The UCLA experience. Disasters 1983;7:8–11.
Johnson DE, Williams RG, Burke DS, Murray BE: Observations on medical care in a refugee camp in Thailand. Military Med 1981;146:842–45.
Kastner R: Training of expatriate refugee health workers: Principles and practices. Disasters 1983;7:41–43.
League of Red Cross Societies: Red Cross Disaster Relief Handbook. Geneva, ICRC, 1976.
Levy BS: Working in a camp for Cambodian refugees. New Engl J Med 1981;304:1440–44.
Levy BS, Susott DC: Years of Horror, Days of Hope: Responding to the Cambodian Refugee Crisis. New York, Associated Faculty Press, 1986.
Li TC, Kris M, Weiner D, Jones TC: Medicine in a disrupted society: The role of the academic medical center. Am J Med 1981;70:998–99.
Logue JN, Melick ME, Hansen H: Research issues and directions in the epidemiology of health effects of disasters. Epidemiol Rev 1981;3:140–62.
Loizos P: The Heart Grown Bitter. London, Cambridge University Press, 1981.
Manning D: Disaster Technology: An Annotated Bibliography. London, London Technical Group, 1973.
McMahon R et al: On Being in Charge. A Guide for Middle-Level Management in Primary Health Care. Geneva, World Health Organization, 1980.
Montague J, Montague S, Cebula D et al: Primary Health Care Bibliography and Resource Directory. Geneva, World Federation of Public Health Associations, 1984.
Morley D: Pediatric Priorities in the Developing World. London, Butterworth, 1973.
Morley D, Rohde JE, Williams G: Practicing Health for All. Oxford, Oxford University Press, 1983.
Newland K: Refugees: The New International Politics of Displacement. Worldwatch Paper 43. Washington, DC, Worldwatch Institute, 1981.
Olness K: Health outreach to a refugee camp: Perspectives for would-be volunteers. Pediatrics 1981;67:523–29.
OXFAM Medical Unit: OXFAM's Practical Guide to Refugee Health Care. London, OXFAM, 1983.
PAHO: Emergency Health Management after Natural Disaster. PAHO Sci Pub 407. Washington, DC, Pan American Health Organization, 1981.

Sandler RH: Medical help for developing nations (letter). JAMA 1984;252:766.
Seaman JA: Medical Care in Refugee Camps. Disasters 1981;5:173–336.
Simmonds SP: Curative medicine or community health? Appropriate health services with refugees. J Trop Med Hyg 1980; 83:49–52.
Simmonds SP: Refugees, health and development. Trans R Soc Trop Med Hyg 1984; 78:726–33.
Simmonds SP, Gabaudan M: Refugee Camp Health Care: Selected Annotated References. Ross Institute Bulletin 14. London, London School of Tropical Medicine and Hygiene, 1982.
Simmonds SP, Shears P: Changing perspectives in health care in Africa. In: Refugee Report 1984, London, British Refugee Council, 1984, pp 31–33.
Simmonds SP, Vaughan P, Gunn SW (eds): Refugee Community Health Care. Oxford, Oxford University Press, 1983.
Smilkstein G: Refugees in Thailand and short-term medical aid. JAMA 1981; 245:1052–54.
Somali Ministry of Health, Refugee Health Unit: Guidelines for Health Care in Refugee Camps of the Somali Democratic Republic. Oxford, OXFAM Press, 1982.
Stein BN: Refugee research bibliography. International Migration Review 1981; 15:331–93.
Tayler AJ: The who and what of training for disaster relief. Disasters 1983;7:37–40.
Taylor CE: Changing patterns in international health: Motivation and relationships. Am J Public Health 1979;69:803–108.
UN High Commission on Refugees: Handbook for Emergencies. Geneva, United Nations High Commission on Refugees, 1982.
Un Protein-Calorie Advisory Group: A Guide to Food and Health Relief Operations for Disasters. New York, United Nations, 1977.
Vanderkooi M, Translators W: Village Medical Manual. Waxwal, NC, JAARS Printshop, 1985.
Waddel WH, Pierre-Leoni RG, Suter E (eds): International Health Perspectives: An Introduction in Five Volumes. New York, Springer, 1977.
Walsh JA, Warren KS: Selective primary health care: An interim strategy for disease control in developing countries. N Engl J Med 1979; 301:967–74.
Walsh JA, Warren KS: Strategies for Primary Health Care. Technologies Appropriate for the Control of Disease in the Developing World. Chicago, University of Chicago Press, 1986.
Walt G, Vaughan P: An Introduction to the Primary Health Care Approach in Developing Countries: A Review with Selected Annotated References. Ross Institute Publication 13. London, London School of Tropical Medicine and Hygiene, 1981.
Werner D: Where There Is No Doctor. Palo Alto, Hesperian Foundation, 1977.
WHO: World Health Statistics Annual. Geneva, World Health Organization, 1982.

2
Epidemiology and Health Planning

JOAN KREISS

ROLE OF EPIDEMIOLOGY

Epidemiology is the study of health and disease patterns in human populations. Whereas the practicing doctor or nurse diagnoses and treats a disease in an individual patient, the epidemiologist, by assessing the health problems of a group of individuals, makes a community diagnosis and recommends interventions that will improve the health of a community as a whole.

In countries with a sophisticated level of health care, the public health system is often far removed from medical services that provide individual health care, and the average health practitioner may be unaware of, or take for granted, the safeguards that exist to protect the health of the community. This is not the case in a refugee camp. In a refugee setting there is often a low general level of health, many serious disease problems, and limited resources (supplies and trained personnel); therefore, every health worker must take an epidemiologic approach. The emphasis should be on major health problems of the community rather than the individual patient, and on preventive measures rather than curative medicine.

An epidemiologic approach can serve a number of purposes. First, it describes the health status of a community. By examining the frequency and distribution of health problems, an epidemiologic study provides clues to understanding the cause(s) of disease. This, in turn, leads to rational interventions for preventing disease or providing effective treatment. Take as an example an episode from a Somali refugee camp. A community health worker in a health post noticed a sudden and dramatic increase in the number of cases of diarrhea. Looking at his health post records, he found that these patients tended to come from one geographic section of the camp. A rapid community survey was conducted and it was determined that the onset of the diarrhea epidemic coincided with the opening of a new well; the cases were clustered about this water source. Analysis of the well water demonstrated an excessively high fecal coliform count and the well was closed. In this case, an epidemiologic approach was used to identify a health problem, describe its characteristics, pinpoint a cause, and find a solution.

Another crucial role that epidemiology plays in a refugee camp setting is in planning health care services. The first step in this process is to assess the health needs of the community based on an understanding of the demographic characteristics of the population and its patterns of disease morbidity and mortality. The second step is to determine how to use the limited available resources to make the greatest impact.

Table 2-1 illustrates one systematic method of determining priorities (also see Chapter 9). Each major health problem is ranked according to its frequency (incidence or prevalence), its seriousness (case fatality rate or disability), and the availability of effective and inexpensive control measures (treatment or prevention). Each variable is assigned a 1+ to 4+ rating, and the total score for a given disease is the product of the three variables. Table 2-1 lists five diseases and indicates how they might be ranked in a refugee camp. Measles is a disease that spreads rapidly through nonimmune children in a crowded community, has a high mortality rate in malnourished individuals, and is readily prevented by an effective and inexpensive vaccine. Thus, the control of measles (and other immunization-preventable diseases) should be a high public health priority. Cancer, on the other hand, although a serious condition, requires costly chemotherapeutic drugs, radiation therapy equipment, or surgical expertise for treatment, none of which is available in most refugee camps; it is therefore assigned a low priority.

During the process of priority assessment, it is important to maintain a dialogue with the community. A good way to initiate the process is to ask representatives from the refugee population to develop a list of medical problems thought to be of most importance to the com-

Table 2-1. Establishing Public Health Priorities for Community Health Care

Health Problem	Frequency ×	Seriousness ×	Feasible Control Measures	=	Total Score
Measles	++	+++	++++		24
Diarrhea	++++	++	+++		24
Tuberculosis	++	+++	+++		18
Scabies	+++	+	+++		9
Cancer	+	++++	+		4

munity. A relief team's determination of health care needs may differ markedly from the perceived needs of community leaders, traditional healers, or indigenous health workers. Medical projects that lack community support are rarely successful.

Once priorities have been established, strategies to control the most significant health problems can be planned and carried out. Each major intervention may be accompanied by an epidemiologic evaluation to assess whether or not the desired impact is being achieved. For example, the efficacy of a supplementary feeding program for malnourished children may be evaluated by weekly weight measurements of the enrolled children (to ensure that their nutritional status is improving) and periodic nutritional surveys of the community (to ensure that the target population of malnourished children is being reached by the feeding center).

Table 2-2 shows the results of two nutritional surveys carried out in Somali refugee camps. The surveys documented a significant drop in malnutrition rates in two of three regions, which was attributed to a supplementary food program. In the third region, the malnutrition rate remained high, thus prompting an attempt to solve the logistical problems that were interfering with reliable food distribution to the refugee camps.

MEASURES OF DISEASE FREQUENCY IN POPULATIONS

General Rate

Epidemiologists often use rates to describe how commonly a disease or other physiologic condition occurs in a community. A rate is a measure of risk or frequency; that is, rate equals

$$\frac{\text{Total number of events}}{\text{Total population at risk} \times \text{some given time} \times 10^x}$$

All rates have three essential elements: the **event** (i.e., disease cases, deaths); the midinterval **population** in which the events occur; and the **time** interval during which the events take place. For convenience, rates are expressed in terms of number of cases occurring per 1000 (or 10,000, million, etc.) in the population. This factor is chosen so that the rate is expressed with at least one digit to the left of the decimal point.

Table 2-2. Prevalence of Moderate and Severe Malnutrition in Refugee Children, Somalia, May and September 1980

	Prevalence in May 1980, %		Prevalence in September 1980, %	
Region	Moderate[a]	Severe[b]	Moderate[a]	Severe[b]
Wagooyl Galbeed	22.2	6.2	6.0	0.5
Hiran	23.8	3.7	1.0	8.0
Gedo	19.2	2.5	15.0	3.0

[a]Moderate PEM: 71 to 80 percent of median weight for height.
[b]Severe PEM: ≤70 percent of median weight for height.

From Follow-up on refugees—Somalia. MMWR 1981;30:85.

Rates may be inaccurate because of numerator errors or denominator errors. The major problems in determining the number of events (the numerator) are incomplete reporting or counting and inaccurate diagnoses. In a refugee camp, the population denominator usually presents greater problems. The general difficulty in obtaining reliable census figures may be compounded by political opposition to accurate refugee counts and in-and-out migration for those camps with unrestricted passage.

Prevalence and Incidence

The two most commonly used rates are prevalence and incidence. Point prevalence is a measure of the **existing** cases of a disease in a population at a given point in time. Point prevalence equals

$$\frac{\text{Number of existing cases of a disease}}{\text{Total population}} \times 10^x \text{ at a point in time}$$

Period prevalence expresses the number of existing cases over a specified period of time, such as one year.

Incidence is a measure of the number of **new** cases of a disease in a population over a given time period. Incidence equals

$$\frac{\text{Number of new cases of a disease}}{\text{Population at risk}} \times 10^x \text{ over a given time period}$$

Prevalence depends not only on how commonly a disease occurs but on how long the disease lasts until recovery or death and on the migration of ill persons into and out of the community (see Figure 2-1). Prevalence varies directly with incidence and disease duration. Under stable conditions in a closed community;

$$\text{Prevalence} = \text{Incidence} \times \text{Duration}$$

It is possible to have a disease of low incidence and high prevalence if the disease duration is long (e.g., leprosy). On the other hand, if a disease is rapidly lethal, the point prevalence will be low even when the disease occurs with high frequency (e.g., during an epidemic of meningococcal meningitis).

In an open community, migration patterns may significantly alter the prevalence of certain conditions. For example, when a refugee camp along the Thai–Kampuchean border opened a tuberculosis treatment center, the prevalence of tuberculosis in the camp rose because Khmers with tuberculosis migrated from the Kampuchean countryside into the camp specifically to seek therapy.

Crude versus Specific Rates

Crude rates are summary rates expressed in terms of a total population. Crude death rate equals

$$\frac{\text{Total number of deaths}}{\text{Total midyear population}} \times 1000 \text{ per year}$$

Crude birth rate equals

$$\frac{\text{Total number of live births}}{\text{Total midyear population}} \times 1000 \text{ per year}$$

Specific rates measure the number of events occurring in a population of a given age, race, or sex. It is important that the denominator includes the appropriate population at risk rather than the total population. Age specific

Figure 2-1. The prevalence pot.

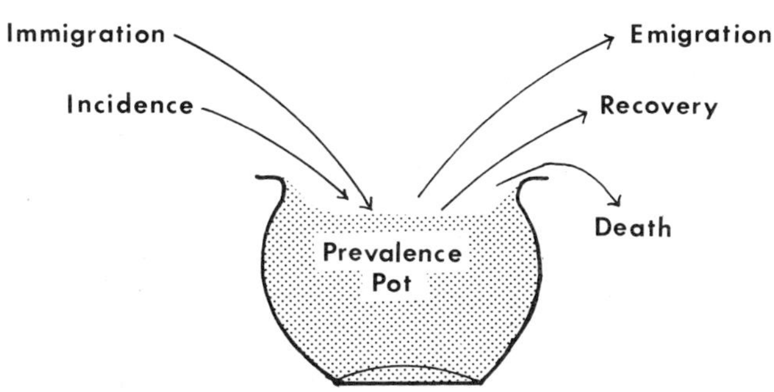

mortality rate (5–9-year-olds) equals

$$\frac{\text{Number of deaths of those aged 5–9}}{\text{Number of 5–9-year-olds}} \times 1000 \text{ per year}$$

Cause and sex-specific death rate (malaria, males) equals

$$\frac{\text{Number of malaria deaths in males}}{\text{Total number of males}} \times 1000 \text{ per year}$$

Other Common Rates

Infant mortality measures the risk of dying during the first year of life among infants born alive:

$$\frac{\text{Number of infant deaths at 0–1 year}}{\text{Number of live births}} \times 1000 \text{ per year}$$

Neonatal mortality measures the risk of an infant dying in the first month of life:

$$\frac{\text{Number of deaths at 0–1 month}}{\text{Number of live births}} \times 1000 \text{ per year}$$

Maternal mortality measures the risk of puerperal (pregnancy-related) death:

$$\frac{\text{Number of puerperal deaths}}{\text{Number of live births}} \times 1000 \text{ per year}$$

The fertility rate is the rate at which women of child-bearing age reproduce:

$$\frac{\text{Number of live births}}{\text{Number of females aged 15–44}} \times 1000 \text{ per year}$$

Case fatality rate measures the risk of death among those with a specific disease, that is the proportion of deaths among cases:

$$\frac{\text{Number of deaths from a given disease}}{\text{Number of cases of the disease}} \times 100$$

The case fatality rate for rabies, a uniformly fatal disease, is 100 percent, whereas the case fatality rate for hepatitis A is less than 1 percent.

Proportionate mortality is the proportion of total deaths that are due to a specific cause:

$$\frac{\text{Number of deaths from a specific disease}}{\text{Total number of deaths from all causes}} \times 100$$

If, for example, 24 deaths are reported in a camp during a one-month period, and six of these are due to diarrhea, then the proportionate mortality due to diarrhea is 25 percent. Because this measure does not require a population census for the denominator (it is not a true rate), it is particularly useful in those refugee camps in which population counts are inaccurate. If reporting of deaths is complete and ascribed causes of death are reliable, proportionate mortality identifies those diseases that contribute most to overall mortality in a community.

EPIDEMIOLOGIC PROFILE OF REFUGEE CAMPS

The vast majority of today's refugees come from underdeveloped countries, and their health problems are similar to those of nonrefugees in the same countries. The precise demographic makeup and health characteristics of each refugee community are unique. However, one can use the general epidemiologic profile of a community in the underdeveloped world as a guideline.

Population Demographics

The age structure of the underdeveloped world is dramatically different from that of the developed world. Figure 2-2 contrasts the triangular population pyramid of the underdeveloped world with the rectangular shape of the developed world. In the former, a high percentage of the population consists of infants and children (20% under 5 years of age; 45% under 15 years of age), and a small percentage are elderly. This pattern may be accentuated in a refugee community, for the elderly are less likely to survive the hardships of migration and may be more likely to stay behind in their homeland.

Some refugee communities feature a distinctive sex distribution, with a relative paucity of adult males. This may be due to a variety of social, economic, and political factors. For example, men may have been killed in war or conscripted from the camps to serve in the military, or they may be seeking work, herding livestock, or farming. In Honduras, a camp of Salvadoran refugees who were supportive of antigovernment guerilla activities contained almost no young men. A nearby camp, largely inhabited by Salvadoran government proponents, contained an abundance of young men.

Figure 2-2. Population pyramids for the developed and developing worlds. Reproduced with permission from Morley D: Paediatric Priorities in the Developing World. London, Butterworths, 1973. p. 62.

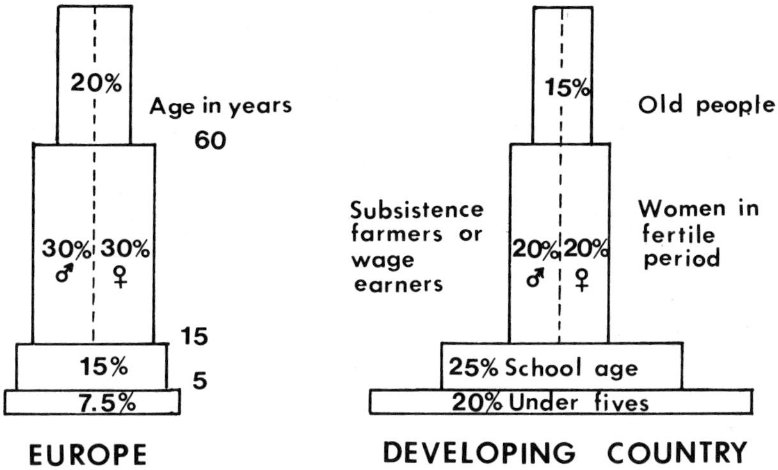

The importance of these demographic characteristics lies in anticipating community needs and planning health services. If young women and children constitute 75 percent or more of a refugee camp's population, then maternal and child health care should be stressed rather than, for example, the care of chronic diseases in the aged. If a camp is situated near a war zone, and if refugees participate in military activities, then surgical facilities for treating land mine injuries and gunshot wounds would have to be established.

Indices of Community Health

A number of basic measurements are used as indicators of the health status of a community. These key rates are often used for comparative purposes from country to country or camp to camp, or to follow a given population serially over time to detect trends or evaluate the impact of health care interventions.

As illustrated in Table 2-3, a community in a poor, rural area tends to have a high crude birth rate, a high crude death rate, and a high infant mortality rate compared with communities in the developed world. In addition, individuals born in the underdeveloped world have a lower life expectancy than individuals in the developed world (40 years versus 70 years). Most of the improved survival in developed countries is a result of decreased infant and child mortality.

Patterns of Morbidity

The illnesses seen with high frequency in refugee camps are very different from those seen

Table 2-3. Basic Indices of Community Health in the Developed Versus the Underdeveloped World

Index	Developed World	Underdeveloped World
Crude birth rate (per 1000 population)	15	45
Crude death rate (per 1000 population)	10	20
Infant mortality rate (per 1000 live births)	10	150

Derived from World Health Statistics Annual. Geneva, World Health Organization, 1983.

in Western societies. They tend to be diseases associated with poverty, crowding, poor hygiene and sanitation, and inadequate nutrition. The diseases that contribute most to morbidity and mortality in refugee camps (and in the underdeveloped world) are infectious in origin. Compared with the chronic diseases that are found in the developed world, these infectious diseases are relatively easy and inexpensive to prevent or treat. Table 2-4 compares the general mortality patterns seen in the developed and the underdeveloped worlds.

Table 2-4. Five Leading Causes of Death in the Developed and Developing Worlds

Developed	Developing
Ischemic heart disease	Respiratory disease
Cancer	Other infectious and parasitic diseases
Cerebrovascular disease	Diarrheal disease
Respiratory disease	Tuberculosis
Accidents, violence	Perinatal deaths

Derived from Demographic Yearbook 1982. New York, United Nations, 1982.

REFUGEE CAMP DEMOGRAPHICS—A PRACTICAL APPROACH

To plan and provide services in a refugee camp, be they health care, education, food supplies, or blanket distribution, one must answer the questions of where, how many, and who (with respect to age and sex) the refugees are.

Making a Map

The first question requires the construction of a map. For some refugee camps, a map may be available from the host government or United Nations High Commission on Refugees. Aerial photographs, though rarely available, are especially useful for counting households in camps that do not have a patterned layout.

If there are no preexisting maps, then a crude map will have to be drawn. For a large camp, an overall map including major landmarks and political divisions of the camp should be drawn first (see Figure 2-3). Next, a more detailed map of each section should be made with the help of the community health workers (see Figure 2-4). The map should include all households, and a numbering system should be devised. If possible, the numbers should be painted on the houses so that a given home can be readily identified. The map

Figure 2-3. Overall sketch of a refugee camp.

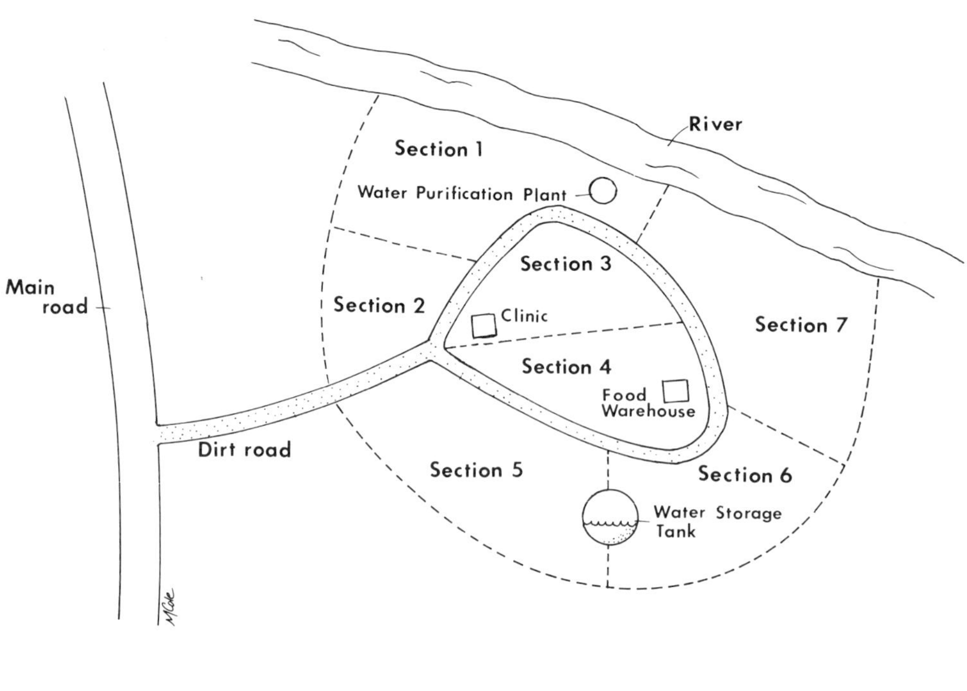

Figure 2-4. Detailed map showing all households.

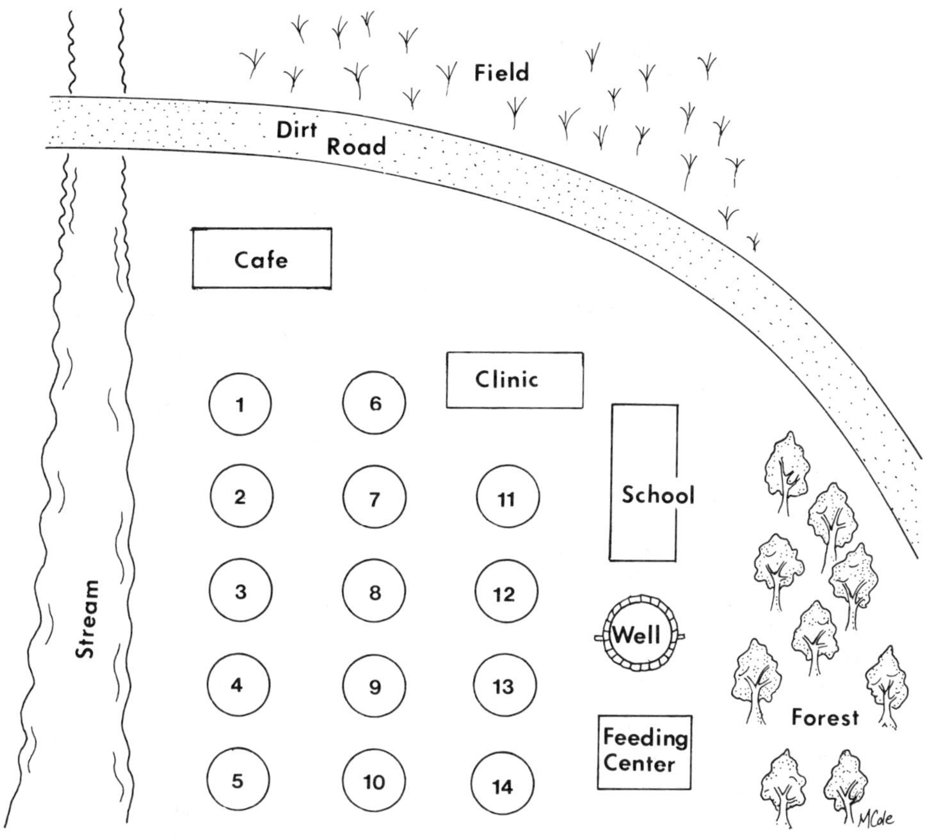

should also include the location of all community buildings (clinics, camp administration offices, schools, warehouses, cultural centers), wells, water storage tanks, community latrines, roads, and key natural landmarks. Such a map is invaluable for determining the total number of households in a camp, performing a random sample during community surveys, ensuring equitable geographic access to health care and other services, and finding and following sick patients, postpartum women, and so on.

Community Census

The number of refugees in a camp and their age/sex distribution are usually determined by conducting a community census. In some camps, this information may already be available through a registration system. For example, in a Khmer transit camp in which refugees are processed for third-country immigration, all individuals are registered and entrance and egress are restricted. In other camps, all families must register in order to receive food rations. The information is often unavailable or unreliable, however, and a census is required.

To conduct an accurate census, considerable advance planning and coordination are needed. A census requires the cooperation of the community. Plans for counting refugees should be discussed in advance with the UNHCR, the host country government, and the political leaders of the camp. There may be political opposition to accurately determining refugee numbers because of the concern that food and other foreign aid will be reduced if the true census number is less than the estimated figure. In other situations, there may be political motivations for deflating refugee numbers (e.g., impact on tourism, foreign relations with neighboring countries). The refugee community should be alerted before the census, and it should be stressed that the census-takers are concerned only with health care issues and have nothing to do with food distribution, repatriation efforts, conscription, or taxes.

There are two types of census to consider—a complete census and a sample census. A complete census attempts to count each individual in the camp and is practicable when a camp is small and personnel are plentiful. When registration of each individual by name is the goal, a complete census is necessary.

A sample census counts only a proportion of refugees in a camp, and the total figures are extrapolated estimates. For example, from an aerial photograph, one determines that there are 2000 dwellings in a camp that is divided into ten equal sections. For a sample census, all 200 households in a randomly selected section are visited and 1000 refugees are counted. The extrapolated estimate of the total camp population is then 10,000. This assumes that the camp is homogeneous and that the sampled section is representative of the entire community. If this is not the case (e.g., refugees of a higher socioeconomic class with a smaller number of individuals per household may tend to live together in one section), then a random sample of households throughout the camp should be used (see the section on Surveys below). A sample census is useful when time, money, or personnel are in short supply; when a rapid preliminary assessment is needed (such as shortly after the opening of a camp); or when a complete listing of refugees by name is not considered essential.

The next step is to determine what information to gather. Data should be collected only if it will be used; the tendency to obtain as much information as possible should be avoided. The successful census is usually one with a simple form and limited questionnaire. For a sample census, the basic information to collect is number, sex, and age of refugees. Figure 2-5 shows an example of a simple form that is easy to complete and allows for rapid extraction of data at the end of the census. For a complete census, a column for names may be added.

Data from a census may be collated in tabular form, and a population pyramid can be constructed. When this was done in a refugee camp on the Kampuchean border shortly after it was opened (see Table 2-5 and Figure 2-6), it was found that the extremes of age were underrepresented in the refugee population compared with the demographic composition of the country of origin. Higher mortality among the elderly and young children, combined with low fertility, resulted in a community made up largely of young adults.

SURVEILLANCE

Surveillance is the ongoing monitoring of the occurrence and distribution of disease in a community. Surveillance contrasts with surveys in two respects: (1) surveillance is a continuous process, whereas a survey collects information at a single point in time; (2) surveillance usually relies on a passive information-gathering system rather than the active data-seeking approach of surveys.

Disease surveillance is an essential component of any health care system. It provides information about morbidity patterns and trends, mortality and natality rates, epidemics,

Figure 2-5. Basic sample form for a census.

	MALES									FEMALES								
Household #	<1	1-4	5-9	10-14	15-24	25-34	35-44	45-54	55+	<1	1-4	5-9	10-14	15-24	25-34	35-44	45-54	55+
1	I	II				I						I			I			I
2				I						I				I			I	
3		I			I					I	I			I				
Total	1	3	0	1	1	1	0	0	0	2	1	1	0	2	1	0	1	1

Table 2-5. Age and Sex Distribution of a Random Sample of Refugees, Sakaeo, 1979

Age, years	Male, No.	Female, No.	Total No. (%)
<1	9	3	12 (4)
1	1	1	2 (1)
2	1	1	2 (1)
3	3	1	4 (1)
4	5	2	7 (2)
5–9	12	19	31 (10)
10–14	24	24	48 (15)
15–24	54	68	122 (38)
25–34	19	24	43 (13)
35–44	12	14	26 (8)
45–54	6	6	12 (4)
55+	5	5	10 (3)
Total	151	168	319 (100)

From Health status of Kampuchean refugees—Sakaeo, Thailand, MMWR. 1979; 28:546.

and clinic or hospital utilization rates—all of which are crucial for assessing health care needs, planning health care services, making rapid interventions when a serious health problem surfaces in a community, and evaluating the impact of medical services on community health.

The first step in a surveillance system, data collection, depends on a good record-keeping system. Standardized recording and reporting forms should be devised for all components of health care delivery (feeding centers, hospitals, maternal-child health centers, adult clinics, etc.). In addition, a method of registering all births and deaths is essential. The forms should be simple, self-explanatory, and easy to fill out. Only essential information should be gathered, and the type of information should reflect the level of sophistication of the health workers, diagnostic methods, and the medical care available. If the diagnosis of malaria is based on symptom complex rather than microscopic examination of a blood smear, for example, the record form should list "fever with chills" rather than *"Plasmodium falciparum"* or even "malaria." Figures 2-7, 2-8, and 2-9 show samples of a clinic register and monthly morbidity and mortality reporting forms that can be readily used by midlevel health workers. If all recording and reporting forms are designed with concern for clarity and ease of

Figure 2-6. Population pyramids for Sakaeo refugee camp (1980), and Kampuchea (1962). Reproduced with permission of the Population Council from Holck SE, Cates W Jr: Fertility and population dynamics in two Kampuchean refugee camps. Stud Fam Plan 1982; 13:121.

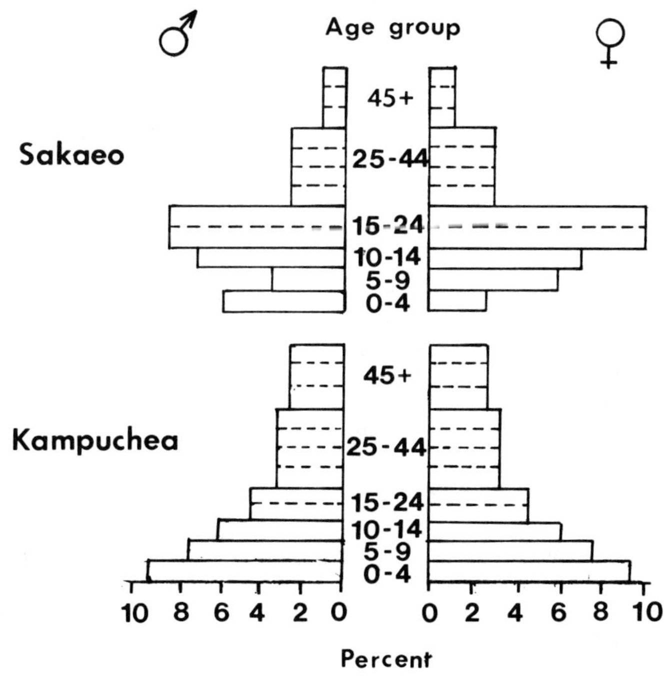

Figure 2-7. Clinic register book sample form.

Name	Address	Age	Sex	Diagnosis	Code	Treatment
Juan Valdez	5-103	5	M	Fever + cough	2	Penicillin
Jose Alvarez	1-211	2	M	Ear infection	10	Ampicillin
Maria Gonzalez	8-73	31	F	Urinary tract infection	15	Ampicillin
Gustavo Ybarra	12-94	1	M	Diarrhea	5	ORS

completion, the problems of underreporting and inaccurate reporting will be minimized.

Once surveillance data have been assembled, they can be converted to tabular or graphic form to facilitate analysis. Graphs are particularly valuable in displaying temporal trends. Although tables can often accommodate more detailed information, a graph gives the observer an immediate visual image of the data. A quick glance at Figure 2-10 readily conveys the dramatic decline in mortality within the first few weeks of the opening of several Thai refugee camps because of the availability of food, shelter, and medical care. In addition to graphs, histograms, bar diagrams, and pie diagrams are all effective for visual display of information.

The final step in a surveillance system is the dissemination and use of collected information. It is particularly important that all health workers who participate in collecting health statistics also be involved in a discussion of the results. A surveillance program will quickly disintegrate if the clinic nurse who completes the monthly morbidity reporting forms fails to understand the utility of the endeavor. If, on the other hand, a graph on the clinic wall charts the decline in diarrhea mortality in response to an aggressive oral rehydration program, or the reduction in measles cases following mass immunization, health workers will not only be encouraged to keep accurate records but will have the satisfaction of seeing the impact of their efforts on community health.

SURVEYS

Surveillance systems have several limitations. First, the collected data may be of questionable reliability when reporting forms are completed carelessly or the information provided is inaccurate. Second, a passive surveillance system may not accurately reflect the pattern of health and disease in the community if health services are underutilized. If most refugees with life-threatening illnesses choose to remain at home to die, a hospital-based mortality reporting system will markedly underestimate the crude death rate of the camp. If most children with severe diarrhea are taken to traditional healers, then diarrhea morbidity reported by a pediatric clinic will be misleadingly low.

Surveys overcome both of these problems. Survey data tend to be more accurate than surveillance data because workers are specifically trained to collect information. Surveys can avoid the problem of utilization bias by obtaining information on specific health attributes from the entire community. Surveys are often used to supplement surveillance data. For example, the surveillance records of a prenatal clinic show that 95 percent of pregnant women attending the clinic take weekly malaria chemoprophylaxis. A survey of all pregnant women in the community, however, indicates that only 40 percent of those surveyed are receiving malaria prophylaxis. This suggests that prenatal care in this camp has failed to reach a significant percentage of pregnant women and a community outreach program may be beneficial.

As described earlier in relation to community censuses, there are two kinds of surveys—a complete survey and a sample survey. Complete surveys are appropriate if the population is small and resources are adequate. Sample surveys have the advantage of being relatively inexpensive in terms of money, time, and personnel. Most communitywide surveys conducted in refugee camps, such as nutritional assessment or immunization coverage, are sample surveys. Care must be taken to ensure that the sample of refugees surveyed is unbiased and that it is representative of the entire

Figure 2-8. Monthly morbidity sample reporting form.

Monthly Clinic Morbidity Surveillance Report

Camp ____________________ Month ________ 198__

Code #	Diagnosis	Number	%
1.	Cough, cold, sore throat		
2.	Fever and cough		
3.	Fever and chills		
4.	Aches and pains		
5.	Diarrhea		
6.	Diarrhea with blood		
7.	Dehydration		
8.	Malnutrition		
9.	Intestinal parasites		
10.	Ear infection		
11.	Eye infection		
12.	Measles		
13.	Whooping cough		
14.	Skin diseases		
15.	Urinary tract infection		
16.	Obstetrical / gynecological		
17.	Venereal disease		
18.	Anemia		
19.	Trauma		
20.	Others		
Total			100 %

(Adapted with permission from Guidelines for Health Care in Refugee Camps of the Somali Democratic Republic. Refugee Health Unit. 1982, p 60.)

population. This is usually accomplished by choosing a random sample.

Basic Random Sampling Techniques

In a simple random sample, each individual or household has an equal chance of being selected. To choose the sample to be surveyed, one starts with a list of all individuals. After calculating the appropriate number of refugees to be surveyed (n), a random number table is used to select n people. As an example, suppose the total population is 59 individuals and 9 are to be selected for a survey. Take a pen

Figure 2-9. Monthly mortality sample reporting form.

DEMOCRATIC REPUBLIC OF SOMALIA, THE MINISTRY OF HEALTH: MONTHLY SURVEILLANCE REPORT – REFUGEE CAMPS

Region ________________ Camp ____________________ Month ____________ 198__

I. Camp Population

a) Total Population (end of previous month) ____________________
b) New arrivals (this month) ____________________
c) Births in camp (this month) ____________________
d) Deaths in camp (this month) ____________________
e) Number of people left camp (this month) ____________________
f) Total camp population (end this month) ____________________

II. Camp Health Personnel

physicians	________	lab. technicians	________
nurses	________	nurse-midwives	________
nurse-auxiliar.	________	TBAs	________
sanitarians	________	CHWs	________
asst. pharmac.	________	Others	________

III. Mortality

Possible cause of death	Age					
	under 1 month	1 - 11 months	1 - 4 years	5 - 14 years	15+ years	Total
Respiratory illness						
Diarrhea						
Measles						
Malnutrition						
Neonatal death						
Maternal death						
Other						
Total						

(Adapted with permission from Guidelines for Health Care in Refugee Camps of the Somali Democratic Republic. Refugee Health Unit. 1982, p 59.)

and blindly pick a starting point on the random number table (Table 2-6)—say the pair of digits that begins with the number at column 6 and row 6, that is, 34. For the 9 people in the survey, read down the column and record the first nine numbers that are less than or equal to 59: 34, 45, 2, 5, 3, 14, 39, 6, and 17.

A simple random sample is often not practicable in a refugee camp because a list of all individuals or houses may not be available. An alternative approach is a systematic random sample in which every k^{th} person is chosen after a starting point has been randomly picked. Suppose we want to interview every third refugee who comes to the adult clinic. Use a random number table to decide whether to start with the first, second, or third patient. If a random number table is not available, the serial number on a currency note can be substituted or a number can be drawn out of a hat.

Picking a sample randomly does not guarantee that it will be representative of the population. By chance, it may turn out that in a random sample of children in a feeding center, only girls are chosen. Stratified random sampling is a technique for avoiding this possibility. First, the population is divided into subgroups, such as males and females, ten-year age groupings, or some other grouping. Then a random sample is selected from each subgroup.

Cluster Samples

Cluster sampling is a method whereby groups or clusters of individuals are selected randomly and then surveyed. Cluster sampling is particularly useful in surveys of large populations, especially those that are geographically dispersed. Suppose we are interested in the nutritional status of children in 100 small nomadic refugee encampments in the Sudan. A simple or systematic random sampling technique would require visiting each of the 100 encampments. With a cluster sampling technique, we could first randomly select a subset of the encampments to visit and limit the survey to these camps. For this reason, cluster surveys can be done more quickly and easily than simple random surveys. They have the additional major advantage of not requiring a census listing of individuals. Because of these factors, cluster surveys have been widely used in refugee camps and in the underdeveloped world.

For example, consider an immunization coverage survey of 50,000 refugees in a camp. The standard sample size for this type of survey is 210 children of the requisite age group (say six months to five years), with 7 individuals chosen from each of 30 clusters. The selection of the sample is done in two stages: first, the random selection of 30 clusters, then

Figure 2-10. Crude mortality rates in three Kampuchean refugee camps, October to December 1979.

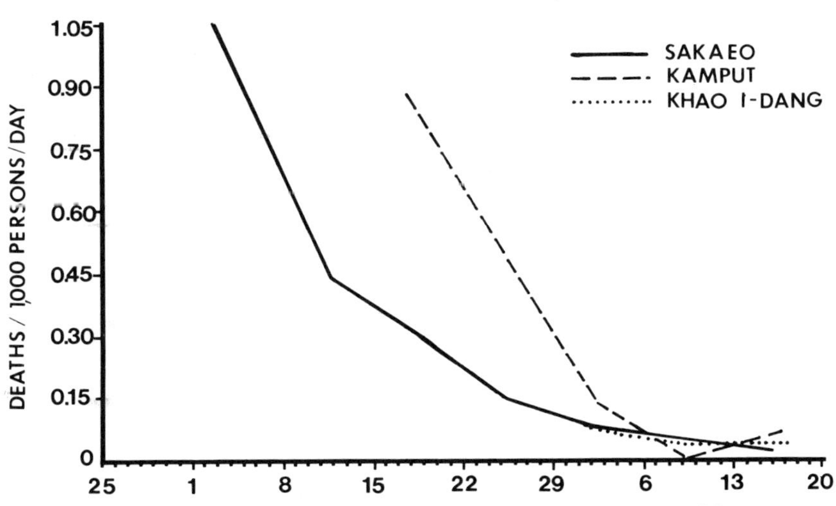

(Follow-up on the health status of Kampuchean refugees—Thailand, November 1979–February 1980. MMWR 1980;29:219.)

Table 2-6. Random Number Table

10 09 73 25 33	76 52 01 35 86	34 67 35 48 76	80 95 90 91 17	39 29 27 49 45
37 54 20 48 05	64 89 47 42 96	24 80 52 40 37	20 63 61 04 02	00 82 29 16 65
08 42 25 89 53	19 64 50 93 03	23 20 90 25 60	15 95 33 47 64	35 08 03 36 06
99 01 90 25 29	09 37 67 07 15	38 31 13 11 65	88 67 67 43 97	04 43 62 76 59
12 80 79 99 70	80 15 73 61 47	64 03 23 66 53	98 95 11 68 77	12 17 17 68 33
66 06 57 47 17	34 07 27 68 50	36 69 73 61 70	65 81 33 98 85	11 19 92 91 70
31 06 01 08 05	45 57 18 24 06	35 30 34 26 14	86 79 90 74 39	23 40 30 97 32
85 26 97 76 02	02 05 16 56 92	68 66 57 48 18	73 05 38 52 47	18 62 38 85 79
63 57 33 21 35	05 32 54 70 48	90 55 35 75 48	28 46 82 87 09	83 49 12 56 24
73 79 64 57 53	03 52 96 47 78	35 80 83 42 82	60 93 52 03 44	35 27 38 84 35
98 52 01 77 67	14 90 56 86 07	22 10 94 05 58	60 97 09 34 33	50 50 07 39 98
11 80 50 54 31	39 80 82 77 32	50 72 56 82 48	29 40 52 42 01	52 77 56 78 51
83 45 29 96 34	06 28 89 80 83	13 74 67 00 78	18 47 54 06 10	68 71 17 78 17
88 68 54 02 00	86 50 75 84 01	36 76 66 79 51	90 36 47 64 93	29 60 91 10 62
99 59 46 73 48	87 51 76 49 69	91 82 60 89 28	93 78 56 13 68	23 47 83 41 13
65 48 11 76 74	17 46 85 09 50	58 04 77 69 74	73 03 95 71 86	40 21 81 65 44
80 12 43 56 35	17 72 70 80 15	45 31 82 23 74	21 11 57 82 53	14 38 55 37 63
74 35 09 98 17	77 40 27 72 14	43 23 60 02 10	45 52 16 42 37	96 28 60 26 55
69 91 62 68 03	66 25 22 91 48	36 93 68 72 03	76 62 11 39 90	94 40 05 64 18
09 89 32 05 05	14 22 56 85 14	46 42 75 67 88	96 29 77 88 22	54 38 21 45 98
91 49 91 45 23	68 47 92 76 86	46 16 28 35 54	94 75 08 99 23	37 08 92 00 48
80 33 69 45 98	26 94 03 68 58	70 29 73 41 35	53 14 03 33 40	42 05 08 23 41
44 10 48 19 49	85 15 74 79 54	32 97 92 65 75	57 60 04 08 81	22 22 20 64 13
12 55 07 37 42	11 10 00 20 40	12 86 07 46 97	96 64 48 94 39	28 70 72 58 15
63 60 64 93 29	16 50 53 44 84	40 21 95 25 63	43 65 17 70 82	07 20 73 17 90
61 19 69 04 46	26 45 74 77 74	51 92 43 37 29	65 39 45 95 93	42 58 26 05 27
15 47 44 52 66	95 27 07 99 53	59 36 78 38 48	82 39 61 01 18	33 21 15 94 66
94 55 72 85 73	67 89 75 43 87	54 62 24 44 31	91 19 04 25 92	92 92 74 59 73
42 48 11 62 13	97 34 40 87 21	16 86 84 87 67	03 07 11 20 59	25 70 14 66 70
23 52 37 83 17	73 20 88 98 37	68 93 59 14 16	26 25 22 96 63	05 52 28 25 62
04 49 35 24 94	75 24 63 38 24	45 86 25 10 25	61 96 27 93 35	65 33 71 24 72
00 54 99 76 54	64 05 18 81 59	96 11 96 38 96	54 69 28 23 91	23 28 72 95 29
35 96 31 53 07	26 89 80 93 54	33 35 13 54 62	77 97 45 00 24	90 10 33 93 33
59 80 80 83 91	45 42 72 68 42	83 60 94 97 00	13 02 12 48 92	78 56 52 01 06
46 05 88 52 36	01 39 09 22 86	77 28 14 40 77	93 91 08 36 47	70 61 74 29 41
32 17 90 05 97	87 37 92 52 41	05 56 70 70 07	86 74 31 71 57	85 39 41 18 38
69 23 46 14 06	20 11 74 52 04	15 95 66 00 00	18 74 39 24 23	97 11 89 63 38
19 56 54 14 30	01 75 87 53 79	40 41 92 15 85	66 67 43 68 06	84 96 28 52 07
45 15 51 49 38	19 47 60 72 46	43 66 79 45 43	59 04 79 00 33	20 82 66 95 41
94 86 43 19 94	36 16 81 08 51	34 88 88 15 53	01 54 03 54 56	05 01 45 11 76
98 08 62 48 26	45 24 02 84 04	44 99 90 88 96	39 09 47 34 07	35 44 13 18 80
33 18 51 62 32	41 94 15 09 49	89 43 54 85 81	88 69 54 19 94	37 54 87 30 43
80 95 10 04 06	96 38 27 07 74	20 15 12 33 87	25 01 62 52 98	94 62 46 11 71
79 75 24 91 40	71 96 12 82 96	69 86 10 25 91	74 85 22 05 39	00 38 75 95 79
18 63 33 25 37	98 14 50 65 71	31 01 02 46 74	05 45 56 14 27	77 93 89 19 36

Table 2-6. Random Number Table

74 02 94 39 02	77 55 73 22 70	97 79 01 71 19	52 52 75 80 21	80 81 45 17 48
54 17 84 56 11	80 99 33 71 43	05 33 51 29 69	56 12 71 92 55	36 04 09 03 24
11 66 44 98 83	52 07 98 48 27	59 38 17 15 39	09 97 33 34 40	88 46 12 33 56
48 32 47 79 28	31 24 96 47 10	02 29 53 68 70	32 30 75 75 46	15 02 00 99 94
69 07 49 41 38	87 63 79 19 76	35 58 40 44 01	10 51 82 16 15	01 84 87 69 38

Reproduced with permission from the Rand Corporation: A Million Random Digits with 100,000 Normal Deviates. NY, The Free Press, 1955, p. 1.

the random selection of 7 children from each cluster. For the first stage, take a map and divide the camp into sections of approximately equal population size, say 100 sections of 100 households each. Randomly select 30 sections using the random number table. For the second stage, select the first household to be visited in a chosen section. If houses are numbered and a list is available, a random number can be picked. If houses are unnumbered, proceed to the geographic center of the section. Determine what direction to proceed in by spinning a bottle on the ground or twirling a pen in the air. Pick a random number between 1 and the total number of houses in the line of direction between the center and the periphery of the section, say 17; then start the survey at the 17th household and collect immunization histories from all the children between six months and five years of age. Proceed to the adjacent household, and continue in this fashion until 7 children have been identified. If the household containing the seventh child includes 2 other children of the appropriate age, the survey should include 9 children from the cluster.

Sample Size Requirements

In planning a survey, it is important to consider the number of individuals who should be included in the sample. If resources were unlimited, the ideal situation would be to include all members of the community. This would provide the greatest precision in terms of survey results. For practical considerations of speed and limited health workers, a small sample size is preferable, but precision suffers. For every sample survey, a compromise between these two considerations is reached.

For a simple random sample, the following formula is used to arrive at the appropriate sample size:

$$n = \frac{t^2pq}{d^2}$$

where n = sample size,
t = confidence limit factor (1.96 for 95% confidence),
p = estimated proportion in the population who have the characteristic being measured (if unknown, use $p = 0.5$),
$q = 1 - p$.
d = precision (usually 0.05 or 0.10)

As an exercise, suppose we decide to assess immunization coverage through a simple random survey:

$$n = \frac{1.96^2(0.5)(0.5)}{0.10^2} = 96$$

If we determined from the survey that 80 percent of young children in the camp had received a complete series of vaccinations, we could calculate the actual precision of our result through the following:

$$d = t\sqrt{\frac{pq}{n}} = 1.96\sqrt{\frac{(0.8)(0.2)}{96}} = 0.08$$

We would express the immunization coverage for the camp as 80 percent ± 8 percent.

The sample size formula above is applicable only to simple random surveys. Cluster surveys require larger sample sizes—for example, 210 children rather than 96 for immunization coverage determinations. Unfortunately, there is no simple way to calculate sample size requirements for cluster surveys. As a very rough rule of thumb, the sampled population in a cluster survey is usually two to three times that of a simple random survey. Before embarking on a cluster survey, however, it is wise, if possible, to consult the literature or an epidemiologist with survey expertise.

Carrying Out a Survey

What follows is a general, step-by-step approach to planning and carrying out a sample survey:

1. The first step is to decide what information the survey will provide. Is the information already available through other means? Will the information be used? How? A questionnaire should be designed which is simple and collects only the essential information. Figures 2-11 and 2-12 show a sample questionnaire and recording form for an under-five-year-old childhood mortality survey.
2. The next step is to decide on the population to be sampled—what age group; males, females, or both; the entire camp or only a particular area?
3. A sample size calculation is computed.
4. The sample of individuals or clusters to be included in the survey is selected.
5. Survey workers, usually chosen from the pool of health workers, are trained. It is important that the entire survey procedure be standardized to the greatest extent possible.
6. The questionnaire is field tested and any changes made before the actual survey begins. This also provides practice for the survey team.
7. The actual survey is taken.
8. The survey data are collated and analyzed.
9. The results are discussed with health care workers, community leaders, international and voluntary agencies, and so on. The conclusions should be used for planning purposes to design strategies to improve the health status of the community.

CONCLUSION

During the last ten years, the number of refugees fleeing political or natural catastrophes

Figure 2-11. Sample questionnaire for under-five childhood mortality survey.

Questionnaire for Under-5 Childhood Mortality Survey

1. Are there any children under 5 years of age currently living in this household? If so, how many?
2. Have any children under 5 years of age in this household died during the past year? If so, how many?
3. How old was each child at the time of death ?
4. Did the child have any of the following during the week before death ?

   Fever with cough ?
   Fever without cough ?
   Diarrhea ?
   Tetanus ?
   Measles ?
   Accident ?

   What other symptoms did the child have ?
   Which of these problems do you think was the cause of death in your child ?
5. Did the child visit the health post during the week before he/she died ?

Figure 2-12. Sample under-five childhood mortality survey recording form.

Under-5 Mortality Survey																	
Household #	# of live children <5	Of deaths in children <5 in past year															
		Age at death							Cause of death							Visit to health post	
		0-30 days	>1 mo -6 mos	>6 mos -1 yr	>1 yr -2 yrs	>2 yrs -3 yrs	>3 yrs -4 yrs	>4 yrs -5 yrs	Fever/cough	Fever/no cough	Diarrhea	Tetanus	Measles	Accident	Other	Yes	No

has increased. Each of the major refugee crises of the past decade (in Thailand, Somalia, Pakistan, Latin America, Ethiopia/Sudan) has been unique, but factors common to all of them have been limited medical resources and severe community health problems. Trained epidemiologists can play an important role in assessing the health problems of refugees and making recommendations regarding priorities and interventions. However, epidemiologists are rarely available on a camp level, and relief organizations that provide medical services in refugee camps often work as autonomous units (often because of unavoidable impediments to communication such as impassable roads or malfunctioning radios). Because of these factors, decisions affecting the health of the community are often made by medical personnel with little formal training or experience in public health approaches. It may be difficult for a nurse or doctor from an intensive care unit in San Francisco to decide whether it would be better to open a ten-bed hospital or to initiate a measles vaccination campaign; whether all clinical malaria should be treated with chloroquine or Fansidar or both; whether vitamin A capsules should be given to all children enrolled in a supplementary feeding program; or whether bloody diarrhea is more likely the result of amebiasis or shigellosis. If all health workers involved in refugee medical care were to take an epidemiologic approach and use the simple epidemiologic tools described in this chapter, the answers to these and similar questions could be more easily found.

SUGGESTED READING

Barker DJP: Practical Epidemiology. Edinburgh, Churchill Livingstone, 1982.

Belete S, Gebre-Medhin M, Hailemariam B et al: Study of shelter population in the Wollo region. J Trop Paediatr & Environ Child Health 1977;23:23–38.

Bennett FJ, Jelliffe DB, Jelliffe EFP, Moffat M: The nutrition and disease pattern of children in a refugee settlement. E African Med J 1968;45:229–46.

Brown JE, Brown RC: The community census as a basis for health programmes. J Trop Paediatr Environ Child Health 1975;21:315–20.
Brown RE, Carroll D, Mulvihill G et al: Field nutrition survey of Nigerian children in Ivory Coast refugee camps. Trop Geogr Med 1974;26:152–56.
Centers for Disease Control: Follow-up on health status of Kampuchean refugees—Thailand November 1979–February 1980. MMWR 1980;29:218–25.
Centers for Disease Control: Follow-up on refugees—Somalia. MMWR 1981;30:85–88.
Centers for Disease Control: Gonococcal infections among Indochinese refugees—Thailand. MMWR 1981;30:355–62.
Centers for Disease Control: Health status of Kampuchean refugees—Sakaeo, Thailand. MMWR 1979;28:545–56.
Foege WH, Hogan RC, Newton LH: Surveillance projects for selected diseases. Int J Epidemiol 1976;5:29–37.
Gardner P, Rohde JE, Majumdar MB: Health priorities among Bangladesh refugees. Lancet 1972;1:834–36.
Gebre-Medhin M, Hay R, Licke Y, Maffi M: III. Initial experience of a consolidated food and nutrition information system. Analysis of data from the Ogaden area. J Trop Paediatr Environ Child Health 1977;23:29–36.
Glass RI, Cates W, Nieburg P: Rapid assessment of health status and preventive-medicine needs of newly arrived Kampuchean refugees—Sa Kaeo, Thailand. Lancet 1980;1:868–72.
Guinena AHI: Protein calorie malnutrition in young refugee children in the Gaza strip. J Trop Paediatr Environ Child Health 1977;23:38–57.
Henderson RH, Sundaresan T: Cluster sampling to assess immunization coverage: A review of experience with a simplified sampling method. Bull WHO 1982;60:253–60.
Holck SE, Cates W: Fertility and population dynamics in two Kampuchean camps. Stud Fam Plan 1982;13:118–24.
Hurwitz ES, Johnson D, Campbell C: Resistance of *Plasmodium falciparum* malaria to sulfadoxine-pyrimethamine (Fansidar) in a refugee camp in Thailand. Lancet 1981;1:1068–70.
Keittivuti B, D'Agnes T, Keittivuti A, Viravaidya M: Prevalence of schistosomiasis and other parasitic diseases among Cambodian refugees residing in Bang-Kaeng holding center, Prachinburi Province, Thailand. Am J Trop Med Hyg 1982;31:988–90.
Lucas AO: Surveillance of communicable diseases in tropical Africa. Int J Epidemiol 1976;5:39–43.
McCusker J: Epidemiology in Community Health. Nairobi, African Medical and Research Foundation, 1978.
Miller DL: Monitoring communicable disease: Vaccination programmes. Int J Epi 1976;5:45–50.
Morley D: Nutritional surveillance of young children in developing countries. Int J Epi 1976;5:51–55.
O'Sullivan G, Ebrahim S, O'Sullivan J, Tafts C: Nutritional status of Laotian refugee children in Ubon camp, Thailand. J Epi Community Health 1980;34:83–86.
Simmonds S, Vaughan P, Gunn SW (eds): Refugee Community Health Care. Oxford, Oxford University Press, 1983.
Somali Refugee Health Unit: Guidelines for Health Care in Refugee Camps of the Somali Democratic Republic. Oxford, OXFAM, 1982.
Swaminathan MC, Vijayaraghavan K, Rao DH: Nutritional status of refugees from Bangladesh. Indian J Med Res 1973;61:278–84.
Wegesa P: The resettlement of refugees and onchocerciasis in Tanzania. E African Med J 1968;45:251–53.
Winardi B, Adhyatma P: Diarrhoeal diseases among refugees in Indonesia. Southeast Asian J Trop Med Pub Health 1982;13:361–65.
World Health Organization: The Place of Epidemiology in Local Health Work. Geneva, WHO, 1982.

3

Environmental Health and Sanitation

RICHARD H. SWENSON
EDWIN SCHODORF

This chapter is divided into three sections. The first provides an overview of environmental health, including environmental health management, in a refugee camp. The second discusses various water and sanitation technologies. The third section presents a detailed checklist of a broad range of public health measures. The checklist may be especially helpful to nonenvironmental health personnel who suddenly find themselves responsible for implementing an environmental health program.

ENVIRONMENTAL HEALTH OVERVIEW AND PROGRAM MANAGEMENT

The field of environmental health is concerned with the question of how external conditions affect living creatures. These conditions include drinking water, waste disposal, vector control, food protection, and housing. Environmental health programs are very important in a refugee setting because camps are typically crowded. Control of water and sanitation can reduce the spread of fecally transmitted disease, prevent vector-borne disease (insect and rodent), and generally make life a bit more bearable (Hawkins 1983; Kroeger 1976). Providing a healthy environment becomes difficult because most refugee camps are located in countries that usually do not have adequate sewage systems or safe water supplies. About 85 percent of rural people in underdeveloped countries lack adequate sanitation facilities (Feachem et al 1980), and according to Ward (1982), "Foul water may well rate as the greatest single source of human disease and misery." Specific environmental actions that can be taken to control or prevent disease are listed in Table 3-1 (Pineo 1981).

Forces Affecting Environmental Health Programs

The success of environmental health programs depends on many factors. As Figure 3-1 illustrates, politics, economics, and sociocultural realities are interrelated and each factor varies in importance from country to country, camp to camp, and over time. Persons attempting to implement water and sanitation programs must recognize each component's importance and incorporate a planning process that is sensitive to these forces. People and personalities often play a greater role in the success of these programs than the selection of a specific technology. This is especially true in the area of sanitation. For example, refugees, host-country officials, and relief workers all have different perceptions of how to dispose of fecal material. There will be no health benefits if latrines are well constructed but not properly maintained (Feachem et al 1980). The human element cannot be overlooked.

Prior planning is essential for realizing the goals of improved health conditions. Unfortunately, disasters usually happen quickly and fall on the least prepared communities. Health workers are therefore pressed to make up for lost time by taking quick action to address the camp's severe environmental health problems as soon as possible. Planning is neglected and obvious mistakes are made. People tend to react rather than act preventively. Even in the developed world, environmental health, which is preventive by nature, is hindered by the much greater emphasis on corrective or curative measures. In underdeveloped countries, such an emphasis, although dramatic, may be disastrous to the overall health of the population.

At the Sakaeo refugee camp in Thailand, environmental health efforts were not given the early priority they deserved. There were eight medical wards, and some medical teams actually searched for patients while the latrines were inadequate for the camp population of more than 28,000. Patients in the hospital wards were being given IVs while just outside piles of feces were accumulating. Garbage services were not organized and no wastewater disposal was provided. This led to a tremendous

Table 3-1. Environmental Action to Control or Prevent Disease

	Changes Needed to Break Cycle					
Disease	Excreta Disposal	Water Purification	Water Avoidance	Food Sanitation	Personal Hygiene	Insect Protection
Vector-borne parasitic diseases						
Malaria						X
Schistosomiasis	X		X			
Filariasis						X
Onchocerciasis						X
Trypanosomiasis						X
Gastrointestinal Infections, Including Intestinal Parasites						
Typhoid fever	X	X		X	X	X
Bacillary and amoebic dysentery	X	X		X		
Hookworm	X					
Ascaris	X	X		X		
Cholera	X	X				
Pinworm	X					
Viral gastroenteritis	X	X		X		
Other Infectious Diseases						
Hepatitis	X	X		X	X	
Trichinosis	X			X		
Trachoma					X	X
Yellow fever						X
Dengue						X

Source: Modified and reproduced with permission from Pineo C. et al: Environmental Sanitation and Integrated Health Delivery Programs, Monograph Series No. 4. Washington, DC, American Public Health Association, 1982.

Figure 3-1. Factors influencing refugee health.

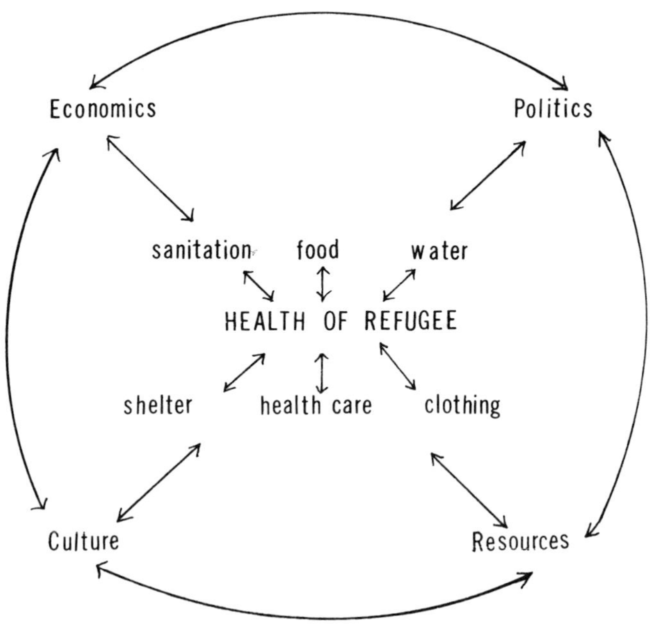

(Reproduced with permission from Simmonds SP: Refugee community health care in the tropics. Transactions of the Royal Society of Tropical Medicine and Hygiene 1984;78:729.)

increase in the fly population, which placed the community at increased risk for communicable disease outbreaks. Wide-scale insecticide spraying was initiated to combat the huge fly problem. Consequently, the flies soon became resistant to all available chemicals. Finally, almost by default, basic sanitation measures were instituted.

Sometimes, even with the best of intentions, circumstances do not permit the institution of a desired environmental health program. For example, sanitary, fly-tight latrines are a camp necessity, yet host-country officials may be reluctant to allow construction of these facilities if they lack the resources to provide similar facilities for their own people. Despite limited resources, cultural and political forces beyond the control of health care workers, and lack of early environmental health planning, good environmental health programs can be implemented with a resultant reduction of illness and death. The UNHCR Handbook for Emergencies (1983) illustrates the "likely relative impact of health measures" on a refugee population (Figure 3-2). Curative care alone cannot be depended on to improve refugees' health status (Grabe 1983).

Program Implementation and Management

Lengthy discussion of the many forces that must be considered before and during program implementation is beyond the scope of this chapter. Discussion is limited to a few topics the authors feel are especially significant to developing an effective, ongoing environmental health program—the philosophy and abilities of volunteers, prioritizing of activities, organization management, the community development approach, and health education.

Volunteer Philosophy and Abilities

Under the present system of refugee health services delivery, expatriate volunteers or employees from international agencies play a key role in shaping the program. Their philosophy and abilities are important. Some of the more successful programs have included the following volunteer attributes:

- Refugees must eventually solve their own problems. The volunteer acts as a caring facilitator who works with the refugees to help them understand what the environmental health problems are and what can be done about them.
- The volunteer is a trainer of trainers. The refugee population is generally more receptive to being led and trained by other refugees. This increases their interest and skills.
- The volunteer is politically astute and is sensitive to the forces existing within the camp and host country. As Peter Okoye, a former

Figure 3-2. Likely relative impact of health measures on a refugee population.

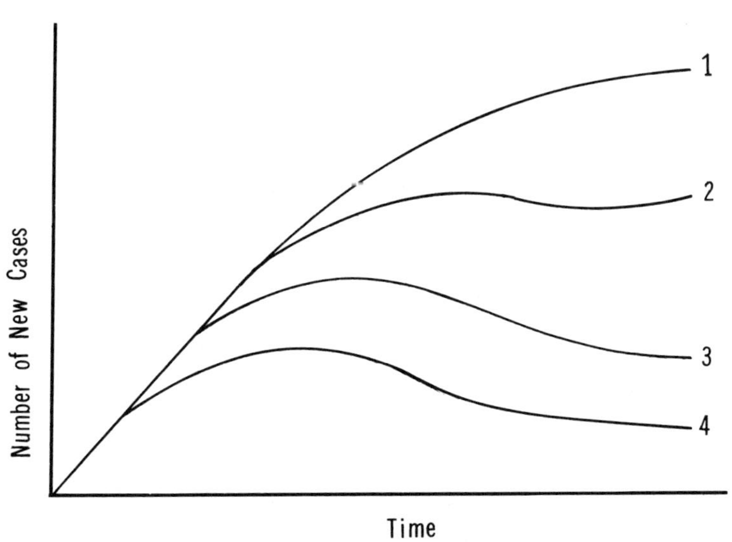

1. Curative care alone; 2. Safe water, enough food (tends to rise again as the environment becomes contaminated); 3. Above, plus proper sanitation and housing; 4. Above, plus active preventive health measures and public health education.
(From UNHCR Handbook for Emergencies, 1982.)

volunteer with Public Health International in the Sudan, said, "There are few written contracts and fewer attorneys in Africa. Agreements to do something are usually based upon friendship, rather than the written word."

- The volunteer possesses knowledge of water and sanitation technology, but emphasizes the "people" solution to problems. Public health volunteers work well with other health care providers and keep track of diseases prevalent in the camp.
- The volunteer is well-organized, flexible, has management abilities, is a good listener, keeps in close touch with the refugees and host-country officials, and writes frequent reports on problems and progress.
- The volunteer has a good sense of the importance of details and a sense of humor.

Prioritizing Activities

Program goals and objectives must be clearly written and then communicated to all affected parties. Prioritizing activities is a critical step. It is at this stage that the originally drafted goals and objectives undergo modification. Commitment and education also take place with the prioritization process. For example, in Wad Kowli, an Ethiopian refugee camp in the Sudan, a group of elders met to discuss the fly infestation problem. They had not been very concerned about the several hundred donkeys wandering about the camp. Once they realized that flies were breeding in the manure, it took only a week to build a fenced area away from the camp for the donkeys, roundup the donkeys, and develop a way to keep the donkey area clean. The elders understood why removing the donkeys from the refugee camp was one of the first priorities.

Establishing priorities at first seems unnecessary when environmental conditions are so poor that cleaning up the camp needs immediate attention. It is because initial conditions can be so overwhelming that clear, detailed planning and mutual support are necessary to implement an effective, well-organized program. Priority ranking can be established in a number of ways. A simple, yet effective, tool is a priority ranking sheet (Table 3-2). This process allows a maximum of input in a short time, and it is easily understood.

Organizational Management

A program can fail even with the best technology, good resources, and support from others. Good organizational management is critical because the job to be done is implemented by others but depends largely on people who understand their responsibilities and are well organized. Good organizational charts that show lines of reporting and linkages for formal communication are essential.

Figure 3-3 represents an ideal public health service delivery system. Note the close association of the environmental health specialist and the public health nurse. This facilitates the transfer of disease monitoring data. The health education component is developed jointly by the nurse and environmental health specialist. Of special importance is the public health advisory council. Here, many of the political, sociocultural, and economic issues are addressed, commitment is gained, and communication is accomplished.

Health Education

Few public health programs that depend on changes in human behavior can be successful without health education. Health education must be incorporated into all other programs and given a high priority. The education should focus on key environmental health

Table 3-2 Simple Method to Prioritize Environmental Health Activities.

Task	Public Health Significance (1–10)	×	Materials Available (1–5)	×	Time Frame (1–5)	×	Manpower Available (1–7)	×	Aesthetics (0–1)	=	Total
Repair privy	10		5		5		7		1		28
Spray for flies	10		2		5		7		1		25
Get water for gardens	5		4		2		7		1		19
Construct garbage pits	9		5		4		7		1		26

Source: Reproduced with permission from Rahe T: Work plan: Mesa Grande Refugee Camp, Honduras, January 1–June 31, 1984 (personal communication).

Figure 3-3. Public health organizational structure in a refugee camp.

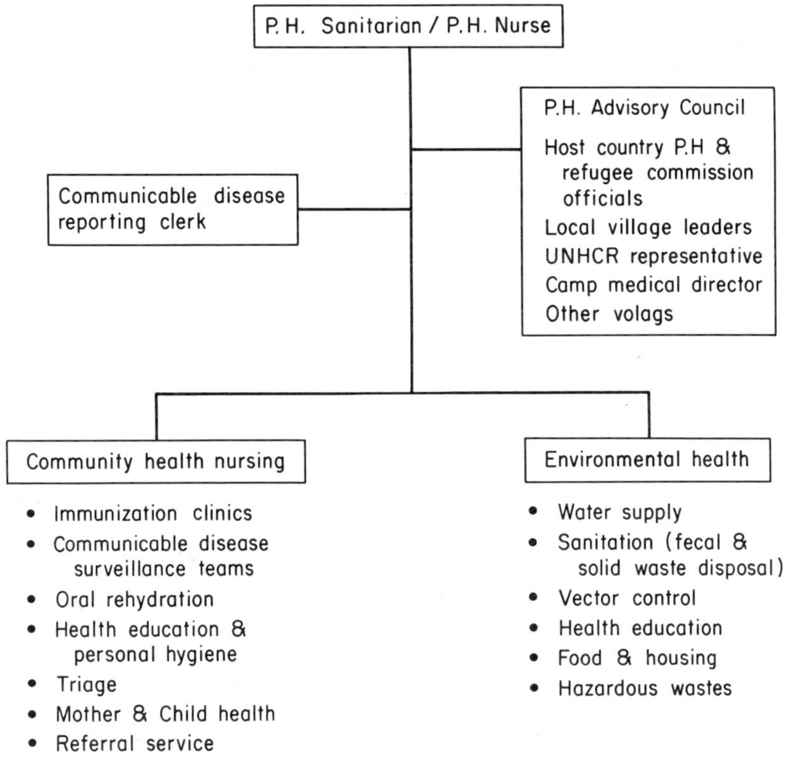

measures and the reason for these measures. Following is a partial list of health education topics:

- How diseases are transmitted by flies, contaminated water, poor personal hygiene, improper sewage disposal, and poor food protection.
- What diseases are present in the camp and how each disease is associated with a particular environmental factor.
- Protection of water supplies by avoidance of contamination by dipping buckets; facts about chlorine in the drinking water; storage of water in the housing unit.
- Safe sewage disposal; the need for handwashing after defecation; proper facilities and how to use and maintain them.
- Food protection by covering food to prevent contamination by flies and dust; rodent and insect infestation and control.
- Personal hygiene; use of soap and water, adequate bathing, and disposal of feces from babies.

Successful environmental health education programs operate on three levels: (1) educating a cadre of refugees to teach other refugees; (2) educating the mass of the refugee population; and (3) educating camp leaders and decision makers. Chapter 4 discusses in more detail the issues of training refugees to be health workers.

Community Development Approach

Water and sanitation activities are, necessarily, project-oriented activities such as building privies, constructing water storage tanks, and establishing garbage collection systems. Certain questions should be asked to determine whether the project has a high potential for failure or success. Ben Wisner has formulated a practical checklist (Timberlake 1985). If the answers to the following questions are positive, the project is likely to be successful:

- Is the project oriented to the needs of the people involved in it?
- Does the project make use of local human

resources including knowledge, cultural values, and organizational structure?

- Is the project based on local natural resources including materials, land, and energy?
- Is the project sustainable over the long term?
- Is external aid provided in reasonable amounts and in such a fashion that the people being helped do not become dependent on it?
- Is the project coordinated with local and regional authorities?
- Are new group alliances being formed through the project?

Once a program is organized and goals and objectives are agreed on, the selection of appropriate technological interventions should be considered.

WATER AND SANITATION TECHNOLOGIES

Camp Site Selection

Water and sanitation technologies are necessarily closely linked with the physical setting of the camp. The need for proper site selection was summarized by Dr. A. G. Rangaraj, UNHCR Medical Coordinator in Southeast Asia, who wrote that "all our sanitation, water supply, and drainage problems in the refugee camps have been, and still are, due to wrong selection of camp sites" (Personal correspondence 1981).

There appears to be a striking propensity to ignore environmental constraints during the site selection process of many refugee camps, even though guidance for siting can be found in World Health Organization (WHO) literature (Assar 1971). Most of the refugee camps in Thailand were placed in areas with insufficient water supplies, poor drainage, and endemic vector control problems. The original Sakaeo camp, for example, was placed in a rice paddy. Although Sakaeo was habitable during the dry season, when the monsoons came, the camp had to be moved to higher ground at great expense. In Sudan, Wad Kowli could be reached only by a three-hour drive over dirt roads. During the rainy season, the camp was virtually inaccessible, causing disruption of food supplies. In addition, Wad Kowli was located along a riverbed that dried up and the salty groundwater was unusable. Water, therefore had to be trucked in.

In Thailand, there were basically two types of camps. The initial sites were along the Laotian and Kampuchean borders. These, for the most part, just "sprang up," often at food distribution areas, water supply locations, or along transportation routes. Because these evolved without prior planning, water and sanitation problems could not be prevented but had to be solved after they occurred. A state of confusion often existed. The second type of camp was a "holding center." These were usually located some distance from the border. They were more organized than the first type of camp, and there was more potential for careful planning.

Water Supply

A plentiful water supply is not enough; water must also be protected from contamination during transportation, storage, and use. Proper disposal of water spilled at the water supply point helps reduce mosquito breeding. When no provision is made to drain spilled water, the water-dispensing points become mudholes.

Cholera, typhoid, hepatitis, and many enteric pathogens can be spread by contaminated water supplies. *Vibrio cholera* was isolated from the bathing waters at the Rangsit Transit Center in Bangkok. The suspected source was sewage seeping into the water lines. Water systems must be inspected, maintained, and tested routinely to avoid such outbreaks.

In a Thai-Kampuchean border camp, water was taken from wells 8 to 12 meters deep. Problems with water procurement, transportation, utilization, and storage were best addressed at the individual or family level, with health education being a critical element. In the better organized camps, the division of labor with water supply management was at a campwide level. In Sakaeo I, drinking water was trucked in from distant sources. Chlorine was added when the water was placed in the trucks, allowing for disinfection during transportation (chlorine should be in the water for 30 minutes for disinfection to occur). Chlorine monitoring teams would "greet" each truck as it entered the camp. The residual chlorine was measured. If it was satisfactory, the truck was allowed to proceed to the distribution points. If too little or no chlorine was found, chlorine would be added and the truck was "quarantined" for 30 minutes. Since truckers were paid by the number of loads, lack of chlorine was rarely a problem. At Sakaeo II (Sakaeo I relocated), wells pumped water directly into storage tanks. Because water was easily contaminated by buckets being dipped into the tanks, chlorine was added to each tank. Bucket dipping was a problem when water supplies were low. Frequently, there were long lines of refugees with their buckets waiting for water. When water came, most of the refugees did not want to wait longer for it to flow from the sanitary spigots, so the tank lids were opened and the dipping began. Because of the heavy use of open buckets for water collection and storage, chlorination and chlorine testing was a must even when the original water supply was excellent.

Excreta Disposal

One of the most important, though difficult, tasks in a refugee camp is the proper disposal of human excreta. Many refugees were rural farmers. Previous sanitary habits of defecation in the open fields had not created a health threat, but in a crowded camp setting, the same habits produced stench, a breeding grounds for flies, and a health hazard.

Overcoming tradition is never an easy task. Selection of an appropriate sanitation system is critical. If refugees do not accept the technology, or are not willing to maintain it, little real health progress can be made. Technology must be chosen to match the physical site conditions including soil type, rainy season water table levels, wind direction, and accessibility. Many of the sanitation systems are discussed in the literature and are presented below. The main caution is, *never initiate construction of a sanitation system without refugee involvement and a clear and acceptable method of maintenance.*

Figure 3-4 (Kalbermatten 1980) illustrates the construction of a typical pit privy. Of special note is the fly-tight lid covering the hole. This is often forgotten, which defeats the well-intended effort to construct the rest of the privy in a fly-tight manner. In Sakaeo I, trench latrines were originally constructed and covered with wooden planks. The planks were nailed tightly together when the wood was still "green." As the planks dried out, gaps appeared between them, making perfect entry points for flies. Eventually, the used planks had to be taken apart and renailed.

Figure 3-5 (Kalbermatten 1980) illustrates the construction of a privy in an area where the water table is high. Here, the privy must be elevated to avoid water entering the pit and causing the contents to overflow. Pit privies and trench latrines with individual compartments provide privacy, which is an important

Figure 3-4. Conventional unimproved pit latrines.

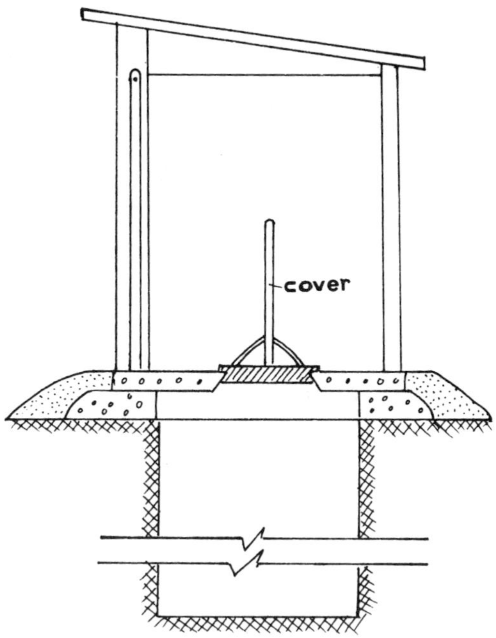

(Adapted with permission from Kalbermatten, et al 1980.)

consideration. In some soils, pits and trenches cave in, so special reinforcement of the earthen walls is required.

Open fields can be used in hot, dry climates, but the fecal matter must be scraped up at least every third day to avoid fly breeding. In Sudan, where the temperatures reach 51°C, there was a common misconception that the exposed feces would quickly dry out and flies would not breed. In reality, flies have no trouble breeding in the fecal matter, even on the hottest days.

Refugees and volunteer staff often dig open pits to dispose of wastewater or waste milk at the feeding centers. As flies need moisture to breed, these are perfect breeding grounds. Figure 3-6 illustrates a simple, but effective, soakaway pit that is sanitary and flyproof.

Figure 3-7 (Kalbermatten 1980) illustrates an aqua-privy system. As feces are deposited in a tank filled with water, a small amount of the water is displaced into a soakaway pit. Eventually, the privy tank must be pumped out. It is important to locate the tanks near roads so they are accessible to the pumper truck. Aqua-privies were installed in Sakaeo II. Four families shared an aqua-privy and were responsible

Figure 3-5. Alternative pit latrine designs.

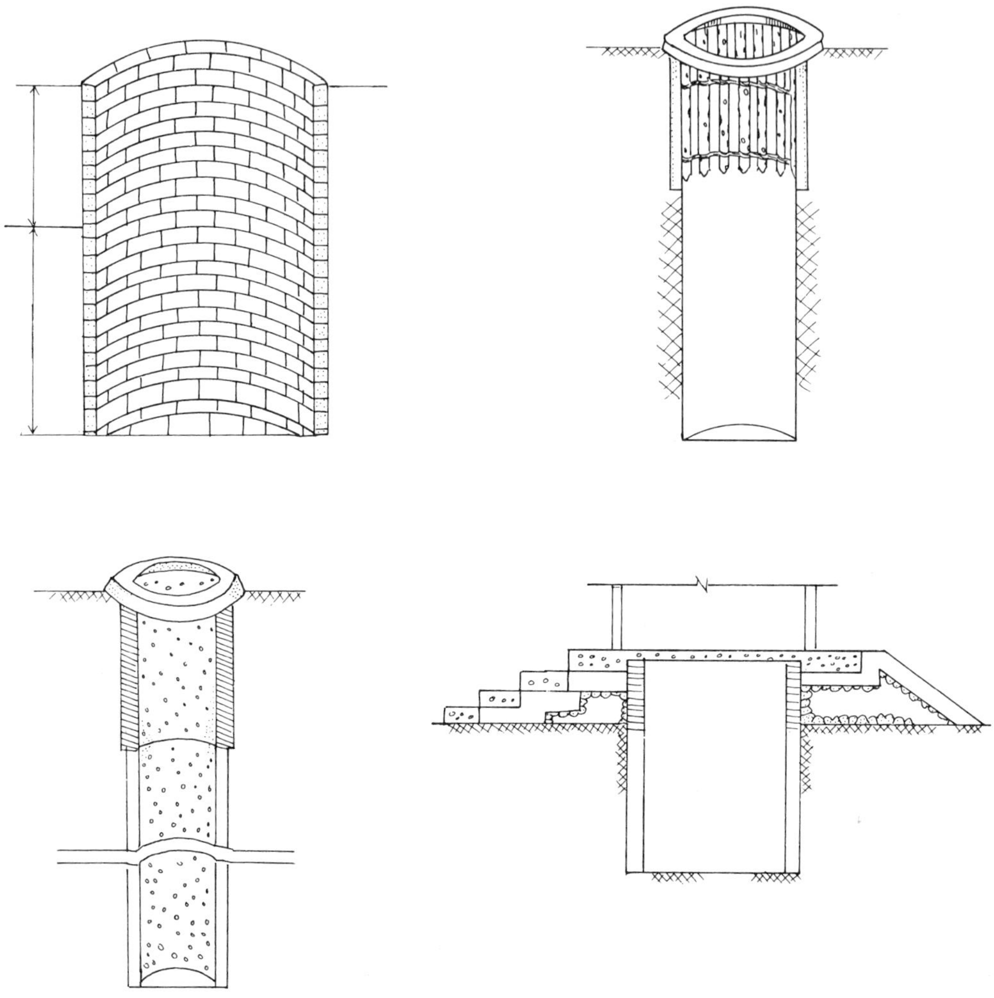

(Adapted with permission from Kalbermatten, et al 1980.)

for its maintenance. Because each privy had few users, maintenance problems were greatly reduced. The system was expensive but proved to be very sanitary.

Communal-type sanitation facilities require maintenance crews to keep the facilities clean. If left unattended, the facilities soon become a health hazard.

Solid Waste Management

Proper refuse collection, storage, and disposal are necessary for control of vector-borne diseases. In the early days of a refugee camp, few items and little rubbish are generated. Soon, however, food scraps appear, hospital and laboratory wastes accumulate, and discarded clothing, building materials, and other debris are strewn about.

In Sakaeo, a modern garbage compactor truck was donated, but because no spare parts were available, it was soon abandoned. It was replaced with a simple, flat-bed truck, which made the rounds of the camp each day and carried the trash and garbage to an approved site away from the camp. In the Sudan, small garbage carts or donkey carts were provided to do the hauling. These methods work well as long

Figure 3-6. Flyproof soakaway pit.

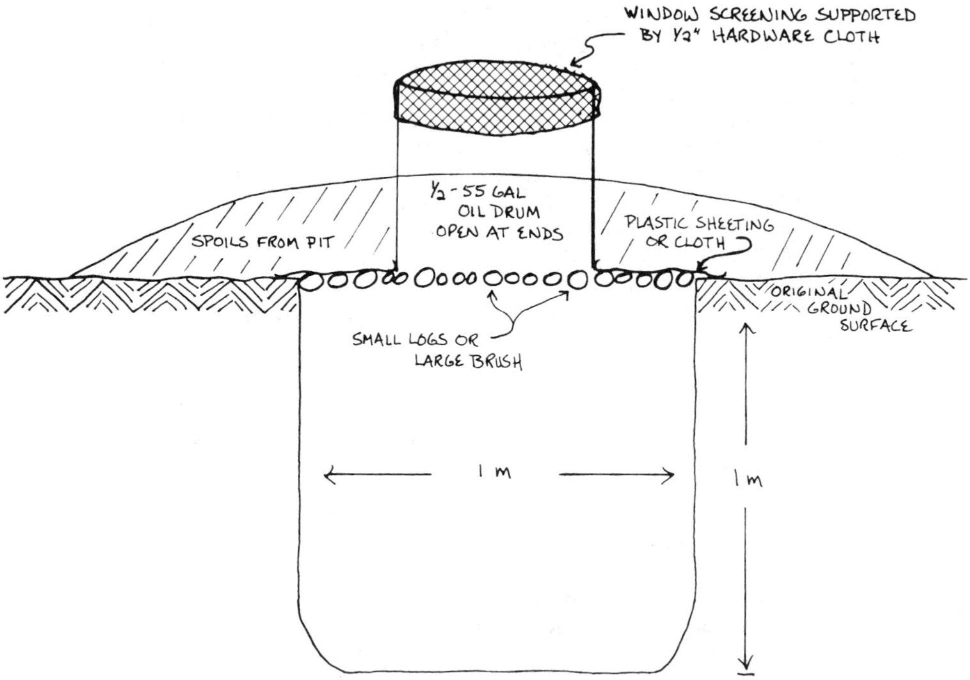

(Drawn by J. Heron, R.S.)

Figure 3-7. Conventional aqua-privy.

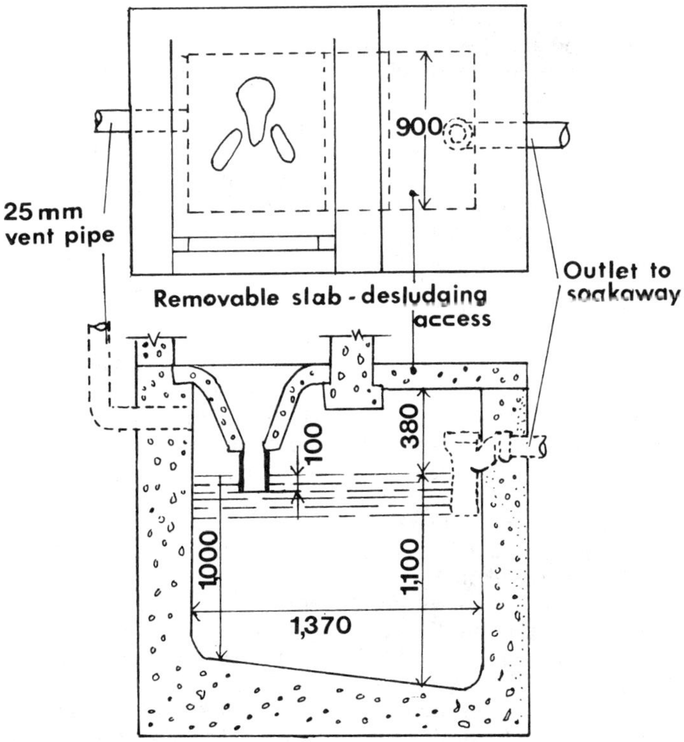

(Adapted with permission from Kalbermatten, et al 1980.)

as the work crews are adequately supervised and have designated areas they are responsible for maintaining.

One of the most critical components of a solid waste management system is the safe disposal of hospital and laboratory-generated wastes. At Sakaeo II, children would find used syringes and play with them. A secure storage system was devised and the refuse was burned each day, thus solving this problem. A simple incinerator was made from a 55-gallon steel drum. Maintenance was easy because there were no moving parts.

Vector Control

The problem of flies, mosquitoes, and rodents can be reduced if proper attention is paid to the previously discussed topics. Use of chemicals should be considered as a last resort. Not only are the chemicals dangerous if improperly applied, but they also give a false sense of security if a vector-borne disease outbreak occurs. Relying on chemicals as a means of standard control during an outbreak can produce resistant vectors. Then the chemicals cannot be relied on to have a quick-kill effect.

Spraying crews must be carefully trained. In the Sudan, one of the authors witnessed the hospital food being sprayed with DDT because there were flies on the food. Needless to say, the food had to be discarded and the spraying crew instructed on proper spraying methods.

Housing

Housing ranges from no shelter at all, to makeshift lean-tos of plastic scrap or straw, to "permanent" duplex-type structures constructed from local materials. Housing should provide protection from rain, heat, and cold and offer privacy.

Fire Safety

Fire is always a serious threat. When straw structures are crowded together, fire spreads quickly, especially on a windy day. Firebreaks created by open space should not be overlooked in camp layout and design. In the Nong Khai camp in Thailand, fire destroyed housing for 17,000 refugees. The hospital in Khao-I-Dang burned to the ground in 15 minutes (there was a fire truck in the camp but the keys were 200 km away in Bangkok). In Wad Kowli, Sudan, a fire started in a crowded area where straw was the major housing material and a strong wind was present. In all three instances, the refugees, knowing the seriousness of the situation better than the volunteer staff, quickly organized and either put the fires out with dirt and by beating it with their hands, or evacuated the premises. Without their quick action, several hundred people might have died. Emergency fire plans and equipment should be on hand at all times. Fires will inevitably occur.

PUBLIC HEALTH CHECKLIST

GENERAL

- A system is in place for surveillance and reporting of communicable diseases. Report forms are standardized. Monthly disease incidence and prevalence rates are calculated.
- Prompt and appropriate investigations are carried out on receipt of communicable disease reports.
- Adequate handwashing facilities are available for hospital and clinic workers.
- Screening and/or nets are available to help protect hospital patients from mosquitoes.
- An adequate immunization program is in place. There is an immunization tracking system.
- A program for screening health problems of children under 12 years of age is in place.
- Adequate emphasis has been placed on education of health workers and the general refugee community regarding the importance of handwashing, breastfeeding, and other public health and preventive medicine principles.
- Birth control information and techniques are available and appropriately disseminated.
- Malnutrition surveys are performed in the camp.
- Supplementary feeding programs are available.
- Maternal-child health clinics are in place and follow the Road to Health chart of height and weight (WHO), provide supplementary feeding and vitamins (when indicated), and provide basic instruction to mothers on sanitation, breastfeeding, and related topics.

DRINKING WATER SUPPLY

- The water supply is free of hazards.
- The water is regularly tested for microorganisms.
- The water meets WHO standards.
- The water is protected from contamination.
- Test kits are available for measuring both free and total chlorine residuals.

• One person is in charge of monitoring water quality. Problems are reported to appropriate, previously identified, officials.

• Adequate quantitites of water are available (approximately 20 liters/person/day depending on the ambient temperature).

• Sewage disposal is located at least 30 meter (100 feet) from water sources.

• Safe and adequate water storage facilities are available.

DRINKING WATER TRANSPORT VEHICLES (if in use)

• The water is chlorinated.

• Free chlorine residual = 0.2 mg/liter if the water is clear.

• The chlorine dosage must be increased to 10 to 20 mg/liter if the water is muddy.

• Each truck load is tested and the results are recorded.

• The load is rejected if chlorine concentration is less than required.

EXCRETA DISPOSAL

• An administrative structure is in place to report and deal with problems.

• An adequate budget is available to purchase disinfectant, brushes, pails, repair materials, and, ideally, toilet paper.

• One person is in charge of overseeing inspection and maintenance.

• At least one privy per 20 refugees is provided.

• Privy facilities afford some privacy.

• Privies are conveniently located.

• Privies are separated from water sources.

• The soil drains well during all seasons, with the sewage system properly designed to overcome any soil limitations.

• Latrines are flyproof and rodent-proof.

• Privies and sewage facilities are inspected daily.

• Facilities are cleaned and disinfected daily.

• Work crews are organized to repair privies.

• Wastewater from bathing and washing is properly disposed of.

• Sewage pumpings are safely disposed of.

• A surveillance system is in place to locate and remove feces from ground surfaces.

SOLID WASTE DISPOSAL

• Disposal sites are safe and properly constructed.

• Covering of the disposal site is done daily or weekly.

• There is no leechate runoff into water ways.

• There are an adequate number of garbage collection containers (one container per 40 refugees).

• Garbage collection crews are available and collection routes are clearly identified.

• Garbage is removed daily (a must in hot climates).

• One person is in charge of garbage collection and disposal.

• Camp cleanup campaigns are scheduled.

• A system for safe disposal of hospital hazardous wastes is in place.

• Control of used syringes is adequate.

VECTOR CONTROL

• Evidence of rodents is checked for regularly.

• Rodent harborages are removed.

• Food storage buildings are rodent-proofed.

• Garbage containers have covers.

• Stagnant water sites (ponding) are searched for and eliminated (mosquitoes breed in stagnant water).

• A system for rapid detection and identification of significant vectors is in place.

• Sanitation measures rather than spraying are relied on for vector control.

• Adequate and appropriate chemicals and equipment are available to spray for flies and mosquitoes in case of emergencies.

FIRE CONTROL

• Buildings are adequately spaced.

• Fire extinguishers are available in kitchens, hospitals, generator buildings, and other major facilities.

• The hospital kitchen is carefully constructed.

• Kitchens and other hazardous areas are inspected frequently.

• Workers in areas with high fire hazard potential are instructed in fire prevention and fire-fighting principles.

• All flammable materials are properly stored.

• Accumulation of potential kindling is avoided.

• Hospital staff have a plan for moving patients safely and extinguishing fires, should they occur.

• Fire drills are conducted.

• A fire-fighting system is in place in the camp including watch towers, fire trucks with properly trained personnel, and a communication system between the areas of highest fire risk and the fire station.

REFERENCES AND SELECTED READING

Assar M: Guide to Sanitation in Natural Disasters. Geneva, World Health Organization, 1971.

Cairncross S, Feachem R: Environmental Health Engineering in the Tropics: An Introductory Text. New York, John Wiley, 1983.

Feachem R et al: Health aspects of excreta and sullage management: A state of the art review. In: Appropriate Technology for Water Supply and Sanitation, vol 3. Washington, DC, The World Bank, 1980, pp v, 159.

Grabe M: Emergency refugee health care. In: Allegra DT, Nieburg P, Grabe M (eds): A Chronical of Experience in the Khmer Assistance Operation 1979–1980. Washington DC, US Department of Health and Human Services, 1983, pp 91–98.

Hawkins P: Environmental health. In: Simmonds S, Vaughan P, Gunn SW (eds): Refugee Community Health Care. Oxford, Oxford University Press, 1983, pp 166–95.

Kalbermatten J et al (eds): A Planner's Guide in Appropriate Technology for Water Supply and Sanitation, vol 2. Washington DC, The World Bank, 1980, pp 85, 90, 108.

Kroeger EK: Disaster management in tropical countries. Tropical Doctor 1976;6:185–86.

Pineo CS, Schnare DW, Miller GW: Environmental Sanitation and Integrated Health Delivery Programs, Monograph Series No 4. Washington, DC, American Public Health Association, 1981, p 5.

Timberlake L: Africa in crises—the causes, the cures of environmental bankruptcy. Earthscan, 1985; pp 218–19.

UN High Commissioner for Refugees: Handbook for Emergencies. Part I: Field Operations. Geneva, UN High Commission for Refugees, 1983, p 72.

Ward B: Low Cost Technology Options for Sanitation: A State of the Art Review and Annotated Bibliography. In Rybezynski W, Chongrak P, McGarry M (eds): Appropriate Technology for Water Supply and Sanitation, vol 4, p 3. Washington DC, International Development Research Center and the World Bank, 1982.

4
Training Refugees to Be Health Workers

RICHARD H. SANDLER

More often than not, health workers from abroad arrive in refugee camp settings with the expectation that they will be providing direct patient care. Although this may be important in an immediate crisis situation, for the medium or long term, direct patient care is less important than the training of refugee health care workers. Such training is vital for the following reasons:

- By training refugees to act as care givers, medical care can be extended to many more people. For example, in one refugee camp clinic a physician saw about 60 out-patients a day. After he trained refugee primary health care workers, more than 300 patients were helped each day.
- Refugee health care providers can often provide superior primary health care because they better understand the language and culture of the patients.
- Trained refugee health workers will often remain in the refugee setting as providers and teachers long after short-term health workers have gone (although a rapid turnover of trained refugees due to resettlement is a large problem in some settlements).

TRAINING PROGRAMS FOR REFUGEE HEALTH WORKERS

Refugee health workers should be trained and integrated into the medical system early in the relief effort to facilitate their maximum use. OXFAM has identified four principal groups of refugees who may be most helpful as health workers:

- Refugees who previously qualified as professional health workers.
- Traditional healers and midwives who might be incorporated into the health care system.
- Nonmedically trained refugees who can be trained as preventive health workers, educators, and basic clinical assistants.
- Nonmedically trained refugees who, after minimal training, can assist with important ancillary health tasks such as waste disposal.

The following are key issues to consider in setting up refugee health worker training programs:

What are the goals of the training program? Different purposes might include training refugee health workers to do the following:

- Augment the functions of the foreign health workers in order to eventually replace them in the camp.
- Function as "barefoot doctors" after repatriation.
- Serve in the host country as health care workers on a long-term basis. If this is the goal, provisions should be made to coordinate training efforts with the host government or, ideally, to have them conduct the training. Refugee health workers who complete their training might receive some form of certification or licensure, thus enabling them to practice legitimately in the host country at a later time.
- Provide occupational therapy or intellectual stimulation for refugees who have little else to do.

What is an appropriate level of care to teach refugee workers? This is difficult to establish. Health care providers from Western countries generally come from sophisticated medical environments. In the refugee setting, most sophisticated medical technology is not available. Often the technologies or drugs available in the early development of a refugee camp or settlement are inappropriate for the setting—for example, a neonatal respirator. A detailed discussion of these complex issues is beyond the scope of this chapter (see Chapter 9), but some major considerations include the following:

- What should be used as a "standard" or "benchmark" against which to judge an "appropriate" level of care? Should the level of health care available in the surrounding village populations be matched? Should the standard be that which existed in the refugees' home country, or that of industrialized nations? Should the short-term limitations of health workers, technology, and financial resources dictate the standard?

• Host countries often object to refugees receiving a higher level of care than the local national population. How should this problem be handled while keeping in mind that the refugee camp exists at the pleasure of the host country?

• To what degree should advanced levels of care be avoided if the highly skilled personnel, medications, equipment, and other resources necessary to maintain that level of care are likely to be less available in the future?

• To what degree should efforts be made to divert well-funded acute care resources to potentially more useful (in overall reduction of morbidity and mortality per dollar or person-hour) nutrition, immunization, sanitation, and other public health programs?

Answers to these questions will vary depending on the refugee setting, resources, educational level of the refugees, and duration of the refugee problem. The best approach might be to avoid the imposition of rigid regulations on situations that are always changing and to reassess priorities at frequent intervals.

To what degree is a "little bit of knowledge a dangerous thing"? Refugee health workers often have had no previous medical training. They may be taught an enormous amount in a short time. The potential for misunderstanding is compounded when the training is conducted in a language that the refugees have varying levels of proficiency in, such as English. Much of Western medical technology is associated with significant risks even when properly used. Might refugee health workers use some of their newly acquired knowledge in a manner that will do more harm than good? In addition to emphasizing the inherent hazards of medicines and techniques, should information about certain medicines or potentially harmful procedures be withheld? Careful attention to the potential hazards of each technique may prevent the initiation of procedures that are more dangerous than helpful.

Do training programs create a privileged class of refugees by providing English instruction and recommendations on behalf of selected refugees to embassies or resettlement agencies?

Should refugees receive financial or other forms of payment? This is a controversial issue, but it is often found that few refugees will work on a regular basis without some financial incentive.

How should refugee health workers be chosen? It may be preferable to have the candidates chosen by the refugee community. Although this may work in an established camp, refugees have often arrived from disparate towns and villages and will have difficulty choosing potential health workers. Werner and Bower (1982) state that the most reliable age groups are the 25 to 40-year-olds. Although this generalization does not always hold true, younger individuals may command less respect, while those over 40 may be somewhat inflexible. The proportion of men and women as workers will be determined, in part, by local custom, but a mix of both is generally advantageous.

Elements of a Successful Training Program

There is no set formula for a successful training program, but the following considerations should be helpful:

• Define program goals and purposes as carefully as possible with the participation of the refugees and local health authorities before training is begun.

• Include the host government and the refugees in the execution of training programs whenever appropriate.

• Base the training program on the actual needs of the camp and use a problem-solving approach.

• Be flexible and change plans according to what does and does not work as camp conditions change.

• Have the refugees themselves conduct the training, in their native language to the extent possible.

• Divide tasks so that individual students will have less material to master.

• Include, as important components of a successful training program, lectures, discussions, handouts, and practical hands-on experience.

• Take into account the existing knowledge of the trainees, and the prevailing traditional and modern local health practices.

• See that relevant medical texts are available. Two helpful books are *Where There Is No Doctor* (Werner 1977; currently available in 28 languages) and *Primary Child Care: A Manual for Health Workers* (King 1978).

- Use a participatory teaching approach that emphasizes culturally appropriate methods such as storytelling, singing, and role-playing. This method teaches the trainees to teach others and creates a "multiplier effect." Involve the students in making their own teaching aids.
- Respect cultural differences and taboos, especially regarding issues such as physical examination of sexual genitalia and discussion of family planning methods.
- Emphasize the basics of public health, including personal hygiene and sanitation, breastfeeding, and the use of oral rehydration solutions.
- Consider establishing a centralized training center where basic vocabulary and information can be provided before more specialized on-the-job clinical training is undertaken.
- Teach trainees to use a limited number of drugs and few, if any, invasive procedures.

Tasks for Refugee Health Workers

The tasks for which refugee health workers should be trained are contingent on many factors including the type of refugee setting (e.g., initial crisis collection camp, transit camp, chronic camp, relocation camp), the educational level of the available workers, cultural taboos, expected time in residence for the health workers, the types of health problems that exist in the camp, and the financial and training resources available. A camp or settlement that has recently been set up to receive large numbers of acutely ill refugees will not be able to engage in extensive training activities. Shortly after the situation stabilizes, however, serious training efforts should begin. Unfortunately, after a camp has been stable for a few years, apathy sets in and training efforts become more difficult.

In November, 1980, the Khao-I-Dang (KID) Holding Center for displaced Khmers in Thailand provided a favorable combination of the above factors when the author conducted a review of all the refugee health worker training activities occurring in the camp. There were 1125 refugee health workers performing approximately 15 different health-related roles. The following were among the health worker roles:

- *Nurses.* About 240 refugee health workers functioned as nurses on the hopital wards. The nature of their tasks and training were highly variable. On some wards, the refugee workers were given extensive responsibility for virtually all aspects of nursing care including starting IVs and delivering IV medication. A nursing school was established and provided an intensive three-month course for about 30 students at a time. The first six weeks were devoted to intensive didactic teaching of anatomy, physiology, microbiology, and pharmacology. The last six weeks provided clinical activity supervised by designated preceptors.
- *Physician's assistants.* Two hospital wards and all but 1 of 12 out-patient departments (OPDs) trained health workers to function as physician's assistants. For example, in one OPD, 12 Khmers served as physician's assistants. Each morning a one-hour didactic session was held. During the day, all of the refugee workers were called together to examine instructive patients. In teams of two, they took vital signs, did a focused history and physical examination, ordered appropriate laboratory tests, and diagnosed and treated the patients. The health workers consulted the supervising physician when patients appeared ill or had vital signs beyond certain age-specified ranges, or when they were uncertain of a diagnosis or therapy. It is very encouraging that after one to two months of training, individuals with no previous medical background were able to deliver quality, out-patient medical care for the vast majority of illnesses seen.
- *Dental workers.* Under the supervision of two dentists, ten refugee health workers provided a wide range of dental services after only four to eight weeks of training. They performed all of the extractions, drillings, fillings, and some of the more complex work such as root canal surgery.
- *Family planning counselors.* Many of the OPDs had full-time family planning refugee health workers. In one OPD, a Khmer man and woman worked as a team. Their activities are described in Chapter 7.
- *Maternal and child health workers.* Each OPD was paired with a maternal and child health (MCH) clinic. Refugee health workers weighed and measured children, plotted the measurements on the "Road to Health Chart," and gave appropriate immunizations. Perhaps most importantly, they taught mothers about such critical topics as personal hygiene and sanitation, breastfeeding, family planning, nutrition, and the use of oral rehydration solutions. An extensive system of home visitors also existed; refugee health workers systemati-

cally went into the homes of other refugees to perform the preceding functions.

• *Communicable disease tracers.* Under the direction of the public health staff, 14 refugee workers systematically looked through the log books of all the hospital wards, laboratories, and OPDs for certain communicable diseases. Each of these was then investigated in the community with appropriate follow-up measures taken. These health workers also made up the basic work force for mass immunization efforts.

• *School health workers.* All 20,000 school children in the refugee camp were methodically screened by 17 refugee health workers for nutrition, hearing, vision, dental, orthopedic, dermatologic, and other problems. The yield of underlying illness was impressive. For example, about 35 percent of the children screened were found to have dental problems.

• *Sanitarians.* Each home was inspected and graded every seven to ten days by a team of 16 refugee workers and one supervising sanitarian. Rodent harborages, garbage, mosquito larvae, and water supplies were all carefully reviewed. Either the occupant, group leader, or section leader was asked to take corrective action when a problem was identified.

• *Laboratory technicians.* One professional laboratory technician trained and supervised 14 health workers in all the basic laboratory services. These included Gram's stains, acid-fast bacillus (AFB) smears, malaria smears, hematocrits, complete blood counts, and stools for ova and parasites. The blood bank was run successfully by two refugees with little supervision.

• *Physical therapists.* Twenty refugee health workers and five physical therapists provided both preventive and therapeutic physical therapy services (see Chapter 21).

• *Elementary school teachers as health educators.* Khmer elementary schoolteachers were given a course one hour a day for one month. Basic preventive medicine principles including hygiene, sanitation, accident prevention, communicable disease control, nutrition, and dental and skin care were taught. The teachers were assisted in developing a health curriculum for the schools.

• *Public health educators.* Refugees were involved in direct public education on certain fundamental public health issues such as personal hygiene, breastfeeding, communicable disease control, and family planning. Methods of reaching the refugee population included use of the mass media (such as the public address system), community meetings, posters, and, occasionally, slides and films.

• *Rural health workers.* A two-month intensive rural health worker program was begun using *Where There Is No Doctor* (Werner 1977) as a text. The entire book was later translated into Khmer. The course was originally established to train refugees in the border camps using a model similar to the "barefoot doctor" program developed in China. The expectation was that the trained refugees would return to Kampuchea after completing the course. Unfortunately, this expectation proved to be unrealistic and the course emphasis was changed to focus more on the needs in the refugee camp.

• *Other refugee health roles.* Refugees were trained to provide many other roles such as operating room technicians, lay midwives, and pharmacy technicians.

Training of Khmers was carried out by many different groups. Most of the training occurred on the job and was supplemented by regularly scheduled didactic lectures. Some programs began with a few days to weeks of didactic material. To provide training more efficiently, a few centralized efforts were begun, such as the previously mentioned nursing school.

The type and extent of refugee training will be a function of many factors, with local policies often determining priorities. For example, in Somalia, the Ministry of Health took responsibility for establishing and running the training programs. In Sudan, training was left up to the refugees although some foreign health worker assistance was available. Those from abroad should encourage and support the refugees to take initiative recognizing their long-term role in their own health needs.

REFERENCES AND SUGGESTED READING

Abbat FR: Teaching for Better Learning: A Guide for Teachers of Primary Health Care Staff. Geneva, World Health Organization, 1980.

Bechtel RM (ed): SALUS: Low-Cost Rural Health Care and Health Manpower Training. An Annotated Bibliography with Special Emphasis on Developing Countries. Ottawa, International Development Research Centre, 1981.

Campbell JW (ed): The training and support of primary health care workers. In: Proceedings of the National Council for International Health 1981 International Health Conference. Washington, DC, National Council for International Health, 1981.

Ericsson S, Adjou-Moumouni BSF: Training course for village health workers in Lome, Togo, Regional Training Center. Geneva, World Health Organization, 1979.

Katz FM: Guidelines for evaluating a training program for health personnel. Geneva, World Health Organization, 1978.

King MH, King F, Martodipoero S: Primary Child Care: A Manual for Health Workers, London, Oxford Univ Press 1978.

MEDEX Group: The MEDEX Primary Health Care Series (35 volumes). Honolulu, The MEDEX Group, University of Hawaii, 1983.

Parlato MB, Favin MN: Primary Health Care: Progress and Problems. An Analysis of 52 AID-Assisted Projects. Washington, DC, American Public Health Association, 1981.

Seaman J (ed): Training for disaster management. Disasters 1983;7(1).

Simmonds SP, Vaughan P, Gunn SW (eds): Refugee Community Health Care. New York, Oxford University Press, 1983.

Stinson W, Favin M, Bradford B: Teaching Community Health Workers. Information for Action Series. Washington, DC, World Federation of Public Health Associations, American Public Health Association, 1983.

Storms DM: Training and use of the auxiliary worker: Lesson from developing countries. Washington, DC, American Public Health Association, International Programs, 1979.

Vaughan JP: Barefoot or professional? Community health workers in the Third World: Some important questions concerning their function, utilization, selection, training and evaluation. J Trop Med Hyg 1980;83:3–10.

Werner D: Where There Is No Doctor. Palo Alto, CA, Hesperian Foundation, 1977.

Werner D, Bower B: Helping Health Workers Learn. Palo Alto, CA, Hesperian Foundation, 1982.

World Health Organization: Primary health worker: Working guide. Guidelines for training. Guidelines for adaptation, Rev ed. Geneva, World Health Organization, 1980.

World Health Organization: Training and Utilization of Auxiliary Personnel for Rural Health Teams in Developing Countries. WHO Technical Report Series No 633, Geneva, World Health Organization, 1979.

5
Immunizations for Health Workers

THOMAS C. JONES

If health workers are to provide medical care for refugees, it is essential that they maintain appropriate care of their own health. For some inexplicable reason, that basic requirement is often ignored. It has been observed that health care organizations provide no advice to their medical personnel, furnish misinformation, or, when advice is given, do little to encourage compliance. In addition, health care personnel reject the necessary changes in personal habits that would protect them against diseases such as shigellosis, giardiasis, hepatitis, and malaria.

Health workers' disregard for their own health, or an organization's failure to develop comprehensive health programs for its workers, carries an unacceptably high price tag. The cost in time, money, and energy directed away from the primary goal of refugee health care has been tremendous. One estimate is that approximately 20 percent of health workers are unavailable to provide health care at any given time because of their own ill health. Though health care workers acknowledge this estimate, there is disagreement concerning the measures necessary to decrease this high morbidity.

This chapter provides guidelines for those who want to maintain their health in a potentially contaminated environment. Persistent attention to avoiding contaminated food and water and insect vectors of disease and to getting proper immunizations *does* decrease illness among health workers.

IMMUNIZATIONS

Health workers will be exposed to a wide range of organisms for which no previous immunity has been established. The following sections describe methods of vaccination and chemoprophylaxis, and advice to provide maximum health protection. More detailed information is available in the pamphlet *Health Information for International Travel* (CDC 1984).

Vaccines

Although several vaccines can be administered simultaneously at different sites, typhoid, plague, and cholera vaccines often cause uncomfortable side effects and are best given at different times. If possible, immune globulin should not be given for three months before or less than three weeks after a live virus vaccine. Preliminary data indicate, however, that immune globulin does not interfere with the immune response to oral polio virus vaccine or to yellow fever vaccine. Because several of the vaccines recommended for health workers require multiple doses at intervals of four or more weeks, immunization schedules should be planned as far in advance as possible. Immunocompromised patients should not receive live virus vaccines.

Tetanus and Diphtheria

The organisms that cause tetanus and diphtheria are found throughout the world. Whether traveling or not, everyone should receive a primary series of immunizations against tetanus and diphtheria and a tetanus–diphtheria toxoid booster injection every ten years. Because health workers are at increased risk for minor injury and for exposure to the *Corynebacterium diphtheriae* bacteria, their immunization status should always be current.

Polio

Health workers who have not previously been immunized against polio should receive a primary series of inactivated polio vaccine unless protection is needed within four weeks; in this case a single dose of trivalent oral polio vaccine is recommended. The use of inactivated polio vaccine avoids the low but potential risk of vaccine-related polio that occurs more often in adults who have never received oral live virus polio vaccine. Vaccination with inactivated polio vaccine must be repeated every three years. If a health worker was immunized with a complete primary series of oral polio vaccine more than five years earlier, a booster of the oral vaccine is recommended.

Measles

Many individuals born after 1956 have not had measles. Because this disease is endemic in underdeveloped countries, it is recommended that all health workers and members of their families born after 1956 who have not had a measles vaccination, who received only the inactivated measles vaccine, or who have not had documented measles infection be inoculated before traveling abroad.

Influenza

All health workers should receive a single injection of the current influenza vaccine as risk of exposure to potential epidemics is high. Although the risk of serious influenza disease is low in healthy individuals, the illness will reduce the ability to provide health care to others and may contribute to spread of the infection.

Typhoid

Since typhoid is common in areas of poor sanitation, refugee health workers are at risk. Typhoid vaccine prepared from killed bacteria offers only partial protection and often causes one to two days of pain at the site of injection, sometimes accompanied by fever, malaise, and headache. A single dose is of no value. An oral typhoid vaccine is available in some countries and may be more effective (Jones 1985).

Immune Globulin for Hepatitis

This is recommended for all health workers. It should be taken as close to the time of entry into the refugee setting as possible because the period of maximum benefit occurs soon after the injection and is of short duration (three to six months). The dose is 0.05 ml/kg of standard immune serum globulin (ISG) intramuscularly every three to six months. Alternatively, 0.02 ml/kg can be administered intramuscularly every two months. Local tenderness, the only adverse effect, is decreased with the latter regimen.

Hepatitis B

A recently released vaccine for this disease offers good protection. Health workers have significant contact with blood products and are at higher risk for hepatitis B than the population at large; the vaccine is therefore indicated. Three injections administered over three months provide maximum protection, but if time does not permit completion of the series, two injections provide greater than 80% protection (Szmuness 1981).

Cholera

This vaccine has limited effectiveness and a moderately high incidence of side effects. However, because of the potential albeit low risk of encountering cholera in a refugee camp setting, it is recommended that health workers receive two doses of this vaccine and that booster doses be administered at six-month intervals when practical.

Plague

This vaccination is generally recommended only for health workers who may have contact with wild animals or who will be working in rural areas of Southeast Asia, Africa, or South America where plague is enzootic. Plague vaccine is a killed bacterial preparation, and adverse effects are similar to those of typhoid vaccine.

Meningococcus

Meningococcemia or meningitis is a potential epidemic problem in refugee settings. Health workers should be protected against the A, C, Y, and W135 serotypes. Available in a single dose, this vaccine is safe and effective. The duration of effective protection has not yet been determined.

Yellow Fever Vaccine

This attenuated live virus vaccine, which is prepared in eggs, should be considered whenever health workers travel to infected areas.

These areas include countries in Africa and South America 15 degrees north and south of the equator. The vaccine is effective for ten years.

Rabies

This vaccine is an inactivated virus preparation recommended for health workers anticipating contact with animals or prolonged residence in an area where rabies is a threat. The new human diploid cell rabies vaccine, which is safer and more effective than the duck embryo vaccine, is currently the only one available in the United States (Anderson 1980).

Bacille Calmette Guérin (BCG)

This vaccine against tuberculosis is widely used in Europe. It is approximately 50 percent effective in preventing tuberculosis or decreasing the severity of the illness once contracted. It should be considered for those health workers likely to have contact with patients with active tuberculosis (Jones 1985). This is particularly important in areas such as Southeast Asia where drug-resistant *M. tuberculosis* is common. The vaccine is safe when given to immunocompetent individuals and has few side effects. It reduces the usefulness of purified protein derivative (PPD) skin testing to determine recent exposure to tuberculosis.

Smallpox

This vaccine should no longer be used and is not available.

Malaria Chemoprophylaxis

Malaria prophylaxis is the most important chemoprophylaxis measure available for the worker in malaria-endemic areas. Adults who weigh more than 50 kg should take 500 mg (300 mg base) of chloroquine phosphate weekly, beginning one week before arrival and continuing for six weeks after departing an endemic area.

For elimination of the exoerythrocytic malaria parasite after departure from areas where *Plasmodium vivax* and *Plasmodium ovale* are endemic, many experts prescribe primaquine phosphate, 26.3 mg (15 mg base) daily, during the last two weeks of chloroquine prophylaxis.

Health workers in areas with chloroquine-resistant *P. falciparum* malaria should take the combination of 25 mg of pyrimethamine with 500 mg of sulfadoxine (Fansidar) once a week in addition to chloroquine if no history of drug allergy reactions is present (particularly to sulfa drugs). If there is such a history, doxycycline, 100 mg per day, should be used as malaria prophylaxis (CDC 1985). (Also see the discussion of malaria prophylaxis in Chapter 25.)

Pregnant women should not take pyrimethamine, which is teratogenic in animals. Malaria resistance to both chloroquine and Fansidar has been reported, particularly near the Thailand–Cambodia border and in the Amazon region of Brazil. In such areas, the best regimen has not been defined. Leading the present alternatives is doxycycline 100 mg orally daily (CDC 1985). Diarrhea, vaginitis, and photosensitivity reactions are complications of tetracycline. Workers should check the most current recommendations for malaria prophylaxis in the region to be visited before departure.

HEALTH ADVICE

Most of the diseases acquired by health workers are transmitted either by ingestion of contaminated food or water, or by insect vectors. To avoid these diseases, the worker must be fastidious in taking care of all food and water sources and follow routine precautions against insects.

Avoiding Contaminated Food or Water

In most underdeveloped countries, human feces containing many human pathogens contaminate the water system. What should be done to protect oneself from ingesting this contaminated water? In order of preference, we suggest the following: (1) drink only bottled, previously unopened, processed water or personally collected rain water; (2) drink boiled water; (3) drink chemically treated water. Bottled water is ensured as safe only if it is carbonated; this allows visual confirmation that the bottle has not been opened. Boiled water is also safe. To kill disease-producing microbes, bringing water to a brisk boil is adequate except at high altitudes where more prolonged boiling (five to ten minutes) is required. The most commonly used agents for chemical purification are chlorine and iodine (Jones 1985).

Iodine is more effective than chlorine. The concentration and duration of treatment are critical and vary depending on the degree of fecal contamination. With the variables involved, we find it best to discourage chemical treatment of water as a means of water purification. Freezing water into ice preserves, rather than kills, contaminating microbes. Ice should therefore be avoided unless it has been made with bottled or boiled water.

Vegetables are contaminated by human feces in the fields where they are grown or in marketplaces where they are handled. Various studies have shown that vegetables are heavily contaminated with protozoa and helminth eggs in underdeveloped countries. The health worker should consume ground-grown vegetables or fruits only after they have been thoroughly cooked. Fruits that are tree-grown and can be peeled are safe. Those who are abroad for long periods usually have a place where they can ensure proper preparation of fresh vegetables. The preparation process includes treating the vegetables with a detergent (any laundry soap), soaking them in 5% vinegar for 10 to 15 minutes, then rinsing them in previously boiled water. This process of alkali, dilute acid, and rinsing removes or kills potential human pathogens.

Avoiding Rare or Raw Meat and Fish

Rare or raw meat, fish, or crustacea can be the source of numerous infections. These include *Toxoplasma, Trichinella, Taenia, Clostridia, Salmonella* in meat, and *Paragonimus, Clonorchis, Diphyllobothrium, Capillaria, Ansakis, Angiostrongylus,* and *Vibrio parahaemolyticus* in fish or crustacea, to name some of the more common organisms. In addition, they may be contaminated by all of the organisms in the water during processing or storing. If one is not certain that food has been processed in a manner that eliminates these microbes, the only solution is to cook it until it is well done. Unpasteurized or unsterilized milk products are associated with risk because cattle inspection programs for prevention of brucellosis, salmonellosis, and tuberculosis may not be efficient (Jones 1985).

Avoiding Fecally Contaminated Fresh Water When Swimming

The most important disease acquired from freshwater swimming is schistosomiasis. Health workers in Africa, South America, and certain parts of Asia should be certain that the snail vectors and fecal contamination conditions for transmission of schistosomiasis are absent before they venture into the water. Chlorinated, properly filtered pools, and the ocean beyond the low tide region of a river estuary are safe from this infection.

Decreasing Arthropod Exposure

The frequent occurrence of skin ailments during work abroad is often due to improper protection against biting arthropods including mosquitoes, flies, and ticks (Jones 1985). The best methods for avoiding these pests include wearing adequate protective clothing, using insect repellent, using insecticides in closed areas, and ensuring proper screening from flying insects. Proper clothing is often omitted by the health worker because of the heat in a tropical country. This tendency can be lessened by wearing properly fitting cotton rather than synthetic clothing. Repellents may be ineffective because inadequate amounts are applied to the skin, they are not used because of their unpleasant effects on mucosal surfaces, or they are rendered useless by dilution from sweating or bathing. Only repellents with more than 25 percent diethyltoluamide should be used [those with higher concentration (up to 80%) are used when heavy insect exposure is likely]. The repellent is particularly important in the hours of dusk, when mosquito biting is common. We recommend an insecticide spray for use in sleeping quarters before one retires for the night. The doors or windows of such quarters are often open during the day; insects can enter and become confined within when the screening or mosquito netting is put in place. A short spraying of the room after screening ensures a safe night of sleep. One may leave the room for 10 to 15 minutes after spraying to allow the spray to settle from the air. The same procedure can be used within the mosquito netting over a bed after all openings are tightly closed. Finally, all netting and screening should be checked for holes that render the above measures useless.

HEALTH CARE FOLLOWING RETURN FROM WORK ABROAD

After returning from abroad, or at one- to two-year intervals, health workers should be examined for potential diseases acquired during their work. We suggest a screening physical examination, chest x-ray examination, blood count, stool examination for bacteria and parasites, and liver function tests. A PPD should be done to detect recent conversion from negative to positive. Those workers with symptoms should have a thorough evaluation for tropically acquired diseases, including blood smears and special serologic tests (Jones 1985). With these measures, proper care of health workers is ensured.

REFERENCES AND SUGGESTED READING

Anderson LJ et al: Postexposure trial of a human diploid cell strain rabies vaccine. J Infect Dis 1980;142:133.

Centers for Disease Control: Poliomyelitis prevention. Ann Intern Med 1982;96:630.

Centers for Disease Control: Health Information for International Travel 1984, PHS Document, 1984.

Centers for Disease Control: Morbidity and Mortality, Malaria Chemoprophylaxis. February 1985.

Chin J: Raw milk: A continuing vehicle for the transmission of infectious disease agents in the U.S. J Infect Dis 1982;146:440.

Jones TC: Immunization and travel advice for travelers. In: Remington J., Schwartz M. (eds): Current Topics in Clinical Infectious Diseases. New York, Mc-Graw-Hill, 1985, pp 45–65.

Ried HE: Bites and stings in travelers. Postgrad Med J 1978;51:830.

Szmuness W et al: The immune response of healthy adults to a reduced dose of hepatitis B vaccine. J Med Virol 1981;8:123.

6

Immunization Programs for Refugee Children and Pregnant Women

PHILLIP NIEBURG
TIMOTHY J. DONDERO

Immunizations against childhood diseases are among the most useful and cost-effective prevention measures available in industrialized countries. In underdeveloped countries, where infectious diseases are a more significant factor in childhood mortality, the importance of these vaccines is even greater. Although large-scale childhood immunization programs use considerable resources during their planning and implementation, they are cost-effective when properly carried out (Creese & Henderson 1980). This chapter outlines the principles that can provide the basis for a successful refugee immunization program.

PRIORITY OF IMMUNIZATIONS IN PROGRAMS FOR REFUGEE POPULATIONS

Between one quarter and one third of childhood deaths in underdeveloped countries can be prevented by immunization (Dondero 1983). Refugee children in these countries, living in crowded conditions and frequently malnourished, are at least as vulnerable as other children residing in the same countries and may be at even greater risk of death, particularly from measles. Disease prevention by immunization should therefore receive high priority in any refugee relief program.

Six antigens (measles, polio, pertussis, and bacille Calmette Guérin [BCG] vaccines, and tetanus and diphtheria toxoids) are included in the Expanded Programme on Immunization (EPI) of the World Health Organization (WHO). Other vaccines may become important in specific situations.

Measles vaccine is the most likely of all the EPI vaccines to be life-saving. Because of the severity of measles among malnourished children, measles immunization programs should have very high priority during the early (emergency) phase of refugee relief efforts. Emergency measles immunization programs are warranted whenever large numbers of malnourished children lacking this immunization congregate.

Although the other EPI vaccines are important, they usually should not be included in emergency immunization programs because their administration may delay the provision of measles vaccine. Rather, these other vaccines can be provided later as part of other maternal–child health and disease control programs.

PLANNING AN IMMUNIZATION PROGRAM FOR REFUGEES

Initial Vaccine Distribution

The design of a specific immunization program for a refugee population will depend, to a large extent, on the age and type of refugee settlement. For example, if newly arrived refugees receive health screening as they are processed to enter a camp, it may be feasible to provide measles vaccine to children as part of their processing at the screening site (Allegra et al 1984). On the other hand, if immunization services are to be provided for the first time to an existing refugee camp or population, then a mass communitywide program may be the most effective means of rapidly achieving high immunization coverage.

Supplementary feeding centers or prevention-oriented maternal–child health centers that provide services for a high percentage (i.e., ≥80%) of the target population are excellent alternative bases for immunization programs. Clinics and hospitals are often less desirable bases for populationwide immunization programs because a smaller proportion of the target population may use them.

The malnourished children often found in

hospitals or attending therapeutic feeding centers are probably the highest-priority group among all refugee children for measles immunization. Children at these two sites should receive measles vaccine at the onset of any immunization program; their other immunizations can be deferred until nutritional recovery begins. When feeding centers are used as bases for measles or other immunization programs, it is essential that ongoing feeding programs not be disrupted.

One device that may be used to identify as-yet unimmunized children during a brief, communitywide immunization campaign is gentian violet to mark a designated fingernail of children who have already been immunized. Outreach workers seeking unimmunized children in the community on the second or third day of the campaign can quickly identify them by the absence of the violet stain on the designated fingernail.

Planning should include consideration of refrigeration during storage and transport, as well as vaccine delivery methods. Because of the risk of transmission of hepatitis B and other diseases associated with reuse of needles and syringes, disposable, single-use materials must be used. Alternatively, adequate provision must be made for reusable needles and syringes as well as for sterilizers and the fuel to operate them. Jet injector guns may be more efficient than needles and syringes when large numbers of children are to be immunized against measles; however, spare parts and experienced staff are required for maintenance and effective use of jet injectors. Fifty-dose vials of measles vaccine are preferred for mass programs, especially when jet injectors are used.

A communitywide campaign should be preceded by intensive publicity on the need for and target age ranges for immunizations. The information can be disseminated by community leaders and health center or school staff or at food distribution sites and supplementary feeding centers.

Subsequent or Ongoing Vaccine Distribution

Children requiring immunizations after an initial program include the following:

- Those who were missed during the initial program (including those who received only measles vaccine during an initial program).
- Those who entered the camp(s) since the last program.
- Newborns and other infants who have reached the age when initial or booster doses of vaccine are recommended (e.g., those who initially received measles vaccine at <9 months).

Planning for an ongoing immunization program should take all three groups into account. As with initial immunizations, maternal–child health and supplementary feeding centers with high coverage may be ideal sites for ongoing (maintenance) vaccine distribution. If immunization coverage is not high, or if refrigeration is lacking or uncertain, then subsequent communitywide programs can be planned for one- to four-day periods at intervals of one to three months to reach the three target groups. This latter "pulse" approach has the theoretical advantage of minimizing the exposure of labile vaccines to uncertain refrigeration.

If immunizations are given in a mass program that is not integrated into ongoing health care activities, the involvement of local community leaders and administrative authorities during the planning phase is essential. Without such support, it is impossible to make critical decisions such as selection of immunization center location(s), methods of identifying all children, and suspension of some routine activities (e.g., wood gathering) on "immunization day" to maximize coverage.

Finally, as emphasized by Simmonds et al, refugee immunization programs should be coordinated by—or at least with—host governments and local EPI staff (Simmonds et al 1983). These groups can be of great benefit in arranging for an adequate cold chain and for uniform record keeping. In addition, if the refugee community is involved in the planning, coordination, implementation, and evaluation phases, they can provide leadership and staff to organize and run a program, as well as provide advice on how to present the program to the refugees in the most culturally acceptable way.

VACCINE TRANSPORT STORAGE AND HANDLING—THE "COLD CHAIN"

Because nearly all vaccines are sensitive to heat, and some are sensitive to light, planning for immunization programs must include careful attention to vaccine protection during transport, storage, and use. The system responsible for such attention is called the "cold chain" (EPI 1980).

Proper storage and handling are among the most important aspects of any immunization program. Provision of vaccines inadvertently inactivated by cold chain failure is a waste of resources and gives health workers and refugees alike a false sense of security. If many cases of vaccine-preventable disease occur among improperly immunized children, the refugees may lose confidence in immunization, which could reduce the effectiveness of other preventive health programs and future immunization efforts (Preblud et al 1984b).

Ordering of vaccines and cold chain planning should be done by, or in conjunction with, personnel with cold chain experience. Principles of appropriate vaccine handling are given in Tables 6-1 and 6-2.

DOCUMENTATION OF REFUGEES' IMMUNIZATION STATUS

Planning for documentation of the refugees' immunization status is an important aspect of immunization program planning. Prior records will not be available in most refugee situations. Children should be considered unimmunized unless written records are available.

A permanent immunization record given to families during the immunization program serves several important functions. First, it is useful to health providers to document completion of immunizations. Second, it may be useful to refugee children registering at supplementary feeding sites where proof of immunization is required. Finally, possession of a record may prevent needless duplication of immunizations if, and when, refugees are moved to other camps or are processed for return to their country of origin or permanent resettlement in other countries.

The immunization document should provide space for the date and type of vaccine and the signature or initials of the immunizer. The document should be kept in the possession of the refugee family. A small plastic bag distributed with the card can help improve its durability. Road-to-Health cards (UNICEF), which also allow for nutritional monitoring, have been used in a number of situations. A mass immunization program may provide an ideal opportunity to distribute Road-to-Health cards (Simmonds et al 1983).

INDICATIONS AND CONTRAINDICATIONS FOR IMMUNIZATION OF MALNOURISHED OR ILL CHILDREN

Every opportunity should be taken to immunize refugee children appropriately, but health workers are sometimes hampered in their immunization efforts by unnecessarily strict lists of contraindications.

It is especially important to immunize malnourished children. Malnutrition is **not** a contraindication to the use of any of the EPI antigens. Risk of adverse reaction is **not** in-

Table 6-1. Some Basic Principles of Vaccine Storage, Transport, and Usage

"Cold chain" planning is the single most important aspect of planning an immunization program.
Central and regional storage should include temperature alarm as well as backup generator.
A minimal inventory log should include amounts, batch numbers, arrival and expiration dates, and usage records of vaccines and toxoids. This same log can serve as the refrigerator/temperature log.
Temperatures should be checked and recorded at least twice daily during storage.
DTP vaccine must not be frozen.
Vaccines should not be stored on the doors of refrigerators or with food or beverages (since frequent opening of refrigerators will expose vaccines to higher temperatures).
Vaccines must be kept cool during transport and during use in the field.
Diluents do not require refrigeration during storage; they should be refrigerated (but not frozen) just prior to use, to avoid any reduction in vaccine potency due to mixing with warm diluent.
Oldest vaccines (i.e., those closest to expiration) should be used first. Vaccines beyond their expiration date should be discarded.
Vaccine vials that are taken to immunization sites but are not used or are partly used should be discarded after three such trips *even if properly stored.*
Ampules of measles and BCG vaccines should be covered with aluminum foil during use to protect them from light.

Table 6-2. Temperature Requirements for Vaccine Storage

	Level and Storage Time at				
Vaccine	Central Store (<8 mos)	Regional (<3 mos)	Health Center (<1 mo)	Transport (<1 wk)	Immunization Center (few days)
Measles Oral polio	−15 to −25°C Deep Frozen				In cold box +2 to +8°C
Inactivated polio DPT Tetanus BCG	+2 to +8°C Do not freeze!				

Adapted from United Nations High Commissioner for Refugees: Handbook for Emergencies. Part I: Field Operations, p 94. Geneva, United Nations High Commissioner for Refugees p 94.

creased, and even severely malnourished children will respond with adequate levels of protective antibody (Galazka et al 1984; WHO 1984). For measles vaccine in particular, malnutrition is a positive indication for immunization, since malnourished children who get measles are at high risk for complications and death (see Chapter 27). Measles immunization can be a life-saving measure for these children.

Minor illness is also **not** a contraindication to immunization (Galazka et al 1984; WHO 1984), and the opportunity to immunize a mildly ill child should not be missed. The following WHO guidelines on immunization in underdeveloped countries also apply to refugee children:

- Any decision not to immunize should be made only after serious consideration of the potential consequences to the individual child and to the community.
- It is particularly important to immunize children suffering from malnutrition. Low-grade fever, mild respiratory infection, diarrhea, and other minor illnesses should not be considered as contraindications to immunization of children, regardless of nutritional status.
- Immunization of children who are ill enough to require hospitalization should be deferred for a decision by hospital staff. Any referral data sent to the hospital with such a child should include a notation about the lack of needed immunizations.
- The immunization status of already hospitalized children should be evaluated and they should receive appropriate immunizations at discharge. In some cases, they should be immunized against measles on admission, or while still in the hospital, because of the high risk associated with hospital-acquired measles (Aaby et al 1985). Measles vaccine virus is not transmissible.

ADVERSE EFFECTS

No vaccine is totally without adverse reactions, but the risks of serious complications from the EPI vaccines are far lower than the risks from the natural diseases (Galazka et al 1984; WHO 1984; Table 6-3).

Adverse reactions occur no more frequently in refugee children than in other children. Rare and common adverse effects associated with specific vaccines are listed in Tables 6-3 and 6-4, respectively. Persons responsible for immunization programs should be familiar with the information on adverse reactions provided in the package inserts.

ORGANIZATION OF VACCINE DISTRIBUTION SITES

The flow of children past the immunization team(s) must be controlled. Use of a single entrance point and a single exit point to and from a building or cordoned-off area is helpful, and program staff should regulate the flow of foot traffic at these sites. As few people as possible should be inside the actual immunization area (International Disaster Institute 1982).

Table 6-3. Summary of Less Common Adverse Effects of EPI Vaccines

Vaccine and Reaction	Vaccine Reaction Rate/100,000 Immunizations	Disease Complication Rate/100,000 Cases	Relative Frequency Vaccine/Disease
DTP (Pertussis)			
Brain damage	0.2–0.6	600–2,000	1/1,000–1/10,000
Death	0.2	100–4,000	1/500–1/20,000
Encephalopathy/ encephalitis	0.1–3.0	90–4,000	1/30–1/40,000
Convulsions	0.3–90	600–8,000	1/6.5–1/26,400
Shock	0.5–30	?	?
Measles			
Encephalopathy/ encephalitis	0.1–0.3	50–400	1/165–1/4,000
Panencephalitis (SSPE)	0.05–0.1	0.5–2.0	1/5–1/40
Pneumonia	———	3,800–7,300	———
Convulsions	0.02–190	500–1,000	1/2.6–1/50,000
Death	0.02–0.03	10–25,000	1/330–1/1,250,000
Polio			
Paralytic disease	0.003–0.02	500–1000	1/25,000–1/330,000

Adapted from World Health Organization: Vaccines used in the EPI: Indications and contraindications. WHO Chronicle 1984; 38:95–98.

Table 6-4. Summary of EPI Antigens for Use in Refugee Populations

Infection	Disease Frequency	Disease Severity[a]	Epidemic Potential (4 = highest)	Doses[b]	Age at First Dose	Route[c]	Common Adverse Effects	Usual Efficacy (%)
Measles	High	Mod-high, F	4	1(2)[d]	9 mo	SC	Rash, fever	≥90
Paralytic polio	Low	Mod-high, F	3	3(4)	4–6 wk	PO,IM	Local for IM	≥90
Diphtheria (throat)	Low	High, F	3	3(4)	4–6 wk	IM	Local	≥90
Pertussis	Medium	Variable, F	4	3(4)	4–6 wk	IM	Local, fever	3 doses, 60–90
Tetanus								
Child	Low	High, F	0	3(4)	4–6 week	IM	Local	90
Neonatal (vaccine to pregnant women)	Medium	High, F	0	(2–3 to pregnant women in 2nd or 3rd trimester)		IM		2 doses, 80 3 doses, 98
Childhood Tuberculosis (BCG)	Low	Variable, F	2	1	Birth or later	ID	Adenitis & local	Variable

[a]F = potentially fatal.
[b]Multiple-dose vaccines (polio, DTP) must have at least four weeks between doses.
[c]ID = intradermal; IM = intramuscular; SC = subcutaneous; PO = oral.
[d]If first dose is given before the age of nine months, give second dose after nine months; see the text.

Children should first stop at a screening area where the immunization record is provided or checked. Children with severe illness or with a history of severe vaccine reactions should be referred to a health worker for a specific decision on immunization.

MONITORING THE COVERAGE AND EFFECTIVENESS OF IMMUNIZATION PROGRAMS

Refugee relief operations usually face serious resource limitations; this makes efficient use of available resources essential. In addition, maximum immunization coverage is important to minimize subsequent preventable illness and death. With coverage much below 80 to 90 percent, especially for measles vaccine, more attention must be paid to immunization programs.

The simplest method of assessing the adequacy of immunization coverage is to compare doses of vaccine distributed with the number of children in the target population:

$$\% \text{ coverage} = \frac{\text{Doses of vaccine distributed}}{\text{Children in target population}} \times 100$$

This method requires an accurate count, or estimate, of children in the appropriate age range (which is also needed for other purposes). This method has the disadvantage of not providing characteristics of the unreached population, so retargeting of vaccines is difficult. In addition, it is difficult to assess correctly the coverage of multiple-dose vaccines such as polio and DTP (diphtheria-tetanus-pertussis).

An alternative method, which is preferable if time and resources permit, is to survey children of the appropriate age in the population randomly and collect information from immunization records on all documented immunizations. This can be done for immunization status alone or it can be combined with an assessment of nutrition and other health indicators.

In a refugee camp with a supplementary feeding program that covers a high proportion of the childhood population, program registrants can be surveyed for immunization status as they arrive for feeding. Alternatively, one can survey children's records during general food distribution (Simmonds et al 1983). Finally, one can use an opportunity presented by health screening on entry to camp or on transfer between camps to survey immunization status. These types of surveys should provide immunization coverage rates and other information (age, location, nutritional status, time in camp), which can be used to improve monitoring and subsequent program targeting.

A different type of evaluation is possible if an outbreak (such as measles) occurs in a population that is partially immunized against the disease. By collecting information and comparing the rates of disease in both immunized and unimmunized children, one can confirm a vaccine's efficacy in preventing disease (Orenstein et al 1985). A low vaccine efficacy in this setting indicates the existence of a problem such as failure of the cold chain. This type of assessment should be done with the advice of an experienced immunization consultant.

Finally, learning from experience is at least as important in refugee situations as elsewhere. Because the problems encountered during immunization programs among refugees may be different from those found in the usual underdeveloped country setting, health workers and agencies should record and publish their immunization program experiences, with particular emphasis on "lessons learned."

SPECIFIC EPI VACCINES

Table 6-4 provides specific details on characteristics of the EPI vaccines and their use. Factors peculiar to each vaccine are discussed in the following sections.

Measles Vaccine

The standard EPI recommendation is to give one dose of measles vaccine subcutaneously in the upper deltoid region at the age of nine months, or as soon thereafter as possible.

Measles vaccine should be given before a measles outbreak! By the time cases occurring in a refugee camp come to the attention of health workers, it may be too late to mount an effective, large-scale measles immunization program because many susceptibles have already been exposed and infected. (Measles vaccine may provide some protection if given within 72 hours of exposure. After that time, it will probably be ineffective.)

The usual target age for measles immunization of refugee children is 9 to 59 months of age. The vaccine is relatively ineffective before 9 months of age (because of the persistence of maternal antibody), although some children will become susceptible earlier. This early susceptibility may be particularly likely to occur in malnourished children (Halsey et al 1985).

In exceptional situations, such as when trying to avert an impending epidemic or when a large number of children are severely malnourished, the vaccine may be given to children as young as six months of age. However, in that situation, a second dose of vaccine should be given as soon after nine months as possible.

In situations of unusual disease epidemiology (e.g., where previous geographic isolation of the population has resulted in limited transmission of measles), older children—or even adults—may be susceptible. In this case, the upper age limit for immunization may need to be raised (Allegra et al 1984).

Because of the possibility of lower vaccine efficacy due to inadvertant intramuscular administration, measles vaccine must **not** be given in the buttock; upper arm or anterior thigh are both acceptable sites.

Common side effects are fever and rash, seen seven to ten days after immunization; 5 to 15 percent of children will develop fever of 39.4°C or above at that time (Galazka et al 1984).

Measles vaccine can be given simultaneously with DTP, polio, and BCG vaccines. However, **an initial measles immunization program must never be delayed to await the availability of these other vaccines.**

A decision to mount a large-scale measles immunization program in a refugee camp already experiencing measles should take several factors into account, including the number of susceptible children in the camp and their prior **documented** immunization status, the number and source (acquired inside the camp?) of cases that have already occurred, and the length of time needed to obtain measles vaccine and other necessary supplies. For example, if only one case was found in a child who had just entered a large camp several days before, and if vaccine and jet injectors were immediately available, then an aggressive measles immunization program would be indicated and would have a high probability of success (as measured by saving lives). If, on the other hand, obtaining enough vaccine and supplies would take at least several weeks, and if investigation found that cases had been occurring in the camp for several weeks, the probability of preventing a significant number of measles cases in that camp by immunization would be much lower.

During an outbreak, **any** immediately available measles vaccine should be distributed according to the following priorities:

1. Severely malnourished children under five years of age in therapeutic feeding centers or hospitals.
2. Other malnourished children (<80% of median weight-for-height or with arm circumference <13.5 cm).
3. Other hospitalized children under three years of age.
4. Other children from 9 to 12 months of age.
5. All other children from 12 to 35 months.

If and when additional measles vaccine is available, it should be given promptly to children of the appropriate age groups in nearby camps that are as yet unaffected.

Polio Vaccine

The standard EPI recommendation is to give the initial dose of live oral polio vaccine (OPV) at four to six weeks of age. Two subsequent doses must be given at intervals of four or more weeks.

Both OPV and inactivated polio virus vaccine (IPV) are available. Although WHO recommends OPV use, and many countries prefer it, other countries use IPV. Either vaccine can be given in conjunction with DTP vaccine. OPV is preferred for control of an ongoing epidemic because, in addition to directly protecting immunized individuals, large-scale use of the vaccine virus in a population can also reduce the circulation of the wild (disease-producing) poliovirus.

Breastfeeding does not interfere with OPV immunization (Immunization Practices Advisory Committee 1982).

Diarrhea is not a contraindication to the use of oral polio vaccine. However, because of a possible reduction in effectiveness, doses given during a diarrheal illness should ordinarily not be counted toward the recommended number of doses.

Polio and DTP vaccines follow the same schedule and are most efficiently given at the same time.

If resources are available, a "pre-school" dose may be given at four to six years of age; however, in poor or underdeveloped countries, greater than 95 percent of polio cases occur before this age.

DTP: Diphtheria and Tetanus Toxoids and Pertussis Vaccine

The standard EPI recommendations are to give the initial dose of DTP vaccine intramuscularly at four to six weeks of age. Two subsequent doses must be given at least four weeks apart.

Polio and DTP vaccines follow the same schedule and are most efficiently given at the same time.

Common adverse effects include inflammation at the injection site and fever.

A second or third DTP injection should not be given to a child who has suffered a severe neurologic reaction to the previous dose (see Table 6-4) or who has a progressive or unknown type of neurologic disease. Instead, the pertussis component should be omitted and the diphtheria and tetanus immunizations completed.

If resources are available, a preschool booster dose may be given at four to six years of age.

Tetanus Toxoid for Pregnant Women (to Prevent Neonatal Tetanus)

The standard EPI recommendation for pregnant women is to give two doses of the vaccine intramuscularly, at least four weeks apart, in the late second or third trimester.

Women who have received any **documented** previous dose need receive only one booster dose during pregnancy.

Also important for reducing the risk of neonatal tetanus are improved antenatal and delivery care, with increased supervision of deliveries by trained attendants (Benenson 1985).

Bacille Calmette-Guérin (for Tuberculosis)

The BCG vaccine is only an adjunct to community tuberculosis control programs. For effective control of tuberculosis, active cases in the community must be sought out and treated (see Chapter 33). Examples of successful refugee community programs have been reported (Shears 1984; Rieder 1985).

To facilitate subsequent identification of BCG scars, the vaccine should be applied to the skin site specifically designated by national health policy (International Disaster Institute 1982).

For documentation of a successful BCG "take" to appear on an immunization record, evidence of an appropriate local reaction should be required. Lack of a local reaction indicates vaccine failure and a need for reimmunization.

Common adverse effects include suppurative lymphadenitis, which occurs in up to 1 percent of those receiving BCG (Galazka et al 1984; Cameroon EPI, unpublished).

Tuberculin testing is not required prior to mass BCG immunization (International Disaster Institute 1982).

OTHER VACCINES

Meningococcal Meningitis Vaccine

Outbreaks of meningococcal meningitis have occurred in refugee camps (Preblud et al 1984a). Effective, type-specific vaccines against this disease exist and their use in refugee situations has been discussed (Simmonds et al 1983). In geographic areas where epidemic meningococcal meningitis occurs (such as the African Sahel "meningitis belt"), vaccines may prove effective in refugee settings. In one camp for Ethiopian refugees in Sudan, mass immunization appeared to abort an impending epidemic.

Documentation of meningococcal meningitis vaccine effectiveness in refugee situations outside of recognized high-risk geographic areas is lacking. For this reason, those who use this vaccine in such settings in the near future are encouraged to document and publish their experience carefully.

Hepatitis B Vaccine

Hepatitis B vaccine is potentially useful for preventing vertical (mother-to-newborn) transmission of hepatitis B virus in populations in which this infection is endemic. However, its use is limited by its cost and the need for prior serologic identification of high-risk pregnancies. Therefore, hepatitis B vaccine use in refugee camps cannot be recommended at this time.

Hemophilus Influenzae Vaccine

Hemophilus influenzae vaccine is a recently available, but expensive, vaccine that protects against meningitis and other invasive disease caused by *Hemophilus influenzae* type b. Because the epidemiology of this disease is not yet well-defined among refugees and other children in underdeveloped countries, this vaccine cannot currently be recommended for refugee children.

Cholera and Typhoid Vaccines

The most practical measure for the prevention of cholera and typhoid is water purification by boiling, chlorination, or some other effective method. This approach has the advantage of providing protection against other waterborne diseases as well.

The current cholera and typhoid vaccines are not recommended for outbreak control as they do not prevent the carrier state of these diseases and would thus have no impact on disease transmission. These vaccines share several other characteristics: they are of limited effectiveness (Benenson 1985) and provide only minimal protection against a concentrated or prolonged exposure; two doses are required for initial immunization; and reactions occur frequently and may be severe. Finally, administering these vaccines may provide a false sense of security and divert attention away from more appropriate disease control activities such as provision of safe water, oral rehydration programs, and disease surveillance.

These vaccines are rarely, if ever, indicated for use among refugees, and no example of their successful use in refugee populations has been documented. The resources necessary for a cholera or typhoid vaccine program would probably be better spent on improving environmental sanitation (Benenson 1985) (e.g., through distribution of soap for handwashing or teaching methods of safe food preparation).

Other Vaccines Currently Under Development

Several vaccines currently under development may prove useful in future refugee situations. These include vaccines against rotavirus, malaria, and improved vaccines against cholera and typhoid.

SUMMARY

Measles immunization is a high priority in all refugee health programs and should be implemented as soon as possible, before cases are identified in a population. Other childhood vaccines (polio, DTP, BCG) are also cost-effective health measures, and their use should begin as soon as the emergency phase of relief ends. Maintenance of cold chain integrity is a crucial aspect of planning and operating an immunization program. Neither mild illness nor malnutrition is a contraindication to immunization; in fact, the latter is an absolute indication for measles vaccination. Evaluation of the coverage of immunization programs is a high priority.

REFERENCES

Aaby P, Bukh J, Lisse IM et al: Introduction of measles into a highly immunized West African community: The role of health care institutions. J Epidemiol Community Health 1985;39:113–6.

Allegra DT, Glass RI, Nieburg P et al: Rapid health screening as an epidemiologic tool in refugee camps. In Allegra DT, Nieburg P, Grabe M (eds): Emergency Refugee Health Care, pp 171–76. Atlanta, Centers for Disease Control, 1984.

Benenson AS: Control of Communicable Diseases in Man. 14th ed., pp 78–9, 389, 424. Washington DC, American Public Health Association, 1985.

Creese AL, Henderson RH: Cost-benefit analysis and immunization programmes in developing countries. Bull WHO 1980;58:491–97.

Dondero TJ: Impact of vaccine-preventable diseases in developing countries. Presented at the 113th annual meeting of the American Public Health Association, Dallas, Nov. 14–17, 1983.

Expanded Program on Immunization: The Cold Chain. Module III. Washington DC/Geneva, Pan American Health Organization /World Health Organization, 1980.

Galazka AM, Lauer BA, Henderson RH et al: Indications and contraindications for vaccines used in the Expanded Programme on Immunization. Bull WHO 1984;62:357–66.

Halsey NA, Boulos R, Mode F et al: Response to measles vaccine in Haitian infants 6 to 12 months old. Influence of maternal antibodies, malnutrition, and concurrent illness. New Engl J Med 1985;313:544–49.

Immunization Practices Advisory Committee (ACIP): Poliomyelitis prevention. MMWR 1982;31:22–34.

International Disaster Institute: Vaccines and vaccinations. Disasters 1982;5:255–58.

Orenstein WA, Bernier RH, Dondero TJ et al: Field evaluation of vaccine efficacy. Bull WHO 1985;63:1055–68.

Preblud SR, Horan JM, Davis CE: Meningococcal disease among Khmer refugees in Thailand. In Allegra DT,

Nieburg P, Grabe M (eds): Emergency Refugee Health Care, pp 65–69. Atlanta, Centers for Disease Control 1984a.

Preblud SR, Nieburg P, Allegra DT: Vaccination programs for refugees. In Allegra DT, Nieburg P, Grabe M (eds): Emergency Refugee Health Care, pp 135–40. Atlanta, Centers for Disease Control, 1984b.

Rieder HL: Tuberculosis in an Indochinese refugee camp: Epidemiology, management, and therapeutic results. Tubercle 1985;66:179–86.

Shears P: Tuberculosis control in Somali refugee camps. Tubercle 1984;65:111–16.

Simmonds S, Vaughn P, Gunn SW: Refugee Community Health Care. Oxford, Oxford University Press, 1983.

Sisk JE, Sanders CR: Analyzing the cost-effectiveness and cost-benefit of vaccines. World Health Forum 1983;4:83–88.

United Nations High Commissioner for Refugees: Handbook for Emergencies. Part I: Field Operations. Geneva, United Nations High Commissioner for Refugees, 1982.

World Health Organization: Vaccines used in the EPI: Indications and contraindications. WHO Chronicle 1984; 38:95–98.

7
Family Planning

RICHARD H. SANDLER
JOE WRAY

> Family planning can help prevent many unnecessary deaths among women and children. Few public health measures can have so great an effect in a relatively short time as the implementation of a family planning program providing easy access to effective methods of contraception.
>
> (Rosenfield & Wray 1981)

Clear evidence is now available to confirm the truth of the above quotation for underdeveloped and developed nations alike, although the effects are more striking for lower socioeconomic groups and in underdeveloped nations. Among refugee populations, highly vulnerable for many reasons, the effects of birth spacing are likely to be especially important, and access to family planning services is a high priority. The data have been concisely reviewed by Maine (1981) and Maine and McNamara (1985), who make the following observations:

- There is increased infant and child mortality among children with birth intervals of less than two years.
- There is increased infant and child mortality among families with more than three children.
- Increased maternal mortality occurs when parity is greater than three.
- Increased maternal mortality is associated with pregnancy under the age of 20 years or over the age of 35 years.

When legal and effective family planning services are unavailable, many women are forced to seek illegal abortions to terminate unwanted pregnancies, resulting in morbidity and mortality from infection, hemorrhage, and other complications.

WORLD POPULATION GROWTH

It took more than 1 million years for the population of the world to reach 1 billion, 120 years to add the second billion, 42 years to add the third billion, and 15 years to add the fourth. The present world population is about 4.8 billion and it is expected to grow to 10 billion by 2050. Of the expected 10 billion, the population of underdeveloped nations will more than double from the present 3.5 billion to 8.5 billion, while the population of industrialized nations will increase from 1.3 billion to 1.5 billion.

FAMILY PLANNING POLICY

The International Conference on Family Planning in the 1980s, held in Jakarta in 1981, issued a statement that included two important points:

- Family planning is an essential component of any broad-based development strategy that seeks to improve the quality of life for both individuals and communities.
- Family planning is a basic human right. Governments should be encouraged to translate this right into realistic policies and programs that meet the needs of their people.

Other useful policies were stated by the government of India in 1968:

- The community must feel the need for family planning services if they are to be accepted.
- Parents must decide the number of children they want.
- People should be approached through communication channels they respect, such as recognized and trusted leaders.
- Family planning programs should not offend the religious and moral values of the population.
- Services should be made available to the people as near to their doorsteps as possible.
- Family planning efforts should be made an integral part of medical and public health services.

Special Considerations for Refugee Camps

Among the factors operating in the refugee setting that have a bearing on family planning policy are the following:

- The need to consider the policies and politics of the host country, the United Nations High Commissioner on Refugees (UNHCR), and other agencies.
- The risk of coercion by host-country authorities who may want, either overtly or covertly, to limit the size of the refugee population in their country.
- The often captive nature of the refugees in the camp.
- The physical and emotional trauma they may have suffered before reaching the camp, as well as the uncertainty about their future.
- The frequently transient nature of the refugee population, and the concomitant difficulty in obtaining adequate data upon which to base plans for programs and provide proper continuity of care.

Arguments Against Family Planning

There are valid reasons for people to want family planning measures, but health workers must also be sensitive to arguments against these measures. Rawson-Jones and Salkeld (1971) mention a number of these:

- Children are often economically valuable.
- Children share the workload.
- Children can assist their elderly or sick parents.
- Children can add to parental prestige.
- A large number of children can compensate for high childhood mortality.
- A large number of children can increase the likelihood that a male will survive to inherit the family's resources and continue the family line.

Although these points are not always relevant to refugee populations, it is worth noting that they are arguments in favor of having children but not necessarily against proper spacing, timing, or other benefits promoted by family planning programs.

Various groups have charged that family planning measures have been used as a form of genocide against certain groups or that certain contraceptive measures, or the mere concept of family planning, violates religious beliefs and cultural norms. These issues merit consideration in refugee programs as in any other program.

Progress in family planning over the long term depends on concurrent improvements in such fields as health, nutrition, education, and employment. Dr. K. Singh from India's Ministry of Family Planning has stated that "the path to family planning in every country lies through the eradication of poverty which, in fact, has historically been the main cause of overpopulation. . . . It has truly been said that the best contraceptive is development" (Banerji 1976).

DESIGNING A FAMILY PLANNING PROGRAM

As with other aspects of health care planning and service delivery for refugees, there are many important factors to consider when designing a family planning program, including the following:

- The nature of the population problem in the camp or settlement. For example, what are the present birth, death, and fertility rates? What population trends can be discerned? (See Chapter 2 for a discussion of how to gather this information.)
- The relevant UNHCR and host-government policies in place.
- The traditional values and birth control methods of the refugee population.
- The availability of supplies and trained personnel.

Family Planning "No-Nos"

Mandatory, coercive, or manipulative schemes of population control should be avoided. Two examples may suffice to illustrate this point.

In 1980, a voluntary agency that was providing medical care in a Kampuchean refugee camp in Thailand offered a chicken to any woman of childbearing age who accepted a Depo-Provera injection. The women were not informed of the true nature of the injection, but were told that it was a "vitamin shot." No history, physical examination, or laboratory tests were obtained. Aside from the possible side effects on the individual women, the results were distrust of voluntary agencies in general and of family planning efforts in particular.

The second example is a vignette from India (Banerji 1976). A district revenue official received orders from his superiors to procure vasectomy cases or face dire consequences. The official approached a landless laborer with the promise of a land allocation if he agreed to a vasectomy. The laborer had only one son, but the prospect of getting land was such a temptation that he acquiesced. To the laborer's dismay, soon after the vasectomy he discovered that he had been cheated, for the land promised was never to be given. Confounding his misfortune, the laborer's only son developed a high fever several months later and died. It is not surprising that family planning efforts lost favor in the laborer's village because of this episode.

Risk-Benefit Analysis of Different Family Planning Methods

Potts and co-workers (1978) have reviewed the relative risks and benefits of various family planning methods in underdeveloped nations using both a computer model and best available empiric data. Table 7-1 summarizes the projected annual mortality per 100,000 non-sterile women, and puts "bottom line" values on the risks and benefits of reversible fertility control methods in underdeveloped countries. The results are not always as one would expect. For example, if only the risks of the different methods are compared, the zero direct risk to the mother from condom use seems very attractive. However, the overall user risk of death for this method is projected to be about twice as high as for intrauterine devices (IUDs) or oral contraceptives because condoms are less effective for preventing pregnancy than IUDs or oral contraceptives. The mortality from these excess pregnancies is greater than the user risk with IUDs or oral contraceptives (OCs).

It is evident that family planning measures, including those considered more dangerous, are not as hazardous as pregnancy. This is more starkly illustrated in Figure 7-1, which compares the risks of OC use and pregnancy in developing nations. Another means of assessing the risks associated with contraceptive technology is to compare them with everyday

Table 7-1. Risks and Benefits of Fertility Control in Least Developed Countries (Number/100,000 non-sterile women)

	No Method	Oral Contraception	IUD	Tubectomy	Barrier
Deaths directly from use of method	—	0.8	1	3.5[a]	0
Pregnancies	40,000	1600	1100	60	7,600
Deaths from pregnancy for method failures (method failure rate × deaths/pregnancy)	210	8	6	0.3	38
Total deaths from method use	210	9	7	3.8	38
Advantage to user compared to use of no method (total risk of death from this method, compared to risk of death using no method)	—	23:1	30:1	53:1	6:1
Total mortality risk of method if combined with legal abortion for method failures (assuming mortality from legal abortions = 10/100,000)	4	1	1	3.6	0.8
Advantage to user[b] (considering only mortality risk) of combining legal abortion with the method, compared to use of the method alone	210:4	9:1	7:1	3.8:3.6	38:0.8
Advantage to user[b] (considering only mortality risk) of combining legal abortion with the method compared to use of no method	—	210:1	210:1	210:3.6	210:0.8

[a]Assumes the risk associated with the procedure (35/100,000) is divided over ten years.
[b](Note, the important moral considerations are not addressed by this analysis.)

Figure 7-1. Comparison of maternal deaths from oral contraceptive use, versus deaths from pregnancy and childbirth.

Of 15,000 women who become pregnant, this many are likely to die from problems of pregnancy or childbirth.	Of 15,000 women who take birth control pills, only 1 is likely to die from problems related to having taken the pills.
+ +	+

Conclusion:
IT IS USUALLY MUCH SAFER TO TAKE THE PILL THAN TO BECOME PREGNANT.

(Adapted with permission from Werner D: Where There Is No Doctor. Palo Alto, CA, Hesperian Foundation, 1977.)

risks. For example, Table 7-2 illustrates the risks of common daily activities, family planning measures, and pregnancy in developed nations.

A summary of the effectiveness of the various contraceptive methods is also contained in Table 7-1. Although after weighing the implications this may be rejected, it can be seen that barrier methods combined with legal early abortion may offer the safest family planning combination.

Surgical methods for family planning include vasectomy and tubectomy. Each poses a slightly higher patient risk initially, but if this risk is "amortized" over a few years the safety is comparable to oral contraceptives and IUDs.

TRAINING HEALTH WORKERS IN FAMILY PLANNING SERVICES

Extensive experience in the training of nonphysician health workers for delivery of family planning services in underdeveloped countries has been summarized and cataloged by Wortman (1975). Competence of these personnel is largely determined by the quality of leadership and supervision and the availability of appropriate referral backup, continued training, and support.

Figure 7-2 outlines various family planning skills, arranged by order of complexity. Extensive experience demonstrates that all medium and lower-level skills required can be well performed by properly trained health workers. The few programs that have used specially trained health workers for surgical sterilization have also reported satisfactory results.

PATIENT WORKUP

The patient workup carried out before choosing a contraceptive method should ideally include a thorough history and physical examination. When resources permit, an acceptable approach in a refugee camp might be the one adopted by the International Rescue Committee in the outpatient department at Khao-I-Dang Holding Center in Thailand.

A simple questionnaire (Figure 7-3) was first filled out by the patient with the help of either a male or female health worker specifically trained in birth control methods and counseling. Then, blood pressure, scleral icterus, and varicose veins were checked in a brief physical examination. A urinalysis was done for evidence of pregnancy, diabetes, or kidney disease. If any of the history, physical, or laboratory tests were positive for possible risk factors, a doctor or nurse clinician was consulted. Otherwise, the health worker carefully explained the options to the patient, and together they decided on the optimal method.

Note that such a workup, though desirable, is not necessarily required. For example, the International Planned Parenthood Foundation (IPPF) asserted in 1973 that oral contraceptives could be distributed without a history or

Table 7-2. Putting the Risks in Perspective

	Chance of Death in a Year
Motorcycling	1 in 50
Smoking, 1 pack a day	1 in 200
Horse racing	1 in 750
Automobile driving	1 in 6,000
Power boating	1 in 6,000
Rock climbing	1 in 7,500
Playing football	1 in 25,000
Canoeing	1 in 100,000
Using tampons	1 in 350,000
Using Rely tampons	1 in 50,000
Preventing pregnancy	
Oral contraception (nonsmoker)	1 in 63,000
Oral contraception (smoker)	1 in 16,000
Using IUDs	1 in 100,000
Using barrier methods	None
Using natural methods	None
Undergoing sterilization	
laparoscopic tubal ligation	1 in 10,000
hysterectomy	1 in 1,600
vasectomy	None
Injectable progesterone contraception	1 in 10,000
Pregnancy	
Continuing pregnancy	1 in 10,000
Terminating pregnancy	
Illegal abortion	1 in 3,000
Legal abortion	
Before 9 weeks	1 in 400,000
Between 9–12 weeks	1 in 100,000
Between 13–16 weeks	1 in 25,000
After 16 weeks	1 in 10,000

References

Cates W. Putting the risks in perspective. Contraceptive Technology Update 1980 Nov; 1:111.

Dinman BD: The reality and acceptance of risk. JAMA 244:1226–28, 1980.

Tietze C: New estimates of mortality associated with fertility control. Fam Plann Persp 9:74–76, 1977.

National Center for Health Statistics, Final Mortality Statistics, United States, 1976–78.

Center for Disease Control: Abortion-related mortality, United States, 1976–1978.

Reproduced with permission from: Hatcher RA, Stewart GK, Stewart F, Guest F, Josephs N, Dale J (eds): Contraceptive Technology 1982–1983. New York, Irvington Publishers, 1982, page 7.

physical examination. IPPF stated that even store proprietors could be used for such distribution. Although the conclusions are surprising to Western clinicians, the IPPF pointed out that when properly trained health workers are not available for the task, the risks associated with supplying oral contraceptives in underdeveloped countries are small compared with the risks associated with childbirth, high parity, or short birth intervals.

Figure 7-2. Pyramid of family planning tasks. The tasks performed by paramedicals, auxiliaries, and traditional workers range from simple to complex. Few nonphysician personnel are found in the upper ranges.

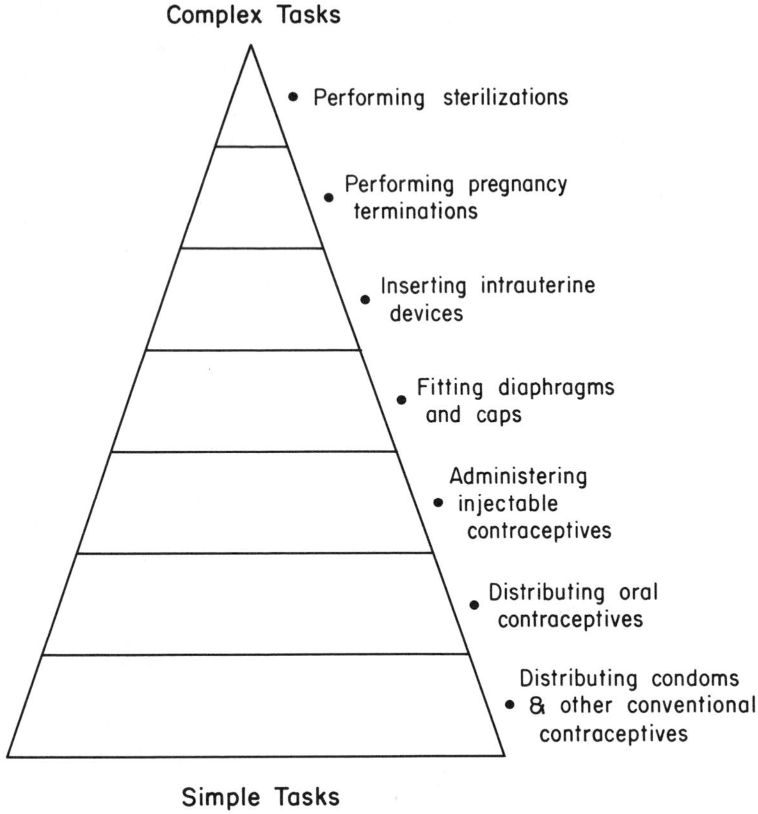

(Reproduced with permission from Wortman J: Training nonphysicians in family planning services. Population Reports, Series J, No 6, Sept. 1975, p J-91.)

PATIENT EDUCATION

Studies confirm that most women do not want to give birth each year, nor do most desire to be pregnant while under 16 years or over 35 years of age. A WHO study of 21,000 women in India, Iran, Lebanon, the Philippines, and Turkey (Omran & Standley 1976) determined that about 90 percent of the women knew the following:

- The health of the child and the mother are better if the child is born three years after the previous birth rather than after only a one-year interval.
- The health of the mother and the child are better if the family is small.
- Family planning improves the health of women and children.

Women, therefore, are often receptive to family planning information.

To be useful, family planning information should be (1) accurate, (2) stated in clear and simple language, (3) slowly and patiently provided, (4) liberally illustrated with clear drawings, (5) packaged in a manner that is appropriate to the religious and cultural mores, and (6) taught by appropriate personnel—not only properly trained, but of the proper age, sex, and status. For example, a 16-year-old male health worker would be a less-than-ideal choice to provide family planning instructions to a 30-year-old woman. Similarly, a young

Figure 7-3. Checklist used by auxiliary midwives in Thailand for screening oral contraceptive candidates before providing them with pills.

	Yes	No
History: ask if the patient has had a history of any of the following:		
Yellow skin or yellow eyes		
Mass in the breast		
Discharge from the nipple		
Swelling or severe pains in the legs		
Severe chest pains		
Unusual shortness of breath after exertion		
Severe headaches		
Excessive menstrual periods		
Increased frequency of menstrual periods		
Bleeding after sexual intercourse		
Examination. Check the following:		
Yellow skin and yellow eye color		
Mass in the breast		
Nipple discharge		
Varicose veins in the legs		
Blood pressure (yes = above 120)		
Pulse (yes = above 120)		
Urine for sugar		
Urine for protein		

(Reproduced with permission from Wortman J: Training nonphysicians in family planning services. Population Reports, Series J, No 6, Sept. 1975, p J-92.)

woman might not be the best educator for the middle aged male.

The need for accurate information is clear from an episode that occurred in a Khmer refugee camp. During one week, three women presented to an outpatient department with the complaint of being pregnant despite using oral contraceptives. Each stated that they had taken the oral contraceptives as instructed. After further investigation, it was determined that all three had been given their pills by the same health worker. The pills were on a card with three horizontal rows of oral contraceptives and a fourth row of placebo tablets. When taken properly from left to right, the patient would receive the appropriate pill each day during a 28-day cycle. Unfortunately, the health worker had incorrectly instructed the women to take the pills from top to bottom, which resulted in the ingestion of a placebo every fourth day.

In refugee camps where population density is great, it may be more cost-effective to arrange for home visitors to explain and provide contraceptive options to those seeking services than to rely on group meetings. For example, Chen and Chow (1973) reported a 6.8 percent IUD acceptance rate in Taiwan with home visitors, versus a 2.4 percent acceptor rate from group meetings for a cost per acceptor of $0.75 and $1.70, respectively.

METHODS OF CONTRACEPTION

Health care workers in refugee camps are often called on to prescribe and provide contraceptive technology for refugees and to train auxiliary workers in their use. The relative risks and efficacy of a wide range of methods are mentioned here, but only a few of the more widely available methods are discussed in detail.

Surgical Sterilization

A detailed review of surgical sterilization is beyond the scope of this chapter but can be found in the Population Reports (series C and D for female and male sterilization, respectively).

Vasectomy offers the advantage of being an effective and permanent method of family planning and requires only a simple outpatient procedure. However, given political sensitivities and the uncertain future for refugees, surgical sterilization methods are often inappropriate in refugee settings.

Breastfeeding

In addition to being the best form of nutrition for infants, breastfeeding is useful for increasing the time between pregnancies (McCann et al 1981). Although it is an imperfect method, about 75% of lactating women will have four or more months of freedom from pregnancy while lactating. Numerous studies have suggested that the mechanism responsible for this effect is probably an increased level of serum prolactin, which acts to delay reestablishment of ovulation.

Intrauterine Devices

The major advantages of IUDs, like injectable progesterones, are that the method offers long-term effectiveness after insertion and is reversible. Table 7-3 lists overall complication and pregnancy rates and other useful information on various IUDs. These figures are based on use in industrialized countries.

Oral Contraceptives

Potts reports that in both developed and underdeveloped countries the only consistently important variables affecting the safety of oral contraceptive use are the user's age and presence or absence of associated risk factors, the most important of which is smoking. It does not require medical qualification to elicit either of these factors from a potential user (Potts 1978). The risk of death related to oral contraceptive use increases sharply for smokers, and women over 40 years of age (Figure 7-4).

Table 7-4 outlines the contraindications of combined estrogen and progestin oral contraceptives. Once the decision to use oral contraceptives has been made and if one has a choice, what is the most sensible oral contraceptive to begin with? Most experienced clinicians begin with a combination containing progestin plus 50 μg or less of estrogen. The so-called mini-pill, which contains progestin without estrogen, may be the initial oral contraceptive of choice for some women because it has fewer serious side effects, but the risk of pregnancy is somewhat higher than with the combination tablet.

A variety of side effects may be observed with oral contraceptive use, many of which will resolve spontaneously after the first two or three cycles. Following are the most common adverse reactions and their management (Hatcher et al 1983; Dickey 1980):

- *Spotting.* For some women under 30, one or two days of spotting per cycle may be acceptable. Early or late spotting can sometimes be controlled by having the patient take the oral contraceptive at exactly the same time each day. Low dose estrogen preparations appear to be associated with higher rates of spotting and breakthrough bleeding early in the cycle, so if these problems persist after three months, higher-dose estrogen pills can be tried.
- *Failure to have withdrawal bleeding.* Pregnancy should be ruled out by physical examination or by urine pregnancy tests, if available. A basal rectal temperature of less than 36°C for two consecutive mornings may be presumptive evidence that a patient is not pregnant (Dickey 1980). Missed menses can initially be managed by switching to an oral contraceptive with a higher progestin content. If the symptoms persist, a pill with more estrogen can be tried.
- *Cyclic weight gain due to fluid retention.* This type of weight gain usually increases later in the cycle. It can be minimized by using a lower dose of estrogen.
- *Hypertension.* With mild hypertension, a lower dose of estrogen can be tried initially, but if the hypertension persists, an estrogen-free oral contractive should be used.
- *Oily skin and acne.* These can be decreased by using a low-progestin, low-androgen oral contraceptive, preferably with 50 μg of estrogen.
- *Hirsutism.* A low-androgenic-activity oral contraceptive with 50 μg or less of estrogen will help minimize this problem.
- *Depression.* This can become severe or may improve remarkably while using oral contraceptives. Some women use oral contraceptives for years and only realize retrospectively after discontinuing their use how depressed they had been while taking them. Management of depression in oral contraceptive users is further complicated by the fact that it can be due to high progestin levels, high estrogen levels, or even low estrogen levels. If decreasing the estrogen content of the oral contraceptive does

Table 7-3. Overview of IUD Effectiveness and Complications[a]

Device	Size	Material	Cost (each)	Year Introduced	Manufacturer or Distributor	Pregnancy Rate, per 100 woman-years	Expulsion Rate, per 100 woman-years	Removal Rate, per 100 woman-years	12-Month Continuation Rate
Lippes Loop[b]	A (small)	Polyethylene Ba Impregnated nylon tail	$6.45	1964	Ortho	8.0	6.9	11.7	63.6
	B					5.8	6.5	21.1	59.2
	C					4.1	5.3	19.2	62.8
	D (large)					3.6	3.6	19.5	65.6
Saf-T-Coil[c]	Nulliparous	Polyethylene Ba impreg. Nylon tail	$5.50	1967	Julius Schmid	0.1	10.0	15.4	78.3
	Multiparous					1.3	11.4	10.0	74.1
T-Cu 200[d]	One size	Polythylene Fine copper nylon tail		1978	Population Council	1.5	5.3	7.2	80.9
7-Cu 200[d]	One size	Polyethylene fine copper nylon tail	$12.96	1973	G. D. Searle	1.5	3.3	4.2	87.6
Progestasert-T[e]	One size	Polyethylele T with polymeric membrane; nylon tail	$14.50	1976	Alza Corp.	2.5 (nulliparous)	7.5		
						1.9 (multiparous)	3.1	9.7	79.1

[a]IUDs currently marketed in the United States or FDA approved.
[b]Tietze C.: Evaluation of intrauterine devices: Ninth progress report, Cooperative Statistical Program. Studies in Family Planning No 55, July 1970.
[c]Cumulative experience of 16 published reports summarizing 586,497 woman-months of use of multiparous Saf-T-Coils by 35,125 women and of 3 published reports summarizing 11,993 woman-months of use of nulliparous Saf-T-Coils by 1658 women (available on request).
[d]Orlans BF: Intrauterine devices, Population Reports Series B, No 1; Dec. 1973. Event rates for the Cu-T and the Cu-7 are averages taken from Table 2 of this publication. These studies summarize 101,334 woman-months of use of the Cu-7 and 80,802 months of use of the Cu-T.
[e]"Erickson R et al: Advances in Planned Parenthood 1976; 11:167–76. Event rates based on 5495 women using Progestasert-Ts for 45,848 woman-months.

Reproduced with permission from Hatcher RA, Stewart GK, Guest F, Josephs N, Dale J: Contraceptive Technology 1982–1983. New York, Irvington Publishers, 1983, p 77.

Figure 7-4. Smoking and the pill: Age is the key

Can a heavy smoker safely be given the Pill? Maybe. The key to increased risk of heart attack, stroke or death in women who both smoke heavily and use the Pill is *AGE*.

A woman under 30 years of age can take the Pill with little risk, even if she smokes heavily. In Pill users under 30 years of age, the risk of death is only slightly higher in smokers than in nonsmokers. But a woman over 30 is taking risks if she both smokes and takes the Pill. In Pill users over 30 the risk soars to three or four times higher in smokers than in nonsmokers. Women over 40 have more of a chance of dying from the effects of both smoking and taking the Pill than from childbirth.

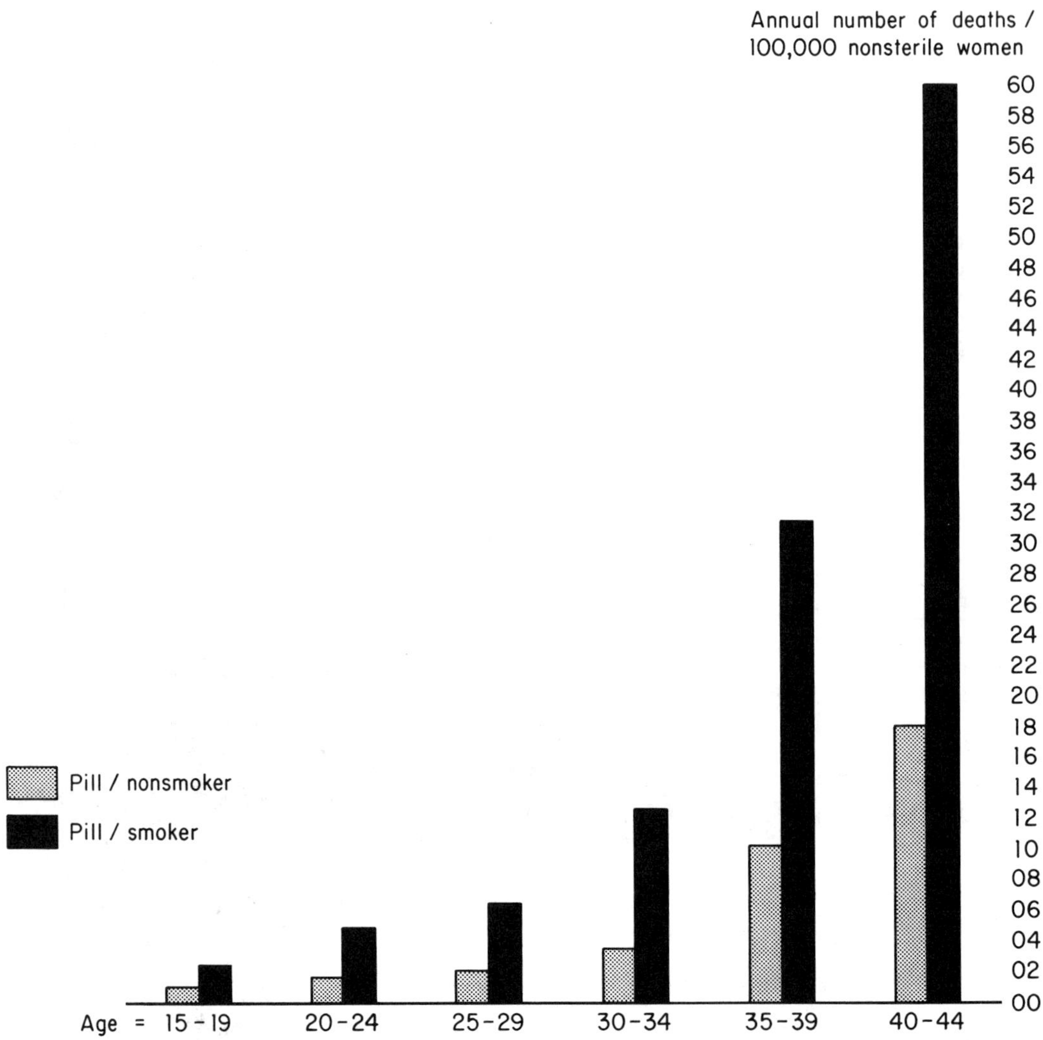

(Reproduced with permission from Hatcher RA, Stewart F, Guest F, Josephs N, Dale J: Contraceptive Technology 1982–1983. New York, Irvington Publishers, 1982, p 51.)

Table 7-4. Contraindications to Combined Birth Control Pills Containing Both an Estrogen and a Progestin

Absolute Contraindications	Strong Relative Contraindications	Other Relative Contraindications
Thromboembolic disorder (or history thereof)	Severe headaches, particularly vascular or migraine[a]	Termination of term pregnancy within past 10–14 days[a]
Cerebrovascular accident (or history thereof)	Hypertension with resting diastolic BP of 90 or greater on three or more separate visits, or an accurate measurement of 110 or more on a single visit[a]	Weight gain of 10 pounds or more while on the pill[a]
Coronary artery disease (or history thereof)	Diabetes[a]	Failure to have established regular menstrual cycles[a]
Known impaired liver function at present time	Prediabetes or a strong family history of diabetes	Patient with profile suggestive of anovulation and infertility problems: late onset of menses and very irregular, painless menses[a]
Hepatic adenoma (or history thereof)	Gallbladder disease, including cholecystectomy[a]	Cardiac or renal disease (or history thereof)[a]
Malignancy of breast or reproductive system (or history thereof)	Previous cholestasis during pregnancy, congenital hyperbilirubin (Gilbert's disease)	Conditions likely to make patient's following of pill instructions unreliable (mental retardation, major psychiatric problems, alcoholism, history of repeatedly taking pills incorrectly)[a]
Known pregnancy	Mononucleosis, acute phase	Lactation (oral contraceptives may be initiated as weaning begins and may be an aid in decreasing the flow of milk)[a]
	Sickle cell disease (SS) or sickle C disease (SC)[a]	May initiate the pill for women with these problems and observe carefully for worsening or improvement of the problem:
	Undiagnosed, abnormal vaginal bleeding[a]	Depression[a]
	Elective surgery planned in next 4 weeks, or major surgery requiring immobilization[a]	Hypertension with resting diastolic BP at a single visit of 90–99[a]
	Long-leg casts or major injury to lower leg	Chloasma or hair loss related to pregnancy (or history thereof)[a]
	Age over 40 years	Asthma[a]
	Age over 35 years and a history of heavy smoking[a]	Epilepsy[a]
	Impaired liver function within past year	Uterine fibromyomata[a]
		Acne
		Varicose veins[a]
		History of hepatitis, but now normal liver function tests for at least one year

[a]This refers to a contraindication to estrogen-containing pills, which may *not* be a contraindication to progestin-only pills or may be less of a contraindication to progestin-only pills than to combined pills.

[b]In some patients this should be listed as an absolute contraindication to use of the pill depending on the definition of "abnormal." If the patient's bleeding pattern is truly abnormal and of unknown cause, do not prescribe birth control pills.

(Reproduced with permission from Hatcher RA, Stewart GK, Stewart F, Guest F, Josephs N, Dale J: Contraceptive Technology 1982–1983. New York, Irvington Publishers, 1982, p 37.)

not control the symptoms, a pill with progestin alone can be used. Depression symptoms can sometimes be diminished by increasing the estrogen dosage. Vitamin B_6 at a dose of 25 mg/day has been advocated for treatment of oral contraceptive-related depression.

Injectable Medroxyprogesterone (Depo-Provera)

Depo-Provera is a long-acting, injectable progestin contraceptive. The important advantage of this method is that the patient does not have to remember to take a pill each day or reach for a device such as a condom. It is also a possible solution for the woman who does not want to become pregnant but whose husband does not want contraception to be used.

What are the possible risks of Depo-Provera? Not infrequently, breakthrough bleeding occurs. It has been noted that many of the women receiving Depo-Provera do not recover fertility for many months and occasionally for years after the injection. Therefore, women who might want to become fertile within the next 6 to 12 months should consider another method of contraception.

Depo-Provera should not be given to pregnant women. Preliminary data suggest that about 4.7 of each 1000 fetuses exposed during the first trimester will suffer some type of limb hypoplasia compared to a risk of about 1:1000 for unexposed fetuses. Also reported is a possible increase in congenital heart defects among those infants similarly exposed. Careful history and urine testing should help to reduce the risk of a gravid female receiving Depo-Provera.

Based on animal data, certain investigators have raised the possibility of increased risk of breast, ovarian, and uterine malignancies with Depo-Provera. However, at least one recent study of 5000 women, with 4 to 13 years of follow-up, failed to show any increased risk of these cancers (Liang 1983).

The dose of Depo-Provera is usually 150 mg IM every three months. The drug is supplied in 5-ml vials of 100 mg/ml, and 2.5-ml vials of 400 mg/ml.

REFERENCES AND SELECTED READING

Banerji D: Forcible sterilization in family planning. Economic and Political Weekly 1976; 11:665–68.

Belmont L, Marolla FA: Birth order, family size, and intelligence. Science 1973; 182:1096–101.

Chen HC, Chow LP: Strategies for the introduction of contraceptive methods: The Taiwan experience. In Duncan GW, Hilton EJ, Kreager P, Lumsdaine AA (eds): Fertility Control Methods: Strategies for Introduction. New York, Academic Press, 1973.

Clausen AW: Population growth and economic and social development. Address to the International Population Conference, Washington, DC, World Bank, Aug. 1984.

Cochrane SH: Fertility and Education: What Do We Really Know? Baltimore, Johns Hopkins University Press, 1978.

Dickey RP: Managing Contraceptive Pill Patients. Minneapolis, Creative Infomatics Inc, 1980.

El-Bushra J, Fordham J, Martius H, Stella R: Working with Youth: Some Out-of-School Approaches to Population, Family Life, and Sex Education. London, International Planned Parenthood Federation, 1978.

Hatcher, RA: Contraceptive Technology 1982–1983. New York, Irving Publishers, 1983.

Holck SE, Cates W.: Fertility and population dynamics in two Kampuchean refugee camps. International Family Planning Perspectives, 1982; 8:84–92.

Huber, SC, Piotrow, PT, et al: Contraceptive distribution: Taking supplies to villages and households. Population Reports 1975; J5.

Kendall M.: The world fertility survey: Current status and findings. Population Reports, 1979; M3:73–104.

Kleinman, RL (ed): Family Planning Handbook for Doctors. London, International Planned Parenthood Federation, 1980.

Kleinman, RL: Vasectomy. London, International Planned Parenthood Federation, 1972.

Liang, AP et al: Risk of breast, uterine corpus, and ovarian cancer in women receiving medroxyprogesterone injections. JAMA 1983; 249:2909–912.

Maine D: Family Planning: Its Impact on the Health of Women and Children. New York, Center for Population and Family Health, Columbia University, 1981.

Maine D, McNamara R: Birth Spacing and Child Survival. New York, Center for Population and Family Health, Columbia University, 1985.

Mauldin WP: The determinants of fertility decline in developing countries: An overview of the available empirical evidence. International Family Planning Perspectives, 1982; 8:116–20.

McCann MF, Liskin LS, Piotrow PT et al: Breastfeeding, fertility, and family planning. Population Reports 1981; Series J: 526–75.

Minkin S: Depo-Provera: A Critical Analysis. San Francisco, Institute for Food and Development Policy, 1980.
Newton JR: Managing Patients with Intrauterine Devices. Minneapolis, Creative Infomatics Inc, 1980.
Nortman D: Parental Age as a Factor in Pregnancy Outcomes. Reports on Population/Family Planning No 16. New York, The Population Council, 1974.
Omran AR, Standley CC (eds): Family Patterns and Health: An International Collaborative Study in India, Iran, Lebanon, Philippines, and Turkey. Geneva, World Health Organization, 1976.
Pebley AR, Brackett JW: The relationship of contraceptive availability to contraceptive use. International Family Planning Perspectives 1982; 8:84–92.
Potts M, Speidel JJ, Kesel E: Relative risks of various means of fertility control when used in less-developed countries. In Sciarra JJ, Zatuchni GI, Speidel JJ (eds): Risks, Benefits, and Controversies in Fertility Control. PARFR Series on Fertility and Regulation. Hagerstown, MD, Harper & Row, 1978.
Puffer RR, Serrano CV: Birthweight, Maternal Age, and Birth Order: Three Important Determinants in Infant Mortality. Scientific Publication No 294. Washington, DC, Pan American Health Organization, 1975.
Rawson-Jones D, Salkeld G: Communicating Family Planning. London, International Planned Parenthood Federation, 1971.
Rodriguez G: Family planning availability and contraceptive practice. Family Planning Perspectives 1979; 11:51–56, 58–63, 67–70.
Rosenfield A, Maine D: Maternal mortality—A neglected tragedy. Lancet 1985; 11:83–85.
Rosenfield A, Maine D, Gorosh ME: Nonclinical distribution of the pill in the developing world. International Family Planning Perspectives 1980; 6:130–36.
Rosenfield A, Wray JD: Conclusion. In Maine D: Family Planning: Its Impact on the Health of Women and Children, New York, Center for Population and Family Health, Columbia University, pp 49–50, 1981.
Sai FT: Some Ethical Issues in Family Planning. London, International Planned Parenthood Federation, 1976.
Sciarra JJ, Zatuchni GI, Speidel JJ (eds): Risks, Benefits, and Controversies in Fertility Control. Hagerstown, MD, Harper & Row, 1978.
Singh K: Population, Poverty, and the Future of India. New Delhi, National Institute of Family Planning, 1975.
Sweeney WO: Media communications in population/family planning programs; A review. Population Reports 1975; J16.
Watson WB: An historical overview. In Watson WB (ed): Family Planning in the Developing World: A Review of Progress. New York, Population Council, 1977.
Westoff CF, Pebley AR: Alternative measures of unmet need for family planning in developing countries. International Family Planning Perspectives 1981; 7:126.
World Bank: World Development Report 1984. Washington, DC, World Bank, 1984.
World Health Organization: Evaluation of Family Planning in Health Services. WHO Technical Report Series No 569, Geneva, World Health Organization, 1975.
World Health Organization: Primary Health Care. (Report of the International Conference on Primary Health Care, Alma-Ata, USSR) Geneva, World Health Organization, 1978.
Wortman J: Training nonphysicians in family planning services. Population Reports 1975; J6.
Wortman J, Piotrow PT: Vasectomy: Old and new techniques. Population Reports 1973; D1.
Wray JD: Population Pressure on Families: Family Size and Child Spacing. Reports on Population/Family Planning No 9, New York, The Population Council, 1971.

8
Refugee Health Care Issues from a Nursing Perspective

MIRIAM GILDAY

This chapter is intended as a stepping-off point to an experience for which one cannot fully prepare. One's nursing education and past experience are the best preparation because, although circumstances differ, the basic principles of health care are the same. The most important assets needed for working successfully in a refugee setting are patience, flexibility, and imagination.

Nurses are generalists. They are concerned with all aspects of health care: physical, emotional, spiritual, political, and economic. In addition, they are concerned with people of all age groups and with the special health care needs that accompany each phase of life. Nurses providing health care in refugee camps will find many challenges in each of these areas.

One of the first things to become clear to any health care provider working in a refugee camp is that there are no well-defined job descriptions. The overwhelming nature of refugee health problems and the limited number of staff available necessitate a blurring of roles and an overlapping of functions between disciplines to meet the varied and complex health care needs. Health care providers should take a broad view of health that includes family, community, and the physical as well as economic and political environment. This means that, in addition to establishing health care programs, providing health education, and performing direct patient care, nurses will find they must be concerned with the problems of sanitation; with the acquisition of food, clean water, and medical supplies; with the design and construction of wards and clinics; and with the provision of housing and basic necessities for the camp population. It is important to maintain a broad view of the problems at hand so that the health care provided will be effective and appropriately directed.

PREPARATION

Because of the critical nature of most refugee situations, a nurse may be asked to leave home on short notice with little preparation time. Some steps can be taken, however, to increase confidence and effectiveness in this new and unusual situation.

Request information from your sponsoring agency, including background information on the factors leading up to the refugee situation; a description of the political and economic structure of the camp, including factors controlling the delivery of health care; and contact with nurses who have recently returned from the camp to which you have been assigned. This information is helpful in gaining an understanding of the specific health needs and nursing demands in the particular refugee setting.

Review a number of topics, including nutrition, particularly deficiency diseases and their management; conditions common to refugee populations, including diarrheal diseases, malaria, tuberculosis, pneumonia, intestinal parasites, skin infections, anxiety, and depression; pharmacology, especially commonly used antibiotics and the medications used for the treatment of the above-mentioned diseases; and immunizations and the diseases they prevent.

In choosing reference books to bring to the camp, consider their weight and portability as well as the quantity and appropriateness of the information they contain. Rorabaugh (1983) suggests bringing an out-of-date nursing text that illustrates such things as sterilization techniques, manual suction, and chest tube drainage systems that do not rely on modern technology or electricity.

In addition to books, it is helpful to have as much of your own assessment equipment as possible. Stethoscopes, blood pressure cuffs, thermometers, and measuring tapes may all be in short supply. A good flashlight with a supply of heavy-duty batteries and a replacement bulb is essential. And, if you are bringing an otoophthalmoscope, be sure it is battery-operated and includes a supply of replacement batteries, bulbs, and ear tips.

One challenge that is difficult to prepare for—but crucial to the success of all health care efforts—is the issue of culture. A chapter in this manual is devoted entirely to a discussion of cultural adjustment (see Chapter 11). Nurses are in a unique position to have a positive long-term effect on the health care practices of a refugee population. This is possible only when health education and health care programs are culturally appropriate and respect the beliefs and practices of the people for whom they are designed to serve. This is not easy, as some of our most basic attitudes toward health care and our beliefs about life and death are often called into question. Sensitivity toward the patient's culture and an awareness of one's own cultural biases are necessary for success in cross-cultural nursing.

Designing culturally appropriate programs can be achieved only when the refugees themselves are involved in every step of the planning, development, and implementation of these programs. Refugee health workers and camp community leaders should be given as much responsibility as possible in meeting the camp's health care needs. In addition, if traditional healers are present in camp, they should be included in health care planning. Traditional healers have much to contribute to the physical and emotional well-being of their people; they are respected members of the community. Designing health care programs to include traditional practitioners whenever possible enhances the credibility of health care and prevents patients from being forced to choose between their own traditions and Western health care.

Regardless of preparation, the situation encountered on arrival can be overwhelming. Wards and clinics with dirt floors and leaking roofs, no running water or electricity, inadequate supplies, and many seriously ill patients may seem completely unmanageable. Camps and settlements that are just being established may lack structures to house patients and the most basic medicines and supplies. A plan of action based on a problem-solving approach is helpful if anything is to be accomplished under such difficult circumstances. As Simmonds (1981) suggests, the basic elements of the nursing process provide an excellent guide for establishing an organized approach. Assessing, planning, implementing, and evaluating on an ongoing basis in collaboration with all health workers, camp leaders, and host-country officials provide the framework for effective health care.

WORKING WITH INTERPRETERS

Inability to communicate is one of the biggest barriers to be overcome in establishing effective health care programs in a refugee setting. Health care providers are often recruited on short notice and rarely have time to learn the language of the refugees. Most communication will be carried on through an interpreter. It is crucial, therefore, to be attentive to the nonverbal communication exhibited by both the interpreter and the patient, which will signal their understanding. Accurate communication can be difficult and time-consuming.

ESTABLISHING WARDS AND CLINICS

The priorities to consider in the establishment and operation of wards and clinics in a refugee setting are so basic they may not be obvious to health workers who are accustomed to working with a highly structured and complex health care system. The following review of the essential considerations may be useful.

Building Construction

Roofs of all structures should be waterproof. If construction materials are not waterproof, roofs can be lined with plastic sheeting when it is available. Tin may be used for more permanent structures, as it is waterproof and requires less maintenance; however, it can make the building very hot. Large windows and doors should be included in the design to provide good ventilation and light. Because windows may simply be openings cut in the walls, a shutter that can be closed against blowing dust and cold nights is beneficial.

An isolation area will be needed on in-patient wards. Air currents should be considered in its design. It should be as separate as possible from the rest of the ward, with separate handwashing and waste disposal facilities.

Sanitation

Latrines and areas for waste disposal should be close enough to the building for patient and staff use, but situated so as to minimize odors and flies in the ward.

A mechanism that provides a flow of water, but minimizes its consumption, will be needed for handwashing in the absence of plentiful running water. One method is to fill covered containers with water and add a low concentration of inexpensive soap or disinfectant, which permits washing without the need for rinsing. The solution can then be poured over the hands and collected in pots or trash cans for later disposal.

Water

Because local water supplies are generally limited and contaminated, water may have to be brought in at considerable expense. The amount of water required to fill the needs of patients, staff, and ward maintenance must be determined and an allotment system established. Equipment for boiling drinking water may also be required.

Patient Supplies

When possible, in-patient wards should provide patients with some basic necessities such as cots, mosquito nets, mats, blankets, eating utensils, bedpans when needed, a wash basin, and a container for storing drinking water at the bedside.

Ward Supplies and Medications

Availability of basic supplies such as soap, dressing, medications, needles, and syringes will vary, but intravenous fluids and oxygen may not be available at all. As a rule, there will be little surplus, and supplies must be used sparingly. Supplies should be kept in a clean, dry place where they are not easily accessible to anyone but staff. An inventory should be taken regularly to monitor usage and to maintain adequate stock. All staff members should be impressed with the fact that supplies are scarce and that they must guard against waste and overuse.

Drugs may be supplied by many different nations under varying brand names and with labels that are difficult to read. Staff should be alerted to look for the generic drug name and for varied strengths.

Like general supplies, medications should be kept in a dry and secure place, inventoried regularly, and carefully monitored. Refugee health workers may be under considerable pressure to take medications home from wards and clinics. This can result in both injuries from improper drug use and medication shortages in the wards. Refugee health workers should be instructed on the actions of medications and the indications for their use, as well as the dangers that result from their indiscriminate use.

Staffing

The experience and expertise of staff members will vary widely, as will their length of stay. Short-term commitments are approximately three to six months; stays of six months or longer are usually considered long term. In addition, health professionals from many nations often work in conjunction to provide health care in a particular refugee camp or settlement. With such a rapid turnover rate, and the variety of backgrounds and attitudes among staff members, it is often difficult to maintain well-organized programs and a cohesive, efficient staff.

The nature of refugee health needs and the shortage of staff make traditional role delineations impractical. Division of responsibilities for the various aspects of patient care and program administration should, therefore, be based on the experience, special talents, and interests of individual staff members. In this way, each staff member's particular abilities will be fully utilized and programs will run more smoothly.

The coordination and administration of health programs, ideally, should be carried out by long-term staff members who have expertise in the particular service being provided. Nurses are often well-equipped to handle these responsibilities because many nurses remain in the camp longer and are experienced in all aspects of patient care.

Coordination between disciplines may work well for some programs. Whatever the arrangement, it is essential that at least one person understand all aspects of the particular program and accept responsibility for it so that the program does not become disorganized with every staff change.

For staff members to work as a team, individual flexibility and good communication based on mutual respect are necessary. The best way to maintain good communication is to schedule regular staff meetings to evaluate programs, share ideas and information, and discuss problems. Decisions that affect patient care, program management, and staffing should be made at these meetings, with staff members having an equal voice in decisions that affect their program or work schedule. Frequent meetings allow for discussion of problems as they arise and give staff members the opportunity to express their feelings. This can enhance understanding and may prevent increasing tension, which can divide a staff.

There will always be problems to discuss, but it is a mistake to focus only on the negative. Some staff meeting time should be devoted to the recognition of program accomplishments and of individual contributions that might otherwise go unnoticed. Mutual support and appreciation will help to balance frustration and decrease the stress that most staff members experience.

Staff scheduling should probably be done by a long-term staff member who understands the program or ward needs, but general decisions about scheduling should be made by the entire staff. Schedules should be based on both the needs of the patients and a realistic appraisal of the consecutive number of days staff members can work, how often they can be rotated, and how much time off is required to keep the staff functioning effectively. Guidelines concerning days off and holiday time may be provided by the employing agency. Once staffing needs have been determined, it may be best for a nurse to take responsibility for the nursing schedule and for a physician to take responsibility for the physicians' schedule. Scheduling must be somewhat flexible because illness among staff members is common, particularly during their first few weeks.

Often medical professionals are not needed to carry out many of the tasks in a basic health care program. As a result, there will be times when nonmedical workers are called on or volunteer to help in health care programs. Nonmedical workers can be a great asset to an overburdened staff and should be included in the schedule as appropriate.

The majority of health care staff members will be refugee health workers trained by the professional staff. Refugee health workers are trained to meet both short-term and long-term needs (see Chapter 4). Health workers from among the camp's refugee population do not have to overcome the barriers of language and culture and are best-equipped to translate Western medicine into culturally acceptable terms. They can accurately assess the health needs and desires of their people, and they can help develop programs that will work within the defined limits of the refugee setting.

Enabling refugees to assume responsibility for their own well-being can help to restore the confidence and self-esteem that may have been damaged by their present situation. Every nurse must be ready to assume the role of teacher and guide rather than primary caregiver. As Simmonds (1981) points out, setting up health care programs that depend heavily on the presence of expatriate staff creates dependence on outside help, which may not always be available. Thus, no long-term benefits are achieved.

The number of staff needed and the organization of tasks and responsibilities depend on the goals and resources of the facility or program. Older, respected members of the refugee community can be helpful in planning health care and will be effective in assuming positions of leadership and authority. Because women are usually responsible for the health care of the family, efforts should be made to reach out to them by including them in training programs and in the planning and implementation of health care.

Language ability is helpful for those refugee health workers who must work directly with expatriate staff. Basic mathematical skills and the ability to read labels are assets for those who will be administering medications. In the absence of these skills, drugs can be separated and labeled with symbols. They can then be ordered by symbol and volume, rather than by name and dose.

For in-patient wards it is helpful to draw the following staff from among the refugee population: interpreters; an admissions clerk; patient care providers; a pharmacy and supply aide, wet nurses, if patients include infants whose mothers cannot feed them; cooks, if food is prepared on the ward; a ward manager; and cleaners. Out-patient clinics usually require a registrar, intake workers, primary health care providers, a medication dispenser, cleaners, and a night guard. Home visits for patient follow-up can be made by clinic staff or, if available, public health workers.

A public health program that can monitor general health needs and provide health education and prevention programs is essential for the health of the whole camp and should be established as quickly as possible. All refugee health workers, regardless of their particular jobs, should be encouraged to share health care knowledge with patients and their families. Regular meetings including both professional and refugee health workers will promote understanding and give refugee health workers the opportunity to evaluate programs and share their ideas and suggestions.

It is important for nurses and other professional staff to remember that their refugee colleagues live with the same levels of stress and uncertainty as the rest of the refugee population. Their ability to concentrate and perform effectively may be hampered, at times, by anxiety and depression. Professional staff may have to provide a great deal of encouragement and moral support during such difficult times.

Record Keeping

Some type of simple health record, containing a growth chart for children and information regarding immunizations, special health problems, and diseases treated, should be provided whenever possible. Such records facilitate health care delivery and promote continuity of care when the refugee moves to another location. Storing records in wards or clinics is usually impractical. Instead, patients should be given their health records with instructions to present them when they seek health care. Records can be made from heavy paper or cardboard and placed in an envelope or plastic bag. A careful explanation of the purpose and importance of the records may minimize their loss.

When children are admitted to wards without their parents, all available information about their identity and the names and location of family members should be recorded and kept to facilitate family reunification.

Statistics of morbidity and mortality should be gathered by health care staff so that disease patterns can be mapped and health programs evaluated. This information can be used in the development of new programs and in the allocation of funds for the support of health care projects.

Protocols

The rapid turnover of health care staff makes it advisable to have as many details of health care as possible in writing. Treatment protocols based on what is appropriate and practical within the camp are helpful for both professional staff and refugee health workers. Documenting programs that work well and outlining necessary procedures save time and effort when new staff arrive. Interpreters can translate protocols into the language of the refugee health workers.

SPECIAL CONSIDERATIONS

Supply Shortages

Medications and supplies are costly and often in short supply or difficult to acquire. Out-of-date drugs that can still produce benefit without causing adverse effects should be used if replacement stocks are not available. Medications that come in ampules intended for one-time use are often too valuable to discard. The open ampules can be covered with gauze or cotton, or the remaining medication can be drawn up into a syringe and kept sterile until it is needed again.

The use of intravenous fluids, when available, should be restricted to those patients who cannot otherwise be managed. Therapy should be discontinued as soon as it is possible to administer fluids orally or by nasogastric tube (see Chapter 15). This approach will conserve limited supplies, and help to minimize adverse effects such as infection, phlebitis, and fluid overload, which can be especially difficult to manage in a refugee setting. It is also important to limit the use of intravenous fluids and parenteral medications to discourage the belief that fluids and medicine are more beneficial when given by injection. When this idea is prevalent, it can lead to serious consequences resulting from the inappropriate use of medications purchased on the black market or taken from wards and clinics.

Limited supplies may make it impossible to change intravenous bottles and tubing as often as recommended, especially for infants and small children who may receive only small amounts of fluid each day. Practical routines for intravenous use must be established, based on the availability of supplies. One bottle of intravenous fluid can be used for more than one patient by using fresh tubing for each patient and careful aseptic technique. Heparin locks can be used for patients who require intravenous medications but not fluid therapy. Venous cutdowns and central lines are usually not practical because of the high risk of infection.

If a patient with a heparin lock or intravenous infusion suddenly develops a fever, the intravenous solution and equipment should be suspected. If no other cause for the fever can be found, the intravenous site should be changed and the fluid and tubing or heparin lock discarded.

Disposable plastics such as feeding tubes and suction catheters can be cleaned with soap and water and boiled for reuse. Some disposable syringes can be boiled and used several times for giving injections. Disposable syringes can also be used for measuring and administering oral medications, particularly small doses required by infants and children. Disposable needles are more difficult to reuse because they become dull quickly, but they can be sharpened and resterilized.

It is more practical to take axillary temperatures than oral or rectal temperatures, in most cases, because thermometers are often scarce and adequate cleaning between patients may not be possible.

Lack of Electricity

The most serious problem posed by the absence of electrical power is inadequate lighting. Examinations that do not require privacy can be performed outdoors or under windows. Flashlights can be used for close examination and can also be shone on microscope mirrors. Locally available lanterns should be kept on the wards to provide light at night.

Lack of Modern Equipment

The absence of pumps and suction machines makes it difficult to manage patients with pneumothorax, empyema, or intestinal obstructions that require gastric decompression. With some basic supplies, however, a water seal drainage system, or a Wangensteen suction apparatus can be set up to take the place of more complex equipment.

The water seal system (see Figure 8-1B) allows air and fluid to leave the pleural space (aided by gravity) while it prevents air from traveling back up the drainage tube. This system works well for a simple pneumothorax and for draining pus or fluid from the pleural space.

To set up water seal drainage, the chest tube is connected to a length of flexible tubing, the

Figure 8-1. A water seal drainage system: (*A*) a Wangensteen apparatus; (*B*) a water seal system.

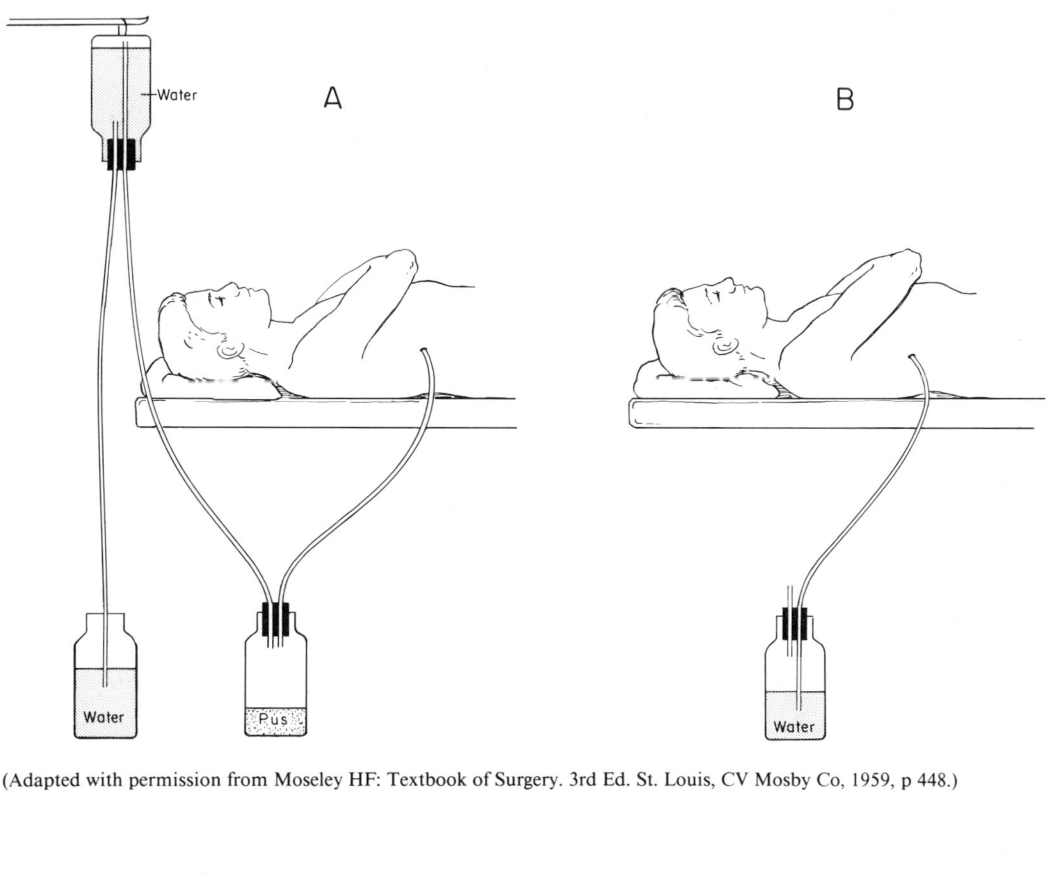

(Adapted with permission from Moseley HF: Textbook of Surgery. 3rd Ed. St. Louis, CV Mosby Co, 1959, p 448.)

other end of which is placed in a container partially filled with boiled water. The end of the drainage tube must be kept below the water level and the container must be kept lower than the patient's chest. The top of the container can be left open if a vented cap is not available, but the opening should be covered with gauze or thin cloth to prevent dirt and insects from entering.

If the pneumothorax fails to resolve or if the fluid in the pleural space is too thick to drain by gravity, a Wangensteen apparatus (see Figure 8-1*A*) can provide suction. This system is more difficult to set up because it requires equipment. The biggest challenge is in improvising the various components of the system if they are not available. Several lengths of flexible tubing, plastic or glass containers, and two-holed airtight stoppers will be needed.

To set up a Wangensteen apparatus, the collection bottle is placed on the floor. This bottle must have an airtight stopper with two openings—one to receive the drainage tube from the patient and the other for the tube that leads to the second bottle in the system. The second bottle, which is nearly filled with boiled water, is suspended upside down from a hook or pole. The tubing from the drainage bottle must be connected to an airway in the stopper of the second bottle. This airway must extend above the water level. A second tube exits the stopper of the second bottle and leads to a third bottle, which is placed on the floor. The third bottle may be left open. The water in the second bottle flowing through the tube to the third bottle produces a negative pressure in the system. When the second bottle is almost empty, the tube between the first and second bottles must be clamped while the second bottle is refilled. A regulating clamp can be placed on the tube leading to the third bottle to control the rate of water flow and to prevent the second bottle from emptying too rapidly. If increased suction is needed, the second bottle can be raised and the regulating clamp removed.

Wangensteen suction can be used in the same way for gastric decompression by attaching the apparatus to a nasogastric tube. If the necessary containers are not available in the refugee camp, it may be possible to purchase them locally, as some hospitals within the host country may use this equipment. It is also possible to improvise the equipment if intravenous solutions are being supplied in glass bottles. Used bottles with intact stoppers and used intravenous tubing make ideal substitutes. If containers are difficult to obtain, a two-bottle setup can be used by eliminating the first bottle, particularly if the system is being used for the evacuation of air from the pleural space. A two-bottle system may not work as well for the evacuation of thick liquids since the effect of gravity between the patient and the first bottle is lost.

The lack of an autoclave makes adequate sterilization of surgical equipment difficult. Cleaning with soap and water, boiling, soaking in disinfectants, and exposing equipment to sunlight are alternatives that can be used in most settings.

Pressure cookers, if available, can be used as autoclaves. A small amount of water is placed in the bottom of the pot. Linens, equipment, and even surgical packs are placed on a wire rack above the water level. The water will evaporate and leave the items inside the pot dry. It is difficult to be certain how much time and what temperature are needed to sterilize various items since pressure cookers are not designed for this purpose. The only way to be certain that sterility has been achieved is to use sterility indicators, which come in several forms for use in autoclaving.

Privacy

In the absence of an enclosed examining area, privacy can be achieved by hanging sheets of colored plastic or cloth around the patient and examining through clothing when necessary. When possible, examiners should be of the same sex as patients.

Families on the Ward

It is often a cultural norm for families to stay on in-patient wards with sick relatives. Although this may cause crowding and some confusion, the family can be a great asset to overburdened staff by providing the patient with personal care and attention. In addition, family members can be taught to perform many specific treatments required by the patient, including administering oral medications. Thus, patients receive caring and personal attention despite staff shortages, and families are given the opportunity to learn about health care.

Premature Infants

Keeping small infants warm is difficult even in tropical countries. Hats made of the warmest available material can cut down on heat loss from the scalp. Infants should be kept with their mothers, whenever possible, because close body contact is an excellent means of keeping infants warm. When infants require close observation, or when mothers are unable to care for them, they may be placed in baskets and kept warm by padded warm water bottles, plastic gloves filled with warm water, or heated intravenous bottles. Infants can also be placed in plastic basins, which are then placed in larger basins filled with warm water, thus producing an incubator effect. The sun can be used for warmth and for phototherapy for jaundiced infants. Be sure to keep infants covered with mosquito netting at all times.

Infants who are unable to nurse can be tube-fed, or milk can be dripped into the infant's mouth from a syringe. The use of infant bottles is not usually recommended because of the dangers presented by inadequate cleaning and lack of appropriate infant formulas. Breast milk, which protects the gastrointestinal tract and boosts the infant's immunity to disease, should be used whenever possible.

Wards and clinics providing care for infants should employ wet nurses for the feeding of infants who cannot be breastfed by their mothers. This not only provides the infant with the safest and most beneficial food possible, it also reinforces that breast milk is the best food for babies. Wet nurses should be given additional food whenever possible to increase their intake of protein, calcium, and vitamins.

Fever Management

Aspirin and acetaminophen may be plentiful but, as with other medications, supplies may not be dependable or available to patients outside the refugee camp setting. Fever management should, therefore, include the removal of blankets and excess clothing, protection from the sun, sponge bathing, an increase in fluid intake, and the use of antipyretics when available. In this way, patients and their families can learn to treat fever effectively without medicines or professional help.

A careful explanation of this type of fever management is important because many people believe that covering a fever victim with warm clothing and blankets is the best treatment. Fear of pneumonia and other adverse effects may prevent families from accepting this "new" treatment until they have observed its benefits firsthand. Staff should also explain that fever may help the body to fight infections.

Wound Care

Caring for wounds in a refugee camp is often complicated by limited supplies. Ordinary soap and water can replace special cleansing solutions. Inexpensive antiseptics, such as hydrogen peroxide and gentian violet, can be used instead of more expensive antibiotic creams. If dressing materials are in short supply, bandages can be made from cloth, using white cotton whenever possible.

Most dressings, even those intended to be disposable, can be reused after being washed, boiled, and dried in the sun. Exposing wounds to air and sunlight usually aids healing. Uncovered wounds should be carefully protected from insects.

Yeast infections such as thrush, and gram-positive skin infections such as impetigo, can be treated effectively with gentian violet (Bergersen & Goth 1979). When using hydrogen peroxide for wound cleaning, be certain to check the concentration, as it may vary from 3 to 25 percent. Even the standard 3 percent concentration should be diluted before use.

Bedridden and Comatose Patients

The patient who is on prolonged bed rest is especially challenging because of the difficulty of preventing associated complications. Although staffing may be limited, the patient's family and friends can be taught to perform much of the patient's care, and the conscious patient can be encouraged to take an active part in preventing complications. Family members can learn chest physiotherapy and postural drainage, range-of-motion exercises, skin care (including massage), the importance of frequent position change, and maintenance of adequate nutrition and hydration. They can also learn to give gavage feedings and to administer medications.

In the absence of mattresses, padding for beds can be made from cloth. If packing materials such as foam rubber or Styrofoam chips are available, they can be covered with cloth and used to cushion bony prominences. Improvised footboards, shoes, and cloth rolls help to prevent hand and foot deformities.

Removal of airway secretions can be accomplished by several methods in the absence of electrical suction machines. A bulb syringe is most useful for clearing the nose and mouth. A regular syringe can be connected to a suction catheter, a feeding tube, or a piece of small-gauge, soft rubber tubing and used for deeper suctioning. A DeLee mucus trap (see Figure 8-2) also provides well-controlled suctioning. Werner (1977) suggests using a small syringe without the needle to aspirate the nares of young children.

Mothers can learn to make saline nose drops for loosening nasal secretions by adding one-half teaspoon of salt to one cup of boiled water. In dry climates, deep airway congestion can be improved by improvising a mist tent using a pot of steaming water and a piece of heavy cloth or plastic. This is also helpful for children with croup. The child in this type of mist tent should be held by an adult, and care must be taken to avoid burns.

Triage

In very critical situations, when camps are overcrowded with large numbers of seriously ill people and staff and supplies are limited, decisions may have to be made about who will receive treatment, and even who will receive a share of available food and water. It may be possible to include only severely underweight patients in feeding programs, and medicines may have to be given on the basis of who is most likely to benefit from them. This is probably the most frustrating and difficult situation the staff must face. Discussion of feelings and mutual support among staff is crucial to cope with these issues on a daily basis.

Death

Every culture has its own rituals and customs surrounding death (see Chapter 11). In addition to dealing with our own feelings about death, it is important to provide families with the opportunity to carry out those practices that are important to them when a family member dies. On in-patient wards, it is helpful to have a quiet place set aside where families can mourn, the body can be prepared by them

Figure 8-2. Using a DeLee mucus trap for suctioning.

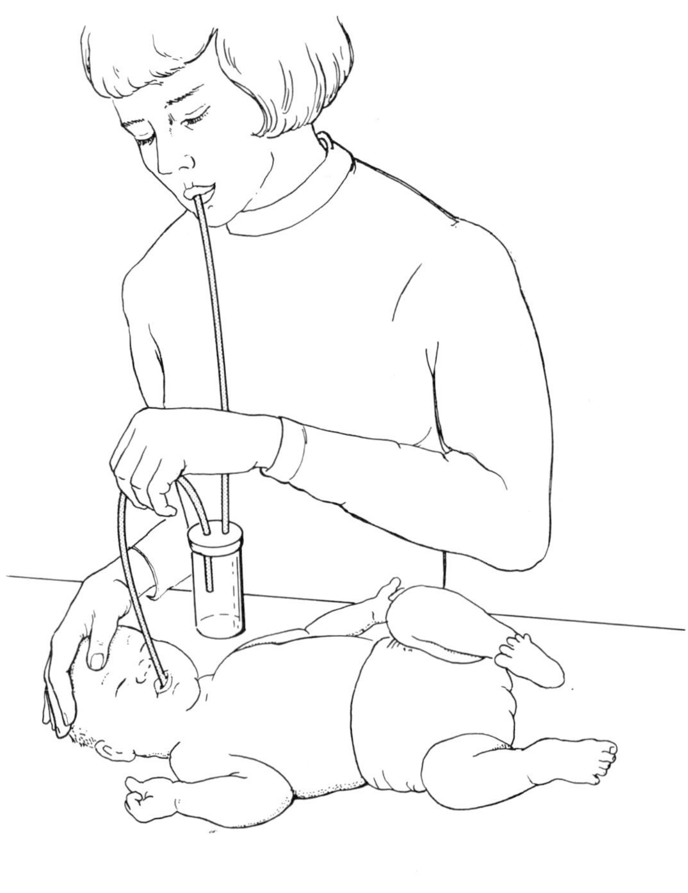

for cremation or burial, and religious services can be held. Final disposition of the body will depend on health regulations in the camp as well as the customs of the people.

ADMINISTRATIVE AND FUNDING ISSUES

Because of the unstable nature of refugee camps, both long-term and short-term planning must be flexible and sensitive to changing needs if programs are to be effective and available funds well used. Keeping agency officials up-to-date on current programs and changing health care needs in the camp or settlement is an important part of the activities of every health care worker. Reports that assess and statistically evaluate programs, written collaboratively by lay and professional staff, should be sent to agency officials at regular intervals. Although it is difficult to find time to write such reports, this is one way that health care providers in the field can have an impact on program funding.

CONCLUSION

The challenges of refugee health care are matched and often surpassed by the rich rewards of traveling, learning about other cultures, working within an international community, and helping people whose needs go far beyond basic health concerns. Refugee health care presents limitless opportunities for creative practice and for personal growth.

REFERENCES AND SELECTED READING

Aguilera D, Messick J: Crisis Intervention: Theory and Methodology. St Louis, Mosby, 1974.
Bergersen B, Goth A: Pharmacology in Nursing. St Louis, CV Mosby, 1979.
Boyer-Chuanroong L: Health promotion in a Cambodian refugee camp: A child-to-child approach. J Sch Health 1984;54(7):253–55.
Harman P: Measuring malnutrition in nutritional emergencies. Nurs Times 1981;(Jan 8):65–69.
King F, Martodipoero S: Primary Child Care: A Manual for Health Workers. London, Oxford University Press, 1978.
Morrow H: The fundamental influence of political, social, and economic factors on health and health care. Int Nurs Rev 1982; 29(6):183–86.
Peel S: Selective feeding procedures. Disasters 1977;1(3).
Rorabaugh MA: The pediatric nurse practitioner in Southeast Asia: A personal account. Pediatr Nurs 1983;9(4):263–66.
Shillington P: Working at a camp in Thailand. Nurs Times 1981; (Jan 8):69–73.
Simmonds S: Feeding the hungry. Nurs Times 1981;(Jan 8):57–62.
Skeet M: Traditional medicine. Nurs Times 1981;(April 2):583–88.
Ulin P: International nursing challenges. Nurs Outlook 1982; (Nov/Dec):5311–315.
Werner D: Where There Is No Doctor: A Village Healthcare Handbook. Palo Alto, CA, Hesperian Foundation, 1977.

9

Setting Priorities and the Level of Health Care in a Refugee Camp

SANDRA GOVE
ABDIKAMAL ALI-SALAD

Setting priorities and establishing the level of care to be delivered in a refugee camp are difficult tasks for the health team and program administrators. Conflicts can occur, particularly when clinicians with little public health experience attempt to duplicate health care services they have been trained to deliver, which usually maximize individual patient health care. Conflicts can be minimized if health care professionals work as a team and give priority to interventions that are likely to reduce morbidity and mortality with the available resources. Resources and health team efforts must be carefully divided among interventions according to their expected results and costs (in time, personnel, and material resources). Once immediate emergency health problems are under control, the level of health care provided should be one that can be sustained. This is often facilitated by standardizing services and treatment guidelines between camps. Where feasible, treatment guidelines for the refugees should be consistent with those established for the local population. Early and continuous involvement of the government health service is important. Where possible, it should be involved in setting the guidelines and implementing programs for health care in the refugee camps.

The early introduction of a surveillance system and the use of simple surveys to identify the leading causes of illness and death can provide vital data to direct clinical and public health activities. Chapter 2 describes the use of epidemiologic data to identify disease problems and determine priorities for the allocation of health care resources.

BASIC INTERVENTIONS IN NEWLY ESTABLISHED CAMPS

In a newly established refugee camp, many of the first health care priorities are not included in the usual training and experience of many doctors and nurses. Adequate food, water, sanitation, and shelter must be ensured. Immediate medical priorities should include rapid immunization of children against measles. Epidemics of measles with high fatality rates can, and often do, occur as new arrivals crowd into camps where immunization programs have been delayed. To begin curative medical care without these basic preventive interventions invites futility. For example, medical staff may have to treat hundreds of patients with diarrhea as a result of contaminated water supplies, or watch children die from measles, despite antibiotics for their pneumonia, because of a failure to immunize. All too often, emergency medical teams leave vaccine procurement and maintenance of the cold chain to in-country systems or other agencies that may not be prepared for rapid response; thus, new arrivals may go unprotected. Once guidelines for preventive programs have been established, care must be taken to implement them effectively.

Many aspects of the physical setting, including shelter, food, and water, are not only outside of the usual expertise of clinicians, but may be the responsibility of other agencies or ministries. In these instances, the role of medical personnel includes education, organization, and advocacy. Advocacy and any interventions which will promote an adequate general ration cannot be overemphasized. This is the key factor in reducing mortality rates in malnourished populations. Medical care is of comparatively limited benefit until a minimum level of nutritional adequacy is established.

Reducing Mortality

Although each refugee health emergency will have special characteristics, Table 9-1 lists common categories of mortality encountered in refugee populations and the key interventions to limit them. These interventions can be

Table 9-1. Major Contributors to Death in Refugees in Underdeveloped Countries and Key Interventions to Limit Mortality

Disease	Key Interventions
Children	
Malnutrition	Adequate food supply Nutrition education Supplementary feeding Prevention of low birth weight with antenatal care and nutrition
Diarrheal disease	Oral rehydration therapy and continued feeding Improved nutrition Environmental sanitation Clean water in adequate quantities Measles immunization Promotion of breastfeeding Antibiotic therapy for dysentery
Acute respiratory infections	Improved nutrition Measles and pertussis immunizations Antibiotic therapy for pneumonia
Malaria	Therapy for malaria Prophylaxis, if high risk Environmental sanitation
Neonatal tetanus	Good umbilical cord care Tetanus immunization
Measles	Measles immunization
Tuberculosis	Case finding and treatment (of adults); BCG
Adults	
Tuberculosis	Case finding and treatment
Maternal death	Improved prenatal care, especially treatment of anemia Improved intraparum care and postpartum management of hemorrhage and sepsis
Acute bacterial infections	Antibiotic treatment

sustained by properly trained refugee health workers (see Chapter 4). Such training is often the only plausible way to deliver an appropriate mix of preventive and curative medical care to a large refugee population. Simple preventive and curative care, with minimal diagnostic aids, can be effective and will substantially reduce morbidity and mortality. Refugee health workers can be trained to deliver this care, thus multiplying many times the beneficial effects of health care. Clinicians often discover new skills as educators and program managers as they implement immunization, oral rehydration, antenatal, and other community-based programs that reach beyond the clinic to the entire population at risk.

It is within the context of a core of carefully selected interventions to reduce morbidity and mortality, that the clinician must gauge how elaborate the management of each disorder should be, without detracting from other life-saving work. When resources are limited, overly elaborate curative services often detract from public health interventions that are generally more effective in the overall reduction of suffering and death (see Table 9-2). To remain effective, programs must be well-supervised and adequately supplied with staff and equipment and with continued in-service training.

Conflicts do occur. Clinicians have been heard to sigh, "I guess I'm just curative," while program administrators despair that camp hospitals are thriving while children remain unimmunized and salvageable refugees languish in tents or huts.

Table 9-2. Introducing Programs in a New Refugee Camp: An Example

Phase of Program	Specific Programs Initiated
First phase	Clean water in adequate supply Sanitation Minimization of crowding Adequate shelter Immunization of children Adequate general ration with supplementary feeding Simplified clinical management of major causes of morbidity and mortality (emphasis on ORT, empiric protocols for management of pneumonia) Simple disease surveillance system Rapid management of disease outbreaks Health worker training Community involvement and education
Second phase	Antenatal program Traditional birth attendant training Tuberculosis case finding and treatment Referral system for hospital care Minor surgery Eye program

Setting the Level of Clinical Care

How far you should go with clinical care, after basic interventions are functioning well, depends on many factors. Answering the following questions may help to gauge what the level of clinical care should be in a particular refugee setting:

- Is the refugee camp temporary, or is it likely to become a long-term settlement?
- What level of care is available to the local national population?
- Is the host government willing to support refugee health care by providing national staff doctors, nurses, pharmacists, and sanitarians, or will long-term expatriate assistance be necessary until refugee health workers can be adequately trained?
- What is the time frame for private voluntary agencies, UNHCR, and government agencies to provide funding for health care in the refugee camp?
- What hospital care is available in the area for refugee referrals? Can this be augmented, or must secondary care be provided within the refugee camp itself?
- Can the clinical care being provided be taught to national or refugee staff? What level of care will continue after foreign health workers leave the area?

Simple, standardized treatment protocols are critical for effective health worker training programs. If expatriate medical personnel administer a technically advanced and expensive form of health care that cannot be sustained after their departure, health workers will have to be retrained and refugees may experience disappointment in the care they subsequently receive. Technologically advanced care can also create an uncomfortable discrepancy between services available to the national population and the refugee population and may lead to resentment, political difficulties, and attempts to divert resources (see Chapter 10 and 11). Local governments do not wish to see their own population suffer from inadequate food, water, and medical care while international interest and support are being delivered to the refugees. The enthusiasm and interests of agencies for the relief effort must be tempered by consideration for the local situation, particularly if refugees will be residents of the host country for a long time.

Sustainability is of key importance when deciding on the wisdom of an intervention, particulary after the acute emergency phase of operations. By seeing one's role as that of an educator and a clinician, and by anticipating one's own departure, it is easier to limit programs and approaches to those that may be sustainable. Although most refugee camps are set up as temporary facilities, many last for years after outside health teams have withdrawn. Whereas logistics may be the only limit to the resources available during an acute emergency, financial and staffing shortages may soon be felt as world attention turns to the next disaster.

Refugee camps provide clinicians with the necessity and the opportunity to learn to make do with less. For many clinical conditions, treatment will be limited to second-line drugs and few, or no, diagnostic aids. Drug formularies that are limited to only the essential drugs should be respected and used whenever possible. Essential drug programs have much to offer underdeveloped countries that cannot afford to buy large amounts of diversified drugs or train health workers in their use.

Often, nursing care will consist of what can

be taught to paraprofessional workers or family members. Many seriously ill patients who could be saved with more intensive medical facilities or in a modern hospital will die. This situation haunts some clinicians. However, it sometimes makes sense to do less for a single moribund patient if a less complicated intervention will free resources to save more lives. These can be very difficult personal and professional experiences for clinicians who have been trained to do the maximum for every individual who comes to them for care. Referral of cases with life-threatening illness to a national hospital may be possible. This approach is usually superior to establishing special hospitals for refugees that consume immense resources and are rarely sustained after expatriate help is withdrawn. Where feasible, supplies and trained personnel can be assigned to a regional hospital if its use for refugee referral care is permitted.

Too often, medical staff are polarized and decision making is impaired by strong disagreements on issues such as preventive versus curative, the epidemiologic approach versus clinical intervention, hospitals versus primary health care, and so on. Usually, both approaches in question are necessary to varying degrees. After immunization, many of the most effective primary health care interventions are, in fact, curative. Good sanitation, clean water, breastfeeding, proper weaning, and safe food preparation can prevent many episodes of diarrhea, but the major breakthrough in reducing mortality from diarrheal diseases is oral rehydration therapy which, technically, is curative. Readily available antimalarial drugs can minimize mortality from malaria. Antibiotic treatment based on simple empiric protocols can save the lives of many children and adults with pneumonia. Finding, and curing, active tuberculosis cases is the only effective way to prevent infection. Although antenatal preventive measures can reduce anemia, and training can prepare birth attendants to help control postpartum hemorrhage, many maternal deaths from hemorrhage cannot be averted without hospital obstetric backup for primary health care services (Rosenfield & Maine 1985).

THE PRIMARY HEALTH CARE MOVEMENT AND REFUGEE MEDICAL CARE

Many health workers in poor or underdeveloped countries see their work as part of the worldwide movement for "Health for All by the Year 2000." Current approaches to primary health care have followed an increasing awareness of the failure of hospital-based medicine (often concentrated in capital cities) to benefit the majority of the population in underdeveloped countries, particularly in rural areas. At the International Conference on Primary Health Care at Alma-Ata in 1978 (sponsored by WHO and UNICEF), essential elements of primary health care were identified as follows:

> Primary health care is essential health care made universally accessible to individuals and families in the community by means acceptable to them, through their full participation, and at a cost that the community and country can afford. It forms an integral part both of the country's health system, of which it is the nucleus, and the overall social and economic development of the community.
>
> Primary health care addresses the main health problems in the community providing preventive, curative, and rehabilitative services accordingly. Since these services reflect and evolve from the economic conditions and social values of the country and its communities, they will vary by country and community but will include at least: promotion of proper nutrition and an adequate supply of safe water; basic sanitation; maternal and child care, including family planning; immunization against the major infectious diseases; prevention and control of locally endemic diseases; education concerning health problems and methods of preventing and controlling them; and appropriate treatment for common diseases and injuries (WHO & UNICEF 1978).

The relevance of a primary health care approach in the care of refugees has been advocated for several years (UNHCR 1982; Simmonds et al 1983, 1985) based on its successful use in Somalia, Angola, Zaire, Ethiopia, and other refugee camp settings. Often, it is the only feasible way for a small professional medical staff to care for large refugee populations.

> The health services provided to the refugees should be based on the concept of primary health care. . . . The refugees must be given responsibility for their own health. Outside health workers must understand the refugees' own concepts of health and disease. From the beginning, services should be developed and operated with, rather than for, the refugees. If not, the services will be less effective, may be distrusted by the refugees, and are likely to collapse when key outside personnel leave. . . . Strong emphasis should be placed on the training and upgrading of medical skills of selected refugees. . . . Even refugees with no prior experience can be very effective health workers following basic on-the-spot instruction in a few relevant tasks (UNHCR 1982).

Clinicians, particularly those trained in internal medicine, may be struck by the lack of emphasis on adult health within many primary health care programs (with the exception of maternal care). The mother and child orientation is firmly established in the child survival orientation of many of the private, government, and multinational agencies involved in refugee health care. This prior definition of health priorities by assistance agencies sometimes conflicts with a family's or community's own priorities for health care.

REFUGEE HEALTH CARE IN SOMALIA

Refugee health care in Somalia provides a good example of interventions that were purposefully gauged to those deemed appropriate for the Somali people and that could be sustained by the national health staff after outside agencies departed. Early in the relief effort, the policy of the Refugee Health Unit (RHU), within the Ministry of Health, was to turn the refugee crisis into an asset for Somalia by instituting a system of primary health care that could be transferred to the national population. Working in a setting generally lacking in trained medical personnel, material resources, and logistical support, reliance on simple care delivered by community health workers and traditional birth attendants proved sensible. Subsequently, the formulary of essential drugs and guidelines for medical care (RHU 1983) have been, in large part, transferred to primary health care programs for the national population. Training has been shared with the national programs by the transfer of experienced nurses and doctors to regional primary health care programs where many work on district primary health care teams supervising village health workers or as regional primary health care coordinators or central staff. The refugee camps have been used as a setting to train nurses and midwives from the national programs.

Setting health care priorities in this way often caused conflict between the RHU and foreign relief agencies that wanted to "do their own thing" and provide whatever level and form of care they felt necessary. Many health workers had worked in Thailand, where more elaborate curative services were offered in field hospitals within the refugee camps. If these groups had been allowed to continue without guidelines, the national staff and refugee health workers would have been trained in methods, and with supplies, that could not have been continued after the agencies handed operations over to the national staff. Instead, Somalia has been left with a functioning primary health care system that can be sustained without foreign health teams. Almost 3000 community health workers and traditional birth attendants are now supervised by national staff doctors and nurses in 39 camps. In addition, the Ministry of Health has been strengthened in its ability to administer an effective primary health care program.

The RHU in Somalia is unique in the guidance and coordination provided from within the Ministry of Health to international agencies and the degree of government contribution to the medical care of the refugees. Although this government contribution may not be duplicated in countries where the refugee population is ethnically distinct from the host-country population, the processes of setting health care priorities to address prevalent health problems and providing a level of health care that can be sustained should be ongoing in refugee health care.

REFERENCES AND SELECTED READING

Bossert TJ, Parker DA: The political and administrative context of primary health care in the third world. Soc Sci Med 1984;18:693–702.

Joseph SC, Russell SS: Is primary care the wave of the future? Soc Sci Med 1980;14C:137–44.

Refugee Health Unit, Somali Ministry of Health: Guidelines for Health Care in Refugee Camps. London, OXFAM, 1983.

Rosenfield A, Maine D: Maternal mortality—A neglected tragedy? Lancet 1985;1:83–85.

Simmonds SP et al: Refugee Community Health Care. Oxford, Oxford University Press, 1983.

Simmonds SP et al: Training refugees for primary health care. World Health Forum 1985;6:235–36.

United Nations High Commissioner for Refugees: Handbook for Emergencies. Part I: Field Operations. United Nations High Commissioner for Refugees, Geneva, 1982.

World Health Organization and UNICEF: Primary Health Care. Geneva, World Health Organization, 1978.

10
Economic and Political Considerations Relevant to Refugee Health Care

BARRY N. STEIN

Refugee problems are caused by political factors often exacerbated by economic factors. The response to a refugee crisis will be affected by political and economic considerations that may limit or enhance the assistance given to the refugees. Although humanitarian concerns play a large role in the reaction to a refugee emergency, the role of political factors will always be significant and often dominant. In this chapter, we will examine how several of these factors influence refugee health care.

ECONOMIC CONSIDERATIONS

The countries of origin, and of refuge, for most refugees are poor or underdeveloped—often the poorest of the poor. The international community does not have to respond to refugee flows or disasters in North America or Europe because those industrial societies can shoulder their own burdens. The situations that concern the international community are mostly in the Third, and even in the Fourth, Worlds ("Third World" is the term commonly used to refer to the underdeveloped economies of Africa, Asia, and Latin America; the "Fourth World" is a world of exceptional poverty within parts of the Third World).

The World Bank lists 35 countries that have low-income economies in which per capita income is $400 (U.S. dollars) or less per year. Twenty four of these 35 poorest countries are currently, or were recently, involved with refugees as host countries, source countries, or both. Virtually all of the major refugee flows are in the Fourth World, with refugee camps typically located on the periphery of the host country in regions that are disadvantaged in transportation, economic development, and services.

In Fourth World circumstances, any aid, despite its humanitarian or life-saving purpose, can create immediate disparities between two groups of poor people—the refugees and the local poor. The mandate and motivation of many aid agencies and volunteers is focused on refugees. As a result, the status of refugees compared with many of the equally poor hosts can be a course of great tension and resentment. These economic factors can be easily transformed into political constraints on health care when a host government sets limits on the level (often that available to the local poor) and visibility of refugee health care; insists that access be equal for refugees and local nationals; or requires the creation of separate, equivalent programs for their citizens.

MANAGEMENT IN REFUGEE CAMPS

The number of potential participants in a refugee emergency is staggering. Among the first to arrive are the private voluntary agencies, some of which already have ongoing programs in the host country. As numerous agencies converge, obvious problems arise in establishing which needs should be served by which agencies, in providing logistical support, and in communication between voluntary and government agencies. The member agencies of the International Red Cross, including the International Committee of the Red Cross (ICRC) and the League of Red Cross Societies (LRCS), are usually involved. United Nations (UN) agencies usually present include the United Nations High Commissioner for Refugees (UNHCR), World Food Program (WFP), Food and Agriculture Organization (FAO), United Nations Disaster Relief Organization (UNDRO), World Health Organization (WHO), and the United Nations Children's Fund (UNICEF). Each of these organizations has its own guidelines for program implementation, but few provide for multiagency planning and program integration in the field. Added to this bureaucratic maze are a variety of bilateral donor countries (primarily North American and West European countries) that may have many agencies within their own governmental structure to assist in disaster and refugee situations. Finally, the sovereign host governments ultimately set the stage for receiving assistance and establish the ground rules for all international aid.

As a sovereign country, the host government has the authority to determine the rules under which assistance will be given to the refugees. It is exceptionally difficult for international agencies and bilateral donors to take any action against the expressed wishes of a host. In 1979 it took months of negotiation and requests before agencies such as UNICEF, OXFAM, and ICRC received permission to visit Cambodia, and ten months elapsed before an aid program could begin. Once programs begin, they may be neglected by the host government, strictly controlled, or subjected to shifting and conflicting policies. Many host governments are not experienced with emergency programs and change their policies as the crisis evolves.

The mix of agencies involved in a refugee crisis will change as the crisis develops. Some agencies, such as ICRC, are mandated to act in the early stages of a crisis but consider leaving as the situation continues and achieves some stability. Other agencies are slower to arrive in the field but are more likely to remain for the duration.

Two prominent actors in refugee emergency situations are UNHCR and ICRC. Though both are based in Geneva, Switzerland, UNHCR is an international organization within the UN system whereas ICRC is a Swiss organization with the International Red Cross movement. Both have grown considerably over the past two decades as a result of their involvement in Third World crises. They often cooperate but their different mandates sometimes allow one to operate in situations where the other might be restricted. UNHCR's mandate, as modified over the years, is to work with refugees or those in a refugeelike situation. In most cases, this limits UNHCR to working outside of the refugees' country of origin except in cases that involve voluntary repatriation. Thus, the UNHCR is not a primary actor in cases of civil or internal strife such as in Lebanon, Ethiopia, Cambodia, or El Salvador. ICRC's mandate includes the protection of civilians in wartime, allowing action in such cases. Both organizations are limited by the requirement to gain the assent of a host government before they can set up operations. The Red Cross, however, has a broad right of initiative and several times has been able to take action in places where "the authorities had refrained from requesting aid from any other organization" (ICRC and LRCS 1981).

UNHCR operates through a central office in Geneva, which is divided into regional bureaus and has branch offices in many parts of the world. UNHCR considers itself an operational agency but generally subcontracts actual operations to other international organizations, governmental units, and voluntary agencies. Although UNHCR ideally should coordinate the programs of its partners as well as those of other agencies involved in a crisis, its effectiveness in this area has been the subject of much criticism in recent years. This criticism is sometimes unwarranted because expectations regarding UNHCR's authority are often not matched by a delegation of responsibility from the host government to UNHCR. In other situations, however, a lack of assertiveness and a hesitant, overly cautious approach have left UNHCR unprepared and unable to coordinate effectively (Shawcross 1980). In response to these criticisms, UNHCR established an emergency unit and training programs in emergency management.

ICRC also operates from a central office in Geneva but does not have a system of permanent branch offices through out the world. ICRC employs a system that sends delegates to refugee situations and works closely with other units of the International Red Cross movement, particularly the League of Red Cross Societies and its constituent national societies.

POLITICAL CONSIDERATIONS

There is no simple way to describe the interplay of political factors and assistance that affect the refugee situation. The possible responses range from a sympathetic embrace of the refugees and their cause to sympathy with their persecutors and even participation in their persecution. For example, refugees such as the Afghans in Pakistan are welcomed as coreligionists and ethnic kin, whereas the Salvadorans in Honduras are viewed as the enemy and have been attacked by the Honduran military. Even more complex is the situation of Palestinian refugees whose cause has been endorsed and supported by Arab governments, but whose camps have been attacked by those very governments.

A major complication arises when refugee camps are used, or suspected of being used, to support a guerrilla movement as a training base, a source of recruits, or a locale for rest and recuperation. Refugee camps may be used as guerrilla bases either with or without the assent of the host country. In either case, however, consequences can be serious.

During the 1960s, invasions by Tutsi refugees trying to retake control of Rwanda brought several host governments close to conflict with that country. In response, the Organization of African Unity resolved that refugee camps ought to be moved away from the border of refugees' homeland as soon as possible. In more recent years, attacks on refugee camps have affected the national territories and military forces of many host countries including Thailand, Mexico, Pakistan, Angola, Somalia, and countries in the Middle East. Attempts to segregate civilian refugee encampments from warrior camps, and to protect innocent camps, have been notably unsuccessful.

Politics of Funding Relief Efforts

Virtually all funding of refugee relief efforts is voluntary. Although funds are available for relief in national budgets and in reserve in international organizations, the allocation of those funds to a particular emergency remains voluntary. Typically, international organizations such as UNHCR, WFP, WHO, and UNICEF have an emergency reserve to permit immediate action in a crisis. If the situation is widespread or drawn out, however, it becomes necessary to turn to donor nations, usually by means of a pledging conference, to acquire the funds needed to continue relief efforts.

Continuation of funding for a relief program is never certain. One hotly debated issue in refugee assistance is whether aid itself has a "magnet effect," which increases the number of refugees by attracting those seeking material or service benefits rather than those fleeing from persecution or catastrophe. The actual existence of a magnet effect has not been proven, but concern about its existence influences policy.

Politics plays a significant role in whether a crisis is ignored or highlighted. The recent famine in Ethiopia was well-known but world attention was scant because of a deliberate downplaying of the situation by the Ethiopian government. Further, Western governments were reluctant to spotlight a situation that would create a need to assist an unfriendly government. With the relief effort, it has been argued that aid has been used as a weapon in Ethiopia's civil strife and that the government's failure to respond to the famine is evidence of the failure of its revolutionary values. This is reminiscent of the situation in Cambodia in 1979, when the Vietnamese-controlled Cambodians delayed the start of famine relief for political reasons. Shawcross (1980) observed, "The Phnom Penh government was extremely reluctant to allow any food to be pushed across the border at first because that is where the Khmer Rouge had their installations. Last summer the Khmer Rouge had been pretty well defeated. . . . Now, because of the international food aid across the border, they are rejuvenated."

Voluntary agencies attempting to steer a humanitarian course through the obstacles of civil strife, refugee warrior communities, and major power involvement can have great difficulties in establishing and operating programs. Host governments or source governments such as Burundi, Ethiopia, or Cambodia may insist that aid be restricted geographically or be provided only to certain friendly parties rather than be distributed to all who are ready.

VOLUNTARY AGENCY FUNDING AND OPERATIONS

Voluntary agencies probably have a better record of maintaining a consistent interest in humanitarian assistance than governmental and international agencies. In many relief situations, voluntary agencies are the first to arrive, partly because they may already be present to carry out development or missionary programs, and because they generally respond to human suffering regardless of the political cause. Several features of voluntary agency response can affect operations in the field. These features include a lack of analysis and evaluation, a resistance to criticism, and fund-raising constraints.

Voluntary agencies devote little time or effort to analysis and evaluation of concluded efforts. The emphasis is on meeting the next emergency rather than learning from the past. "As a result, mistakes are repeated again and again from one disaster to another" (Shawcross 1984).

In part, this failure to learn comes from a basic orientation common to humanitarian assistance that "because a program has good intentions, it will necessarily have good results"

(Taylor & Cuny 1979). Many volunteers reflect this attitude in their resistance to direction and coordination; they believe that because they are doing something good they can behave as they wish (Naponick 1980).

Although voluntary agencies can respond quickly to emergencies, they are unable to remain in the field for long periods unless they engage in fund raising. To stir public interest in a crisis, most agencies reinforce stereotypes rather than engage in education. The focus in most appeals is on sick and starving children and the need for food. Naponick (1980) observed, "You all want something that is visible . . . your own building with one of your workers pictured outside holding a starving child. It is easier to raise funds to feed children than to do sanitation work." Agencies seek to promote an image of efficiency and low overhead and stress that donations are converted into food rather than going to bureaucratic expenses.

Fund-raising methods have an impact on how money is spent in the field. Agencies that feel they have made promises in the course of fund raising may earmark contributions for certain purposes such as refugee children and food and medical programs. In this context, providing care to poor members of the host population or working on low-visibility, low-glamour projects such as water supplies and sanitation (which are often highly cost-effective means of saving lives) may be seen as beyond an agency's mandate.

REFUGEE PARTICIPATION

A constant theme in refugee literature is the need for refugee participation in the design and operation of programs for their benefit. UNHCR's *Handbook for Emergencies* (1982) states that "refugees must be given responsibility for their own health and therefore be directly involved on the development and provision of health services." Perhaps nowhere else in the field of refugee assistance is there a greater gap between theory and practice.

Host government authorities tend to be notably reluctant to allow aliens, who are often unwelcome guests, to share in the decision making and operations of refugee camps and settlements. Further, faced with this reluctance, many assistance agencies who believe in refugee participation fail to promote the idea strongly.

Relations between refugees and camp administrators are often tense and even hostile. Host-country personnel are not always of the highest caliber because relief work is outside of normal career lines, usually in remote areas with few amenities. Low priority is placed on directing competent administrators to what are essentially regarded as ephemeral refugee settlements. Instead, "surplus" personnel or individuals not considered sufficiently competent to operate in other branches of the civil service are sent (Rogge 1985). Such personnel often have a strong desire to control refugees and a need to regiment activities and aid distribution. Over the years, along with many stories of hospitality and generosity, there have been endless stories of problems and abuse. In Tanzania, Gasarasi (1984) noted that, "The spirit of the Refugee Control Act [of 1965] has predominantly been a disciplining one. As a result, it has in most cases produced authoritarian settlement commandants who have often developed antagonistic relations with the refugees. Cases abound where refugees of various settlements have lodged complaints about frequent ill-treatment by these settlement authorities."

The situation is not one-sided, however. Refugees can be unrealistic and demanding regarding aid. Rogge (1985) reported a situation in the Sudan in which refugees refused to clear land because they were under the impression that refugees were not supposed to work and that their status as refugees gave them the right to be maintained as long as they were refugees. Refugees often focus on their own suffering and demand that something be done for them. They are suspicious of requests for proof of suffering before aid is provided. Refugees who are assured of full rations may see little reason to participate in maintenance or self-help activities to improve the camp. They may see themselves as disadvantaged victims being used for the benefit of the host country. For its part, the host often sees the refugees as ungrateful, spoon-fed, passively dependent, unproductive, and demanding.

VULNERABLE REFUGEES

The population structure of a refugee camp will vary greatly depending on the conditions under which it was established. Some refugee flows are a mass exodus in which whole families or villages flee together; others consist of a sizable, but steady, flow over many months or longer; in other cases, refugees may trickle out with occasional episodic spurts. Thus, some camps will be able to replicate social structures fairly quickly, whereas others will be so highly fragmented that replication is not really possible.

Not all refugees go to camps. It is common for refugees to adopt a family-splitting strategy whereby stronger family members manage on their own outside of the camp while weaker members are left to be fed and cared for by assistance agencies (Harrell-Bond 1985). An abnormally high proportion of widows, children, the sick, the physically disabled, and the malnourished may be present. A survey in the Sudan concluded that one third of the refugees in Suki camp were classifiable as "vulnerable" (Chambers 1985). Christensen (1982), reporting on refugee camps in Somalia and later in Pakistan (Christensen 1983, 1984), found that the refugee camp population was highly stratified in terms of access to food. Three categories were distinguished: a group of 10 to 15 percent made up primarily of leaders (section leaders, deputies, village headmen, maliks) and their followers who had a surplus of food; a second group of some 70 percent who had sufficient food; and, at the bottom, a group of 10 to 15 percent composed of the disadvantaged and vulnerable refugees, as well as those on bad terms with the refugee leaders, who had little or no food. The percentages for each group varied from refugee situation to situation and from camp to camp, but the structure of the groupings was relatively constant.

Where refugees are involved in a guerrilla struggle, few able-bodied men may be present. Occasionally, such as on the Thailand-Cambodia border, camps may be controlled by a "liberation" movement. There may be periods of fighting and of forced recruitment of young men. In such situations, the presence of international personnel can have a substantial deterrent and protective effect.

CONCLUSION

Health care in refugee camps takes place in a highly charged political and economic environment. It requires sensitivity to the economic and political needs of the host country, as well as an overriding concern for those who are vulnerable among the refugees and the host population.

REFERENCES

Chambers R: Hidden losers? The impact of rural refugees and refugee programs on the poorer of their hosts. Intern Migration Rev 1986; 20:245–63.

Christensen H: Afghan Refugees in Pakistan: From Emergency Towards Self-Reliance: A Report on the Food Relief Situation and Related Socioeconomic Aspects. Geneva, UN Research Institute for Social Development Report No 84.2, 1984.

Christensen H: Survival Strategies for and by Camp Refugees: Report on a Six Week Exploratory Sociological Field Study into the Food Situation of Refugees in Camps in Somalia. Geneva, UN Research Institute for Social Development Report No 82.3, 1982.

Christensen H: Sustaining Afghan Refugees in Pakistan: Report on the Food Situation and Related Social Aspects. Geneva, UN Research Institute for Social Development Report No 83.3, 1983.

Gasarasi CP: The Tripartite Approach to the Resettlement and Integration of Rural Refugees in Tanzania. Uppsala, Scandinavian Institute of African Studies Report No 71, 1984.

Harrell-Bond B: Imposing Aid: Emergency Assistance to Refugees. Oxford, Oxford University Press, 1985.

Naponick J: Frustration and progress in coordination. In Cambodian Refugee Relief: Lessons Learned and Future Directions, Washington DC, National Council for International Health Workshop Proceedings, 1980.

Rogge JR: Too Many, Too Long: Sudan's 20 Year Refugee Dilemma. Totowa, Rowman & Allanheld, 1985.

Shawcross W: Politics of the relief effort. In Cambodian Refugee Relief: Lessons Learned and Future Directions, Washington DC, National Council for International Health Workshop Proceedings, 1980.

Shawcross W: The Quality of Mercy: Cambodia, Holocaust and Modern Conscience. New York, Simon & Schuster, 1984.

Taylor A, Cuny F: The evaluation of humanitarian assistance. Disasters 1979;3(1).

United Nations High Commissioner for Refugees: Handbook for Emergencies: Part I: Field Operations. Geneva, United Nations High Commissioner for Refugees, 1982.

11

Customs, Culture, and Religion in Refugee Health Care

WOLFGANG F. BULLE

This chapter is intended as a brief guide for health professionals who are assigned on short notice to a country with different customs, manners, and cultural values. With a sense of curiosity, a good bit of patience, a sense of humor, a nonjudgmental attitude, and a willingness to adjust to different ways of life and work, one can function effectively.

To appreciate and participate effectively in a new culture, health workers must accept three important guidelines: (1) that they are both foreigners and guests; (2) that they must leave behind "cultural" baggage—their own way of looking at things, of thinking, of behaving, and of communicating; and (3) that they must learn how to identify, and then to conform with, the norms that people in the host country have established for their interpersonal conduct.

There is one special word of advice for those who work with refugees or victims of major disasters. For people whose means of existence has been lost or put in jeopardy, traditional values and cultural norms take on special importance; their observance and nurture are possibly the only remaining means for hope to be grasped as a viable alternative to prevailing despair. Recognizing this and giving informed, active support to maintaining and strengthening time-honored customs is likely to go far toward helping to restore dignity and self-respect and to ensuring the active participation of the refugee population in relief measures.

CUSTOMS AND MANNERS

A few samples of general rules of conduct observed in most Asian and African countries might alert you to common customs and social proscriptions:

- Give, receive, and touch things only with your right hand, especially in countries where people eat with their fingers.
- Among Buddhists, and in many other cultures, the head is considered the seat of the soul and the feet, the lowliest and dirtiest part of the body. Do not pat even the smallest child on his head. When seated in a chair, plant your soles firmly on the floor and keep them there. Do not cross your legs, and do not point your feet, especially not the soles, at another person.
- Do not praise the beauty of small children. Fear of the jealousy of the gods or "the evil eye" is not limited to Asia and Africa, but persists to this day among some rural communities in Europe.
- For a similar reason, step across, not on, the threshold of a home, shrine, temple, or mosque. The threshold is the protective barrier against evil forces. It might be guarded by a friendly spirit, special blessings, or an embedded verse from the Koran.
- Particularly in the Middle East and Latin American countries, but also in parts of Asia, be careful about expressing your admiration of an adornment or piece of art to avoid the embarrassment of having it presented to you as a gift.
- In lodging, transportation, and personal attire, it is advantageous to be inconspicuous as well as practical. Dress should be as formal as, but more modest than, that customarily worn by local officials. Safari suits, bush coats, or short-sleeved shirts have become common work attire. Women may find long skirts or dresses preferable to trousers. Shorts are unacceptable for women and, with few exceptions, are reminders of colonial days if worn by men. Mimicry of native dress looks ridiculous and should be avoided. Women should be aware that in Islamic countries, shoulders and

Excerpted from *Changing Cultures? Some Suggestions to Smooth the Way,* a document prepared by Dr. Bulle for CDC's International Health Program Office (Crisis Response Activity).

legs should be covered. Trousers for women are not commonly acceptable and, depending on the country, a scarf might be required to cover the head.

COMMUNICATION

Language

If you speak only English, Spanish, or French, you can survive. Knowledge of the local language, however, will broaden the scope of your activities and perceptions immeasurably. The first step should be to delineate clearly for one's self the restrictions imposed by a language barrier; the next step should be to set priorities on how to deal with the limitations. Body language, nonverbal signals, and recognition of social and cultural values are of greater importance than the ability to communicate verbally. However, it will make a great deal of difference in your interpersonal relationships if you have even a rudimentary vocabulary; the ability to ask a few basic questions, especially greeting and thanking people; and the ability to offer a personal apology for having to use an interpreter. People invariably respond very positively to attempts to speak their language, and you can be certain that nobody will laugh at your imperfections. In addition to creating better relationships, study of the local language can provide fascinating insights into the culture and help in understanding the people.

Interpreters

Dependence on an interpreter is a tedious and, occasionally, difficult job that demands persistence and patience. It is essential to find a person who is able to interpret meaning as well as words. It is also important to establish a rapport between you and your interpreter, you and your audience, and your interpreter and your audience. Winfield (1962) has specified four simple rules for effective use of an interpreter:

- Talk slowly and have each sentence or paragraph interpreted.
- Use simple vocabulary. Replace three- and four-syllable words with shorter, more common ones.
- Maintain a simple, clear sentence structure.
- Stay psychologically on the job while the interpreter is speaking. Do not cut yourself out of the communication circuit by showing lack of interest while the interpreter speaks.

It is essential that you and your interpreter function as a team. A relationship must be established prior to any joint appearance at a meeting, public address, or public health assessment. It is important for the interpreter to know in advance the essence of what is to be discussed or transmitted. At meetings with officials, even if they speak English, it is important to have someone along who is familiar with cultural connotations, nuance, and idioms. Encourage the interpreter to interject explanations or clarification of terms when necessary. Thank your interpreter in private for his or her assistance and to elicit feedback as to what you might be able to do to make future presentations or meetings more effective. Another important function of a competent interpreter is described by Gudykunst and Kim (1964):

> In cultures where a third person role is customary (e.g., in Thailand, business transactions between two persons are frequently conducted indirectly by means of a go-between), the interpreter's role may become a very active one, to the consternation of the American who is likely to interpret it as inefficiency or perhaps disloyalty.

In rural areas, it might be best to avoid using a college graduate or a person from the capital to interpret; depend instead on a local teacher or some other English-, French-, or Spanish-speaking person who is known by the people and familiar with local dialects and customs. The following illustrates the point:

> A foreign nurse working at a rural clinic in Africa is told by her interpreter that a pediatric patient is suffering from chronic constipation. As the child is obviously dehydrated, she inquires about details and is finally told; "Well, he defecates at least 10 times a day and it's all bloody." Problem: The interpreter came from an area with a different dialect and in the local language, the terms use for diarrhea and constipation could be differentiated only by a slight tonal inflection.

At times, at least until one gets to know a local official or academician personally, it might not be a bad idea to address him one degree above the one he holds. The term "Your Excellency" is usually reserved for heads of state, ambassadors, and generals. A corporal will be delighted to be addressed at least as sergeant, a captain as colonel, physicians in teaching hospitals as professor. It may be even more important never to omit the prefix Mr., Mrs., or Miss when addressing less sophisticated individuals. In French-speaking countries, address all women as *"mademoiselle,"* never as *"mam'selle,"* and only older women as *"madame."* In turn, do not embarrass servants or waiters with the Americanisms, "Yes, sir" or "No, Ma'am."

One should not be too quick to use first names. The offer cannot be refused, but Europeans and many Africans find it awkward; and for Latins and Asians, it is impossible to deal with.

Greetings

In most societies, greetings between co-workers, acquaintances and friends, and greetings when introduced to officials, are a much more important part of interpersonal communication than is customary in the United States. "Observe and do likewise" is a good rule to follow. One is well advised to take time for exchange of a few pleasantries. The common, hurried American greetings (e.g., "hi," "see you," or "how are you?") without waiting for or expecting a response may be misunderstood as lack of sincerity. Except among many Asian societies where physical contact is avoided, shaking hands is a custom to which you will have to become accustomed. Unless advised differently, the following forms of greeting are suggested:

- In countries in which hand shaking is customary, on entering a home, shake hands, even with persons you may have seen only a few hours earlier.
- Upon entering an office or a place where a social or business gathering that includes up to 15 persons is taking place, shake hands with everyone present.
- In larger groups, it is customary to stop at each small group and shake hands with each person present.
- To offer a general greeting and begin a conversation with one or two persons and ignore the rest is considered bad manners.
- When leaving, the same round of handshakes is expected, rather than just expressing your thanks to the host and quietly taking your departure, as is customary in the United States.

Nonverbal Communication

As mentioned earlier, even a limited knowledge of the local language will be extremely helpful. Of equal importance is an appreciation of nonverbal cues that may convey even more than spoken words. This includes facial expressions, body distance, eye contact, hand gestures, body posture, head movements, and the like. There is no need to copy everything you see, but to avoid miscommunication and unintended offense, it is important to learn what such gestures communicate.

A Peace Corps training notebook on Ghana explains the meaning of 61 different gestures. They range from scratching one's throat (i.e., "I want a bribe") to the left index finger pointed down in traffic (i.e., "Police check ahead"). It would be futile to try to become familiar with all such gestures, but it is important to know of their existence and to keep asking questions about their significance. It is essential, however, for a newcomer to control hand and body movements until he or she has made sure that they do not connotate a meaning different from what is intended. It is both instructive and amusing to watch how nationals interact in support or contradiction of what is being said aloud. Below are a few examples:

- In most countries of the Middle East, keeping eye contact during a discussion is a sign of sincerity, while the cocktail party "wandering eye" of many Americans is considered rude. On the other hand, in Africa and many Oriental cultures, lowered eyes indicate an attitude of respect.
- In many parts of the world, a nodding head does not indicate concurrence, but shaking one's head from side to side does.
- A women should not be surprised about catcalls, or worse, if she waits at a bus stop with her hands on her hips. In many countries that posture means just one thing.
- In Europe, if one tries to order a beer in a noisy resturant by raising an index finger to indicate "one," the waiter will probably bring two. When counting on the fingers, "one" is generally indicated by the thumb. In many countries, the American finger count for "two" (first and second fingers in a V-shape) may be offensive and should be avoided.
- American men frequently appear at a loss for what to do with their hands so tend to put them in their pockets. While abroad, do not. In the presence of women or a senior official, hands in pockets may be considered, at best, boorish conduct, or a sign of defiance or personal insecurity.
- Frequently, laughter is not a sign of fun but evidence of embarrassment or physical pain.

This list could be extended *ad infinitum* with illustrations of tragic-comic misunderstandings, but it should be remembered that nonverbal communication plays a major role in cross-cultural understanding, and one should pursue local significance with perpetual curiosity and be prepared for surprises.

RELIGION AND HEALTH CARE

In contrast to the materialistic worldview of industrialized societies, religious faith and belief in supernatural forces continue to dominate the individual and communal lives of most peoples in the developing world. Interaction with people confronted by existential threats calls for at least a basic comprehension of their life philosophy. Such understanding is essential for strengthening indigenous self-help efforts, for establishing effective relief actions in accordance with local value systems, and for facilitating local acceptance of public health measures.

In 1971, Fred Cuny of INTERTECT was involved in establishing settlements for refugees from East Pakistan (now Bangladesh) in India. Latrines were a major sanitation problem, especially getting people to use them. Designs were constantly upgraded to make the latrines usable, safe, and clean. A model was finally developed that seemed to work, but relief workers were perplexed when, in one camp where they had built a battery of toilets, only those on one side were used. After some investigation, it was learned that the unused latrines were facing West—in the direction of Mecca—and therefore the Muslim refugees refused to use them. During that same refugee assistance effort, in another location, a similar situation was encountered in a Hindu camp. In that case, the unused toilets were facing a sacred banyan tree.

Traditional Religions

Geographic distribution of traditional religions far exceeds the population groups officially identified as adherents of traditional beliefs; even among devout converts to Islam or Christianity, many traditional practices and superstitions are retained for generations. Evil spirits, for example, continue to be thought the chief cause of illness, not only in Africa but also throughout the Muslim world.

When disaster or war force people to leave their ancestral homes, traditional religious rites, seemingly long forgotten, may regain prominence; and religious leaders are likely to reassume positions of unchallenged authority.

In Africa, there exists a common belief in a distant supreme god and creator who is called Faro by the Bambaras, Chuku by the Ibos, Ngai by the Kikuyus, or Nkulunkulu by the Zulus. This supreme deity is not directly accessible. Sacrifices are not generally offered to him but, in extreme circumstances, prayers are directed to him. There is recourse in daily affairs, however, to secondary gods and to the spirits of departed ancestors who, being spirits, are closer to the gods and able to intercede with them.

The basis of African religious values is the concept of the unity of life and time. Past, present, and future blend harmoniously, and there is no clear distinction between animate and inanimate, natural and supernatural, conscious and unconscious. Essential to this view of the world is the belief that there is continuous communication between the dead, the living, and those yet to be born. To Africans, ancestral spirits are ever present in human affairs and they are looked on as the guardians of the established order (Lambo 1978). Religious practices are primarily concerned with maintaining harmony with nature and within society, in good harvests, progeny, and social stability. The dignity of the individual, valued above all else, can be realized only in relationship and solidarity with family, clan, and ethnic group. Initiation of adolescents into the community of men is another characteristic of group solidarity. Many of the myths of traditional religion, the magic arts, and soothsaying, are based on natural forces. These beliefs are deeply ingrained and are rarely, as mentioned, totally replaced by conversion to Islam or Christianity.

Hinduism

A religion having evolved during the last 5000 years, Hinduism (Woodward 1984, 1985) emphasizes *dharma* (good works and obedience to the laws and customs of caste) and its resulting ritual, mystical contemplation, and ascetic practices. The geographic distribution of Hinduism includes India, Nepal, Bhutan, Sri Lanka, Indonesia, Bali, Malaysia, Mauritius, Fiji, and other countries of Indian immigration.

Hinduism contains a wide range of diverse cults, doctrines, and philosophical and religious systems. Religious rituals represent an important part of daily life from cleansing of the body and prayers, to home sacrifices, to the special ceremonies governing births, marriages, and deaths. The strongest unifying force in Hinduism is its holy writings: the *Vedas* (ca. 1200 B.C.), the *Upanishads* (ca. 800 B.C.), and the *Bhagavad-Gita* (ca. 300 B.C.), often referred to as the gospel of Hinduism. The core of Hindu belief is the conviction that the world and everything in it are subject to an eternal process of change. One of the three paths of liberation is the way of knowledge through the discipline of yoga, the complete purification and unification of mind, body, and spirit. The second path is devotion to the gods, represented primarily by Vishnu, Shiva, Kali, and Krishna. The third and most difficult path is good works and obedience to the laws and customs of one's caste.

The caste system is deeply rooted in religion, tradition, and ancient history. The hope of the lower-caste Hindus is to be reborn into a higher caste in the next life. The ultimate goal is to escape *samsara,* the wheel of rebirth, altogether and achieve the bliss of eternal absorption into Brahma, the ultimate ground of all being. In the face of disaster, the passive acceptance of suffering as inevitable *karma* (fate, laws governing the cycle of rebirth) by some high-caste officials can be very irritating to Western relief workers. It helps to recognize the attitude for what it represents and to be aware that Indians know how to deal with this attitude and can be trusted to work their way around such individuals.

Buddhism

In brief, Buddhism is a world-denying religion which holds that suffering is inherent in life and one can be liberated from it by mental and moral self-purification. Buddhism is predominant in Burma, Thailand, Laos, Kampuchea, Vietnam, Nepal, India, Bhutan, Sikkim, Sri Lanka, and other parts of central and eastern Asia.

Buddhism grew out of the life and teachings of Siddhartha Gautama (563–483? B.C.) in India. He emerged, after years of withdrawal and the practice of various forms of yoga, as "the Buddha" (the Enlightened One), having rejected much of Hindu thought and values, including the caste system. In his earliest lessons *(sutras)* he asserted that everything is appearance, nothing is real, and the chief reason for suffering is the ego, which may strive for personal satisfaction and happiness. By extinguishing all desires, one can attain enlightenment and, eventually, escape from the wheel of existence and ascend into nirvana. To achieve this, the Buddha taught an eightfold path: right seeing, right purpose, right speech, right action, right livelihood, right effort, right mindedness, and right meditation.

Buddhists tend to be pacifists but, when forced to defend their country, can justify killing on the ground that victorious bad men multiply bad *karma* in the world. In spite of their lack of an active ethic and their denial of the reality of the physical world, Buddhists are unlikely to withdraw into passive endurance when confronted with a communal disaster and, with their ethic of practiced compassion, they can be counted on to be diligent and resourceful relief workers.

Islam

Faith is belief without reason—a maxim that creates a conflict for many followers of most of the world's major religions. For Muslims, whether laborers or intellectuals, this does not represent a problem. Islamic philosophy is deeply rooted in the minds, hearts, and behavior of its adherents. Islamic belief pervades every facet of life from birth to death, and Muslims believe that their destiny is subject solely to the will of Allah. Even in the case of unexpected personal misfortune or communal disaster, the cause is accepted invariably as the will of Allah as punishment for inadequate fidelity. The Koran is held to be the final and complete work of God. Muslims accept and revere all of the major prophets from Abraham to Jesus, with Muhammed being "the latest and greatest."

Forty-seven nations from Senegal to Bangladesh, and from Turkey to Indonesia, are either entirely or predominantly Muslim. For anyone assigned to these countries, or to allow better interpretation of international news reports, a basic understanding of Islam is essential.

Common Features

One aspect most peoples of the Third World have in common, irrespective of individual religious persuasion, is reverence for old age. This is explicit in the Buddhist and Hindu emphasis on spiritual development that grows stronger the longer one lives and in Taoism, in which old age is proof of sanctity; it is equally true in patriarchal Muslim and other societies. Two of the greatest tragedies experienced by refugees in major disasters and emergencies are (1) the frequently disproportionate high loss of life among the elderly (the often harsh conditions of life in developing countries enforces the view that wives and children are "replaceable") and, even worse, (2) being forced to abandon the land and the graves of their ancestors, both of which represent the roots and the promise of continuity of past and future life.

Writing about Vietnamese refugees, Fitzgerald (1972) describes the experience of losing their homes, an account that would be equally valid for most Africans, Asians, and Pacific Islanders:

> It is the social death caused by destruction of the family that is of overriding importance. . . . The land and the family were the two sources of national, as well as personal, identity. Ancestor worshippers, the Vietnamese saw themselves as more than separate egos, as part of a continuum of life. As they took life from the earth and from the ancestors, so they could find immortality in their children, who in their turn would take their place on the earth. To leave the land and the family forever was therefore to lose their place in the universe and to suffer a permanent, collective death.

In the refugee setting, it may be helpful to encourage and assist the early reinstitution of indigenous worship practices, to carefully protect people against any efforts at proselytization, and to involve indigenous health practitioners actively in health service programs.

Media reports about international relief operations tend to convey an impression of an unfeeling attitude or indifference among Third World peoples regarding the misfortunes of others, leaving the perception that compassionate concern for people in need is solely a Judeo-Christian virtue. Nothing could be further from the truth. The degree of hospitality offered to outsiders in the Middle East, Asia, the Pacific, or Africa far exceeds that in Western countries. Among Muslims, individual mosque communities look after all their needy members. Beggars are usually found only in places frequented by tourists or where urban conditions have broken down the cohesion of the Muslim community. The same holds true for the extended family systems common to almost all developing countries. However, as a result of development of African history and culture, care and compassion for the suffering of others are generally confined to members of one's own clan. For some of the "otherworldly" religions of the East, death is but a transitional stage (but do not try to convince an Indian mother of that after the loss of her child!), and suffering is a way to acquire merits for one's next incarnation. Neither death nor suffering should be rashly interfered with. Buddha originated the ethic of compassion, which was subsequently accepted into Hindusim and most other eastern religious teachings as well. All of these religions place high value on deeds of charity and good works.

The guiding principle for the foreign technical adviser is unquestioning respect of local religious practices including festivals and any other spiritual observances. For advice on these matters, it is best to seek out local people, rather than one's national counterpart. If he has been brought up in the capital, he may have little knowledge of rural customs or, in embarrassment, may make light of local beliefs as "primitive superstitions."

INTERACTION WITH DISASTER VICTIMS AND REFUGEES

One need not visit the scene of a major disaster or see the average refugee camp, but has only to review the current literature on emergency relief to realize that such operations represent a paternalism of the most arrogant kind. An abundance of books and other publications on most aspects of disaster and refugee relief include almost no descriptions of emotional trauma or the hopes held and lost, from the viewpoint of the victims. No commercial enterprise expects to succeed without devoting time and money to active consumer research. Although refugee relief has become a multimillion-dollar endeavor, those providing crisis assistance have not yet listened to the people they intend to help, nor included them as active participants in planning and executing relief measures.

One effort to initiate change, under the sponsorship of a number of foundations and private and government agencies, has been a five-day symposium on "Giving Refugees a Voice," which was held in March 1984, in Oxford, England (Disasters 1984). The 174 participants represented African refugees brought to the United Kingdom directly from various camps, host and donor governments, national and international agencies, relief workers, and academics. Their chief objectives were to exchange and compare individual experiences and viewpoints, and to prepare recommendations for presentation to the Second International Conference on Assistance to Refugees in Africa (ICARA II) held in Geneva in July

1985. The opinions expressed and concerns exchanged were refreshingly frank. The following are some representative comments from refugee and host government spokespersons:

> I would hope that experts will never again have the effrontery . . . to discuss refugees without refugees being present. . . . Refugee work remains, perhaps, the last bastion of the ultraconservative approach to aid and development. It is hard to think of another area where the blinkered nonsense of "we know what's best for them" approach survives so unchallenged.

> [That] we were capable of managing our own affairs before [becoming refugees] still applies now. The fact that our status has changed does not mean that our abilities have gone down.

> National sensitivities are a problem not only for Africa, but the poorer you are, the prouder you are, the more you feel sensitive about dignity and about sovereignty and about independence.

> In any organization there are problems of accountability and control over funds and personnel, but there is far more waste by expatriates who are unwilling to use the skills of the refugees.

> One of the basic needs of a refugee is . . . hope, and the key to hope lies in education. . . . It is one way of giving them . . . moral or mental stability and security. . . . hope is one of the greatest gifts we can give refugees.

> . . . The reason why it is so difficult to assist refugees is that they are not recognized as having any responsibility for their affairs at the beginning. . . . Refugees must not be settled, but must be allowed to try to settle themselves.

As is apparent from these quotes, the role of the foreign expert is not to bring solutions, but to assist the host country professionals (especially those found among the victim population) in their search for indigenous solutions (van Huyck 1978). Irrespective of one's expertise and good intentions, one should not lose sight of the fact that one comes as an intruder whose help may or may not be wanted. Also, one comes as a neophyte and not, no matter what one's personal background might be, as a disaster expert. The only experts of this disaster are the people who had the endurance and courage to survive it. Refugees may feel resentful of undue outside interference and of the prevailing notion that they are unable to cope. Consider the following example:

> Asaba is a town on the west bank of the Niger River which had suffered considerable destruction and hardship during the 1967–1970 civil war. On the basis of a survey showing a high degree of health and nutrition problems, both the Federal and State Ministries of Health requested placement of a Red Cross medical team to the area. It took some time to free up, equip, and house a qualified, largely expatriate group in the area. When they were finally able to go to work, they discovered village volunteers and local government health workers already competently conducting maternal–child health clinics and nutrition programs with outside assistance. Local resilience and initiative had been greatly underestimated.

If at all possible, the initial visit to a disaster site or group of recently arrived refugees should be low-key and confined to a small team of two or three persons. If a helicopter has to be used, it should be put down at some distance well out of sight. Avoid being accompanied by reporters, photographers, or a military escort. If the latter is deemed essential, leave them guarding the helicopter or landrover.

The objectives of the initial contact with the refugees will focus on an eyeball appraisal of emergency needs, establishment of contact with the group and its leadership, inquiry into what help may be needed most, discussion regarding a follow-up survey, and solicitation of local participation in the assessment of existing problems and priorities.

Following a meeting with both official and traditional community leaders, it is advisable to call for an open gathering to give others the opportunity to express their views. Any group initiative or new leadership that may have emerged from the disaster experience can be identified at that time, together with any indigenous health workers and healers. Outsiders may be surprised by the diversity of talent and resourcefulness present among even the poorest communities. For the sake of efficiency and, more important, for the restoration of dignity, it is vital that refugees be made full participants from the outset in the assessment of needs, disease surveillance, and provision of emergency aid. Only such assistance as one is personally able to guarantee should be offered, and the follow-up should be as prompt as possible. Beyond that, assurance of personal concern and sincerity in expressing a desire to help is all that is expected.

The second visit, which includes initiation of health and nutritional status assessment and establishment of surveillance system, must be coordinated with food distribution, emergency medical aid, or other relief provisions. Without these, the health questionnaires, anthropometric measurements, and physical examinations can easily become suspect as academic exercises devoid of any real interest in the welfare of the victim population.

Team work with disaster victims or refugees is generally not difficult and invariably becomes an enriching experience. Exceptions are encountered among refugees who have survived prolonged famine, or among those who have been exposed to terror. Encounters with victims of such extreme suffering were common during the height of the civil war in Nigeria, in the early weeks of the Khmer refugee emergency in Thailand, and among survivors of the current famine in Ethiopia, the Sudan, and other Sahelian countries. The utter silence among listless children and the frozen faces of adults carry their own story of abandoned hope.

The outsider, whether national or foreign, cannot expect to be able to gauge or comprehend what victims of severe disasters have experienced. There is little, therefore, that he or she can accomplish alone. The key is to work through indigenous leaders and other community representatives in triage, assessing needs, or establishing local treatment or feeding centers.

From the very outset of a relief intervention, no matter how pressing day-to-day activities might be, long-term goals and objectives that will lead to ultimate resolution of prevailing emergency problems should be established. These goals should be based on local cultural values and realistic expectations of the affected people and their potential for self-help. Participatory management of daily activities by the refugee population, with maximal transfer of authority to local hands, will ensure that the "victims'" voices will be heard in decision making.

Finally, it should be remembered that in almost all Third World societies, it is customary to show hospitality to a visitor. Even under the most appalling circumstances, food, drink, or a token gift is offered. This represents an important emphasis on self-respect; it is an offer, irrespective of time, pressure, or personal embarrassment, which dare not be turned down. If one responds with a corresponding gift next time around, so much the better.

REFERENCES AND SUGGESTED READING

Allegra DT, Nieburg P, Grabe M (eds): Emergency Refugee Health Care: A Chronical of the Khmer Refugee Assistance Operation 1979–1980. Washington, DC, USDHHS-CDC Pub 554-436/15386,1984.
Brislin WB: Cross-cultural encounters, p 372. New York, Pergamon Press, 1982.
Center for International and Area Studies: Intercultural Communicating, pp 23–25. Provo, Brigham Young University, 1982.
Disasters, London. 1984;8(4):261–72.
Fitzgerald F: Fire in the Lake, pp 429–30. Boston, Little Brown & Co, 1927.
Gudykunst WB, Kim YY: Communication with Strangers, p 277. Reading, MA, Addison-Wesley, 1984.
Haddad Y: The Islamic alternative. The Link; Americans for Middle East Understanding Inc, 1982;15:4.
Lambo TA: Psychotherapy in Africa. Human Nature 1978;(March):164–68.
Leivesly S: Psychological response to disaster. In Seaman et al (eds): Epidemiology of Natural Disasters, p 123. Basel, Karger, 1984.
Mortimer E: Faith and Power: The Politics of Islam. New York, Vintage Books, 1982.
Rosenblatt R: Defenders of the faith. Time Magazine 1984;(Nov 12).
Smith WC: Islam in Modern History. Princeton, Princeton University Press, 1957.
Thomas P: Hindu Religion, Customs and Manners. Bombay, DP Taraporevala Sons, Ltd, 1952.
van Huyck AP: As quoted in David IR: The role of technology in international disaster assistance, NAS-NRC Report, 1978;18.
Winfield L: Living Overseas, p 167. Washington DC, Public Affairs Press, 1962.
Woodward KL: Religions of Asia. Modern Maturity 1984;(Dec).
Woodward KL: Religions of Asia. Modern Maturity 1985;(Jan).

II

SPECIALTY CONSIDERATIONS IN PATIENT CARE

12
Tropical Pediatrics

KAREN OLNESS

This chapter emphasizes basic considerations for health providers who do not ordinarily care for children. After a review of the essentials of physical examination, an annotated list of common pitfalls in tropical pediatrics is given.

The most frequent causes of pediatric mortality in refugee settings are dehydration, malnutrition, and pneumonia. Other frequent causes of illness include measles, pertussis, cerebral malaria, dengue-shock syndrome, sepsis, and asthma. Pediatric deaths in field-hospital settings more often relate to absence of proper supportive care, such as airway suctioning and fluid maintenance, than to lack of drugs or knowledge. Health providers must consider the most efficient allocation of support staff (including parents), and drug, or other limitations before embarking on heroic interventions. A practical cardiopulmonary resuscitation protocol based on available resources should be developed and, when appropriate, all involved staff trained in its application (see the section on cardiopulmonary resuscitation).

The environmental stress of a disaster or refugee situation is devastating for children as well as for adults. A gentle health care provider can symbolize a measure of security important to children out of their usual living environment. Rapport is facilitated, despite language barriers, by providing a few colorful or interesting toylike objects. Such pleasant diversions appeal to children who are anxious about an encounter with a strange adult. If children are old enough to speak, it is helpful to talk with them about their likes and interests or activities.

Special mention should be made of newborn care. It is most important to keep neonates warm (though not too warm). The signs of sepsis in newborns are notoriously subtle, including poor feeding or brief apnea and bradycardia episodes. Hypoglycemia with or without hypocalcemia are common problems in stressed newborns. Both may manifest with jitteriness or seizures.

THE PHYSICAL EXAMINATION

Measurement of height and weight is essential in the examination of children, even when the clinic visit is for acute illness. Children can be measured while they lie on a measuring board or with a measuring tape while they stand straight against a wall. Hanging scales are most practical for weighing young children. Acquisition of reliable scales should be a high priority for pediatric health work in the refugee setting. (See Chapter 14 for height and weight tables.)

It is important to pay attention to the order in which the physical examination of children is performed. With experience and an organized approach, the health provider can note many of the most important physical examination findings in a few moments. The often practiced "head to toe" method used for adults is somewhat less useful for infants and toddlers. This is because ear and throat examinations often make children cry, thus making auscultation of the heart and lungs, and palpation of the abdomen much more difficult. The following order of examination of pediatric patients is suggested. Begin with careful observation while you attempt to gain the child's confidence; then listen to the heart, lungs, and abdomen; feel the abdomen; and, finally, look into the ears and mouth.

Observation is the single most important step, especially for infants. Parents should undress their children and hold them for as much of the examination as possible. While observing the child, it is helpful to ask oneself a series of questions by system, such as the following:

- General. Is the child playful, alert, and well-appearing, or is the child ill-appearing, obtunded, or poorly nourished? Are tears present (good hydration)?
- Skin and hair. Are any redness, rashes, swelling, petechiae, or bruises present? Is there lightening of the hair roots, suggestive of past or present malnutrition?

- Central nervous system (CNS). Is the child irritable or lethargic? Is the fontanel flat? Is the neck being held stiffly? Are all four extremities moving adequately and equally?
- Ears. Does the child dig at or pull on the ears? Is there any drainage?
- Respiratory. Is there any stridor or wheezing? Are there signs of respiratory distress such as rapid respiratory rate, nasal flaring, or intercostal retractions?
- Gastrointestinal. Is there any abdominal distention? Does the skin turgor appear normal? Is there frequent vomiting or diarrhea?

The signs of dehydration on physical examination include increased heart rate, decreased blood pressure (often a late finding in children), sunken eyes and fontanel, poor skin turgor (hyponatremic dehydration), doughy skin (hypernatremic dehydration), dry lips and mouth, and absence of tears (see Chapter 15).

Meningitis may be difficult to discern, especially in infants and toddlers (see Chapter 30). It is preferable to evaluate neck stiffness indirectly by encouraging children to follow an appealing object with their eyes and head, rather than attempting to move the neck passively. A bulging fontanel may be absent in a dehydrated child. Kernig's sign may be helpful in older children. To elicit this, the child lies supine with knee and leg flexed so the thigh is perpendicular to the trunk. The examiner then attempts to extend the knee. If this maneuver is painful, then meningeal irritation may be present.

Lower respiratory illnesses, especially pneumonia (see Chapter 32) and asthma, are very common in disaster situations. It is important to differentiate between the inspiratory stridor of epiglottitis, croup, or diphtheria, and the expiratory wheezing of asthma or foreign body aspiration. The examiner should learn to recognize the difference between fine and coarse inspiratory rales, and should realize that children with pneumonia often consciously suppress coughs because they are painful.

The chest walls of children are thinner than those of adults, which permits better sound transmission. The novice often believes extra sounds in the chest to be from pneumonia when, in fact, they are transmitted coarse upper-airway sounds. One helpful technique for distinguishing between coarse transmitted upper-airway sounds and actual lower-airway rales or rhonchi is to put the stethoscope in front of the child's mouth or on the side of the neck where the upper-airway sounds can best be heard. The examiner should then "inch" the stethoscope down. If the advential sounds heard from the chest are actually emanating from the upper airway, the examiner will note them to be of the same quality as that heard from the throat, but softer.

Otoscopy is often best deferred until the end of the examination. To diagnose otitis media, loss of the light reflex and loss of the normal shiny quality of the eardrum can be appreciated with a standard otoscope. If the child is crying, erythema by itself is an unreliable sign of otitis. Pneumatic otoscopy is a simple, low-technology procedure to determine if the eardrum is mobile . If it is not, then fluid may be present (acutely or chronically) or the eardrum may be scarred. To use a pneumatic otoscope, a tube is fitted into the head of a standard otoscope and an air seal is obtained using a properly fitted ear speculum. Using a rubber bulb or the examiner's mouth, a pulse of air is delivered into the ear canal while the eardrum is observed for movement.

It is important to look for dental caries and abscesses because they may be responsible for facial edema and submandibular adenopathy (see Chapter 19).

If symptoms are poorly described and physical findings uncertain, a period spent watching the child move about, eat, drink, or breathe may be helpful in clarifying the cause. Premedication prior to visiting the clinic is common, and some unexplained symptoms (such as dilated pupils, oculogyric crises, or dry mouth) may be an effect of those drugs.

PITFALLS IN PEDIATRICS

A few of the most common pitfalls in tropical pediatrics are the following:

- Failure to recognize cross-cultural issues in malnutrition and in the provision of preventive services. It is essential that pediatric health practitioners have a knowledge of local child-rearing traditions, taboos toward food or medical practices, birth control, and so on.
- "Shotgunning" with antibiotics. Because of limited laboratory facilities, "shotgunning" is a constant temptation. Not only do health workers use antibiotics improperly, but parents often purchase antibiotics on the local market and administer them for days or weeks before consulting a physician. Intractable diarrhea, overgrowth of resistant organisms, pan-

cytopenia, and allergic reactions are some of the troubling consequences of such practices. Once a decision has been made that the use of an antibiotic is justified, it should be used for at least five days to minimize treatment failures and overgrowth of resistant organisms.

- Failure to use oral rehydration. In general, oral rehydration is as effective as and safer, less expensive, easier to use, and more comfortable for the patient than parenteral rehydration (see Chapter 15).
- Failure to give potassium supplements to children suffering from diarrhea. Inadequate potassium replacement is the most common cause of abdominal distention and ileus in the dehydrated child treated with intravenous fluids. Normal saline, or glucose with water, is inadequate. Chapter 15 discusses the proper composition of rehydration solutions.
- Treating diarrhea with starvation, antispasmodics, or routine antibiotics. Increased morbidity from diarrheal illnesses after such interventions have been demonstrated, especially when the children are malnourished.
- Waiting for laboratory confirmation of diseases before initiating treatment. One must assess the skills of the laboratory technicians before depending on laboratory tests. When acute malaria, meningitis, or other serious illness is suspected, treatment delays can be fatal. If rapid, reliable laboratory results are unavailable, it may be necessary to initiate treatment on the basis of clinical judgment.
- Failure to stress supportive care in tetanus and diphtheria. Many patients begin to recover from tetanus and diphtheria only to succumb to a preventable complication such as aspiration pneumonia. When used, feeding tubes must be carefully place, and tracheostomy tubes carefully watched.
- Administration of antihelminthics and purges to acutely ill or emaciated children. In general, the benefit of antihelminthics and purges is not worth the significant risks of toxicity and bowel obstruction or volvulus (from impacted worms). It is better to use such drugs after the child's constitutional status has improved.
- Administration of steroids to patients with tuberculosis, amebiasis, or strongyloidiasis. Steroids should be used with extreme caution in patients with tuberculosis, amebiasis, or strongyloidiasis as the resultant immunosuppression can lead to dangerous acceleration of their disease.
- Assumption that skin testing materials for tuberculosis are reliable. If skin tests for tuberculosis are routinely negative, it is likely that the testing material is inactive.
- Failure to consider the negative nutritional side effects of drugs. For example, children taking INH for tuberculosis may require pyridoxine (vitamin B) supplementation.
- Failure to recognize the risk of hemolytic anemia when using certain drugs in children with glucose-6-phosphate dehydrogenase deficiency (G-6-PD). This deficiency of the red blood cells is usually an X-chromosome-linked disorder; therefore, males are more commonly affected. The incidence of hemolytic anemia ranges up to 40 percent in certain populations. Greeks, southern Italians, Sephardic Jews, Filipinos, southern Chinese, blacks, and Thais are among the most commonly affected groups. Hemolytic anemia can occur spontaneously or as a result of the use of certain drugs; antimalarials (especially primaquine), antipyretics, sulfonamides, and naphthaquinolones have been implicated most frequently. Definitive testing will usually be unavailable in refugee camps, so history and epidemiologic information must be relied on to suggest which patients may be at higher risk. If a hemolytic crisis should occur, recovery is the rule.
- Failure to consider effects of malnutrition on pharmacokinetics. For example, acetaminophen is not recommended in malnourished children because of toxicity due to delayed metabolism.
- Unawareness of the need for cool storage of certain drugs. The drugs commonly requiring cool storage are listed in Chapter 23, and the importance of maintaining a "cold chain" for proper vaccine storage is discussed in Chapter 6.
- Improper use of blood transfusions. Health workers are often tempted to give large amounts of blood rapidly to treat the profound anemias that can develop from severe malnutrition. These anemias can usually be corrected with iron supplements, vitamins, and nutritional support, alone. Occasionally, a child will present with cardiovascular decompensation secondary to severe anemia from malnutrition. Generally, dehydration and beriberi should be treated first but, if necessary, blood in small amounts can be given slowly. It is best to keep in mind that it takes many months for children to reach this state, and rapid transfusions can lead to irreversible congestive heart failure and death. At this time there are significant risks of AIDS and hepatitis transmission from transfusions of blood products in many developing nations. Therefore, in general

transfusions should be given only for acute severe blood loss or other true life-saving indications.

• Unwillingness to use a feeding tube for malnourished children who will not eat or drink. The feeding tube is a simple, safe method for providing needed fluid and nutrition to the child unable or unwilling to eat or drink. Aspiration must be guarded against.

• Improper care due to ignorance. Ignorance is a common and preventable cause of many pediatric illnesses. An effort should be made to give careful instructions to family members. Dietary instruction is particularly important to prevent recurrences of malnutrition.

• Failure to recognize the important parent surrogate role of older siblings and relatives. Seven- or eight-year-old children may spend more time parenting the infant or toddler than the parents do. It is important that these young caretakers be recognized and included in education programs. *Child to Child* is a useful guide to teaching young surrogate parents (Aarons & Hawes 1979).

CARDIOPULMONARY RESUSCITATION IN CHILDREN

Children frequently die from dehydration, malnutrition, and pneumonias. They also die from measles, pertussis, cerebral malaria, dengue-shock syndrome, sepsis, and asthma. They may die from Reye's syndrome triggered by the use of aspirin in treating influenza. Causes of death often relate more to the absence of supportive care, such as suction and maintenance fluids, than to lack of drugs or knowledge.

When a child's illness progresses to respiratory or cardiac arrest, the most important immediate measures are establishment of an airway, the delivery of air, the performing of closed chest message, and the provision of appropriate fluids. Although intensive chemotherapeutic resuscitation will rarely be practical in refugee camps, the essentials are included below for completeness. This section, by Dr. Theresa A. Baker, is reprinted with the permission of the Research Foundation, St. Louis Park Medical Center, Minneapolis, Minnesota.

CAUSES OF ARREST

Cardiopulmonary arrest in children can result from a number of causes. Usually the initial failure is, or stems from, a blocked airway as in croup, epiglottitis, status asthmaticus, or foreign body aspiration. With progressive respiratory failure and its accompanying hypoxia, cardiac arrest is imminent. Other causes of respiratory arrest include drug ingestion and drowning.

A primary cardiac arrest in a child without congenital heart disease or myocarditis is rare. However, some children have undetected cardiac disease that leads to sudden death. In addition, blood dyscrasias are associated with sudden death, and acute dehydration from severe gastroenteritis can cause circulatory failure and death. There are many other causes. The important thing is to get a good history to help determine the best management of each case. Myocardial infarction and pulmonary edema, which are common in adults, are unlikely to be the cause of cardiac arrest in children.

BASIC LIFE SUPPORT

As in resuscitating any patient, the airway must first be opened. This is done by extending the neck. In this position, the mandible is pulled upward, thus lifting the tongue and epiglottis off the posterior wall of the pharynx. In a child, the head is relative large with respect to the body. The occipital area extends more posteriorly than in an adult, and with the head extended, the shoulders tend to lift off the table. A towel or blanket should be placed under the shoulders. Also, in a child less than 6 months old, the structures in the neck are soft and pliable. If the head is extended too far, the posterior structures will obstruct the airway as they are bent forward.

Once it is established that there is no spontaneous respirations, the child should be ventilated. In an infant, the mouth of the rescuer goes over both the mouth and nose of the infant. In an older child, the mouth-to-mouth technique is used as in an adult. A child's tidal lung volume is approximately 10 ml/kg. Therefore, in a small child, only small puffs are needed to ventilate adequately. In a larger child, a full 800 ml or more may be necessary. An experienced rescuer can tell from the compliance of the airway and lungs how much to ventilate. The chest should be noted to rise and fall with respiration. Four quick breaths are given to expand the lungs, not allowing them to completely deflate between breaths. In children, cardiopulmonary arrest is usually caused by respiratory failure. Often, the cardiac rate is very slow and the heart will respond quickly to adequate ventilation.

CARDIAC MASSAGE

There should be no delay in giving the first two steps of CPR and then doing an adequate assessment of circulation before going on to the third step, which is establishing circulation. An apical pulse in a small child, or the carotid pulse in a larger child, is checked. If no pulse is felt, then external cardiac massage must begin.

During resuscitation, the hands of the rescuer

must be placed with regard to the position of the heart of the child. The younger the child, the higher the position of the heart in relation to the sternum. In a newborn, the heart is directly under the mid-sternum. Also, the liver assumes a cephalad position in the infant and small child, making it more susceptible to laceration from the xyphoid process. In an infant, two fingers are placed over the mid-sternum and the force is applied directly posteriorly. In a larger child, compression may be accomplished with one hand placed on the mid-or lower one third of the sternum. In a large child, the standard adult technique with two hands is used, with the heel of one hand pressing the heel of the other. The fingers are kept off of the chest wall to prevent rib fractures, and pressure is applied directly downward over the lower half of the sternum approximately 2 cm above the xyphoid process.

The suggested rate of compression is 80 to 100 times per minute for infants, and 60 times per minute for older children. In one-person infant rescue, ventilation is performed every five compressions. The breaths are interposed with the compressions so that there is no pause in circulation. In an older child, two breaths are given after 15 compressions, as for an adult. Two-person rescue is also the same as for an adult, with one ventilation every five compressions. The only exception to these ratios is in a newborn, where noncompliant lungs may require a faster ventilatory rate to lower carbon dioxide levels and relieve hypoxia. They may be ventilated as frequently as every three beats, or approximately 30 times per minute.

ADVANCED LIFE SUPPORT

A child can be adequately ventilated with an oral airway and a mask. Because of the various sizes of children, a variety of oral airways ranging from a number 0 to number 5 should be available. Oral airways should only be used in a comatose patient because they can stimulate vomiting. The airway is inserted with the tip pointing upward along the palate, and is then rotated back behind the tongue to rest in the posterior pharynx.

One fairly easy way to ventilate a child is by using a face mask. If the mask is properly applied, air can be given to the patient from the rescuer's mouth. A clear mask is recommended so that any vomitus or secretions can be seen and suctioned promptly. Masks come in a number of shapes and sizes so a variety should be available. A nasogastric tube may help relieve gastric distention which is common in small children. Care must be taken to suction any vomitus from the oropharynx, and the stomach should be emptied, if necessary.

If available, an endotracheal tube can be inserted. A pipe cleaner or copper tubing may be used as a trocar to add stability during intubation. In infants and children under 8 years of age, an uncuffed tube is recommended. Larger children require a cuffed endotracheal tube. Care must be taken not to overextend the child's neck. Visualization of the epiglottis is best done by sliding a blade over the tongue, placing upward traction on the blade, and exposing the vocal cords. Applying gentle pressure on the tracheal rings may allow easier insertion of the tube. The tube is advanced along the side of the oropharynx and directed, visually, into the larynx. After checking for adequate ventilation of both lungs, the person in charge of ventilation should secure the tube in the proper position.

INTRAVENOUS SUPPORT

An intravenous line should be established as soon as possible. This can be the most difficult job during advanced life support, especially in a child who has arrested due to circulatory failure from severe dehydration. Any size IV is better than no IV; even a scalp vein needle is useful. Peripheral veins should be checked, including those on the scalp considering the fact that, with external cardiac massage, the head is receiving a good share of the output. If a surface peripheral vein cannot be found, femoral veins or a saphenous cutdown may be necessary (see Chapter 16). Subclavian or internal jugular vein catheterization should be done only by experienced personnel. For fluid choice and dose, see Chapter 15.

DRUG THERAPY

Once an IV line is established, drugs may be administered with doses based on weight. Children metabolize drugs at different rates. An infant may require a higher dose per kilogram than an adult. Emergency facilities should keep a list of emergency drugs and the recommended doses for children.

With proper ventilation, sodium bicarbonate can be used to combat metabolic acidosis. Also, when used with epinephrine, sodium bicarbonate may convert asystole to fibrillation. The recommended therapy is 1 to 2 mEq/kg per dose. The larger doses are more likely to be used in depressed newborns who have a large base deficit. In infants, sodium bicarbonate should be diluted at least 1:1 with D5W. Too much bicarbonate may lead to metabolic alkalosis and a hyperosmolar state in the postresuscitation period. Once an adequate cardiac output and blood volume are established, the body can clear excess organic acids. Total correction of the base deficit is not recommended.

Epinephrine may help convert cardiac asystole by restoring electrical activity, or it may improve contractility. It lowers the defibrillation threshold making electrical countershock more effective in establishing sinus rhythm. The dose of epinephrine is 0.01 ml/kg. It can be given IV, or may be instilled directly into the endotracheal tube.

Lidocaine is used to treat ventricular arrhythmias which may result from hypoxia. In toxic doses, lidocaine can cause central nervous system depression or seizures, depressed myocardial function, and vasodilation. The dose in children is 1 mg/kg as an intravenous bolus. This may be followed by an intravenous infusion of 20 to 50 mcg/kg per minute.

Isoproterenol is a beta agonist which increases cardiac output. An advantage in pediatric patients is that it does not cause peripheral vasoconstriction, particularly in the renal arteries which are very sensitive to vasoconstrictive agents. Isoproterenol is used to treat sinus bradycardia with hypotension or complete heart block. The dose is titrated intravenously at 0.1 to 0.5 mcg/kg/minute to maintain the blood pressure and pulse in a desired range. Toxic signs include premature ventricular contractions or tachycardia.

Atropine is helpful in treating symptomatic bradycardia because of its vagolytic activity. The dose is 0.01 mg/kg given intravenously or via the endotracheal tube.

Dopamine is used to treat hypotension and its effects are dose related. At 1 to 2 mcg/kg/minute, there is increased renal blood flow, glomerular filtration rate, urine output, and sodium excretion. At 2 to 10 mcg/kg minute, there is increased cardiac output. At 10 to 20 mcg/kg/minute, vasoconstriction causes the blood pressure to rise. Renal vasoconstriction occurs with doses greater than 20 mcg/kg/minute.

Naloxone can be used to reverse respiratory failure from ingestion of even small amounts of drugs such as diphenoxylate with atropine (Lomotil), codeine, or hydrocodone bitartrate cough preparations (Tussionex), paregoric, meperidine hydrochloride (Demerol), or methadone. It is useful in babies born shortly after their mothers have been given meperidine or other narcotics. The dose is 0.01 to 0.05 mg/kg IM.

REFERENCES AND SUGGESTED READING

Aarons A, Hawes H: Child to Child. London, MacMillan Press, 1979.
Balldin B, Hart R, Huenges R et al: Child Health. A Manual for Medical Assistants and Other Rural Health Workers. Nairobi, African Medical and Research Foundation, 1975.
Behrman RE, Vaughan VC, Nelson WE: Nelson Textbook of Pediatrics. Philadelphia, WB Saunders, 1983.
Biller JA, Yeager AM: The Harriet Lane Handbook. Chicago, Year Book Medical Publishers, 1981.
Chandler WU: Investing in Children. Worldwatch Paper 64. Washington, DC, Worldwatch Institute, 1985.
Cole-King S: Approaches to the Evaluation of Maternal and Child Health Care in the Context of Primary Health Care. Geneva, World Health Organization, 1979.
Jelliffe DB, Jelliffe EFP (eds): Advances in International Maternal and Child Health, Vol 5. New York, Oxford University Press, 1985.
Jelliffee DB, Stanfield JP: Diseases of Children in the Subtropics and Tropics. London, Edward Arnold, 1978.
King MH, King F, Martodipoero S: Primary Child Care: A Manual for Health Workers. London, Oxford University Press, 1978.
Mosely WH, Chen L (eds): Child Survival: Strategies for Research. Population and Development Review, Supplement to Vol. 10, 1984.
Olness K: Practical Pediatrics in Less-Developed Countries. Eden Prairie, MN, The Garden, 1980.
Peter G, Giebink GS, Hall CB, Plotkin SA (eds): Report of the Committee on Infectious Diseases. 12th ed. Elk Grove Village, IL, American Academy of Pediatrics, 1986.

13
Prevention of Malnutrition and Supplementary Feeding Programs

ROY E. BROWN
ANGELA BERRY

Health status is directly correlated with nutritional status, and it is impossible to provide adequate medical care without ensuring provision of appropriate nutritional intake. If one were to allocate resources among primary medical care, prevention programs, sanitation, and nutrition, a rational order of priorities would rank nutrition at the top and individual medical care at the bottom (de Ville de Goyet & Lechat 1977). Among the numerous factors that must be considered in preventing malnutrition and achieving a sound health status, the provision of food and water must not be neglected. The initial health and nutritional status of a group of displaced persons or refugees will reflect their health status and events that occurred before the onset of general relief efforts, including the causes and duration of their flight, the availability of food and water along the way, and the effects of exposure to weather and infectious diseases.

Through training and experience, medical workers are typically oriented to the diagnosis and management of the individual patient. The classic medical approach begins by obtaining relevant background information, including major complaints and the historical data that contributed to the current situation, followed by a clinical examination, and the appropriate laboratory tests to arrive at a differential diagnosis. Finally, the process proceeds with the provision of specific therapy or elements necessary for good medical management. When faced with the overall management of refugees, it is essential to shift the medical orientation from the individual to the community. This major modification toward mass management involves careful planning.

To prevent malnutrition and provide food for large populations, a careful phasing of support efforts is necessary. A planning committee must be created to assist with general registration of the population. The committee should include logistics experts, nutrition advisers, and refugee representatives. The planning committee should welcome the participation of agencies such as the UNHCR, World Food Program (WFP), UNICEF, and WHO as well as representatives from the local or national government and other bilateral agencies. The nutrition advisers must consider locally available foods with an early concentration on provision of the minimum calories necessary for survival (about 1500 calories per person per day). The registration process involves listing the entire population, providing an identification wrist band and family card, and dividing refugees into those who are obviously vulnerable and those who appear to be fairly well-nourished. Immediate arrangements for food, water, and proper sanitation, and identification of the vulnerable categories are the critical first steps in the relief effort.

Early in the general organizational plan, serious thought must be given to provision of essential logistical support for the supply of adequate food and water. To accommodate the planning, control, management, and accountability for a mass feeding operation, it may be necessary to establish a separate emergency logistical unit that is distinct from the medical effort but maintains a close liaison with all aspects of the refugee support system.

Certain preliminary data are vital to initiate the supply process—for example, an initial estimate of the number of refugees and the anticipated duration of the catastrophe. While data are being gathered, the preliminary phase requires the identification of all locally available sources of food and water, the provision of shelter against rain or sun, and local fuel supplies for subsequent food preparation.

Once the maintenance phase of operations is entered, a more careful demographic profile is performed. This should include age and nutritional status. Community surveys of anthropometric measurements are the most useful means of malnutrition surveillance in the refugee community. A random sample survey using 30 clusters of seven children each is one rapid method (see Chapter 2). Both demographic information and nutritional status should be updated periodically, and the likely duration of the refugee situation reestimated.

Five additional epidemiologic indicators may be useful:

- Birth weight under 2500 g may be associated with maternal malnutrition.
- Elevated mortality rates in the one- to four-year-olds (and perhaps most sensitively in the one- to two-year-olds) suggest an increased prevalence of protein energy malnutrition (PEM) in the community because malnutrition, directly or indirectly, is often the major cause of death after weaning from the breast.
- Incidence rates of nutritional deficiency diseases reported by clinics and hospitals may indicate changes in PEM trends.
- Community food consumption surveys (usually compiled from diet histories) may suggest nutritional deficiencies. Such surveys are also helpful for understanding traditional weaning practices within the community.
- Delayed age of menarche is a fairly reliable indicator of PEM prevalence. However, this may not be a useful parameter in a refugee camp because ages are often unknown.

The advisers in nutrition will have to consider such important factors as local food habits, cultural determinants, preferred methods of food preparation, nutritional content of the feeding package, and the type of food purchases available locally.

Because all feeding operations are considered personnel intensive, it is important to identify group leaders who can assist with recruitment of refugee volunteers to assist in the feeding process. With the help of interpreters, language barriers can be overcome. The staff for food distribution and emergency logistical support units will comprise both trained professionals and locally trained volunteers. Regardless of previous training, all staff members may require some fundamental training.

Crowd control, particularly with a population under stress, is important because refugees are generally unaccustomed to waiting in line for food and water. If the population has not eaten for some time, the sight of food may result in pushing and injury to the weak. Lengths of fence and rope may be used to establish lines for food and water distribution. Local volunteers can serve as guards, monitors, food preparers, and supervisors of registration and screening.

In the early phases of mass feeding operations, imported food will most often be required. This may involve ocean or rail shipping, port or central warehousing of supplies, transporting by truck, secondary warehousing close to the population being fed, establishing check points, monitoring, and a system of accounting for transported goods to reduce loss. A ten-day cycle of commodities, including imported and locally available food, should be established. Once a system of basic rations for the refugees is established, an identification system for those participating, and triage to set priorities of those requiring special rations, should be organized. As individual food preparation is the direction of feeding programs, it is important to identify those who can prepare their own food. Also needed are a method for identifying newcomers and procedures to follow in the case of lost identification cards or wrist bands. It is important to introduce a cross-reference system to facilitate coordination of services for those requiring special food provision and medical attention.

A good relationship must be established with the local and national government representatives who may already have policies and guidelines for mass feeding operations. Liaison with support agencies is also critical for long-term logistical support. Local leaders from within the group can assist with identifying volunteer workers for routine tasks and translators. If it becomes apparent that support will be necessary for a prolonged period of time, the logistical unit must plan and arrange the long-term systems. These systems include educating and training staff in the prevention of malnutrition and general rehabilitation of the population at risk. Such efforts should be based on a self-help philosophy, to form a pattern of increasing participation from the affected population.

To avoid dependency, a commitment to move away from relief and toward development activities is important. A transfer of decision-making responsibility to the refugees should be encouraged early in the process. Refugees should be trained for all appropriate activities with special emphasis on food production, health and nutrition education, and primary health care services (Brown 1972; Simmonds 1984).

GENERAL RATIONS

The program responsible for providing food to the total refugee population—the "general" or "basic" ration program—will form the foundation of all other health and nutrition-related activities. Although coordinating agencies will most often be responsible for this program, medical agencies should not overlook its importance. Where a ration is lacking in certain nutrients, deficiency diseases and a possible lowered resistance to infection will occur. Where supply problems are encountered, food shortages will eventually result in PEM (seen earliest among children). When camp distribution systems are unfair, certain groups, especially the vulnerable families, will become nutritionally at risk (Christensen 1982). If the general ration program is inadequate, supplementary feeding of vulnerable groups will become a "Band-Aid" effort that will keep certain people alive but never truly rehabilitate them.

Despite its importance, little research has been done on what constitutes an "adequate" diet for refugee populations. Standard rations have been arbitrarily established on recommended daily allowances of macronutrients and micronutrients, with little or no consideration that individual nutritional needs differ greatly with regard to age, sex, level of activity, climate, and health status. Similarly, family and community needs vary with demographic distribution, environment, and general health status. Up to now, such variations have rarely been considered in food ration design.

The medical staff in refugee camps should have input on food planning and policy decisions. This is most easily facilitated by a nutrition coordinator, who should be a nutritionist or a medical person with nutrition expertise. The nutrition coordinator establishes standard procedures for feeding programs and for program monitoring and evaluation, and serves as a liaison between medical and food policy groups. A central food coordinating committee should be established with medical representation as well. Those responsible for food provision, whether from the United Nations (UN), host-country government, or donor groups, should be regularly informed of the quantity and types of food required, and of the impact of programs on the prevalence of malnutrition and deficiency diseases.

Ration design may not always be based on the nutritional needs of particular groups, but rather on what is available from donor contributions and local purchases, and what is feasible to deliver. Because of the practical considerations of intracamp distribution, a ration is devised on a per-person, per-day basis with the assumption that, through sharing within the family, individual needs will be met. Hence, a standard ration per person per day can be outlined as follows:

- 400 to 500 g cereals (rice, wheat, maize, sorghum, etc.).
- 40 to 60 g pulses (beans, lentils, peas).
- 20 to 30 g oil (vegetable oil, butter oil, edible fat).

The primary consideration is to provide sufficient calories. Nutritionists generally designate a ration of 1500 kcal per person per day for survival, 1800 kcal per person per day for subsistence, and 2000 kcal per person per day for long-term maintenance. During acute emergencies, logistical difficulties often result in the distribution of a survival ration. Ironically, a major factor that influences the mass movement of people is often a recent history of food deprivation, which results in impaired nutritional status and greatest nutritional need at the start of relief operations. Clearly, the early introduction of a rehabilitation ration (at least 2000 kcal/person/day) should be the aim at the beginning of relief efforts. Thereafter, evaluation of health status (incidence of infection, morbidity and mortality rates, and prevalence of malnutrition) and environmental considerations (income, market availability, and food production) should figure in the reassessment of the community's caloric requirements.

The standard ration provides between 1800 and 2000 kcal/person/day. In most situations, spices or condiments are included, with a minimum of 5 to 10 g of salt/person/day being an essential provision. The number of ration items can be as many as 20 (as supplied in some refugee camps in Southeast Asia), or as few as three to five items (as supplied in most refugee camps in Africa). This difference generally reflects the ability to purchase locally available fresh foods and the self-sufficiency of the program.

Foods that are sometimes used to supplement the standard ration include canned, fresh, or dried meat and fish; vegetables; fruits; and special foods such as corn-soya milk powder (CSM), fish protein concentrate (FPC), and other donated items. Dried skim milk powder

(DSM) has been used in general distribution for nomadic populations (as in Somalia), but the appropriateness of this product has been disputed. DSM is useful for incorporation into porridge, soup, or other foods as a protein supplement. However, because of the potential danger of artificial formula being substituted for breast milk, any type of bottle and nipple that can be used for feeding should be discouraged. In general, the distribution of milk in both dried and liquid form should be avoided as indiscriminate use in unsanitary conditions and among groups lacking knowledge in proper methods of reconstitution can lead to increased prevalence of diarrhea and, consequently, increased malnutrition. The exception to this may be in a controlled setting, such as a supplementary feeding program, in which high-energy milk is consumed "on-the-spot."

Where refugees subsist on the standard ration (cereals, pulses, oil) alone, with no supplementation of fresh foods, certain deficiency diseases can be expected. Compared with the recommended daily allowances for an adult (FAO Handbook 1974), the standard ration is devoid of vitamins A and C, supplies 25 percent of the calcium requirement, is below the requirements for riboflavin, niacin, folic acid, and thiamine (if polished cereals are provided), and provides minimal levels of bioavailable iron.

A deficient ration is a particular problem when family purchase of supplementary fresh foods is restricted as in drought-affected areas or isolated or remote locations, among groups with no access to money, or where, for political reasons, market activity or personal movement is restricted. For example, in 1982, when a restriction on market activity was introduced in a Cambodian refugee camp on the Thai border, an outbreak of beriberi was reported (Nieburg 1985). When similar market restrictions were imposed in Somalia in 1982, an outbreak of scurvy was reported (Magan et al 1983). In Sudan, where an isolated refugee population subsisted on only the standard ration, as many as 22 percent of the population were affected by scurvy (Berry 1985, unpublished communication). Another outbreak of scurvy was reported under similar conditions in one refugee camp in northern Somalia in August 1985, when 25 percent of the population was affected. Vitamin A deficiency, manifested as xerophthalmia, affected an estimated 7 to 9 percent of Ethiopian refugee children in refugee camps in Sudan early in 1985 (Helen Keller Institute 1985).

Clearly, there is a need to evaluate the nutritional content of any ration to guarantee that all essential nutrients can be obtained by those who consume the ration. Fresh vegetables, particularly those of the dark-green leafy variety that contain many micronutrients usually missing from the standard ration, represent a basic provision. It is important, especially in long-term refugee operations, that seeds and gardening implements be distributed as soon as possible.

Food procurement, shipment, and delivery is most often the responsibility of coordinating agencies such as UNHCR, WFP, or a designated voluntary agency. Distribution on the camp level may be under the supervision of governmental representatives or elected or appointed refugee leaders. In most circumstances, dry rations are distributed on a weekly or ten-day cycle. However, during emergencies or initial phases of organized movement when refugees do not have cooking utensils, or in transit centers, a soup kitchen may be established to serve or distribute cooked food such as soup, porridge, and bread. Whenever possible, however, dry ration distribution is preferable as experience has shown that allowing refugees to prepare their own food best meets individual nutritional needs (Devadas et al 1977).

Distribution systems vary, but the main goal is to ensure that the full ration reaches the intended recipient. Factors to be considered include the following:

- Crowd control.
- Regular distributions. Ideally, rations should be distributed every ten days. Less frequent allocations of large quantities of food supplies can pose storage problems within the refugee family's living quarters. As most refugees have few, if any, resouces or surplus food, a late distribution of even one day can result in severe food shortages in the home. If distributions are irregular, hoarding of food may result. Individuals may eat less than their nutritional needs dictate in order to save food in anticipation of shortages. Eventually, this can contribute to chronic malnutrition, particularly where hierarchical patterns of intrahousehold food allocation are evident.
- Information. Refugees should be informed of the exact items and amounts of food to which they are entitled. This can be done by

displaying ration amounts on a blackboard and by informing refugee leaders, community health workers, and translators, thereby creating a community-based monitoring system to support fair distribution.

• Standardized measurement equipment. Measuring containers and scales will assist in accurate allocations. A container that measures one person's ten-day ration of cereals or beans allows easy counting for family members.

• Payment of workers. After the emergency phase of relief operations, self-help schemes, in which workers are expected to volunteer their services to distribute food, often result in workers helping themselves to extra rations. Usually, some kind of "skim-off" procedure develops, with a small (but perhaps crucial) proportion being taken from every ration. Either the most desirable items, such as meat, or the most easily sold items, such as oil, will be the most withheld. It is preferable to use some form of payment to compensate these workers for their labor.

• An accurate population census, registration, and identification system. Medical agencies shoud verify estimates of refugee numbers with UNHCR, government representatives, and public health program staff. Where discrepancies between official and actual population figures exist, difficulty with accurate food distribution may result. Some people mistakenly believe that an inflated population census will lead to food surpluses for refugee families. Instead, inflated figures generally lead to black market systems being established. Black markets result in a greater incentive for food diversion and often lead to underrationing of families (Christensen 1982). This problem was illustrated in a Laotian refugee camp in 1982, where an estimated 8000 extra rations were provided, yet a higher prevalence of malnutrition was reported among children than in other camps in Thailand.

Refugee populations are not static. All births should be reported and reflected in the amount of food distributed to families. This additional ration will serve as a supplement for lactating mothers (as the newborn will not need solid food until the fourth to sixth month) and will ensure that expanding families do not experience diminished ration supply. The report of death, however, should perhaps not be immediately reflected in a population census if it affects food distribution. Families may be reluctant to report deaths if they know that food ration withdrawal will result. Such failure to report deaths leads to inaccurate mortality statistics and an incorrect assessment of overall health status.

RATION UTILIZATION

The most efficient system of ration distribution will have little impact on the nutritional status of refugee populations if the refugees cannot, or will not, use the ration. What refugees actually consume in the home is often overlooked during planning. Consideration must be given to the appropriateness of the food provided in terms of cultural acceptability, in-home preparation, and socioeconomic factors such as intrafamily food allocation, needs and incentives for trade, and access to income and markets (Brown 1976).

It may seem surprising that hungry people will refuse to eat unfamiliar food. However, food plays a central role in cultural and religious traditions, and since refugees are already adapting to a new and sometimes hostile environment, the provision of familiar food may greatly assist in their adjustment. This applies particularly to the staple, which provides the bulk of calories. For example, in response to an outbreak of beriberi in refugee camps in Thailand, undermilled rice was substituted for white rice in the ration. Undermilled rice (halfway between white and brown) has sufficient thiamine content to eradicate beriberi and, most important, was acceptable to the population. In contrast, Cambodian refugees associated brown rice with an oppressive regime and low social status. Had brown rice been provided, they would have traded it away for a smaller volume of white rice.

The form in which food is distributed can have major implications for its utilization. Refugees in Somalia had traditional pounding equipment for maize, but the equipment was not appropriate for the whole wheat that was distributed; the cereal required boiling for hours, which greatly reduced its nutritional content. Similarly, when commercial-type refined wheat flour (appropriate for baking) was provided for refugees in Sudan, it could not be made into porridge because the high gluten content resulted in a dish that had the consistency of glue. If whole cereals are provided, appropriate grinding facilities must be made accessible to the population. This is especially important when food for children and weaning infants is being prepared. Consideration of traditional food preparation practices must be included in food planning procedures.

Access to fuel is a factor that influences the volume and frequency of meals prepared by the family. If fuel is not included in the ration, it may be either bought (draining economic resources) or gathered. Fuel gathering may reduce the amount of time spent in child care and food preparation, has a calorie cost in energy used, and may have a serious impact on the environment.

The provision of cooking utensils is another important factor related to food preparation that should not be overlooked.

Refugee families are most often from disrupted groups and have a disproportionate number of single-headed households, a lack of extended family, and few economic resources. Food rations may often be the only source of income, making barter and trade of food items a common practice in refugee camps. Such trade is often frowned on by donor communities, which need to account for donations. Evidence of such items within commercial markets may prove an embarrassment. Such trade is unavoidable, however, if items such as spices and condiments, fuel, clothing, soap, and other necessities are not provided in sufficient quantities. For example, it can be argued that tea has no nutritional value and hence shoud be excluded from a ration. In some communities, however, tea represents a very important focus for social interaction and the refugees may trade away needed food rations to obtain it. Including tea in the ration, therefore, would yield indirect nutritional benefit by eliminating the need to barter away food.

The best method for assessing the adequacy and impact of the general ration program is surveillance of the health and nutritional status of the population. An increase of malnutrition among children, or evidence of deficiency diseases, is a definite warning that problems exist. To identify exactly where problems are occurring requires carefully analyzing the ration content, monitoring the efficiency of the distribution system, and assessing the use of food in the home.

Nutritional problems may surface first among the traditionally vulnerable families; thus, focusing evaluation on such selected households can support a system of early warning. Vulnerable groups with decreased access to food include single-parent families (particularly those headed by women); families belonging to minority ethnic groups (or tribes) or minority or religious groups; the unaccompanied elderly; and groups of women without accompanying men. These groups may represent the most socially disadvantaged members of refugee populations, often most vulnerable because they represent those in the lowest economic bracket.

Continuous evaluation of the adequacy of the general ration program is important, as the quantity and quality of the food supply, and the identified vulnerable members of the population, may vary over time. To analyze the adequacy of the ration content, attention must be given to the demographic composition of the population. For example, a ration that contains 2000 kcal/person/day may be adequate for a Cambodian refugee population of which 80 percent are women and children, but it will be inadequate for a camp of Vietnamese refugees a majority of whom are young men between the ages of 16 and 30 years. The ration may provide sufficient iron for the Vietnamese population but would be inadequate in iron for the Cambodian group. Knowledge of the demographic composition of a population permits a more accurate assessment of dietary and ration needs (Table 13-1).

An evaluation of the ration content must include inspection of goods to ensure that they are fit for human consumption. Bulk supplies of food are subject to deterioration, particularly if stored for prolonged periods in hot and humid conditions, and certain toxins may develop that are dangerous if consumed. Cereals and pulses should be inspected for molds. Oil is subject to rancidity and, if spoiled, can have adverse physical effects. A simple field test for rancidity is to taste a small quantity; if it irritates the throat, it is rancid and unfit for human consumption. This test can also be applied to dried milk.

Evaluation of distribution and utilization can best be made through systematic monitoring techniques. Random sample surveys may be done on a selection of families to assess household stocks, and simple questionnaires can be distributed to determine how food is being used (Christensen 1982). Such information will prove extremely valuable when changes or improvements in the general ration program are contemplated.

Table 13-1. A Sample of Food Ration Needs Analysis According to Demographic Distribution[a]

Age (years)/Sex Group	Percentage of Population		Average kcal Needs per day		Fraction Ration Needs (kcal/day)
Cambodian Refugee Population					
<5	20	×	800	=	160
5–14	35	×	1500	=	525
14–44 female (40% pregnant or lactating)	20	×	2800	=	560
14–44 male	10	×	3500	=	350
45+	15	×	2400	=	360
		Total ration needs		=	1955 kcal/day
Vietnamese Refugee Population					
5	10	×	800	=	80
5–14	20	×	1500	=	300
14–44 female (40% pregnant or lactating)	10	×	2300	=	230
14–44 male	50	×	3500	=	1750
45+	10	×	2400	=	240
		Total ration needs		=	2600 kcal/day

[a]Average caloric needs per day are based on FAO/WHO recommended daily allowances and represent estimates that might vary according to the actual distribution of ages within categories. A similar formula may be used for all nutrients to determine more accurately the needs of refugee groups. It should be noted that demographic differences within families occur and must be considered to meet individual needs.

SUPPLEMENTARY FEEDING PROGRAMS

A supplementary feeding program (SFP), sometimes referred to as a selective feeding program, is intended for those individuals who are considered at high risk or more vulnerable to malnutrition (Simmonds et al 1983). The purpose of an SFP is to provide nutritional protection to selected groups based on their particular nutritional needs (Henderson & Biellik 1983; de Ville de Goyet et al 1978). The additional nutrients are required because certain subgroups do not have access to a varied diet. SFPs must ensure that the targeted group receives adequate caloric intake and the essential mineral, vitamin, and protein requirements. An SFP is intended to be a short-term, remedial measure to reach the most nutritionally vulnerable (Taylor 1983). In some instances, an SFP is intended to treat certain individuals with malnutrition and to rehabilitate those persons who arrived in a malnourished state. The aim is to provide additional high-energy (350 to 500 Kcal), high-protein (approximately 15 g), low-bulk food, once or twice a day, as a supplement to the general feeding program (Simmonds et al 1982).

DETECTION OF MALNUTRITION

Anthropometric Measurements

In addition to the initial registration process, there should be a system for identifying vulnerable groups, and a subsequent triage process. For preschool-aged children, mid-upper-arm circumference (MUAC) can be employed for malnutrition screening. Those with an MUAC of less than 12.5 cm are considered extremely wasted, and those with an MUAC of less than 13.5 cm are moderately wasted (see Table 13-2). The MUAC is a rapid screening system that can be easily taught to nonprofessional workers (O'Sullivan et al 1980). (See Chapter 14.)

When the ages of the children being evaluated are unknown, the weight-for-height index can be employed, and this is the preferred index for detecting children in imminent danger (Simmonds et al 1983). Weight-for-height (W/H) should be determined and recorded for children under 115 cm in height. W/H can be used as an indicator for the nutritional status of the entire refugee population (Waterlow et al 1977). (See Chapter 14.)

Table 13-2. Detection of Malnutrition Through MUAC Measurements

Nutritional Status (Weight for Height Standard, %)	MUAC, cm
Mildly malnourished (80 to 90)	12.5–13.5
Moderately malnourished (70 to 79)	11.5–12.5
Severely malnourished (less than 70)	less than 11.5

For weighing, portable spring scales with clear markings are recommended. It is important that the measurer check that the scale rests on zero before each child is weighed. Standardization of the scale with a known weight is important. Spare scales should be available. Up to 25 kg, weight can be recorded to the nearest 0.1 kg using a Salter scale.

In general, children over 85 cm in height can be measured standing, while smaller children are measured in the recumbent position. Height is measured to the nearest 0.5 cm on a slide measuring board with a fixed base.

A newly developed method for assessing W/H requires a multicolored chart. The chart includes a number of columns, each marked with a particular weight and color. After the children are weighed, they are placed in front of the column with the applicable weight. If the child is wasted, the red section of the column will show above the top of the head; if the W/H index is greater than 90 percent of the reference, the top of the head will remain in the green section of the column (Nabarro & McNab 1980). Those who are severely wasted are less than 70 percent of the reference; these children should usually be referred for intensive feeding. Those who are less than 80 or 85 percent of the W/H reference are considered eligible for SFP.

Data are usually collected on the nutritional status of preschool children (under 110 to 115 cm in height) as they are the most easily identified vulnerable group (Simmonds et al 1983). These data can help in estimating the extent and severity of malnutrition in the entire population and subsequent program planning. Care must be taken when interpreting the level of severe malnutrition in those under five years of age because a high mortality rate among this group may artificially reduce the estimated prevalence of malnutrition.

Weight loss that results from decreased nutritional intake is referred to as wasting, whereas a decline in the rate of increase in height is referred to as stunting. Negligible, or low, weight gain is referred to as growth faltering. Wasted children are at greater risk of death and infectious diseases than those with normal measurements due to impaired resistance (Brown 1977b). The prevalence of undernutrition is highest among children from the poorest families in the refugee population (Simmonds et al 1983).

In addition to anthropometric measurements, several physical signs are indicators of nutritional status. Pitting ankle edema is easily detected and is a sign of hypoalbuminemia. Severe pallor indicates anemia and can be detected by examination of the mucous membranes of the conjunctiva, mouth, nail beds, and palms. Night blindness is usually easy to detect and is early evidence of vitamin A deficiency.

Surveillance

Supplementary food programs have the additional objective of establishing procedures for ongoing surveillance of the nutritional status of the entire population. Periodic surveys are the most efficient method to determine the general nutritional status, to identify the most malnourished groups, and to monitor the effectiveness of the nutritional program (Miller et al 1977; Taylor 1983).

Once the decision to have an SFP is made, policy guidelines must be established by the planning committee as to who should be included in the program. The number of people in the SFP will be determined by both need and available resources. Groups eligible for admission to the SFP might include children under five years of age whose W/H is equal to or less than 80 percent of the reference, pregnant women, lactating mothers, patients with clinical illnesses such as tuberculosis, and, if resources permit, elderly individuals and those with clinical signs of undernutrition.

In general, SFPs are considered preventive programs, intended to keep the moderately malnourished group from becoming severely malnourished. In contrast, therapeutic feeding programs are strictly for life-saving and rehabilitation purposes and are directed toward the most severely malnourished individuals (see Chapter 14).

Survey Sample

When a community wide nutritional survey is undertaken, it is easier if a sample of children is selected for measurement. It is essential that a random and well-scattered sample be selected. A small cross-sectional study should include approximately 100 males and 100 females with both infants and one- to three-year-olds represented. If cluster sampling is employed, an inclusion of 30 clusters of seven children each will provide acceptably reliable measurements and estimates of nutritional status (Graitcer 1981). Either the MUAC or the W/H method permits rapid assessment of subjects (Simmonds et al 1983).

FOODS USED FOR SUPPLEMENTARY FEEDING PROGRAMS

Foods commonly used for SFPs include the following:

- Corn-soya milk (CSM). CSM provides 370 kcal and 20 g of protein per 100 g of the powdered form. CSM is prepared by mixing one part powder with two to three parts water, and cooking it for five to ten minutes. Usually, one-tenth part of sugar is added for taste and one-tenth part oil for additional calories. Instant corn-soya milk (ICSM) provides 380 kcal and 20 g of protein per 100 g of ICSM powder. ICSM is mixed in equal parts with hot water (since it is precooked and sweetened). Additional sugar and oil can be added if available.
- Wheat-soya blend (WSB). WSB provides 360 kcal and 20 g of protein per 100 g of WSB powder. WSB is prepared by mixing one part WSB powder with ten parts water, bringing it to a boil, and cooking it for five to ten minutes. Sugar is added for taste.
- Dried skim milk (DSM). DSM provides 35 g of protein per 100 g of powder and can be added to other food preparations as a protein complement. It is imperative that DSM be vitamin A enriched. DSM should usually not be reconstituted as milk, but it should be added to other foods in the powdered form.
- Fish protein concentrate (FPC). FPC is a high-protein source containing 65 g protein per 100 g FPC powder. FPC can be added to other foods.

OTHER CONSIDERATIONS FOR SUPPLEMENTARY FEEDING PROGRAMS

Although there are many similarities between refugee communities and stable communities in underdeveloped countries, certain important differences deserve attention (Dick & Simmonds 1983). Similarities may include crowded living conditions, inadequate water and sanitation facilities, and a high prevalence of malnutrition and infectious diseases. However, most reports indicate that refugees demonstrate quantitatively more severe health and nutrition problems, have fewer available resources, and usually have their food supplies controlled by others (Dick 1984).

A major focus of social interaction in any society involves the preparation and consumption of food. When control of food is taken away from refugees, social and cultural disruptions that can adversely affect health may occur. Serious consideration should therefore be given to reducing the refugees' complete dependence on others for food. This process might begin by modifying a strictly relief operation and seeking more development-oriented solutions for health, nutrition, and environmental problems (Simmonds 1984).

Supplementary feeding programs should include a system to identify individuals with the greatest nutritional needs. Even well-designed and operated SFPs, however, are often unable to provide for the most vulnerable (Taylor 1983; O'Sullivan et al 1980). Among alternative program designs might be the targeting of vulnerable families, instead of individuals, for SFPs. Another consideration might be to provide an increase in rations for all individuals identified as vulnerable, rather than institute a separate SFP. It can be argued that everyone in a refugee situation is vulnerable. However, because resources to care for refugees are always limited, some process of targeting additional food is needed.

PREVENTION OF MALNUTRITION

Clinical undernutrition is the result of many factors. SFPs represent only one aspect for improving overall nutritional status. Other important measures include public health programs, promotion of breastfeeding, provision of appropriate weaning foods, prevention of infectious and other diseases through primary health services, and health and nutrition education. To reduce refugee dependence, the nutrition planning group should transfer responsibility for decision making to the refugees and encourage development activities. Training refugees in primary health care activities such as ORT, immunization, early treatment of illnesses, surveillance, and monitoring, and assisting refugees to produce their own food, will result in improvement in the overall health status of the refugees.

Breastfeeding

Universal and prolonged breastfeeding is a major component in the prevention of malnutrition among infants and children. Iron deficiency is less common in breast-fed infants because iron is more efficiently absorbed from breast milk (Jelliffe & Jelliffe 1978). In addition, the protective effect of breast milk against various infections has been well-documented. Morbidity and mortality rates are lower for infants receiving breast milk than for those receiving artificial formula or other milk products (Jelliffe 1970). In most parts of the world where displaced persons are found, breastfeeding is considered essential for health; the infant who cannot be provided with breast milk is in serious jeopardy of malnutrition or recurrent, and fatal, gastroenteritis.

It is extremely important that every pregnant and lactating woman be adequately fed. It is far simpler, and less expensive, to provide a supplemented adult ration to properly nourish a lactating mother than it is to provide an artificial formula or weanling diet to an infant.

If a mother is seriously ill, dies in childbirth, or abandons her children, female relatives often assume breastfeeding the infant until weaning is possible (Brown 1977a). This process is relatively simple if the wetnurse has had a recent birth and is lactating adequately. However, even women who are not lactating can be induced to do so if they have the interest and motivation (Jelliffe & Jelliffe 1978; Brown 1977a). The requirements for relactation are the same as those for successful lactation, they include the following:

- An adequately nourished woman who is interested in nursing.
- A baby with a good sucking reflex.
- An emotional support system.

A woman may be healthy and wish to breastfeed, but may still encounter difficulty at the outset. The success of relactation often depends on a support network (husband, grandmother, a midwife or nurse, physician, a close friend or relative) for encouragement, instruction, assistance, and advice (Jelliffe & Jelliffe 1974).

Reports from many parts of the world describe the initiation of relactation in a nonlactating, nonpostpartum woman as merely putting the infant to the breast and allowing him or her to suckle (Newton 1970; Cohen 1971; Jelliffe & Jelliffe 1972). Suckling stimulates nerve endings that cause the anterior pituitary gland to produce prolactin. Prolactin acts directly on the breast to stimulate the production and secretion of milk. Suckling also stimulates the posterior pituitary gland, which causes the release of the hormone oxytocin. Oxytocin acts on the small muscle (myoepithelial) cells surrounding the milk-producing ducts. This action forces milk to the terminal ducts and is known as the "let down reflex," or the milk ejection reflex (Jelliffe & Jelliffe 1972).

A variety of chemicals have been used to promote relactation. For example, chlorpromazine has been a useful adjunct in the induction of lactation (Brown 1977a) when given in dosages as low as 25 mg three times a day for seven to ten days.

Weaning Foods

The process of weaning is the substitution of solid foods, or special infant foods, for breast milk. When an infant is gaining weight adequately, weaning should not be initiated until the age of approximately six months (Brown 1978). When an infant is not thriving, it is recommended that weaning foods be introduced at the time of growth faltering. The major problem associated with weaning in refugee camps is that there is a marked increase in the incidence of acute diarrheal diseases with associated debilitation, dehydration, and nutritional hazards that lead to death when food other than breast milk is given to infants. Weanling diarrhea is a well-documented phenomenon (Gordon et al 1963).

It is important to evaluate culturally related food habits for each population group. One should identify which foods are considered acceptable as weaning foods, and when selected foods are to be introduced into the infant's diet. These foods should be prepared under as sanitary conditions as possible.

Grinding facilities can play a vital role in the

preparation of weaning foods. Local staple foods, such as cereals and pulses, can be finely ground and served as porridge. Cups and spoons can be more easily cleaned than narrow-necked bottles and should be used to introduce weaning foods.

Feeding Problems

Breastfeeding should be continued during the weaning process and for as long as possible. Infants who develop diarrhea should neither be taken off the breast nor have their semisolid foods reduced, but should be given oral rehydration solution (ORS) (see Chapters 15 and 34). Locally prepared double mixes, triple mixes, and multimixes made of vegetable and animal proteins may represent the solution to weaning problems (Andersen 1976; Cameron & Hofvander 1983).

When an infant or child is too weak to accept the foods offered, a nasogastric tube can be used to provide liquid feeding or ORS. If available, packets of ORS can be reconstituted with clean water (Hirschhorn 1980). If commercially prepared packets are not available, health workers and parents can easily be taught how to prepare a home mixture. ORS should be given in addition to their regular diet to infants or children with frequent watery stools. Gastroenteritis, in conjunction with moderate or severe malnutrition, is extremely dangerous for the young child (Chen & Scrimshaw 1983). If diarrhea continues, or if food and ORS are not well-tolerated, early referral to the medical backup team is essential.

When anemia is widespread, as documented by a high prevalence of severe pallor, a tablet or liquid form of supplemental iron should be provided weekly or biweekly to children attending the SFP. Malaria and intestinal parasites should also be considered in conjunction with anemia. If malaria is highly endemic (see Chapter 25), chloroquine prophylaxis can be introduced as part of the SFP for young children and pregnant women.

If vitamin A deficiency is prevalent (see Chapter 18), distribution of vitamin A or multivitamin capsules should be considered. Xerophthalmia is often associated with the risk of blindness among refugee children, particularly if measles exists in the community. As a prophylactic measure, a massive dose of vitamin A (200,000 IU for children one to five years of age; 100,000 IU to infants less than one year of age) should be adminstered every six months. In communities where foods rich in vitamin A are not part of the diet, a prophylactic dose of vitamin A should be administered to all children every three months (Helen Keller International 1985).

Refugees often have a lowered resistance to certain communicable diseases. Mass immunization programs may be coordinated with SFP or other feeding programs. All of the recommended interventions can be easily administered if logistics are carefully planned, trained personnel are available, and regular supply shipments can be arranged. In general, the interventions recommended are relatively inexpensive and cost-effective in the long run.

REFERENCES AND SUGGESTED READING

Anderson MA, Grewal T: Nutrition Planning in the Developing World. New York, CARE, 1976.
Beaton GH, Bengoa JM, (eds): Nutrition in Preventive Medicine. Geneva, World Health Organization, 1976.
Brown RE: Some nutritional considerations in times of major catastrophe. Clin Pediatr 1972;11:334.
Brown RE: Group feeding in normal and emergency situations. In McLaren D (ed): Nutrition in the Community. New York, John Wiley & Sons, 1976.
Brown RE: Relactation: An overview. Pediatrics 1977a;60:116.
Brown RE: Interaction of nutrition and infection in clinical practice. Pediatr Clin North Am 1977b;24:241.
Brown RE: Weaning foods in developing countries. Am J Clin Nutrit 1978;31:2066.
Cameron M, Hofvander Y: Manual on Feeding Infants and Young Children. Oxford, Oxford University Press, 1983.
Chen LC, Scrimshaw NS (eds): Diarrhea and Malnutrition: Interactions, Mechanisms, and Interventions. New York, Plenum Press, 1983.
Christensen H: Survival Strategies for and by Camp Refugees. Geneva, UN Research Institute for Social Development, 1982.
Cohen R: Breastfeeding without pregnancy. Pediatrics 1971;48:996.
Devadas RP, Kamalanathan G, Kandiah M, Kupputhai, U: Studies on special nutrition programme III "Spot feeding" vs. "Take home feeding." Indian J Nutrit Dietetics 1977;14:193.
de Ville de Goyet C, Lechat MF: Priorities in health activities in refugee camps. Rev Epidemiol Sante Publique 1977;25:99.

de Ville de Goyet, Seaman J, Geijer U: The Management of Nutritional Emergencies in Large Populations. Geneva, World Health Organization, 1978.
Dick B, Simmonds S: Refugee health care—Similar but different? Disasters 1983;7:291.
Dick B: Diseases of refugees—Causes, effects, and controls. Trans Roy Soc Trop Med Hyg 1984;78:734.
FAO/WHO: Handbook on Human Nutritional Requirements. FAO Nutrition Studies No 28; WHO Monograph Series No 61, Geneva, World Health Organization, 1974.
Gordon JE, Chitkara ID, Wyon JB: Weanling diarrhea. Am J Med Sci 1963;245:345.
Graitcer PL: A Manual for the Basic Assessment of Nutritional Status in Potential Crisis Situations. Atlanta, Centers for Disease Control, 1981.
Helen Keller International Inc.: Report of Vitamin A Deficiency in Ethiopian Children. New York, Helen Keller International, 1985.
Henderson PL, Biellik RJ: Comparative nutrition and health services for victims and drought and hostilities in the Ogaden, Somalia, and Ethiopia 1980–1981. Int J Health Serv 1983;13:289.
Hirschhorn N: The treatment of acute diarrhoea in children: A historical and physiological perspective. Am J Clin Nutrit 1980;33:637.
Jelliffe DB: Diarrhoeal disease of early childhood. In Woodruff A. W. (ed): Alimentary and Haematological Aspects of Tropical Disease. London, Edward Arnold Ltd, 1970.
Jelliffe DB, Jelliffe EFP: Nonpuerperal induced lactation. Pediatrics 1972;50:171.
Jelliffe DB, Jelliffe EFP: Confidence and the science of lactation. J Pediatr 1974;84:762.
Jelliffe DB, Jelliffe EFP: Human Milk in the Modern World. Oxford, Oxford University Press, 1978.
Magan AM, Warsame M et al: An outbreak of scurvy in Somali refugee camps. Disasters 1983;17:2.
McNeilly AS, Thorner MO, Volans G et al: Metoclopramide and prolactin. Br Med J 1974;2:729.
Miller DC, Nichaman MZ, Lane JM: Simplified field assessment of nutritional status in early childhood: Practical suggestions for developing countries. Bull WHO 1977;55:79.
Nabarro D, McNab S: A simple new technique for identifying thin children. J Trop Med Hyg 1980;83:21.
Newton M: Breastfeeding by adoptive mothers. JAMA 1970;212:1967.
Nieberg P, Allegra DT: Emergency refugee health care: A chronicle of experience in Khmer assistance operation, 1979–1980. Epilogue 1985;187.
O'Sullivan G, Ebrahim S, O'Sullivan J et al: Nutritional status of Laotian refugee children in Ubon Camp, Thailand. J Epidem Cummun Health 1980;34:83.
OXFAM Health Unit: OXFAM's Practical Guide to Selective Feeding Programmes. OXFAM's Practical Guide No 1, Oxford, OXFAM, 1984. Based on Peel S (revised by Lusty T, Diskett P): Selective Feeding Procedures. Oxford, OXFAM, 1977.
Protein-Calorie Advisory Group of the UN: A Guide to Food and Health Relief Operations for Disasters. New York, United Nations, 1977.
Simmonds S, Gabaudan M: Refugee Camp Health Care: Selected Annotated References. Ross Institute Publication No 14, London, London School of Trop Med & Hyg, 1982.
Simmonds SP: Refugees, health, and development. Trans Roy Soc Trop Med Hyg 1984;78:726.
Simmonds SP, Vaughan P, Gunn SW (eds): Refugee Community Health Care. Oxford, Oxford University Press, 1983.
Taylor WR: An evaluation of supplementary feeding in Somali refugee camps. Int J Epidemiol 1983;12:433.
United Nations High Commissioner for Refugees: Handbook for Emergencies, Part I: Field Operations. Geneva, United Nations High Commissioner for Refugees, 1982.
Waterlow JC, Buzina R, Keller W et al: The presentation and use of height and weight data for comparing the nutritional status of groups of children under the age of 10 years. Bull WHO, 1977;55:489.
World Health Organization: Guidelines for Training Community Health Workers in Nutrition. WHO Publication No 59, Geneva, World Health Organization, 1981.
World Health Organization: The Treatment and Management of Severe Protein-Energy Malnutrition. Geneva, World Health Organization, 1981.

14

Diagnosis and Treatment of Severe Malnutrition

RICHARD H. SANDLER,
WILLIAM C. MACLEAN, JR.

Malnutrition, directly or indirectly, is often the major cause of childhood death in acute care refugee situations. Presently in the Sudan, acute malnutrition in emergency camps (less than 80% of standard weight for height) is found in 14 to 52 percent of all refugee children (Berry 1985). In some underdeveloped nations, four out of five young children have some degree of malnutrition, the majority becoming undernourished during weaning from breastmilk. A 1973 study in Latin America found malnutrition to be fully or partially responsible for 57 percent of childhood deaths, while 30 percent died directly from diarrheal illnesses. Measles, pnuemonia, malaria, tuberculosis, and other common childhood illnesses often become killers in the face of malnutrition. Malnutrition early in life can lead to later learning disability (Galler et al 1984).

The direct cause of malnutrition is often poor calorie or protein intake, or both. Infection can also help push a child into a malnourished state by increasing calorie and nitrogen demands. It should be kept in mind, however, that the underlying causes of malnutrition often are not medical but economic, social, and political (Allegra et al 1984; Sen 1981; Brown & Brown 1979).

Classically, two types of severe malnutrition have been described. Marasmus results from inadequate calorie intake, whereas kwashiorkor (KW) is produced by severe protein deficiency. Most patients have some combination of both disorders, therefore, the term "protein energy malnutrition" (PEM) is now generally used.

DIAGNOSIS OF MALNUTRITION

Anthropometric measurements have the advantages of economy, speed, safety, and simplicity appropriate for application by unskilled (but supervised) workers. The edema of KW, however, increases the weight somewhat and leads to underdiagnosis of malnutrition if weight and height are the only variables considered. Therefore, anthropometric measurements, history, physical examination, and laboratory determinations should all be used to help make the diagnosis of malnutrition because greater accuracy results from the combination of data.

The precise criteria to use for diagnosing malnutrition are in dispute (Waterlow 1976; Jelliffe 1966). Table 14-1 summarizes several major anthropometric criteria.

A distinction must be made between "stunting" and "wasting." Stunting refers to a decreased height for age; it is related to chronic marginal undernutrition. Repeated short episodes of PEM with limited catchup growth can also cause stunting. Short periods of PEM can often be compensated for by catchup growth if adequate health and nutrition are present subsequently. Short stature at the time of examination does not necessarily indicate present malnutrition; the child may be growing well when examined, but simply have failed to catch up with his or her reference height. Stunting is seldom seen in infants; when present, it is more likely due to small size at birth than to current PEM. Wasting is diagnosed by finding a decreased weight for height (and decreased weight for age if the height is not proportionately decreased). The presence of wasting suggests acute malnutrition and requires more urgent intervention.

Marasmus occurs most frequently in infants and young toddlers. It is characterized by growth retardation and wasting of muscle and subcutaneous fat, with retention of mental alertness and appetite. The patient often appears anxious. The face looks like that of an old man or woman. The skin has a loose, "baggy pants" appearance. The muscles are

Table 14-1. Methods of Grading PEM Severity

Author	Index	"Normal"	Mild PEM	Moderate PEM	Severe PEM
Gomez et al	Weight for age	100–90[a]	90–75	75–60	60
McLaren & Reed	Weight for height/ age index	110–90[a]	90–85	85–75	75
Kanawati & McLaren	Arm circumference/ head circumference	0.31	0.31–0.28	0.28–0.25	0.25
Waterlow	Height for age	95[a]	95–90	90–85	85
	Weight for height	90[a]	90–80	80–70	70

[a]Percentage of Harvard mean reference values.

(Adapted with permission from Waterlow J C: Classification and definition of protein-energy malnutrition. In Beaton G H, Bengoa J M (eds): Nutrition in Preventive Medicine, p 549. Geneva, World Health Organization, 1976.)

markedly wasted, a sign easily noticeable in the arms, thighs, and buttocks. The patient has no edema or changes in hair color.

Kwashiorkor (KW) occurs most often in older toddlers. In under-developed nations, the incidence peaks a few months after breast-feeding has stopped (at about 18 months of age). There is not complete agreement on the criteria to be used for the diagnosis of KW, but the presence of edema is agreed on by most experts. The edema results from decreased intravascular oncotic pressure, which is caused by hypoalbuminemia. (The edema causes some children to appear less malnourished than they are.) Appearing first in the lower extremities, the edema extends to include the face (causing moon facies), abdomen, and other extremities

Poor appetite with apathy, lethargy, or irritability are often present with KW. Hyperpigmented skin changes occur in areas of irritation (e.g., extensor surfaces of the forearms), followed by a "flaky paint" desquamation and dyspigmentation of the skin. This may progress to a thickened "enamel paint" dermatosis, which peels to leave raw, weeping skin. The hair is often sparse and thin and, if naturally curly, may become straight. In dark-skinned patients, the hair color can change to streaky red or grayish blond. McLaren and co-workers (1967) reported their experience that, for patients with albumin levels below 2 g/dl, 100 percent had edema, 88 percent had hair changes, 76 percent had hepatomegaly, and 52 percent had dermatosis.

Anthropometric Measurements

Anthropometric measurements are probably the most important parameters used to make the diagnosis of PEM, and many different approaches have been used. Length is not a reliable indicator of malnutrition in infants under one year of age. The weight for age method is useful in very small children if scales are available and ages are known (Table 14-2). Although ages are often unknown in underdeveloped countries, an events calendar (Table 14-3) can be used to help discern the age. Another method is to estimate dental age. For example, children with 6 to 18 teeth are in their second dental year (Jelliffe & Jelliffe 1969).

When scales are available, weight for height is the most sensitive method of determining PEM in children over one year of age. Given a child's weight and height, the degree of malnutrition can be determined (Table 14-4).

For the one- to 5-year-old children under 110 cm tall, measurement of the midportion of the upper arm circumference (MUAC) can be used as an indicator of PEM. Muscle and liver tissue lose up to 50 percent of their protein mass in severe PEM. The upper arm (since it is less affected by edema) more accurately reflects this mass change than the lower extremity. The upper arm measurement is relatively constant at a mean value of 16.5 cm from ages one to five years and increases only about 2 percent a year. (Most of these data are based on measurement of the MUAC of the left arm.) A value of 12.5 to 13.5 cm suggests mild to moderate PEM, while less than 12.5 cm usually suggests severe PEM (Cameron & Hafvander 1983). It should be noted that strict comparisons between MUAC and other anthropometric measurements, such as weight for height, must be made with caution. For example, moderate malnutrition was found to correspond to MUAC of less than 12.5 cm and

Table 14-2. Percentage of Reference Weight-for- Age in Kilograms[a]

Age (months)	60%	75%	90%	100%	Age (months)	60%	75%	90%	100%
0	1.9	2.4	2.9	3.2	52	10.1	12.7	15.2	16.9
1	2.5	3.1	3.7	4.1	53	10.3	12.8	15.4	17.1
2	2.9	3.7	4.4	4.9	54	10.3	12.9	15.5	17.2
3	3.4	4.3	5.1	5.7	55	10.4	13.1	15.7	17.4
4	3.8	4.8	5.8	6.4	56	10.6	13.2	15.8	17.6
5	4.2	5.3	6.3	7.0	57	10.6	13.3	15.9	17.7
6	4.5	5.6	6.8	7.5	58	10.7	13.4	16.1	17.9
7	4.8	6.0	7.2	8.0	59	10.8	13.5	16.2	18.0
8	5.1	6.4	7.7	8.5	60	10.9	13.7	16.4	18.2
9	5.3	6.7	8.0	8.9	61	11.0	13.7	16.5	18.3
10	5.5	6.9	8.3	9.2	62	11.1	13.9	16.7	18.5
11	5.8	7.2	8.6	9.6	63	11.2	14.0	16.7	18.6
12	5.9	7.4	8.8	9.8	64	11.3	14.1	16.9	18.8
13	6.1	7.6	9.1	10.1	65	11.4	14.3	17.1	19.0
14	6.2	7.7	9.3	10.3	66	11.5	14.3	17.2	19.1
15	6.4	8.0	9.5	10.6	67	11.6	14.5	17.4	19.3
16	6.5	8.1	9.7	10.8	68	11.6	14.6	17.5	19.4
17	6.6	8.3	9.9	11.0	69	11.8	14.7	17.6	19.6
18	6.7	8.3	10.0	11.1	70	11.9	14.9	17.8	19.8
19	6.8	8.5	10.2	11.3	71	11.9	14.9	17.9	19.9
20	6.9	8.6	10.4	11.5	72	12.1	15.1	18.1	20.1
21	7.0	8.8	10.5	11.7	73	12.2	15.2	18.3	20.3
22	7.1	8.9	10.7	11.9	74	12.3	15.4	18.5	20.5
23	7.3	9.1	10.9	12.1	75	12.4	15.5	18.5	20.6
24	7.3	9.1	10.9	12.1	76	12.5	15.6	18.7	20.8
25	7.4	9.2	11.1	12.3	77	12.6	15.8	18.9	21.0
26	7.5	9.4	11.3	12.5	78	12.7	15.8	19.1	21.2
27	7.6	9.5	11.4	12.7	79	12.8	16.1	19.3	21.4
28	7.7	9.7	11.6	12.9	80	13.0	16.2	19.4	21.6
29	7.9	9.8	11.8	13.1	81	13.0	16.3	19.5	21.7
30	8.0	10.0	12.0	13.3	82	13.1	16.4	19.7	21.9
31	8.1	10.1	12.2	13.5	83	13.3	16.6	19.9	22.1
32	8.2	10.2	12.2	13.6	84	13.4	16.7	20.1	22.3
33	8.3	10.4	12.4	13.8	85	13.6	17.0	20.3	22.6
34	8.4	10.5	12.6	14.0	86	13.7	17.1	20.5	22.8
35	8.5	10.7	12.8	14.2	87	13.8	17.3	20.7	23.0
36	8.6	10.8	13.0	14.4	88	13.9	17.4	20.9	23.2
37	8.7	10.9	13.1	14.5	89	14.0	17.6	21.1	23.4
38	8.8	11.0	13.2	14.7	90	14.2	17.7	21.2	23.6
39	8.9	11.2	13.4	14.9	91	14.3	17.9	21.5	23.9
40	9.0	11.3	13.5	15.0	92	14.5	18.1	21.7	24.1
41	9.1	11.4	13.7	15.2	93	14.6	18.2	21.9	24.3
42	9.2	11.6	13.9	15.4	94	14.8	18.5	22.1	24.6
43	9.3	11.6	14.0	15.5	95	14.9	18.6	22.3	24.8
44	9.4	11.8	14.1	15.7	96	15.1	18.8	22.6	25.1
45	9.5	11.9	14.3	15.9	97	15.2	19.0	22.8	25.3
46	9.6	12.0	14.4	16.0	98	15.4	19.2	23.0	25.6
47	9.7	12.2	14.6	16.2	99	15.5	19.4	23.2	25.8
48	9.8	12.2	14.7	16.3	100	15.7	19.6	23.5	26.1
49	9.9	12.4	14.9	16.5	101	15.8	19.8	23.8	26.4
50	10.0	12.5	14.9	16.6	102	16.0	20.0	23.9	26.6
51	10.1	12.6	15.1	16.8	103	16.1	20.2	24.2	26.9

Table 14-2. Percentage of Reference Weight-for-Age in Kilograms[a] (*Continued*)

Age (months)	60%	75%	90%	100%
104	16.3	20.4	24.5	27.2
105	16.4	20.6	24.7	27.4
106	16.6	20.8	24.9	27.7
107	16.8	21.0	25.2	28.0
108	17.0	21.2	25.5	28.3
109	17.2	21.5	25.7	28.6
110	17.3	21.7	26.0	28.9
111	17.5	21.9	26.3	29.2
112	17.7	22.1	26.6	29.5
113	17.9	22.4	26.8	29.8
114	18.1	22.6	27.1	30.1
115	18.2	22.8	27.4	30.4
116	18.4	23.0	27.6	30.7
117	18.6	23.3	27.9	31.0
118	18.8	23.5	28.2	31.3
119	19.0	23.8	28.5	31.7

[a]Prepared using sex averaged data from: Normalized NCHS/CDC Anthropometric Reference. Atlanta, Georgia, Centers for Disease Control, 1980.

(Adapted with permission from Simmonds S, Vaughan P, Gunn S W (eds): Refugee Community Health Care, pp 313–16. Oxford, Oxford Unversity press, 1983.)

severe malnutrition to less than 11 cm among Ethiopian refugees in Sudan (Berry 1975); hence, a history of prolonged and chronic malnutrition may lower the MUAC cutoff criteria for malnutrition. Arnhold (1969) and Davis (1971) increased the accuracy of the MUAC measurement by assessing arm circumference in relation to height. Table 14-5 shows how to construct and use the measuring stick.

Although less reliable than weight for height determinations, and not as useful for gauging the progress of an individual child once refeeding has begun, the MUAC method has some advantages: untrained health workers can learn to use the method easily; it can be used as a rapid screening assessment and outreach by home visitors; the age does not have to be known; and a scale for measuring the weight is not needed. MUAC measuring tapes can be made easily by coloring plastic strips.

Chest-to-head circumference ratio and skin fold thickness are two other methods that have been used for malnutrition screening. Currently, there is insufficient research on their use, and it appears that the methods mentioned previously are more sensitive for early detection of malnutrition.

It has been noted that young children of any race born anywhere in the world have about the same ratio of weight to height if nutrition and environmental stimulation are supplied equally and infection and stresses are controlled (Cameron & Hofvander 1983). Because these factors are not always controlled equally, modifications of these standards have sometimes been made (Olness et al 1984). For purposes of intercamp and intracamp comparison, however, it is recommended that the U.S. National Center for Health Statistics/WHO standards always be used.

Workup of the Patient with Protein Energy Malnutrition

The workup of patients with malnutrition should include a history, physical examination, and appropriate laboratory determinations when these are available (Table 14-6). Besides anemia and hypoalbuminemia, total lymphocyte count is a useful and easily obtained laboratory measure of malnutrition (Walker & Hendricks 1985). The total lympho-

Table 14-3. Sample Calendar of Local Events[a]

Month	Event
January	Harvest maize
February	Harvest groundnuts School children on holiday
March	Harvest beans
April	Eat flying ants
May	Rains end
June	Eat green maize Independence Day
July	Mango trees bloom School holidays
August	Rains begin
September	Plant maize, beans, groundnuts Start of school year
October	Flight of butterflies
November	Gather and eat caterpillars
December	Christmas month

[a]Movable festivals such as religious feasts, and other well-known events such as visits by politicians, the opening of new buildings, or fires or epidemics, should be inserted for a particular year.

(Reprinted with permission from Cameron M, Hofvander Y: Manual on Feeding Infants and Young Children, p 11. New York, Oxford University Press, 1983.)

Table 14-4. Percentage of Reference Weight-for-Height (Sexes Averaged) in Kilograms[a]

Height (cm)	50%	60%	70%	80%	90%	100%	110%
55	2.3	2.8	3.2	3.7	4.1	4.6	5.1
56	2.4	2.9	3.4	3.8	4.3	4.8	5.3
57	2.6	3.1	3.6	4.1	4.6	5.1	5.6
58	2.7	3.2	3.8	4.3	4.9	5.4	5.9
59	2.8	3.4	3.9	4.5	5.0	5.6	6.2
60	3.0	3.1	4.1	4.7	5.3	5.9	6.5
61	3.1	3.7	4.3	5.0	5.6	6.2	6.8
62	3.3	3.9	4.6	5.2	5.9	6.5	7.2
63	3.4	4.1	4.8	5.4	6.1	6.8	7.5
64	3.6	4.3	5.0	5.7	6.4	7.1	7.8
65	3.7	4.4	5.2	5.9	6.7	7.4	8.1
66	3.8	4.6	5.4	6.2	6.9	7.7	8.5
67	4.0	4.8	5.6	6.4	7.2	8.0	8.8
68	4.1	4.9	5.7	6.6	7.4	8.2	9.0
69	4.3	5.1	6.0	6.8	7.7	8.5	9.4
70	4.4	5.2	6.1	7.0	7.8	8.7	9.6
71	4.5	5.3	6.2	7.1	8.0	8.9	9.8
72	4.6	5.5	6.4	7.4	8.3	9.2	10.1
73	4.7	5.6	6.6	7.5	8.5	9.4	10.3
74	4.8	5.8	6.7	7.7	8.6	9.6	10.6
75	4.9	5.9	6.9	7.8	8.8	9.8	10.8
76	5.0	6.0	7.0	8.0	9.0	10.0	11.0
77	5.2	6.2	7.2	8.2	9.3	10.3	11.3
78	5.3	6.3	7.4	8.4	9.5	10.5	11.6
79	5.4	6.4	7.5	8.6	9.6	10.7	11.8
80	5.5	6.5	7.6	8.7	9.8	10.9	12.0
81	5.6	6.7	7.8	8.9	10.0	11.1	12.2
82	5.7	6.8	7.9	9.0	10.2	11.3	12.4
83	5.8	6.9	8.1	9.2	10.4	11.5	12.7
84	5.9	7.1	8.3	9.4	10.6	11.8	13.0
85	6.0	7.2	8.4	9.6	10.8	12.0	13.2
86	6.1	7.3	8.5	9.8	11.0	12.2	13.4
87	6.2	7.4	8.7	9.9	11.2	12.4	13.6
88	6.3	7.6	8.8	10.1	11.3	12.6	13.9
89	6.4	7.7	9.0	10.3	11.6	12.9	14.2
90	6.5	7.9	9.2	10.5	11.8	13.1	14.4
91	6.6	8.0	9.3	10.6	12.0	13.3	14.6
92	6.8	8.2	9.5	10.9	12.2	13.6	15.0
93	6.9	8.3	9.7	11.0	12.4	13.8	15.2
94	7.0	8.4	9.8	11.2	12.6	14.0	15.4
95	7.2	8.6	10.0	11.4	12.9	14.3	15.7
96	7.3	8.7	10.2	11.6	13.1	14.5	16.0
97	7.4	8.9	10.4	11.8	13.3	14.8	16.3
98	7.5	9.0	10.5	12.0	13.5	15.0	16.5
99	7.7	9.2	10.7	12.2	13.8	15.3	16.8
100	7.8	9.4	10.9	12.5	14.0	15.6	17.2
101	7.9	9.5	11.1	12.6	14.2	15.8	17.4
102	8.1	9.7	11.3	12.9	14.5	16.1	17.1
103	8.2	9.8	11.5	13.1	14.8	16.4	18.0
104	8.4	10.0	11.7	13.4	15.0	16.7	18.4
105	8.5	10.1	11.8	13.5	15.2	16.9	18.6
106	8.6	10.3	12.0	13.8	15.5	17.2	18.9
107	8.8	10.5	12.3	14.0	15.8	17.5	19.3
108	8.9	10.7	12.5	14.2	16.0	17.8	19.6

Table 14-4. Percentage of Reference Weight-for-Height (Sexes Averaged) in Kilograms[a] (*Continued*)

Height (cm)	50%	60%	70%	80%	90%	100%	110%
109	9.1	10.9	12.7	14.5	16.3	18.1	19.9
110	9.2	11.0	12.9	14.7	16.6	18.4	20.2
111	9.4	11.3	13.2	15.0	16.9	18.8	20.7
112	9.6	11.5	13.4	15.3	17.2	19.1	21.0
113	9.7	11.6	13.6	15.5	17.5	19.4	21.3
114	9.9	11.9	13.9	15.8	17.8	19.8	21.8
115	10.1	12.1	14.1	16.1	18.8	20.1	22.1
116	10.3	12.3	14.4	16.4	18.5	20.5	22.6
117	10.4	12.5	14.6	16.6	18.7	20.8	22.9
118	10.6	12.7	14.8	17.0	19.1	21.2	23.3
119	10.8	13.0	15.1	17.3	19.4	21.6	23.8
120	11.0	13.2	15.4	17.6	19.8	22.0	24.2
121	11.2	13.4	15.7	17.9	20.2	22.4	24.6
122	11.4	13.7	16.0	18.2	20.5	22.8	25.1
123	11.7	14.0	16.3	18.6	21.0	23.3	25.6
124	11.9	14.2	16.6	19.0	21.3	23.7	25.3
125	12.1	14.5	16.9	19.4	21.8	24.2	26.6
126	12.4	14.8	17.3	20.0	22.2	24.7	27.2
127	12.6	15.1	17.6	20.2	22.7	25.2	27.7
128	12.9	15.4	18.0	20.6	23.1	25.7	28.3
129	13.1	15.7	18.3	21.0	23.6	26.2	28.8
130	13.4	16.1	18.8	21.4	24.1	26.8	29.5
131	13.7	16.4	19.2	22.0	24.7	27.4	30.1
132	14.0	16.7	19.5	22.3	25.1	27.9	30.7
133	14.3	17.2	20.0	22.9	25.7	28.6	31.5
134	14.6	17.5	20.4	23.4	26.3	29.2	32.1
135	14.9	17.9	21.0	23.8	26.8	29.8	32.8
136	15.3	18.3	21.4	24.4	27.5	30.5	33.6
137	15.6	18.7	21.8	25.0	28.1	31.2	34.3

[a]Prepared using sex averaged data from: Normalized NCHS/CDC Anthropometric Reference. Atlanta, Georgia, Centers for Disease Control, 1980.

(Adapted with permission from Simmonds S, Vaughan P, Gunn, SW (eds): Refugee Community Health Care, pp 309–10. Oxford, Oxford University Press, 1983.)

Table 14-5a. Preparation and Use of the QUAC (Quaker Upper Arm Circumference) Stick for Rapid PEM Detection Using Height and Arm Circumference

To Make the Stick	To Use the Stick
Obtain a straight stick about 140 cm long and 4 cm wide. Plane a flat surface. Tape a centimeter rule to the stick so that it will not move during marking. Mark off two columns of numbers. Use a black pen on the left and a red pen on the right. Measuring from the bottom, mark a line at each level up from the ground, as indicated in Table 14-5b. At each line, write in the proper arm circumference value indicated in Table 14-5b.	The finished stick shows the correlation between centimeters of height and the arm circumference values at which PEM can be diagnosed. With the child standing straight against the stick, measure the mid-upper-arm circumference. Find this measured number on the stick. If the child's height is above the line next to his or her arm circumference, then moderate (black line) or severe (red line) PEM can be diagnosed.

Table 14-5b. QUAC Stick Height/Arm Circumference Values

Location from Bottom of Stick (in cm)	Black Scale (85% of standard)	Location from Bottom of Stick (in cm)	Red Scale (80% of standard)
70	13.25	70	12.2
78	13.5	80	12.75
89	13.75	90	13.0
96	14.0	98	13.25
101	14.25	103	13.5
105	14.5	107.5	13.75
108.5	14.75	110	14.0
112	15	113.5	14.25
117.5	15.5	116	14.5
122	16	118.5	14.75
126	16.5	121	15.0
129	17	125	15.5
132	17.5	129	16

(Table 14-5 adapted with permission from Davis LE: Epidemiology of famine in the Nigerian crisis: Rapid evaluation of malnutrition by height and arm circumference in large populations. Am J Clin Nutr 1971;24:358.)

cyte count (TLC) can be calculated from the formula

$$TLC = \frac{\% \text{ Lymphocytes} \times WBC}{100}$$

where WBC is the total number of white blood cells per deciliter. The normal TLC is over 1500; a TLC under 1000 suggests significant malnutrition.

An identification bracelet with name and registration number should be placed on the wrist or ankle of each child for easy identification. A record card should be kept for each patient, noting initial weight and height, daily weight and temperature, changes of symptoms and signs, laboratory results, a problem list, and treatments. Flowsheets should be maintained for both nutritional orders (Table 14-7) and charting daily intake and output (ideally noting the character and weight of the stools, not just the number).

The parent or guardian should be fully apprised of the child's problems and necessary treatment. Teaching that "food is medicine" will encourage compliance and help reduce the risk of relapse after discharge.

TREATMENT OF SEVERE MALNUTRITION IN A FIELD HOSPITAL

The mortality rate for severe PEM is high. The most common causes of death are fluid and electrolyte imbalance, infection (including measles), hypoglycemia, hypothermia, and congestive heart failure. Knowledge of these hazards will avert many unnecessary deaths.

Initial Priorities of Treatment

The overall brittleness of malnourished children must be emphasized. Interventions should be taken cautiously to help avoid the high mortality too often experienced in the first 24 to 48 hours after treatment is initiated. In the acute situation, treatment of severe dehydration, hypoglycemia,and hypothermia are the most urgent priorities. Provision of energy foods and proteins is next. Also a high priority is treatment of infections, anemia, and vitamin deficiencies. Measles vaccine should be administered as soon as possible because severely malnourished children are at high risk of dying from this disease (see Chapters 6 and 27). Early administration of vitamin A is essential because of the rapidity with which deficiency can cause irreversible damage (see Chapter 18).

Children with KW have increased total body water (TBW), which normalizes with refeeding. Marasmic children have a normal TBW unless they have diarrhea (Picou 1981). Mild to moderate dehydration from diarrhea can be treated with oral rehydration therapy (ORT), as discussed in Chapter 15. Those with severe dehydration may need (cautious) parenteral fluids initially, but can soon be switched to oral therapy. Usually, oral fluids are administered alone for no longer than 12 to 24 hours. Longer

Table 14-6. Key Elements in the Workup of PEM

I. History:
- Diet history to gauge type and severity of malnutrition
- Questions to help gauge hydration and electrolyte status (see Chapter 15)
- System-by-system questions about recent infectious diseases (especially TB) exposure and symptoms of infection
- Questions about night blindness and other specific deficiency syndromes
- Symptoms of congestive heart failure

II. Physical examination:
- Height, weight, and mid-upper-arm circumference. Weight should be measured daily until clear progress is made, then once each week.
- Temperature, pulse, respirations, and blood pressure
- Careful search for signs of infection (including otoscopic exam)
- Conjunctival and skin pallor should be noted, suggesting anemia
- Signs of vitamin deficiency diseases should be looked for

III. Laboratory tests:
- High priority
  - Blood sugar (e.g., by "Dextrostix" finger prick)
  - Potassium, sodium, and other electrolytes if available
  - Hematocrit and/or hemoglobin, with microscopic red blood cell morphology if low
  - Malaria smears
  - Urinalysis
  - Sputum (or gastric washings for those too young to cough effectively) and pus for AFB
  - Sputum and pus for Gram's stains (and cultures if available)
- Second priority
  - White blood cell count with differential (including calculation of total lymphocyte count)
  - Serum albumin and/or total protein
  - Stool for ova and parasites
  - TB skin testing (Note: these can be negative in active infection due to anergy and malnutrition; see Chapter 33.)
  - Chest x-ray (if available and indicated)
  - Stool for pH and reducing substances
- Helpful if available
  - Blood and other cultures if indicated
  - Blood urea nitrogen
  - Serum creatinine
  - Liver enzymes
  - Prothrombin time as an index of liver function (abnormalities are treatable with vitamin K)
  - Magnesium and calcium levels

use only worsens the nutritional status of PEM patients because oral rehydration solution has no protein and few calories (150 ml/kg/day of ORS provides only 12 kcal/kg/day).

Hypoglycemia is often present in severely malnourished patients, especially those with KW. The clinical signs, though nonspecific, include irritability, lethargy, pulse rate elevation or depression, hypothermia, and apnea in infants. A dipstick glucose determination (e.g., Dextrostix) can be checked if available, or a therapeutic trial of glucose can be given. Oral therapy will usually suffice even if diarrhea is present. The WHO ORS solution alone, which supplies only 2 g of carbohydrate per 100 ml, is not optimal therapy for acute hypoglycemia, but additional sugar can be added. Approximately four teaspoons of table sugar per 100 ml yield a 20 percent carbohydrate solution with 10 percent dextrose. If the child is hypo-

Table 14-7. Sample Form for Writing Diet Orders

Date	Formula	Formula strength	Frequency of Feeds	Route (PO or NG)	ml/feed	kcal/kg/day	ml/kg/day	No. of Stools per Day	Stool Volume & Character	Emesis	Comments

tensive or "shocky," an intravenous glucose solution is used because intestinal absorption is poor and rapid expansion of intravascular volume is needed. The intravenous dose is 200 mg/kg of glucose. For example, 2 ml/kg of 10 percent dextrose solution can be given. If the hypoglycemia is so severe that the child is convulsing, 500 to 1000 mg/kg IV of dextrose (2–4 ml/kg of D25W) is given.

The incidence of hypothermia may be very high in children with PEM, especially during the first two or three nights of hospitalization. It can occur even with comfortably warm ambient temperatures. For example, Brenton and co-workers (1967) reported that in Uganda, with lowest daily temperatures between 16 and 18°C (61 to 65°F), 38 percent (23/60) of the malnourished children overall, and 47 percent (21/45) of those children with KW, experienced at least one episode of hypothermia after admission. The best therapeutic intervention is prevention by using blankets and by encouraging parents to sleep close to their children.

Infection is an ever-present risk in the patient with PEM (Scrimshaw et al 1968: Scrimshaw 1981). Although this is an area of dispute, it seems more sensible not to use prophylactic antibiotics (MacLean et al 1980). Overgrowth of resistant organisms, diarrhea, confusion over whether fever is secondary to treatment failure or a drug reaction, and future difficulty in obtaining cultures are some of the complications of prophylactic antibiotic therapy.

In looking for infections, a careful history and physical examination are most important. Upper respiratory tract infections, otitis media, and bacterial pneumonia are the most common illnesses. In endemic areas, malaria should be ruled out with several malaria smears, and prophylaxis should be started. A high level of suspicion should be maintained for tuberculosis (TB), especially miliary and meningitic tuberculosis, because TB is common in PEM patients (see Chapter 33). Urinary tract infections can be screened for with urinalyses and microscopic quantification of bacteriuria (see Chapter 36). Appropriate cultures should be obtained if they are indicated and available.

Intestinal parasites are often pandemic in malnourished refugee populations (see Chapter 35). Treatment, however, is usually a secondary priority and probably should be delayed about one week.

Congestive heart failure (CHF) in PEM patients is most often due to overzealous parenteral rehydration, too rapid an advancement of the diet, or too much salt in the diet. The best treatment is prevention. If CHF is severe, cautious treatment with 1 mg/kg per dose of furosemide (Lasix) can be given intravenously, intramuscularly, or by mouth, and digoxin can be added if necessary. Thiamine deficiency and anemia (see below) are the next two most common causes of CHF in this setting; fortunately, both are readily treatable. Other treatable etiologies include hypokalemia and hypothyroidism.

Severe anemia causing CHF, with hematocrit less than 10 percent or hemoglobin less than 3 g/dl, should be treated with transfusions. Ten millileters per kilogram of typed and crossmatched blood is given, or O negative blood can be used. Packed red blood cells are preferable, but whole blood can be used. There is some danger of volume overload in nondehydrated patients, so transfusions should be given slowly (e.g., over a few hours). Occasionally furosemide may be needed. Iron therapy should be started.

Some experts have suggested more liberal criteria for transfusion. For example, Peel et al (1984) reported their experience in Thailand where transfusion of all patients with hematocrits under 15 percent was thought to decrease mortality significantly.

Diarrhea is frequently present in children with PEM, often caused directly by parasitic, bacterial, or other infectious agents (see Chapter 34). Not uncommon is osmotic diarrhea from malabsorption following acute gastroenteritis. If persistent loose or watery stools are present, consideration should be given to either briefly reducing the concentration of feeds (to keep the fluid volume up and decrease the osmotic load), or to changing from a milk (lactose containing) to a soy formula. Feedings should not be changed if the watery diarrhea occurs during breastfeeding.

The dermatosis of KW will resolve with refeeding. Bacterial superinfections may need to be treated (see Chapter 28). The application of paraffin gauze dressing to raw areas helps relieve pain. Soaking affected areas in 1 percent potassium permanganate solution for ten minutes each day may be helpful. Diaper rash should be left to air dry, although protective barrier creams such as zinc oxide can be tried.

Vitamin Deficiencies

Vitamin deficiencies are usually present along with the PEM. Vitamin A and thiamine are the two most common deficiencies recognized clinically. (As mentioned earlier, vitamin A deficiency should be treated as a medical emergency to prevent irreversible eye damage.) Also often present, but subclinical, are deficiencies of vitamic C, vitamin K, folic acid, vitamin D, and niacin. Vitamin B_{12} deficiency is seen in malnutrition of long duration.

In the refugee setting, it will not be practical to perform laboratory analyses to document the presence of these deficiencies; therefore, presumptive therapy is indicated. Dosages for the treatment of acute vitamin deficiencies in infants and young children are listed in Table 14-8. Therapy for chronic deficiencies is best instituted with properly balanced meals, although multivitamin tablets are often used.

Signs and symptoms of the major vitamin deficiencies are as follows:

- Vitamin A deficiency (see Chapter 18).
- Vitamin B_1 (or thiamine) deficiency. Beriberi is an uncommon deficiency and can manifest in different ways. "Dry" beriberi presents with neuritis leading to limb paralysis, whereas patients with "wet" beriberi present with diffuse edema (anasarca) and congestive heart failure. A moderate form presents with malaise, decreased appetite, and severe weakness, especially of the lower extremities. Infants may have a severe and rapidly progressive form of beriberi. Symptoms may include vocal cord paralysis (hoarseness), ptosis (drooping of the

Table 14-8. Acute Treatment of Specific Deficiencies for Infants and Children with PEM

Deficiency	Dosage
Iron	6 mg/kg/day of elemental iron divided 3 times a day for 3 months to replenish iron stores; then 1 mg/kg/day (up to 15 mg) of iron given as a single dose to help prevent further iron deficiency. Ferrous sulfate salts are better absorbed than the ferric form. Different oral ferrous sulfate preparations include 200-mg tabs (40 mg iron), and 90-mg/5-ml syrup (18 mg iron/5 ml). UNICEF tablets contain 30 mg of elemental iron and 0.1 mg of folic acid. Iron powder can be added to milk.
Folic acid	Oral folic acid 0.25 mg daily for 10 days to replenish stores, then a daily dose to maintain stores of 0.1 mg for infants, and 0.4 mg for patients over 4 years of age, except for pregnant or lactating women, who require 0.8 mg/day. UNICEF tablets contain 30 mg of elemental iron and 0.1 mg of folic acid.
Vitamin A	In addition to treating all patients with signs of xerophthalmia (including night blindness), the Helen Keller Institute recommends that all severely malnourished children and all children with measles should be treated for vitamin A deficiency, whether or not symptoms are apparent. The recommended dose is 200,000 IU orally (well-absorbed) or IM on days 1, 2, and 8. Alternatively, 100,000 IU can be given intramuscularly for the first dose. For prophylaxis of older children and adults 200,000 IU is given every four to six months. Each of the above doses should be halved for children under one year of age. (The WHO also recommends that all women receive 200,000 IU of Vitamin A orally within one month of delivery.)
Vitamin C	500 mg PO daily for 4 weeks (some advocate much larger doses).
Vitamin D	No more than 100,000 to 300,000 IU (2.5–7.5 mg) of cholecalciferol (vitamin D) in single doses of 1000 IU (25μg) daily for 10 to 30 days. Exposure of skin to sunlight.
Vitamin K	1 mg IM each day, for 1 to 3 days.
Thiamine	10 mg IV once, then 10 mg IM twice a day for 3 days, or 10 mg PO 4 times a day for 6 weeks.
Niacin (or niacinamide)	Niacin PO daily, 100 to 300 mg for children, 300 to 500 mg for adults, in divided doses. If PO cannot be tolerated, about 10% of the oral dose can be given *very* slowly IV.

eyelids), and gastrointestinal symptoms (Beaton & Bengoa 1976). Prevention of beriberi can be achieved by undermilling or brief boiling ("parboiling") of rice to ensure a thiamine intake of at least 1 mg daily. Other sources include undermilled cereals, legumes, and green leafy vegetables. Tea and raw fish may have enzymes that destroy thiamine.

• Niacin deficiency. Pellagra, characterized by a bilaterally symmetric rash on skin exposed to sunlight, is often accompanied by severe diarrhea and mental deterioration. Niacin deficiency is found mostly among maize- and sorghum-eating populations and can be prevented with 15 to 20 mg of niacin (nicotinic acid) daily. Sources are legumes and undermilled cereals.

• Vitamin C deficiency. Scurvy is recognized by bluish, spongy, swollen gums, especially over the upper incisors. The large joints may be swollen. Subperiosteal hemorrhages lead to marked bony tenderness, sometimes causing "pseudoparalysis" in infants. The costochondral junctions may be angulated ("scorbutic beads"). Anemia, petechiae, hematuria, melena, and orbital or subdural hemorrhages may be found. Scurvy can be prevented by as little as 10 mg of vitamin C daily—for example, by consuming 15 ml of citrus juice, one quarter of an orange, or 20 g of leafy vegetables. Poor oral hygiene should be considered the cause of gum swelling if the latter does not resolve with 100 to 200 mg/day of vitamin C therapy.

• Vitamin D deficiency. An early sign of rickets is softening of the parietal bones called craniotabes. Palpable enlargement of the costochondral junctions, termed the "rachitic rosary," and thickening of the wrists and ankles are also early signs. Signs of more advanced rickets include flattening of the skull, delayed closure of the anterior fontanel, scoliosis, and kyphosis. Early x-ray signs include cupping and fraying of the distal ends of the ulna and radius. Because exposure to sunlight is the best prevention of vitamin D deficiency, it is uncommon in tropical countries.

Mineral and Electrolyte Deficiencies

Iron stores are most often deficient and should be replenished. Trace minerals are similarly lacking. Consideration can be given to providing additional zinc. Although few data are available, one study (using an uncontrolled and nonblinded therapeutic trial of 25 to 150 μmol/kg/day of zinc) reported benefit for 14 of 16 children recovering from severe malnutrition (Golden & Golden 1981).

Sodium is provided at 2 mEq/kg/day and potassium at 3 mEq/kg/day, except in children with KW; for them, potassium at 5 mEq/kg/day for the first week is more appropriate to help correct the potassium depletion present. High potassium intake is also commonly needed for KW patients during the second and third week of therapy because of the diuresis that accompanies the edema's resolution. Magnesium is also often deficient, and 2 to 3 mEq/kg/day should be supplied.

Choice of Feeding Formula

The progression of feeding formula choice can be divided into five stages:

- Initial oral rehydration therapy.
- Initial use of special formulas in increasing concentrations.
- Change to high-energy formulas.
- Gradual introduction of regular foods.
- Resumption of a full diet.

Oral rehydration therapy is discussed in Chapter 15. The choice of an appropriate formula should be determined by the nutritional needs of the patient, alteration of intestinal function, cost, availability, and local standards. Breast milk is the ideal food for infants, and relactation should be attempted as early as possible (see Chapter 13).

Although exocrine pancreatic function is compromised initially, the digestion of protein is affected less than that of fat and carbohydrate. Protein digestion returns rapidly toward normal, even in severely protein-depleted infants (MacLean et al 1980). This fact should discourage the routine use of free amino acids or protein hydrolysates, especially considering their high cost, scarcity, and high osmolality (which can lead to diarrhea). Ideally, whole protein should be used to supply about 8 percent of the required calories (2 to 3 g/kg/day) since a higher percentage has not been found to hasten recovery.

Malabsorption of fat by malnourished infants can be severe and may last for many months. This probably results more from inadequate bile secretion (leading to decreased micellar solubilization) than from pancreatic insufficiency (Viteri 1981). Therefore, medium-chain triglyceride (MCT) oil can be used, especially for patients with steatorrhea, if at least 3 percent of the energy is supplied by long-chain triglycerides to meet essential fatty acid requirements (Graham et al 1973).

Malabsorption of virtually every carbohydrate has been documented in PEM patients. Brush border lactase is often the lowest in concentration of the disaccharidases, and clinical lactose intolerance is not uncommon in malnourished infants (MacLean et al 1980). Although glucose, maltose, sucrose, and most starches might be better tolerated, at least one recent study (Solomons et al 1984) contradicts the experience of most authors, stating that routine reduction of lactose content from a milk-based diet for severe PEM might offer no advantage.

If lactose intolerance is suspected, two simple tests help to determine if carbohydrate malabsorption might be causing diarrhea. The first is a pH test of the stool, in which a reading of less than 6.0 suggests malabsorption. The second checks for stool-reducing substances by adding a Clinitest tablet directly to liquid stool. Greater than 0.5 percent reducing substances (green, brown, or red) suggests malabsorption.

Based on the above considerations, the best initial feeding might be a commercial lactose-free formula, containing whole protein and a mixture of medium- and long-chain triglycerides. However, such formulas are expensive and usually scarce in refugee camps. Soy formulas are a good second choice if they are available. They are lactose-free, usually well tolerated, less expensive, and more available than the specialty formulas.

More likely to be available is K-Mix II, a standard UNICEF formula with high calorie and potassium content, developed for disaster feeding of large PEM populations. K-Mix II contains lactose in lower concentrations than regular cows' milk formulas, but it might still be enough lactose to cause diarrhea in some PEM patients. K-Mix II formula is made with 17 g of calcium caseinate, 28 g of dried skim milk (DSM), 55 g of sugar, 60 g of edible oil, and vitamin A (see Table 14-9 for volume equivalents of weight). To this is added enough warm, boiled water to make a 1-liter suspension. Each milliliter of K-Mix II contains about 0.03 g of protein and 0.9 kcal of energy.

Table 14-9. Approximate Volume Equivalents of Dried Weight Substances for Mixing

Material	g/ml	g/teaspoon[a]
Calcium caseinate	0.3	1.5
Cereal flour	0.45	2.3
Dried skimmed milk	0.5	2.5
Evaporated milk	1.0	5.0
Full-cream milk powder	0.5	2.5
K-Mix II (unconstituted)	0.8	4.0
Sugar	0.8	4.2
Vegetable oil	0.9	4.5
Water	1.0	5.0
Yogurt	1.0	5.0

[a]The volume of a level teaspoon is 5 ml, while a level tablespoon contains 15 ml.

Breast Milk

The importance of breastfeeding in preventing malnutrition cannot be overemphasized. Breastfed infants rarely become malnourished unless they are ill or the mother is without sufficient milk. The very ill infant is usually too weak to suckle, but can be given breast milk by nasogastric tube. Relactation, outlined in Chapter 13, should be attempted.

Homemade Formulas

In Africa, where the largest population of malnourished refugees exists, commercial formulas are rarely available for relief efforts and homemade formulas are the only option for refeeding. These formulas can be used successfully, but they carry some risk of assorted vitamin and trace mineral deficiencies. In particular, vitamins A, C, and D, along with copper, niacin, magnesium, and zinc may inadvertently be deficient.

In general, any food that is sufficient in concentrated calories and digestible can be used for PEM therapy. Such foods ideally should contain about 0.02 g protein and 0.9 kcal/ml, with 20 to 40 percent of the calories provided by oil. For example, a satisfactory milk-based formula can be made by adding 80 g of dried skimmed milk (DSM), 40 g of sugar, and 50 g of edible oil (see Table 14-9 for volume equivalents of weight) into enough cooled, boiled water to make a 1-liter suspension. This mixture contains about the same concentration of protein and energy as K-Mix II.

Fluid milk can also be used. For cows' or camels' milk, full-strength milk formula is prepared by adding 50 g sugar to 1000 ml of milk. Goats', buffalos', or ewes' milk should be diluted 1:1 with water (500 ml of cooled, boiled water should be added to each 500 ml of milk and 50 g of sugar) since these milks are richer in fat. (Note that goats' milk is deficient in folic acid). If evaporated milk is used, it is diluted 1:1 with water and 50 g of sugar is added per liter (WHO 1981). For infants, breast milk can be used for tube feedings. Because breast milk is higher in carbohydrate content than cows' milk (6.8 versus 4.8 g/100 ml), additional sugar is not required.

Yogurt is well-tolerated and nutritious. Full-strength yogurt feed is made by adding 50 g of sugar to each 1000 ml yogurt.

Formula can also be made from full-cream milk powder. Add 150 g of the powder, 50 g of sugar, and enough cooled, boiled water to make a 1-liter suspension (WHO 1981).

The addition of cereal flour to homemade formulas is often helpful in preventing the oil from rising to the top. About 50 g/liter of any locally available and acceptable cereal flour, such as wheat, rice, millet, or oatmeal flour can be used.

If refrigeration is available, a 12 to 24-hour supply of formula can be mixed at one time. In warm climates without refrigeration, formula should be freshly made every three to four hours to prevent spoilage. Premixed preparations are especially convenient for feeding large numbers of patients.

High-Energy Feeding

After children can tolerate regular full-strength formula feedings well (usually after the sixth or seventh day of treatment), it is helpful to begin high-energy feedings. These are usually a more concentrated form of milk, sugar, and oil. The oil is crucial because it provides more than twice the number of calories per gram that carbohydrates or protein do (9 kcal/g versus 4 kcal/g). Table 14-10 lists the contents of common high-energy formulas.

To ensure a smooth transition to a standard diet, traditional foods should gradually replace high-energy foods from about the third week of treatment. Local foods such as rice, noodles, potatoes, bananas, and other fresh fruits and vegetables, are usually well tolerated.

Specifics of Dietary Treatment

As emphasized earlier, dietary therapy for patients with severe PEM must progress very slowly. The general scheme is to begin with ORS, advance to a half-strength formula, and then to full-strength formulas, high-energy feeds, mashed solids, and finally, to fuller feeds over about a four- to six-week period. For initial feeding, small amounts of formula should be given frequently. For example, feeding should occur every two hours for the first two days, then every three hours for the next three days, and then every four hours.

If infants are too weak to breastfeed, breast milk or formula should be given by cup and spoon, or by nasogastric tube if necessary. Bottle feeding should be avoided since nipples are difficult to clean and parents might interpret the use of bottles by the medical staff as an endorsement of bottle feeding after discharge.

If parenteral therapy is required initially, "complete gut rest" should be avoided. Oral feeding, even if only in small amounts, is required to reverse the intestinal epithelial hypoplasia associated with malnutrition. This is probably caused by the release of pancreatic enzymes and other trophic substrates such as the hormone gastrin, which is stimulated by oral feeding. Also important is the direct trophic effect of ingested nutrients (Greene et al 1975).

MacLean and co-workers (1980) identified

Table 14-10. Preparation of High-Energy Milk Feedings (WHO 1981)

	Ingredients (per liter)			Yield (per liter)	
Name of Formula	Milk or Preparation (g)	Oil (g)	Sugar (g)	Kcal	Protein
Cow or goat	900	55	70	1350	30
Buffalo or ewe	800	30	65	1350	30
Skimmed milk powder	90	85	65	1350	32
Full cream milk powder	120	55	65	1360	30
Evaporated milk	450	50	70	1360	31
K-Mix II	120	85	35	1360	30
Yogurt	900	65	70	1360	30

the following main pitfalls in the oral management of PEM patients:

- Imprecise diet orders reflecting imprecise thinking. The volume of fluid and number of calories must be thought of as the number of milligrams per kilogram per day and the number of kilocalories per kilogram per day. These values are then translated into terms more easily understood by other personnel, such as "half-strength," with specific volumes indicated per feeding. Merely ordering "quarter-strength" or "half-strength" formula without considering the volume and energy received per kilogram per day makes no more sense than treating cystitis with half-strength ampicillin and pneumonia with full-strength ampicillin. The form in Table 14-7 can be helpful for writing diet orders and keeping track of changes made.
- Diets are often advanced too rapidly, with the resulting feeding intolerance mistakenly being attributed to the *source* of protein or carbohydrate used rather than to the *amount* fed. If the volume of a feeding is kept the same but the concentration is advanced in one jump from half-strength to full-strength, the doubling of nutrient and solute loads may cause acute diarrhea secondary to malabsorption. A child who has been tolerating a formula at one level of intake and then develops loose stools following a higher intake is probably receiving an excessive (relative to intestinal tolerance) quantity of food. In this instance, rather than change the type of formula, one should reduce the concentration and advance more slowly.
- Early weight gain is often unrealistically expected. Children with severe PEM may have total body salt and water excess. These children, therefore, may not gain weight during the first few days of therapy. Initial progress should be considered satisfactory as long as steady advancement of feeding is tolerated.

Children with PEM require large amounts of energy (kilocalories) to grow. Reasons for this include the following:

- Caloric needs are underestimated when actual body weight is used to calculate energy needs. A corrected weight (which factors in the ideal body weight) should be used instead.
- PEM patients present with varying degrees of malabsorption.
- Initially, PEM patients make inefficient use of absorbed calories.

Stool volume and character are the most helpful guides to dietary treatment of PEM. The number of stools per day can be misleading and should not be used to guide therapy since they can be frequent but small, green, mucousy (so-called starvation stools). Diets can be advanced for infants who have less than 100–150g of soft stool per day (MacLean et al 1980).

MacLean and co-workers (1980) have outlined an effective refeeding program. The volume of the feedings is chosen to meet daily fluid requirements (see Chapter 15). The formula, which contains high-quality protein, vegetable oil, and glucose, maltose, or sucrose (or a mixture thereof), is initially diluted to deliver 25 to 50 kcal/kg/day. Some milk can also be given. If stool output is acceptable according to the criteria noted above, caloric intake is increased by 25 kcal/kg every other day while total feeding volume is held constant. Formula concentration can be increased progressively from 0.15 kcal/ml to a maximum of about 1.0 kcal/ml. Osmolality is kept below 350 mOsmol/l, when possible, to avoid osmotic diarrhea. Once a concentration of 1.0 kcal/ml is reached, further increases in intake are achieved by increasing the volume of feedings. This progression is continued until acceptable weight gain ensues.

Depending on the age and weight deficit of the child, a weight gain rate of 5 to 10 g/kg/day is satisfactory. The energy intake that will eventually be required to ensure weight gain in infants can be estimated by multiplying their ideal or "standard" weight for height, by 120 kcal/kg/day. For example, consider a severely malnourished child who is 77 cm tall and weighs only 6.1 kg (60% of standard weight for height). The standard (or ideal) weight for 77 cm is 10.1 kg. Therefore, an estimate of the energy (kilocalories/day) that will eventually be required for this child would be 120 kcal/kg/day times his ideal weight (i.e., $120 \times 10.1 = 1200$ kcal/day), rather than 120 kcal/kg/day times his actual weight ($120 \times 6.1 = 730$ kcal/day), a difference of 165 percent.

Other than potassium supplementation, the rate of calorie advancement is the only major difference between the treatment of children with KW and those with marasmus. Once an intake of 75 to 100 kcal/kg/day has been achieved, the diet of children with KW is not advanced further until edema starts to diminish and, if serum albumin measurement is available, until this concentration is near or above 2 g/dl. If more calories are given to the KW patient before these criteria are met, resolution of edema tends to be retarded (Mac-

Lean et al 1980). Children will generally tolerate 75 kcal/kg/day by the end of the eighth day of treatment. Restoration of the serum albumin to normal values usually takes several weeks.

Laboratory facilities for measuring serum albumin may not be available in field hospital settings, but refractometers measuring serum total protein may be present. Although not as helpful as serum albumin measurements, total protein measurements at or above 5 g/dl provide a satisfactory guide to refeedings.

The degree and duration of the nutritional insult and the age of the patient are the most influential factors in determining the severity and prognosis of malnutrition disorders (McCance 1962). With high-energy feedings, most malnourished children recover adequate weight for height after four to six weeks (WHO 1981). Weight for age should not be used as an endpoint since children recovering from PEM commonly have low weight for age due to past stunting.

There are a number of reasons for failure to gain weight (or, for those with edema, failure to make progress toward resolution of the edema) including the following:

1. Inadequate caloric intake.
   - If a child is being treated as an outpatient, poor attendance can be the number-one cause of treatment failure.
   - Formulas may be improperly mixed (too dilute).
   - Feeding may not be given as ordered.
   - Staff error or pilferage may occur.
   - The child may have poor appetite (severe KW patients often need nasogastric tube feeding initially, while marasmic children rarely require this intervention).
   - Not enough calories may have been ordered.
   - Calorie needs should be recalculated periodically to allow for increases in weight.
   - Too few feedings may have been ordered (feeding should be continued day *and* night).
   - Continued advancement of caloric intake to high-energy feedings may not have been undertaken.
2. Undiagnosed chronic infection such as tuberculosis, otitis media, tonsillitis, pneumonia, urinary tract infection, or intestinal parasites. Recent data revealed giardiasis in as many as 80 percent of severely malnourished children in one Somali refugee camp.
3. Occult chronic disease other than infection may be present. Common examples include renal disease, heart disease, and sickle cell or other blood diseases.
4. Appropriate vitamin and mineral supplements have not been provided.

Whenever possible, the psychological needs of malnourished patients should also be attended to. Love and affection should be generously shown by parents and staff. Given the social disruption and presence of many orphans in refugee camps, every effort should be made to ensure that someone is taking responsibility for each child. Nutrition rehabilitation units should have games, toys, books, and other stimulation, when feasible. Caution should be exercised to ensure that these additions, especially the games, do not demand large expenditures of energy from the children.

Many criteria can be used to help decide when children are ready for transfer to an outpatient supplementary feeding program. These include good tolerance of feedings with continued weight gain, weight above the 80th percentile for height, and lack of fever, vomiting, diarrhea, edema, or infections. The patient should appear mentally alert, begin relating to relatives and staff, and engage in age-appropriate physical activities. Finally, they should have at least one healthy family member to care for them on discharge.

Close coordination must exist between the hospital and supplementary feeding center staffs, with the latter providing regular follow-up of PEM patients after discharge. Relapse is common and follow-up at least every two weeks for the first two months following discharge is important. This allows for maintenance of nutritional progress, completion of immunizations, and an opportunity for continued family education on child feeding and rearing, family planning, and personal hygiene (WHO 1981). The hospital ID bracelet should be kept on the child to facilitate identification at the supplementary feeding center.

REFERENCES AND SUGGESTED READING

Allegra DT, Nieburg P, Grabe M (eds): Emergency Refugee Health Care—A Chronicle of the Khmer Refugee-Assistance Operation. Washington, DC, U.S. Department of Health and Human Services, 1984.

Andersen G, Hellsing E, Abrahamsson L et al: Red Cross Food and Nutrition Relief Handbook. Stockholm, Danish, Norwegian and Swedish Red Cross, 1978.

Arnhold R: The arm circumference as a public health index of protein-calorie malnutrition of early childhood. XVII. The QUAC stick: A field measure used by the Quaker Service Team in Nigeria. J Trop Pediatr 1969;15:243–47.
Beaton GH, Bengoa JM (eds): Nutrition in Preventive Medicine. Geneva, World Health Organization, 1976.
Berry A: An assessment of nutritional status of children in refugee settlements, emergency reception centers, and in selected Sudanese villages. Geneva, Nutrition Unit, United Nations High Commmittee on Refugees, 1985.
Bourbour F: Practical techniques for front line health workers for the detection, treatment and prevention of nutritional disorders. J Trop Pediatr 1981;27:114–19.
Brenton DP, Brown RE, Wharton BA: Hypothermia in kwashiorkor. Lancet 1967;1:410–13.
Brown KH, MacLean WC: Nutritional management of acute diarrhea. An appraisal of the alternatives. Pediatrics 1984;73:119–25.
Brown JE, Brown RC: Finding the Causes of Malnutrition. Atlanta, Task Force on World Hunger, 1979.
Cameron M, Hofvander Y: Manual on Feeding Infants and Young Children. New York, Oxford University Press, 1983.
Davis LE: Epidemiology of famine in the Nigerian crisis: Rapid evaluation of malnutrition by height and arm circumference in large populations. Am J Clin Nutr 1971;24:358–64.
De Ville de Goyet C, Seaman J, Geijer U: The Management of Nutritional Emergencies in Large Populations. Geneva, World Health organization, 1978.
FAO: Food Composition Tables for Use in Africa. Rome, Food and Agricultural Organization, 1968.
Galler JR, Ramsey F, Soliamano G: The influence of early malnutrition on subsequent behavioral development. Learning disabilities as a sequel to malnutrition. Pediatr Res 1984;18:309–13.
Golden MH, Golden BE: Effect of zinc supplementation on the dietary intake, rate of weight gain, and energy cost of tissue deposition in children recovering from severe malnutrition. Am J Clin Nutr 1981; 34:900–08.
Graham GG, Baertl JM, Cordano A, Morales E: Lactose-free, medium-chain triglyceride formulas in severe malnutrition. Am J Dis Child 1973;126:330–35.
Greene HL, McCabe DR, Merenstein GB: Protracted diarrhea and malnutrition in infancy: Changes in intestinal morphology and disaccharidase activities during treatment with total intravenous nutrition or oral elemental diets. J Pediatr 1975;87:697–704.
Jelliffe DB: Assessment of the Nutritional Status of the Community. WHO Monograph 53. Geneva, World Health Organization, 1966.
Jelliffe DB: Infant Nutrition in the Subtropics and Tropics. WHO Monograph 29. Geneva, World Health Organization, 1955.
Jelliffe DB, Jelliffe EFP: Breastfeeding: A key measure in large-scale disaster relief. Disasters 1977;1:199–203.
Jelliffe EFP, Jelliffe DB (eds): The arm circumference as a public health index of protein-calorie malnutrition of early childhood. J Trop Pediatr 1969;15:177–260.
Keusch GT, Scrimshaw NS: Selective primary health care: strategies for control of disease in the developing world. XXIII. Control of infection to reduce the prevalence of infantile and childhood malnutrition. Rev Infect Dis 1986;8:273–87.
King M et al: Nutrition for Developing Countries. London, Oxford University Press, 1972.
MacLean WC, Jr, Lopez de Romaña G, Massa E, Graham GG: Nutritional management of chronic diarrhea and malnutrition: Primary reliance on oral feeding. J Pediatr 1980;97:316–23.
McCance RA: Food, growth and time. Lancet 1962;2:621–26, 671–76.
McLaren DS, Pellett PL, Read WC: A simple scoring system for classifying the severe forms of protein-calorie malnutrition in early childhood. Lancet 1967;1:533–35.
Morley D, Woodland M: See How They Grow. Monitoring Child Growth for Appropriate Health Care in Developing Countries. London, MacMillan Publishing Co., 1979.
Olness K: Nutritional consequences of drug therapy. Clin Pediatr 1985;24:417–20.
Olness K, Yip R, Indritz A, Torjesen E: Height and weight status of Indochinese refugee children. An anthropometric study of 1,650 children. Am J Dis Child 1984;138:543–47.
Olson RE (ed): Protein-Calorie Malnutrition. New York, Academic Press, 1975.
Peel S, Allegra DT, Knaub C, Finn D: Nutritional assessment and feeding programs in refugee centers: The Thailand experience. In Allegra DT, Nieburg P, Grabe M (eds): Emergency Refugee Health Care—A Chronicle of Khmer Refugee-Assistance Operation, pp 75–84. Washington, DC, U.S. Department of Health and Human Services, 1984.
Picou DM: Evaluation and treatment of the malnourished child. In Suskind RM: Textbook of Pediatric Nutrition, pp 217–28. New York, Raven Press, 1981.
Protein-Calorie Advisory Group of the United Nations System: A Guide to Food and Health Relief Operations for Disasters. New York, United Nations, 1977.
Scrimshaw NS: Significance of the interactions of nutrition and infection in children. In Suskind RM (ed): Textbook of Pediatric Nutrition, pp 229–40. New York, Raven Press, 1981.
Scrimshaw NS, Taylor CE, Gordon JE: Interactions of Nutrition and Infection. Geneva, World Health Organization, 1968.

Sen AK: Poverty and Famines: An Essay on Entitlement and Deprivation. Oxford, Clarendon Press, 1981.
Shakir A, Morley D: Measuring malnutrition. Lancet 1974;1:758–59.
Simmonds SP, Vaughan P, Gunn SW (eds): Refugee Community Health Care. New York, Oxford University Press, 1983.
Solomons NW, Torun B, Caballero B et al: The effect of dietary lactose on the early recovery from protein-energy malnutrition. I. Clinical and anthropometric indices. Am J Clin Nutr 1984;40:591–600.
Sommer A: Field Guide to the Detection and Control of Xerophthalmia. Geneva, World Health Organization, 1978.
Suskind RM: Textbook of Pediatric Nutrition. New York, Raven Press, 1981.
United Nations Protein–Calorie Advisory Group: A Guide to Food and Health Relief Operations for Disasters. New York, United Nations, 1967.
Viteri F: Primary protein–calorie malnutrition. Clinical, biochemical, and metabolic changes. In Suskind RM (ed): Textbook of Pediatric Nutrition, pp 189–216. New York, Raven Press, 1981.
Walker WA, Hendricks KM: Manual of Pediatric Nutrition. Philadelphia, WB Saunders, 1985.
Waterlow JC: Classification and definition of protein-energy malnutrition. In Beaton GH, Bengoa JM (eds): Nutrition in Preventive Medicine, pp 530–55. Geneva, World Health Organization, 1976.
Wharton B: The Management of Severe Kwashiorkor. London, Teaching Aides at Low Cost, 1969.
WHO: A Growth Chart for International Use. Guidelines for Primary Health Care Personnel. Geneva, World Health Organization, 1978.
WHO: Control of Nutritional Anemia with Special Reference to Iron Deficiency. WHO Technical Report 580. Geneva, World Health Organization, 1975.
WHO: The Treatment and Management of Severe Protein-Energy Malnutrition. Geneva, World Health Organization, 1981.

15
Fluid and Electrolyte Therapy

RICHARD H. SANDLER
WILLIAM C. MACLEAN, JR.

The death rate from diarrheal illnesses in refugee camps can be staggering. In many underdeveloped nations, about one in ten children succumbs to diarrhea before his or her fifth birthday; infants and toddlers are at special risk. For children under two, about 10 percent of diarrheal episodes lead to dehydration, and 10 percent of these are life-threatening (Parker et al 1984). Worldwide, this results in about 5 million deaths annually. With proper therapy, however, mortality from severe dehydration can be reduced from over 25 percent to below 1 percent.

ORAL REHYDRATION THERAPY

The single most important tool for reducing the high mortality of diarrheal diseases is the aggressive, early use of oral rehydration therapy. Formerly, it was thought that children with diarrhea had poor absorption of liquids and needed "complete gut rest." There is now solid evidence that this is not true for most patients (Parker et al 1984; Hirschhorn et al 1980; Santosham et al 1982b). Except for the patient in shock, if glucose, salt, and water are given in the proper proportions, active glucose transport and, with it, electrolyte and water absorption are well maintained in the small bowel.

The effectiveness of oral rehydration therapy (ORT) was clearly demonstrated in a West Bengal refugee camp during the 1971 Bangladesh war. During a raging cholera epidemic, there was a 25 percent mortality rate when only intravenous therapy was available. Case fatality decreased to 3.6 percent when ORT was introduced.

The health needs of refugees are better served with ORT than with intravenous rehydration. First, ORT is effective, simple, safe, and inexpensive. Second, it can be easily taught to health workers who then educate the community. Third, once they are learned, ORT skills can be used in a camp setting or wherever refugees settle. And fourth, ORT can be used not only to treat, but also to prevent dehydration safely and easily. Therefore, ORT should be used routinely for all but those severely dehydrated and in shock, patients with ileus (absent bowel sounds and abdominal distention), those with persistent severe vomiting, and obtunded patients with a questionable gag reflex.

The following are some highlights of recent research that supports the above recommendations:

- Pizarro, Posada, and Mata (1983a) reported their experience of orally rehydrating 242 infants in Costa Rica. The mean level of dehydrations was 5 percent and the average time for complete rehydration was 7.5 hours. Only 3 percent of these children required intravenous fluids. In another article, Pizarro and colleagues (1983b) detailed the effectiveness of ORT in treating hypernatremic (N = 61) and hyponatremic (N = 33) dehydration. Seizures occurred in 8 percent (5/61) of the hypernatremic infants, compared to a 14 percent (6/43) convulsion rate previously encountered when intravenous therapy was used.

- A prospective, controlled study by Santosham and co-workers (1982b) examined ORT versus intravenous therapy in 146 moderate to severely dehydrated children aged three months to two years in the United States and Panama. Eleven of the children considered to be severely dehydrated on admission initially received intravenous therapy. This was changed to ORT after the blood pressure and pulse returned to normal. One of 101 children randomized to the ORT group required additional intravenous therapy. The only three patients with complications (seizures, hydrothorax after subclavian line placement, and phlebitis) were in the subgroup receiving intravenous therapy.

- Tamer and colleagues (1985) carried out a prospective, randomized trial of ORT versus intravenous therapy with 100 dehydrated, acidotic, but well-nourished infants in the United States. Ninety-four percent were successfully rehydrated with ORT alone. Compared to the intravenous rehydration group, the patients given ORT had a faster correction of acidosis.

Composition of ORT

Premeasured, sealed packages of the recommended WHO oral rehydration salt and glucose mixture (ORS) are distributed by UNICEF. Prior to 1984, each package contained 3.5 g of table salt (NaCl), 2.5 g of baking soda ($NaHCO_3$), 1.5 g of potassium chloride, and 20 g of glucose to be dissolved in 1 liter of potable drinking water. This yielded a solution containing 90 mEq Na^+, 20 mEq K^+, 80 mEq Cl^-, 30 mEq HCO_3^-, and 80 kcal of glucose in each liter (1 mEq is equivalent to 1 m Osmol for these univalent ions).

In 1984, WHO recommended substituting 1.9 g/liter of trisodium citrate dihydrate for the 2.5 g of sodium bicarbonate, which led to a longer shelf-life and reduced stool volume by as much as 46 percent (Parker et al 1984). The older ORS packets work very well, however, and are recommended until existing stocks are used up. As a guide for those mixing ORS, the volume of each of the above components is listed in Table 15-1.

The sodium concentration of diarrheal stools varies greatly. Secretory diarrheal stools (e.g., cholera) contain 60 mEq/liter up to 120 mEq/liter of sodium. The sodium content of malabsorptive diarrheal stools (e.g., rotavirus) is much lower, usually less than 40 mEq/liter. The sodium concentration of WHO ORS solution was originally chosen to replace the high sodium losses seen with cholera.

Table 15-1. Dry Volumes of ORS Components (To Make 1-liter Oral Rehydration Solution)

Substance	Weight (g)	Approximate Dry Volume (cc)[a]
NaCl	3.5	2.5
KCl	1.5	2
Plus either		
Trisodium citrate dihydrate	2.9	3
or		
$NaHCO_3$	2.5	2.5
Plus either		
Glucose	20	25
or		
Sucrose (table sugar)	40	35

[a]Very dependent on crystal size. The values given are the actual measured volumes of medium-sized crystals.

Finberg (1982) and others have pointed out that 90 mEq/liter of sodium may be too much salt for noncholera patients. The present WHO recommendation for maintenance fluids after rehydration is to alternate two parts ORS with one part low-salt liquid. This yields an average sodium concentration of about 60 mEq/liter.

Diarrheal stools contain from 10 to 80 mEq of potassium per liter. Therefore, children dehydrated from diarrhea are usually potassium depleted. Hypokalemia is the major cause of ileus and abdominal distention in these children.

It is standard practice in developed nations to withhold potassium supplementation of intravenous rehydration solutions until the patient urinates. However, it would be impractical to attempt distribution of ORS packets without potassium. Because renal failure is rare in acutely dehydrated patients, ORS with potassium can almost always be used safely.

There is presently no controversy about whether properly mixed, standard ORS solutions are effective. Some, however, have raised questions about the safety and efficacy of homemade ORS concoctions. Possible risks from homemade sugar and salt solutions include acidosis, hypokalemia, and hyponatremia from lack of bicarbonate, potassium, and sodium, respectively. Hypernatremia can result from too much salt or too little water if those who have no precise measuring instruments merely "pinch or scoop" the salt.

At present, firm data do not exist to assess the magnitude of the risks from homemade ORS solutions precisely. Parker and co-workers (1984) recently reviewed the relevant literature and made the following suggestions:

- Acidosis does not appear to be a significant problem for dehydrated children treated with ORS without bicarbonate. This is probably because renal function remains intact until dehydration becomes severe.
- Hypokalemia can develop, but local foods rich in potassium can help to prevent it.
- Neither hyponatremia nor hypernatremia has been a significant problem with home-measured salt and sugar solutions, but the po-

tential for harm can be minimized by careful measurement of ingredients.

- Forty grams of sucrose (table sugar) may be an acceptable substitute for the 20 g of glucose per liter in the standard ORS solution. Note that, although there is some evidence to support this conclusion, it appears more prudent to avoid adding the less absorbable sugars (like the fructose in sucrose) to diseased intestines.
- Thirty grams of rice powder per liter may be as safe and effective as 40 g of sucrose for ORS. (This can be prepared by grinding either dry grains of rice or popped, unhusked rice.)
- Studies from Singapore suggest that rice water (water drained from cooked rice) alone, or with added salts, may be as safe and effective as the WHO ORS formula. However, rice water's concentration of electrolytes and carbohydrates can vary greatly.

The conclusion regarding home-mixed ORS solution is that suboptimal oral therapy is better than no therapy at all. However, because of the uncertainties involved and the potential for harm caused by improperly mixed solutions, it is best to secure WHO ORS premixed packages. Failing this, the clinician should try to provide premixed packets, even if they must be premixed and packaged in the out-patient clinic (Parker et al 1984).

With or without premixed packets, the proper concentration of ORS ingredients will be obtained only if the correct amount of water is used for mixing. Families often have little concept of how much a liter is. There are many ways to circumvent this problem. For example, 1-liter mixing containers can be provided, or families can be taught to use commonly available vessels such as standard glasses or beer bottles. If these are not the correct size, a mark can be made on them to indicate 1 liter, or locally packaged ORS can be made especially for mixing in a widely available, odd-sized vessel. Finally, special spoons can be distributed to help families measure rehydration salts and glucose.

It is recommended that the water used for ORT be boiled first even though boiling consumes precious fuel and can delay administration while the water cools. Nonboiled water was used successfully in one comparative study (Parker et al 1984). Boiled or not, ORT solutions are a good medium for bacterial growth. Solutions should be mixed fresh daily and unused portions discarded after 24 hours.

Training for the Use of ORT

It has been clearly shown that careful, individual instruction for mixing ORS is beneficial. Especially important is actual demonstration of the mixing technique. For example, in one study in Nepal where women were initially instructed to use a pinch of salt and a scoop of sugar, 25 percent of the 56 women mixed solutions with too much salt. But when a second group received more extensive training and closer supervision, none mixed solutions that were too salty. One useful technique for helping mothers to avoid mixing too salty a solution is to teach that the mixture should not taste saltier than tears. Table 15-2 summarizes an excellent method used to teach ORT to fifth graders in Indonesia that can be adapted for refugee camp use.

How to Use ORT

The WHO recommends that undiluted ORS (90 mEq sodium/liter) be used to completely rehydrate patients (or perhaps slightly overhydrate as indicated by minimal periorbital edema). Since "straight" WHO ORS solution may be too salty for maintenance fluid administration after deficits have been replaced (Finberg et al 1982), WHO recommends maintaining hydration by alternating two parts ORS solution with one part of a less salty fluid such as breast milk, water, or a carbonated beverage.

It is important to keep in mind that feeding, especially breast feeding, should be restarted along with fluid therapy as soon as possible (see Chapters 13, 14, and 34). If the mother's milk is insufficient, treat the child and feed the mother (see Chapter 13 for a discussion of relactation).

The techniques of giving oral rehydration fluids are straightforward. Giving frequent sips is superior to infrequent feedings of large volumes, and sips should be offered every five minutes around the clock for severely dehydrated children. Vomiting, unless severe, does not preclude the use of ORT because there is usually a net retention of the solution. For the vomiting child, oral fluids given at the rate of one teaspoon (5 ml) every minute are usually well tolerated. Although this seems like a slow rate, it delivers adequate hourly volumes (300 ml). Oral rehydration fluids are usually given with a spoon instead of a bottle (spoons are easier to clean and the hazard of encouraging bottle feeding is avoided). A weak child will

Table 15-2. Lessons for Teaching about Diarrhea[a]

Basic Learning Objective	Demonstration/Discussion	Homework
Diarrhea is any liquid stool—leads to loss of body water	Soil in bottle; add water, looks like diarrhea; the water makes the diarrhea.	Discuss "what is diarrhea" with parents and neighbors.
Water loss causes weakness or death.	Freshly watered plant and chronically unwatered plant (wilted).	Discuss importance of water to living things—drought. Discuss how lack of water can cause death.
Make special drink of water, salt, and sugar.	Using drinking glass and teaspoon, each child prepares proper salt-sugar hydration mixture. Drinks to taste and describes saltiness (less salty than tears).	Demonstrate at home to parents and neighbors. Ask them to make and taste the mixture.
Give one glassful of liquid for each liquid stool passed.	Clay pot (with painted face) full of water, hole in bottom (matchstick size); catch water coming out and replace—one glass out, one glass in, pot stays full and "healthy."	Measure water entering and leaving a full rice terrace; small fish pond, or home water reservoir; inflow stops, goes dry. Demonstrate/discuss this principle—input must equal output.
Eat extra food to make body strong—helps intestine recover from illness.	Poster of breastfeeding mother. Discuss role of food in giving strength and need for extra during illness.	Discuss Koranic charge to breastfeed for two years. Discuss fasting and its harmful effects (well known because of Muslim fasting month). Ill person is excused from religious fasts—child with diarrhea should similarly not fast.

[a]Five half-hour lessons are taught in sequence on separate days to primary school children and include specific tasks to be done at home. In addition, the main objectives are illustrated in a children's story aimed at the reading level of forth- and fifth-grade children and used in ithe language-reading class.

(Used in the Comprehensive Community Health Care Education Program, Indonesia. Reproduced with permission from Rohde JE, Sadjimin T: Elementary-school pupils as educators: Role of school health programmes in primary health care. Lancet 1980; 1(8182):1350–352.)

usually swallow reflexively if ORT is squirted directly into the mouth using a plastic dropper or a 5-ml syringe. A nasogastric or orogastric tube may be used to administer ORT to moribund patients, but caution must be exercised to prevent aspiration. The proper volume of ORT can be estimated using the methods outlined in the next section, but thirst will usually serve as an adequate guide.

Often, a large diarrheal stool follows initiation of ORT. This may cause parents or health workers to believe mistakenly that the ORT is worsening the diarrhea. Instead, fluid entering the stomach causes a reflex evacuation of the colon (gastrocolic reflex). Diarrhea is increased with ORT only if too great a carbohydrate concentration is used.

CALCULATING FLUID AND ELECTROLYTE REQUIREMENTS

For patients with adequate renal function, thirst can help to guide fluid therapy and detailed calculations are less necessary. Severely dehydrated patients require more careful evaluation and aggressive intervention.

Fluid and electrolyte management has three components: replacement of dehydration deficits, replacement of ongoing losses due to diarrhea and vomiting, and "maintenance requirements" (including normal urine, stool, sweating, and respiratory tract losses). Stated mathematically,

$$T_x = D + L + M$$

where T_x represents the overall fluid therapy requirements, D stands for fluid and electrolyte deficits from dehydration, L denotes continuing fluid and electrolyte losses from diarrhea and vomiting, and M represents maintenance intake requirements.

The most accurate fluid calculations are based on the patient's estimated body weight before becoming dehydrated. However, since fluid calculations serve only as an initial rough estimate, it is satisfactory to use the child's present weight.

Estimating Fluids and Electrolyte Deficits

With a focused history and physical, the degree and type of dehydration can be estimated. As noted earlier, less precision is demanded if renal function is intact and oral rehydration therapy is used. Laboratory facilities are often primative or nonexistent in refugee camps, but some helpful laboratory determinations are listed in Table 15-3.

Useful historical data to obtain in the workup of patients with dehydration include the following:

- Intake of fluids—how much of what kind
- Urine, stool, and vomitus output
- Recent previous weight (to estimate weight change)

For example, a child who consumed large amounts of sweetened condensed milk would be likely to have hypertonic dehydration. There is some concern that these patients not be rehydrated rapidly with hypotonic solutions because cerebral edema, seizures, and death may result. Breast-fed infants are more likely to have hyponatremia and hypokalemia since breast milk has a low electrolyte content.

Physical examination is important in assessing fluid and electrolyte losses. Table 15-4 summarizes some physical findings seen with varying degrees of dehydration. These signs vary with the degree of dehydration, the type of accompanying salt losses, and the rapidity with which depletion occurred. One difficulty is that marasmic children often look dehydrated when, in fact, they are not. A trial of fluid therapy is often the only way to sort this out.

Tables 15-5, 15-6, 15-7, and 15-8 can help in the assessment of fluid and electrolyte deficits. Table 15-5 shows the concentration of electrolyte deficits that result from losses of different body fluids. Table 15-6 lists the changes seen with isonatremic, hyponatremic, and hypernatremic dehydration, and Table 15-7 notes the signs associated with other electrolyte abnormalities. Table 15-8 provides an estimate of total body fluid and electrolyte deficits in infants with varying types of dehydration.

Ongoing Losses

In general, replacement for continuing fluid and electrolyte losses can be calculated on a milliliter for milliliter, milliequivalent for milliequivalent basis. Table 15-9 can be used to estimate diarrheal stool volumes. In patients with massive continuing losses such as those with cholera, measurement of these losses is important. A "cholera cot," made by cutting a round hole in the middle of a canvas cot, can be used for this purpose. The patient's rectum is positioned over the hole and a collection bucket is placed under the hole.

Burn patients experience enormous fluid and heat losses. The Parkland formula states

Table 15-3. Laboratory Data Useful in Planning Fluid and Electrolyte Therapy

Often available in refugee camps	Less often available	Usually not available
Urine specific gravity	Serum sodium, potassium, chloride, and bicarbonate	Blood urea nitrogen (BUN)
Urine dipstick for glucose and ketones	Serum total protein (or albumin)	Serum creatinine
Urine microscopic examination	Serum osmolarity (freezing point depression)	Arterial blood gases
Hemoglobin and/or hematocrit		Serum calcium and magnesium
Blood glucose (e.g., Dextrostix)		

Table 15-4. Physical Examination Signs of Dehydration

Estimate of Weight Loss (%)	Net Water Deficit (ml/kg)	Severity of Dehydration	Clinical Data
<5	~30	Minimal	Thirst
5	50	Mild	Dry mucous membranes Decreased tears Has not voided for 4–8 hours
6–9	60–90	Moderate	Poor skin turgor Sunken fontanel Tachycardia Absent tears Has not voided for over 8 hours
10 and above	100 and up	Severe	Apprehensive, ill appearing Very dry mucous membranes Decreased blood pressure Feeble or absent pulse No urine

that fluid losses from second- and third-degree burns are about 4 ml/kg/day per percentage of body surface area burned. The latter can be estimated from Figure 15-1. For example, a 10-kg, two-year-old child with a second-degree burn of the entire front half of one leg would have fluid losses from the burn of (0.5 of the leg) × (15% of the body) × (4 ml/kg/day) × (10 kg), or about 300 ml for the first day. The second day's fluid losses average about 50 to 75 percent of that experienced on the first day.

Table 15-5. Electrolyte Composition of Body Fluid Losses

	Electrolyte Loss (mEq/liter)		
Fluid	Sodium	Potassium	Chloride
Gastric	20–80	5–20	100–150
Pancreatic	120–140	5–15	90–120
Small intestine	100–140	5–15	90–130
Bile	120–140	5–15	80–120
Ileostomy	45–135	3–15	20–115
Diarrheal			
Noncholera	10–90	10–80	10–110
Cholera	80–140	10–50	70–115
Sweat	10–30	3–10	10–35
Burns	140	5	110

Maintenance Requirements

In the tropics, dehydration occurs more rapidly than in temperate climates since higher ambient temperatures lead to more rapid insensible fluid loss. Long-standing depletion of electrolytes, especially potassium, is more common in malnourished populations.

Many different formulas have been developed to estimate maintenance fluid requirements, and each approximation is useful as a starting point to be adjusted frequently after judging clinical response. One standard method (Segar 1972) states that for each of the first 10 kg of body weight, a child requires 100 ml/kg/day. For each of the next 10 kg of body weight, another 50 ml/kg/day is required. For each kilogram over 20, another 20 ml/kg/day is added to maintenance fluid requirements.

For example, a 24-kg child without fever or other complicating factors has about the following daily fluid requirement: Maintenance fluids

$$
\begin{aligned}
(\text{ml/day}) &= (10\ \text{kg} \times 100\ \text{ml/kg/day}) + \\
&\quad (10\ \text{kg} \times 50\ \text{ml/kg/day}) + \\
&\quad (4\ \text{kg} \times 20\ \text{ml/kg/day}) \\
M &= 1580\ \text{ml/day}
\end{aligned}
$$

Table 15-6. Changes of Physical Findings Seen with Moderately Severe Dehydration as a Function of Serum Sodium Concentration

	Change with Different Types of Dehydration		
Biologic Characteristic	Isonatremic	Hyponatremic	Hypernatremic
Sodium loss in proportion to water	Proportionate	Increased	Decreased
Extracellular fluid volume decrease	Marked	Severe	Moderate
Intracellular fluid volume	Maintained	Increased	Decreased
Skin			
Temperature	Cool	Cool	Cool or warm
Turgor	Poor	Poor	Fair
Feel	Dry	Clammy	Thickened,doughy
Mucous membranes	Dry	Slightly moist	Parched
Neurologic status	Lethargic	Comatose	Irritable

(Adapted with permission of the publisher from Robson AM: Parenteral fluid therapy. In Behrman RE, Vaughan VC, Nelson WE: Nelson Textbook of Pediatrics, p 234. Philadelphia, WB Saunders Co, 1983.)

An alternative formula for calculation of maintenance requirements is given by Weil and Bailie (1977):

$$M \text{ (ml/kg/day)} = 95 - (3 \times \text{age in years})$$

Although this formula is easier to use in calculating fluid requirements of children, it tends to somewhat underestimate the fluid needs of infants and is not valid for patients over 18 years of age. Whichever formula is used, estimated "maintenance" fluids often need to be altered (see Table 15-10); for example, increased by about 10 percent for each degree centigrade of fever.

TREATMENT OF SEVERE DEHYDRATION

ORT is the treatment of choice for all but those patients in shock, with ileus, or with persistent severe vomiting. However, in shock, significant amounts of fluid might be absorbed from

Table 15-7. Signs Suggestive of Acid/Base Disturbances or Increased or Decreased Concentration of Specific Ions

Condition	Signs
Acidosis	Respiration depth and rate increased (Kussmaul breathing)
Alkalosis	Respiration depth and rate decreased, tetany
Hypokalemia	Intestinal ileus, muscle weakness, decreased deep tendon reflexes
Hyperkalemia	Cardiac ECG changes (peaked tall T waves, shortened Q-T interval, widened QRS), ventricular asystole or fibrillation, rarely flaccid muscle paralysis
Hypocalcemia	Tetany, seizures, jitteriness
Hypercalcemia	Constipation, anorexia, nausea and vomiting, abdominal pain, ileus, decreased muscle tone
Hypomagnesemia	Anorexia, nausea, vomiting, lethargy, weakness, tetany.
Hypermagnesemia	Absent deep tendon reflexes, hypotension, respiratory depression, lethargy, cardiac arrest

Table 15-8 Probable Total Body Deficits of Water and Electrolytes in Infants with Moderately Severe (10%) Dehydration

Condition	Deficit (mEq per kg body weight)[a]		
	Sodium	Potassium	Chloride
Fasting and thirst	5–7	1–2	4–6
Diarrhea			
Isonatremic	8–10	8–10	8–10
Hypernatremic	2–4	0–4	8–10
Hyponatremic	10–12	8–10	10–12
Pyloric stenosis	8–10	10–12	10–12
Diabetic ketoacidosis	8–10	5–7	6–8

[a]Water deficit for 10 percent dehydration = 100 ml/kg.

(Adapted with permission of the publisher from Robson AM: Parenteral fluid therapy. In Behrman RE, Vaughan VC, Nelson WE: Nelson Textbook of Pediatrics, p 232. Philadelphia, WB Saunders Co, 1983.)

Table 15-9. Estimating Diarrheal Stool Volumes

Type of Stool	Approximate Stool Volume (ml/kg/day)
"Mild" diarrhea	25–35
"Moderate" diarrhea	35–50
"Severe" diarrhea	60–75
Cholera	100–300

the gastrointestinal tract and some clinicians suggest that ORT be considered even here (through a nasogastric tube with aspiration precautions).

Dehydration with shock is a medical emergency and time should not be wasting attempting a venous cutdown. One or more large-bore needles should be aseptically placed as quickly as possible into a large vein, the peritoneal space, or the tibial intramedullary space. The following is a list of veins in order of priority, that can be used when intravenous therapy is elected:

- Peripheral arm veins
- Peripheral lower extremity veins
- External jugular veins
- Femoral veins
- Scalp veins in infants
- Internal jugular veins in children or adults
- Subclavian veins in adults

Emergency tibial intramedullary infusion is rapid, safe, effective, and easy to perform (Kanter et al 1986). Using the anterior approach, it only takes a few moments to insert

Figure 15-1. Burn assessment chart. The numbers under the figures indicate age; other numbers indicate percentage of body surface.

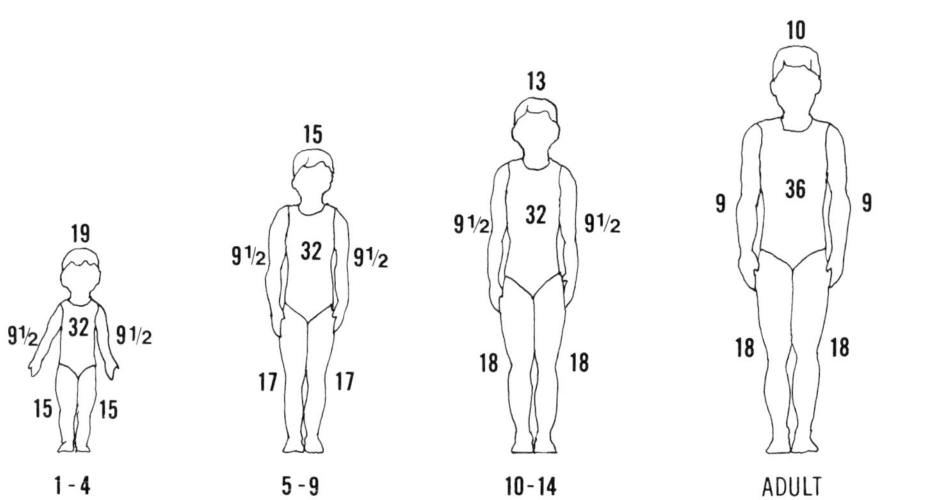

(Adapted with permission of the publisher from Behrman RE, Vaughan VC, Nelson WE: Nelson Textbook of Pediatrics, p 267, Philadelphia, WB Saunders Co, 1983.

Table 15-10. Factors Altering Maintenance Fluid Requirements

Maintenance Fluids Increased With
Fever (increased 10% for each degree centigrade over 37°C)
Heat stress
Increased respiratory rate
Increased renal losses (e.g., diabetes insipidus or uncontrolled diabetes mellitus)
Increased sweating
(Increased vomiting or diarrhea losses. Not included in this chapter under "maintenance," but calculated separately under "losses.")
Maintenance Fluids Decreased With
Decreased renal losses. A fluid challenge should usually be tried to be certain that the anuria or oliguria is not secondary to dehydration.
High humidity environments (e.g., mist tents)
Congestive heart failure
Syndrome of inappropriate antidiuretic hormone (e.g., with meningitis or closed head injuries)

an 18-gauge spinal needle (with the stylet in place) asceptically into the tibial intramedullary space. Once placed, the stylet is removed, and fluid is introduced rapidly through the needle.

Isotonic solutions such as normal saline or Ringers lactate (even through the latter has 4 mEq/liter potassium), are used initially for the severely dehydrated patient, followed in a few hours by one-third to one-half normal saline with 5 percent dextrose. Twenty to 40 mEq/liter of potassium chloride is added after the patient urinates.

A bolus of 10 to 20 ml/kg should be given as rapidly as possible to reestablish the patient's circulatory status. This dose may have to be repeated. Even when a patient appears to have no pulse, it is worth carrying out a rapid infusion trial because in near-terminal dehydrated patients, the heartbeat may be inaudible and the pulses virtually absent.

During therapy, the peripheral and central pulses, along with urine output, are monitored to guide initial infusion rates. Blood pressure is a less helpful guide because peripheral arteries may constrict while strong central pulses are maintained. The patient should be observed for signs of fluid overload such as neck vein distention, periorbital edema, and rales at the lung bases.

Experts disagree over how quickly fluid and electrolyte deficits should be replaced. Traditionally, rehydration has been accomplished over 24 to 48 hours to minimize the risks of congestive heart failure and seizures. Recent evidence suggests, however, that most children will tolerate more rapid rehydration such as over a 6- to 8-hour period. Even the prohibition against rapid rehydration of hypernatremic dehydration is now being questioned. Pizarro and co-workers (1983b) rehydrated 61 hypernatremic infants and children with ORT over an 8-hour period and found essentially the same seizure incidence as for children rehydrated over 24 to 48 hours in a previous study (8% and 14%, respectively). A major advantage of rapid therapy is that patients can be orally rehydrated in an out-patient clinic or, if hospitalized, the length of admission can be shortened.

Sample Calculation

A shocky, 15-kg child is approximately 15 percent dehydrated, and defecating about 25-ml stools approximately once an hour. What should the initial rate of fluid therapy be? What type of solution should be used?

A patient in shock first requires a bolus of fluid to help reestablish adequate circulatory status. With profound dehydration, venous access will be difficult to achieve; if this is the case, the intraperitoneal approach might be chosen. After the lower abdominal wall is thoroughly cleaned, a large-bore needle is placed perpendicularly through the midline, about halfway between the umbilicus and symphysis pubis. After entry, a 20 ml/kg of normal saline (without potassium) bolus is given through the needle, or about 300 ml (15 kg × 20 ml/kg) for this patient. Assuming the child responds well to the bolus, the next fluid therapy rate can be calculated from the formula mentioned earlier:

$$T_x = D + L + M$$

In this example, the values solved separately are as follows:

- (D)eficit = 15 kg × 0.15 = 2250 ml fluid deficit. If the decision is made to rehydrate over eight hours, this translates to about 280 ml/hour for the first eight hours.
- Continuing (L)osses = 25 ml/hour.
- (M)aintenance = (10 kg × 100 ml/kg/day) + (5 kg × 50 ml/kg/day) = 1250 ml/day. This, divided over a 24-hour period, yields a

maintenance requirement of 50 ml/hour (1250 ml/24 hr = 52.1 ml/hr).

Therefore, the child's initial fluid therapy rate, after the bolus, will be

$$T_x = 280 + 25 + 50$$
$$T_x \sim 350 \text{ ml/hr}$$

In this example, what type of fluid should be used? The composition of the bolus has already been noted. For the first few hours, intraperitoneal therapy might be continued or an IV started. The proper choice of IV fluids will depend on the electrolyte composition of the lost fluids and other factors noted above. One-third normal saline in a 5 percent dextrose (D5W) solution is appropriate for most situations, often after normal saline is used for the first few hours. Potassium at 20 to 30 mEq/liter is added after the child urinates. The patient is switched to ORT as soon as possible.

Simplified Table for Fluid Therapy

Table 15-11 provides a simplified approach to fluid therapy designed specifically for nonphysicians who might need to treat patients with parenteral fluids. Given the patient's weight and approximate degree of dehydration, fluid requirements per hour can be read directly

Table 15-11. Simplified Approach to Fluid Therapy: Approximate Fluid Therapy Rates (in ml/hour)

Weight (kg)(1)	Maintenance Fluid Rate (2)	Level of Dehydration 5% (3)	10% (4)	15% (5)	Bolus of Ringer's Lactate or Normal Saline for Severe Dehydration (6)
1	4	10	17	24	15
2	8	20	33	45	30
3	12	30	50	70	45
4	17	40	70	90	60
5	20	50	80	115	75
6	25	60	100	140	90
7	30	75	120	160	105
8	35	85	135	185	120
9	40	100	150	210	135
10	40	100	165	230	150
11	45	115	180	250	165
12	45	120	200	270	180
13	50	130	210	300	200
14	50	140	225	300	210
15	50	145	240	330	225
20	65	190	315	440	300
25	65	220	380	530	375
30	70	250	450	630	450
35	75	300	500	730	525
40	80	330	580	830	600
45	85	370	650	930	675
50	85	400	700	1020	750
55	90	430	780	1120	825
60	100	475	850	1220	900
65	100	500	900	1320	975
70	100	540	975	1400	1050

Column 2 = maintenance, based on 100 ml/kg/d for the first 10 kg, 50 ml/kg/d for the next 10 kg, and 20 ml/kg/d for each kilogram over 20. Columns 3, 4, and 5 = dehydration deficit, replaced over eight hours (maintenance included). Column 6 = fluid bolus for severe dehydration, at 15 ml/kg.

from the table. (The maintenance requirements are calculated from the Segar formula outlined above. Dehydration losses are calculated for replacement over eight hours. The fluid bolus for shocky patients is figured at 15 ml/kg.)

For example, if only maintenance fluids are needed, find the patient's weight in Column 1, and read the maintenance fluid rate (in milliliters per hour) in Column 2. If the patient is mildly, moderately, or severely dehydrated, read the fluid requirement directly from Column 3, 4, or 5, respectively. Note that maintenance requirements are already included in Columns 3, 4, and 5. Patients with profound dehydration and signs of shock should be given a fluid bolus, as indicated in Column 6, followed by the hourly fluid rate indicated in Column 5. Remember that continuing losses must be added to these requirements. Also, see Table 15-10 for factors that increase or decrease maintenance requirments.

Here is one example in the use of Table 15-11. What would be the initial fluid therapy rate for a 10 percent dehydrated, afebrile, 13-kg child with early signs of shock, and approximately 20 ml/hr of continuing stool loss? First, find 13 kg in Column 1. Column 6 shows the fluid bolus volume to be 200 ml of normal saline or Ringer's lactate solution. Column 4 provides the initial hourly maintenance rate of 210 ml/hr (figured to replace the losses over eight hours), to which the continuing losses of 20 ml/hr should be added, for a total of 230 ml/hr after the bolus.

This chapter focuses on the fluid and electrolyte treatment of dehydration. If the patient is hypovolemic from another cause, for example trauma or a gastrointestinal bleed, the same approaches can be used. However, with massive blood loss or septic shock, other options might be considered. For these patients, there is research to support the use of colloid (e.g., 5% albumin) rather than crystalloid (normal saline or Ringer's lactage solution) (Rackow et al 1983). Blood replacement will be needed eventually for patients with massive blood loss.

When all of the calculations are completed, it might be well to remember that a wise nephrologist once said, "The dumbest kidney is smarter than the smartest doctor" in helping to determine the actual fluid needs of the patient. Urine output should be greater than 1 ml/kg/hr, and urine specific gravity less than 1.015. The patient's thirst is also an excellent guide for fluid requirements. Daily weight plus measurements of intake and output should be monitored. A helpful rule is that the patient will lose about 1 kg of body weight for each 7700 calories of body mass consumed. Therefore, if the patient has a 1900 cal/day calculated requirement and is not consuming any food, a 0.250-kg (7700/1900) daily weight loss would be expected. A larger weight loss usually indicates a net loss of water, suggesting that an increase in fluid intake is needed. Conversely, if the patient is gaining more weight than expected, a net fluid gain is evident and fluid therapy may need to be decreased.

REFERENCES

American Academy of Pediatrics, Committee on Nutrition: Use of oral fluid therapy and posttreatment feeding following enteritis in children in a developed country. Pediatrics 1985;75:358–61.

Favin MN, McMurty ME: Oral Rehydration Therapy. Information for Action Resource Guide. Washington, DC, World Federation of Public Health Associations, American Public Health Association, 1983.

Finberg L et al: Oral rehydration for diarrhea. J Pediatr 1982;101:497–99.

Hirschhorn N: Successful ORT. Dialogue on Diarrhoea 1985;22:6.

Hirschhorn N: The treatment of acute diarrhea in children: An historical and physiological perspective. Am J Clin Nutr 1980;33:637–63.

Kanter RK, Zimmerman JJ, Strauss et al: Pediatric emergency intravenous access. Am J Dis Child 1986;140:132–34.

Parker RL, Rinehart W, Piotrow PT et al: Oral Rehydration Therapy for Childhood Diarrhea. Population Reports Series L, No 2, July–August 1984.

Pierce NF, Hirschhorn N: Oral fluid—a simple weapon against dehydration in diarrhoea: How it works and how to use it. WHO Chronicle 1977;31:87–93.

Pizarro D, Posada G, Mata L: Treatment of 242 neonates with dehydrating diarrhea with an oral glucose-electrolyte solution. J Pediatr 1983a;102:153–56.

Pizarro D, Posada G, Villavicencio N et al: Oral rehydration in hypernatremic and hyponatremic diarrheal dehydration. Am J Dis Child 1983b;137:730–34.

Rackow EC, Falk JL, Fein A et al: Fluid resuscitation in circulatory shock: A comparison of the cardiorespiratory effects of albumin, hetastarch, and saline solutions in patients with hypovolemic and septic shock. Critical Care Med 1983;11:839–49.

Rohde JE, Sadjimin T: Elementary-school pupils as educators: Role of school health programmes in primary health care. Lancet 1980;1(8182):1350–52.

Robson AM: Parenteral fluid therapy. In Behrman RE, Vaughan VC, Nelson WE: Nelson Textbook of Pediatrics, pp 228–49. Philadelphia, WB Saunders Co, 1983.

Santosham M, Sack RB, Lochlear E et al (letter): Storing oral rehydration solution. Lancet 1982a:1(8275):797.

Santosham M, Daum RS, Dillman L et al: Oral rehydration therapy of infantile diarrhea: A controlled study of well-nourished children hospitalized in the United States and Panama. N Engl J Med 1982b;306:1070–76.

Segar WE: Parenteral fluid therapy. Curr Probl Pediatr 1972;3:3–40.

Sladen GE, Dawson AN: Interrelationships between the absorption of glucose, sodium, and water by the normal human jejunum. Clin Sci 1969;36:119–32.

Tamer AM, Friedman LB, Maxwell SR et al: Oral rehydration of infants in a large urban US medical center. J Pediatr 1985;107:14–19.

Weil WB, Bailie MD: Fluid and Electrolyte Metabolism in Infants and Children. New York, Grune & Stratton, 1977.

World Health Organization: Treatment and Prevention of Dehydration in Diarrheal Diseases. Geneva, World Health Organization, 1977.

16
Surgical Aspects of Refugee Health Care

L. MASON COBB
WILLIAM P. SCHECTER

Surgical problems of refugees may vary widely from one locale to another. Likewise, the expertise of personnel and available material will vary widely from camp to camp. Therefore, this chapter considers only basic concepts and approaches.

Two types of surgical problems must be addressed in the refugee setting. First, there are situations that can be handled by nonsurgeon physicians with some knowledge and expertise. Second, more serious problems require specialized surgical expertise and resources beyond the scope of the nonsurgeon. When these resources are not immediately available, primary health care workers must attempt to stabilize the patient until transfer is possible.

The health care worker without specialized surgical training requires authoritative texts to handle either of these two types of problems adequately. Texts should cover closed treatment of fractures, basic surgical wound management, and diagnosis of the acute abdomen. A list of books which we have found very useful in surgical practice in underdeveloped countries is included at the end of this chapter.

In the Khmer refugee crisis of 1979, about one third of the major surgical problems were war-related. More than two thirds were non-war-related; possibly half of those problems could have been (or were) managed by nonsurgeons. Therefore, some war injuries will be discussed in this chapter; however, the bulk of this chapter will address the more commonly encountered problems that a nonsurgically trained physician can manage when given the proper guidelines.

EQUIPMENT

Equipment and facilities will vary widely from refugee camp to refugee camp. However, certain very basic tools of the trade are required in any setting. These basic tools are listed in Table 16-1.

Three major classes of drugs form the basic armamentarium for the physician involved in surgical care. Antibiotics are discussed in Chapter 23. The second class of drugs includes sedatives, narcotics, hypnotics, and other unclassified agents that are given in the preoperative setting to make the procedure more comfortable for the patient and more manageable for the operator. Their basic features are described in Table 16-2. The third class of drugs includes regional and local anesthetics. Their uses and properties are shown in Table 16-3. Techniques for the major regional blocks, demonstrated nicely in Hill's *Outpatient Surgery* (1980), should be mastered.

EVALUATION

Successful surgical management requires accurate diagnosis and good surgical technique. Good diagnosis depends on a reliable history, which must be taken despite possible language and cultural barriers. Even though the physical examination may suggest a complete story, a complete regional and systemic history and related review of symptoms are as important for surgical problems as for medical problems.

For trauma victims, for example, a general history should include the mechanism of injury, an estimate of the amount of blood loss at the scene of the accident, a history of previous hospitalizations and operations, a history of medications taken, and a history of allergies. Most refugee patients will not have been immunized against tetanus.

Patients who present with abdominal pain will require an organized history. Did the pain begin suddenly or did it slowly worsen? How long has the pain been present? Is the pain getting better or worse? Where is the pain located? Has it moved? Is the pain constant or does it come and go? Is the pain associated with nausea, vomiting, diarrhea, or hematemesis? Are bowel movements regular and once a day? Is

Table 16-1. Equipment

Syringes and needles from 1 to 60 cc and 18 to 25 gauge
Antiseptic
Sterile towels
Sterile gloves
Dressing supplies
No. 10 and No. 11 scalpel blades, plus a scalpel handle
Suture material (absorbable and nonabsorbable)
Drains (Penrose or rubberband)
Double-edge safety razor and blades
Hemostats (curved and straight)
Sterile gauze sponges
Thumb forceps
Scissors (suture and tissue)
Blood pressure cuff
Elastic bandages
Chest tubes from 20F to 36F
Tubing and bottles or other collection device for chest tube
Large-bore 14 or 16-gauge central venous catheter equipment or cutdown catheters
Iodoform gauze
Laryngoscope and endotracheal tubes
Ambu or Mapleson ventilating bag
Sterilization equipment

the stool brown or is blood or melena present? Is there any history of jaundice, gallbladder disease, or pancreatitis? Is urinary frequency, dysuria, or hematuria present? In women, an accurate menstrual and obstetric history is very important. In particular, the relationship of the abdominal pain to the last menstrual period may give important diagnostic clues. A complete review of systems may pick up unusual causes of abdominal pain.

Perhaps more than in other fields, the physical examination is crucial in surgical problems. Especially important is differentiation of infected from noninfected tissue. In injuries and infections of the extremities, a thorough regional neurovascular and structural examination is important. The differentiation of peritonitis from other causes of pain and tenderness must be made in the abdominal examination. Observing the patient in shock from moment to moment during resuscitation is a life-saving skill. Not only in the refugee setting but in nearly any surgical situation, careful physical assessment before and after surgery is needed for good results.

note the location and condition of the wound. Is the wound tidy or is it filled with dirt, grease, or vegetation? In extremity wounds, a careful examination of the distal blood supply, pulses, and sensory and motor nerve function is essential. In addition, knowledge of the anatomy of the area of injury will allow specific testing of the nerve and muscle–tendon units that may have been damaged.

Thoughtful examination of the acute abdomen is one of the most difficult skills in clinical examination. Ask the patient to cough. Cough tenderness, either localized or generalized, is highly suggestive of peritoneal irritation. Gently scratch the skin in the four abdominal quadrants. Hyperesthesia of the overlying skin may suggest underlying parietal peritoneal irritation. Then, gently percuss the four abdominal quadrants again looking for localized tenderness. Gentle, light abdominal palpation is next, followed by the assessment of rebound tenderness in the four abdominal quadrants. This test is done by gently palpating the abdomen and quickly releasing the palpating hand. The resulting movement of the peritoneum is exquisitely tender in the presence of peritonitis or peritoneal irritation. Only after completion of an organized search for peritoneal irritation should deep palpation of the abdomen be performed. Observation of a distended abdomen, visible peristalsis, hepatosplenomegally, or an intra-abdominal mass may yield important diagnostic clues. Every patient presenting with acute abdominal pain requires a rectal and pelvic examination, if appropriate. Technique and attention to detail are essential to the surgical physical examination. Details of the examination of the acute abdomen are given later.

SURGICAL TECHNIQUE

In the best of all possible worlds, surgical procedures would be performed under absolutely sterile conditions on a well-nourished, normovolemic, nonanemic patient who is medically sophisticated enough to manage his or her surgical wounds successfully in the postoperative period. A clean, stable environment during the recovery period is also desirable. None of these conditions may prevail in the refugee setting. The factor that is controllable, however, is the operator's technique.

Failure to follow sterile precautions is the single greatest contributor to bad results. Sterile technique involves careful cleansing of the

Table 16-2. Preoperative Medications and Sedatives

Agent	Description
Thiamylal (Surital)	
Action	Short-acting barbiturate
Route	IV
Dose	Children: 2–5 mg/kg Adults: 150–200 mg
Duration	10 minutes
Advantages	Rapid onset Predictable response Wide margin of safety
Cautions	Dose should not be repeated more than one time Intubation equipment should be available for respiratory depression Should not be given to patients with a full stomach
Thiopental (Pentothal)	
Action	Short-acting barbiturate
Route	IV
Dose	Children: 2–5 mg/kg. Give lower dose first and increase as needed. Adults: 3–5 mg/kg up to 200 mg (dose may be increased until the blink reflex is lost)
Duration	5–10 minutes
Advantages	Rapidly acting Safe if overdosage is not given
Cautions	Do not use in acute intermittent porphyria Prepare to deal with respiratory depression
Methohexital (Brevital)	
Action	Ultra-short-acting barbiturate
Route	IM, PO, or per rectum
Dose	Same as for thiopental
Duration	10–15 minutes
Advantages	Less drowsiness postprocedure than from most other ultra-short-acting barbiturates Rapid onset IM or by rectum
Caution	Beware of vomiting Be aware of possibility for respiratory and cardiovascular depression Do not use repetitively
Fentanyl (Sublimaze)	
Action	Narcotic analgesic
Route	IV
Dose	0.002–0.05 mg/kg IV or IM; individualize dosage
Duration	15–30 minutes
Advantage	May be reversed with naloxone One of most potent narcotics
Cautions	Respiratory depressant May produce bronchospasm
Naloxone (Narcan)	
Action	Narcotic antagonist; to reverse narcotic overdose
Route	IV
Dose	0.2–0.4 mg May be repeated
Duration	Very short Patient should be observed for reappearance of respiratory depression
Advantage	Offers a rapid method of reversing narcotic overdosage
Caution	See duration
Ketamine	
Action	So-called dissociative anesthetic; no other distinct class
Route	IV or IM
Dose	2 mg/kg IV, over 4 minutes 5–10 mg/kg IM
Duration	15–20 minutes
Advantage	Excellent analgesia with amnesia and little respiratory depression
Caution	Beware of hallucinations; may be used with barbiturate or a benzodiazapine to minimize these Laryngospasm may occur Respiratory depression with too rapid IV administration
Diazepam (Valium)	
Action	Sedative and amnestic
Route	PO, IV, per rectum
Dose	Children: 0.1–0.3 mg/kg Adults: 2.5–10 mg

Table 16-2. Preoperative Medications and Sedatives (*Continued*)

Agent	Description	Agent	Description
		Chloral hydrate	
Duration	15–45 minutes	Route	PO or per rectum
Advantage	Rapid onset IV Good amnestic response IV Works well and fairly rapidly PO	Dose	Children: 50–65 mg/kg Adults: 1–2 g
Caution	Apnea with rapid IV dosage Does not absorb well IM Effect not predictable in children	Duration	30–45 minutes
		Advantages	Very safe
		Caution	Unpredictable sedative effect Respiratory depression a risk with larger doses

Table 16-3. Local Anesthetics

Types of block	
Topical	Works best on mucosal surfaces; several agents
Field	Dermal injection in surrounding area (e.g., scalp, abdominal wall); 0.5–1.0% lidocaine is best
Infiltration	Direct dermal injection. Too deep an injection *beneath* the dermis wastes medication and does not produce anesthesia. Be sure the entire area is injected. Lidocaine is most commonly used, often mixed with epinephrine for improved hemostasis—except local anesthetic injection of distal extremities is done *without* epinephrine.
Regional	Specific nerve blocks give regional anesthesia; most useful on extremities
Recommended Agents	
Lidocaine (Xylocaine)	
Supplied	0.5–2.0%
Route	Infiltration, topical, regional
Maximum dose	4 mg/kg
Onset	Infiltrate, 1 minute Regional, 5–10 minutes
Duration	30–60 minutes
Advantages	Rapid onset Few adverse reactions
Recommended Agents (*Continued*)	
Cautions	Convulsions or hypotension may be seen
Bupivicaine (Marcaine)	
Supplied	0.25–0.75%
Route	Infiltration, regional
Maximum dose	175 mg (adult)
Onset	10–15 minutes
Duration	12–18 hours
Advantages	Long-lasting block (e.g., intercostal blocks, other regional blocks) Good for incisional relief
Cautions	Tremor, convulsions
Tetracaine (Pontocaine)	
Supplied	1 to 3% solution
Route	Topical (spray)
Maximum dose	(may be absorbed) 150 mg Children: 1.5 mg/kg
Onset	Nearly immediate
Duration	2 hours
Advantage	Not irritating to mucosa Rapid onset with good duration
Caution	Very safe; occasional convulsions

operative site with soap and water and then antiseptic solution. Sterile towels or other drapes must be applied in such a way that they do not slide from an unsterile area onto the operative field. Anything crossing the sterile area (including the operator's and the assistants' arms and clothing) must also be sterile. The most difficult aspect of sterile technique is the discipline required to reglove, reprepare the skin, redrape, or discard an instrument if it becomes contaminated. When the operator is exhausted and the workload is particularly heavy, this requirement of proper technique is often abandoned. These breaches of sterile protocol are significant causes of poor operative results due to infection. If an autoclave for instruments and other operative material is not available, instruments should be rinsed with sterile water or saline before being used. If this is not possible, equipment should be boiled for a minimum of five minutes and handled only with other sterile materials to transfer them to the operative field. Alternatives, such as soaking in Cidex or other antiseptic solution, are also effective.

OTHER TECHNIQUES

Other techniques important to proper healing include the following:

1. Adequate debridement of contaminated wounds is essential. A contaminated wound should be debrided liberally except when it is on the face, or great amounts of tension are required for closure. Respect must be given to tendons, nerves, and major blood vessels. When in doubt about the viability of tissue, it is always wise to debride. Sharp debridement (scissors or scalpel) does not leave crushed tissue behind. Even though additional bleeding may be associated with the debridement, it is controllable and, in fact, a sign that viable and clean tissue has been reached. When in doubt, leave heavily contaminated wounds open. A delayed, primary closure may be performed four to five days later if no infection develops.
2. Foreign bodies must not be left within a surgical wound. Bits of bone, dirt, cloth, and other objects must be assiduously irrigated, debrided, or otherwise removed from the wound. Besides poor sterile technique, foreign or dead material is the greatest cause of poor healing. This is especially true of war-related injuries such as shrapnel or bullet wounds. The bullet or shrapnel itself may be left in place if its removal would be complicated or dangerous to important structures, but the wound must be clean and viable.
3. Although a wound may bleed profusely, this bleeding must be controlled without undue damage to the tissue. Wound hematomas provide an excellent culture medium and may lead to infection. If the hematoma is under closed fascia, a compartment syndrome may develop and jeopardize a limb. The application of a hemostat should include as little tissue (other than the bleeding vessel) as possible. Sometimes leaving the hemostat in place for a couple of minutes is all that is required to check the bleeding; a ligature or suture ligature may not be required. If no vessel is clearly visible, but there is a slow ooze, then compression for five minutes by the clock (especially with a warm pack) may be effective in controlling bleeding. In open or infected wounds, or those in which considerable dead space is left behind, a rubber drain (or a finger of a sterile glove) or gauze packing may be left in place and removed when the drainage decreases. Packing should generally be removed within 24 hours, or at least be progressively removed over the course of two to three days.
4. Management of dressings is largely a matter of patient education after the original dressing is applied. This factor may be one of the most difficult to control but also one of the most important.
5. Proper instruction to patients and their families is necessary to ensure proper wound care after a procedure is performed. Traditional remedies that are deleterious to wound healing are sometimes applied. A knowledge of the population's clothing, habits, and health attitudes is important to ensure compliance.

The operator must be sure that postoperative instructions are successfully communicated and that an understanding is reached with the patient. Perhaps the most important factor in the operative process is the patient's perception that the doctor is competent and cares personally about the patient.

ANESTHESIA

Certain procedures, especially extensive procedures or intracavitary surgery, are best done under general or spinal anesthesia. A trained surgeon, if one is available, should perform most such procedures. General anesthesia may be available only in centers where more sophisticated procedures are done. In the United States, regional blocks are not widely used because of the safety and efficiency of general anesthesia in the hospital setting.

Common to all anesthetic techniques are the concepts of resuscitation, homeostasis, and pain relief. Most surgical procedures performed by the physician without specialist training can be done with local or regional anesthesia. Local techniques range from a local field block to peripheral nerve block and, finally, to major nerve plexus blocks. Well-thought-out and well-executed regional anesthesia can be performed quite rapidly and will allow nearly painless surgery in most cases. Refer to Table 16-3 for the more commonly used agents.

Regional blocks or other procedures that require tourniquets and wrapping of an extremity should be avoided in patients with sickle cell anemia or serious overall circulatory compromise. Allergic or other previous severe reaction to regional anesthetic agents is also a contraindication to their use.

Another key to the successful use of local or regional anesthesia is communication with the patient. The operator must maintain complete composure throughout the procedure and communicate with the patient at frequent intervals. Thus, "verbocaine" greatly potentiates the effect of any type of block.

Knowledge of the duration of the agent's action, the effects of overdosage and toxicity and the ability to fit the particular agent to the situation are required for safe and successful use. Although there are situations in which spinal, epidural, sympathetic, or pudendal blocks may be desirable, they are not within the scope of this chapter. Refer to a standard text for such information.

TRAUMA

Trauma has become a subspecialty within surgery. The possible types of trauma that can be encountered in a refugee camp are nearly limitless. Minor trauma can be managed easily. Major trauma requires prompt and skillful stabilization, and definitive management by a trained surgeon. Therefore, both triage and prognostic decisions must be based on the availability of more sophisticated surgical care.

The more common traumatic situations in the refugee experience will be discussed here. Again, reference to a standard surgery text will be necessary for details and for information on management of specific types of injury.

To quote Shakespeare's Hamlet, "The native hue of resolution/is sicklied o'er with the pale cast of thought/ . . . and lose[s] the name of action." The major problem for most physicians who are unfamiliar with trauma management is the delay of forthright action in pursuing diagnosis and treatment. Even for those unfamiliar with trauma or who lack sophisticated resources, certain principles may be applied that will give an accurate diagnosis of the type, extent, and severity of injury, and ways of effectively managing it.

The physician dealing with refugees needs an easy-to-use armamentarium of techniques for diagnosis and emergency treatment of trauma. Following protocols may be unimaginative, but it is often effective in the emergency setting. Tables 16-4, 16-5, and 16-6 present trauma protocols and checklists.

Minor Trauma

By far, the most common injuries incurred are minor and will resolve without the intervention of a physician. In certain injuries, although minor, steps that the physician can take can produce better cosmetic results and ameliorate suffering.

Lacerations

At the time a laceration is evaluated, the tetanus immunization status should be determined (see Chapter 6). The initial evaluation should consider the seriousness of the injury, the time since its occurrence, and how badly it is contaminated. If folk remedies have already been used, their effect on standard medical treatment should be considered. The degree of wound contamination will affect the decision to cover a patient with antibiotics and, in combination with the tetanus status, should determine whether or not active tetanus prophylaxis is required.

Anatomic considerations concern the part of the body injured and the presence of musculotendonous injury, bony injury, or neurovascular injury. It is beyond the scope of this chapter to discuss specific treatments for these more complex injuries. Generally, however, extensor tendon injuries can be managed on an out-patient basis by suturing the tendon together using heavy, nonabsorbable suture and

Table 16-4. Trauma Priorities

Assess
- Vital sign stability, general inspection
- Airway (O_2)—Prong or mask
  - Oral airway
  - Endotracheal tube or tracheostomy (e.g., when stridor, laryngeal or neck edema, or emphysema is present)

Bleeding
- Tamponade
- Immobilize
- Thoracotomy[a] (for crush injury, stab wound with cardiac tamponade, flail chest, history of deceleration injury or hemothorax with persistent hypotension)
- Blood (O negative or unmatched type-specific)[a]
- Crystalloid and colloid—until blood pressure and urine output increase adequately
- IV—cutdown, 12–14 gauge

Cardiovascular
- Monitor
- Closed chest cardiac compressions PRN
- Volume is key

Consciousness—Glasgow coma scale[b]

Eye Opening		Motor Response		Verbal Response	
Spontaneous	4	Obeys commands	6	Orientated	5
To speach	3	Localizes pain	5	Confused	4
To pain	2	Withdraws	4	Inappropriate	3
Nil	1	Abnormal flexion	3	Incomprehensible	2
		Extensor response	2	Nil	1
		Nil	1		

Digestive
- Nasogastric tube if any question of gastrointestinal tract injury, or presence of depressed consciousness

Excretory
- Rectal exam
- Foley urethral catheter if no urine extravasation
- Urethrogram (if indicated)[a]

Fractures
- Evaluate
- "Splint 'em as they lie"

[a]If facilities are available.
[b]The score is the sum of all three sectional scores. A Glasgow scale of 6 for 8 hours carries a high mortality.

splinting for three weeks in the so-called position of function. Flexor tendon repairs require special expertise, but the skin cut can usually be closed primarily, the hand splinted, and elective repair planned.

A wound on the face less than 12 hours old, or on the extremities less than 8 hours old, can be closed safely when seen. Although irrigation, even with a solution containing an antiseptic, is important, sharp debridement is the key to preventing infection. This is best accomplished with small scissors, but a scalpel may be used while holding the tissue to be debrided under tension with thumb forceps. Sharp debridement of the skin should be precisely perpendicular to the plane of the skin, so the apposing edges of the skin fit together without a bevel.

Any dead space should be eliminated with absorbable suture including muscle bellies and fascial planes of muscle. Fatty subcutaneous tissue, especially, must be carefully closed with absorbable suture. The best cosmetic result can be obtained with a deep dermal closure using

Table 16-5. Trauma Checklist

Assess	Do	Complete	Obtain	Remember to check for
Airway	IV	Fracture	Lab	No cervical fx
Oral Airway	No. 12–16	exam	ABG[a,b]	No aortic tear
Oxygen	Foley	splinting	CBC[c]	No hypoxia
Endotracheal tube	(except urethral trauma)	Neuro exam	T&CM 6U[a,j]	No hemoperitoneum
		Consciousness level	Urinalysis	No pneumothorax
Bleeding	Immunization	(Glasgow)	X-Ray[a]	Changes over time
Tamponade	(DT or DPT[f])	Cranial nerves	Skull	
Immobilization	NG[i]	Spinal Cord	Cervical spine	
Thoracotomy[a]	CPR[d]	Motor function	Chest	
Circulation		Screening exam	Abdomen	
Vital signs		Chest: Palpate	Special:	
Monitor:		Auscultate	IVP[h]	
ECG[a,g]		Ventilate	Urethrogram	
CVP[a,e]		Chest tube	Bones	
		Abdomen: Palpate		
		Ausculate		
		Lavage[a]		
		Genitourinary exam		
		Rectal exam		

[a] If facilities are available
[b]ABG = arterial blood gas.
[c]CBC = complete blood count.
[d]CPR = cardiopulmonary resuscitation.
[e]CVP = central venous pressure.
[f]DPT = diphtheria, pertussis, tetanus.
[g]ECG = electrocardiogram.
[h]IVP = intravenous pylogram.
[i]NG = nasogastric tube.
[j]T &CM 6U = type and crossmatch 6 units of blood.

fine surgical absorbable suture in an interrupted fashion, followed by a superficial epidermal closure with a running fine suture.

The dressing is not as important as the instruction to keep the wound clean and dry, and the understanding that, with signs of infection, follow-up and aggressive treatment are needed.

Infected wounds should not be closed primarily, and general principles of drainage of dead space, cleansing of the wound, and appropriate dressings, elevation, immobilization, and antibiotics should be used. This is particularly applicable to hand infections. However, pus tracking down a tendon sheath must be treated aggressively with special drainage techniques. Exquisite pain on slight movement at the joint, swelling, and tenderness along the tendon proximally are suggestive of infection.

Animal bites should generally be debrided very thoroughly and left open. These are packed with saline-moistened gauze at least daily until granulation and epithelialization are established. Such wounds on the face may be closed primarily, and an antibiotic should be given. Recommendations for treatment of rabies are given in Table 16-7.

Septic Surgery

The surgery of the complications of infection constitutes the bulk of the surgical practice in underdeveloped countries. The majority of such cases will be due to bacterial infection. There are three major types of septic complications—drainage; nectrotizing soft tissue infections requiring wide debridement of all involved skin, fat, fascia, and muscle; and infected gangrenous extremities due to diabetes or peripheral vascular disease requiring wide debridement or amputation.

The classic signs of pain, redness, swelling, heat, and impaired function suggest a diagnosis of infection. A history of trauma is often present. Needle aspiration revealing pus may prompt immediate incision and drainage in borderline cases. Other cases will more obvi-

Table 16-6. Specific Procedures

Endotracheal Tube
- Suction available
- Compress larynx
- Beware of cervical spine injury
  - (Use nasotracheal tube if there is a question of cervical spine fracture and spontaneous respirations are present.)

Central venous pressure line
- IV ready
- Dressing ready
- Antibiotic ointment
- Benzoine
- Chest x-ray (portable upright)
- Take great care if patient is agitated

IV
- Proper needles
- IV ready—percutaneous femoral, cephalic, antecubital
- Children—intraosseus
- Cutdown
  - Quickest is saphenous at groin
  - Obtain blood sample

Peritoneal lavage
- Bladder and stomach evacuated
- Lavage specimen sent for
  - Hematocrit
  - White blood cell count
  - Gram stain

Chest tube
- Bottles to suction with chambers filled properly
- Dressing

Pericardiocentesis
- No. 16 angiocath or spinal needle from under xiphoid toward left scapula
- ECG with alligator clip-on needle (lead V precordial)

Facial or head injury
- Assess Glascow Coma Scale
- Assess facial bones
- Assess cranial nerves
- Clean and debride
- Use sutures with long tails in scalp

Fractures
- Splint in position found

Spine fx
- Use "log roll" method to move patient, with doctor at patient's head while traction applied

Nasogastric tube
- Not through the nose with severe facial injury or basilar skull fracture, attach to suction

ously require incision and drainage when first seen. In countries located in the tropical belt, deep-seated muscle infections (tropical pyogenic myositis) may present as swelling and pain without the usual signs of heat and redness. This is because of their deep-seated nature. Experience will make these infections readily identifiable in endemic areas, as they are quite common. They almost always require incision and drainage (I and D) and are usually caused by *Staphylococcus aureus.* If antibiotic supplies are limited, I and D will usually solve the problem. On the other hand, if antibiotic supplies are available, a short course of antibiotics following I and D may lead to more rapid resolution of the surrounding cellulitis.

Physical findings suggesting the possibility of a necrotizing soft tissue infection include bright shiny skin, blistering of the skin, or black areas on the skin, as well as respiratory and hemodynamic instability usually with tachycardia. If the surrounding area of cellulitis rapidly advances in the space of a few hours of observation, a necrotizing soft tissue infection is likely. Patients with such infections require large doses of antibiotics with aerobic, anaerobic, and gram-negative coverage. However, antibiotics alone will not cure this infection. The infection must be cut from the body. This is a major operation requiring general anesthesia and often involving the loss of several units of blood.

The feasibility of aggressive treatment in such an infecton will depend on the hospital facilities and blood resources available, as well as the skill and workload of the medical staff. The management of these cases is labor intensive, as wound care and nutrition are major problems.

Treatment of infected gangrene of the extremities requires amputation. The amputation should initially be a guillotine type. The infected part should be removed and the wound left open to drain. Several days later, after appropriate antibiotic therapy, the patient may be returned to surgery for revision and closure of the stump.

Burns

Many patients with second- and third-degree burns who are treated as in-patients in more sophisticated settings can be handled on an out-patient basis. In general, patients without inhalation injury, and who have less than 25 percent of their body surface area burned, can

Table 16-7. A Guide to Prophylaxis Against Rabies in Exposed Persons

A. General considerations

1. Rabies occurs in many wild animals, bats and domestic animals such as dogs, cats, and cattle, but rarely, if ever, in rodents.
2. A dog or cat that remains healthy for 10 days after a bite does not have rabies, and prophylaxis for a person bitten by that animal is not indicated.
3. A negative fluorescent antibody (FA) examination of an animal brain in an experienced laboratory is reliable evidence that the animal did not have rabies.
4. Saliva of a rabid animal on an open wound (usually a bite) or mucous membrane constitutes exposure to rabies.
5. A decision to initiate postexposure prophylaxis is based on balancing two probabilities: (a) that rabies virus was introduced into an exposed person and (b) that a serious reaction to prophylaxis material might occur.
6. The Centers for Disease Control's approach to rabies postexposure prophylaxis is summarized in Part B. The guidelines illustrated constitute an algorithmic interpretation of the U.S. Public Health Service's official treatment recommendations.

B. Postexposure rabies prophylaxis algorithm — RABIES PROPHYLAXIS

1. Was the person bitten or licked on an open wound or mucous membranes by a possibly rabid animal? → NO → None
   ↓ YES
2. Is rabies known or suspected to be present in the species and area? → NO → None
   ↓ YES
3. Was the animal captured? → NO → 4. Is the animal a dog or cat? → NO → Serum and vaccine
   - 4. ↓ YES → 5. Was the person bitten? → NO → Vaccine
   - 5. ↓ YES → Serum and vaccine
   - 3. ↓ YES → 6.
6. Was the animal a normally behaving vaccinated dog or cat? → YES → 7. Does the animal become ill under observation during next 10 days? → NO → None
   - 7. ↓ YES → 8.
   - 6. ↓ NO → 8.
8. Does laboratory examination of brain by fluorescent antibody confirm rabies? → NO → None
   ↓ YES → Serum and vaccine

Table 16-7. A Guide to Prophylaxis Against Rabies in Exposed Persons (*Continued*)

C. Principles of postexposure prophylaxis

1. Local wound treatment is very important. Thoroughly scrub the wound with soap and water.
2. Indications for immunization, dosages, injection sites, and adverse reactions (see Part B):
   a. For all bite exposures, unless rabies can be excluded, and for all nonbite exposures if the animal is proven to have or is strongly suspected of having rabies, provide both passive and active immunization. Passive immunization is achieved by using either human rabies immune globulin (RIG) (20 IU/kg), or equine antirabies serum (ARS) (40 IU/kg). With either RIG or ARS, infiltrate the wound with up to 50% of the material and give the remainder intramuscularly in the buttocks. RIG eliminates the hazards of sensitivity to horse serum. RIG or ARS is administered only one time, at the initiation of antirabies therapy.

      and

      Rabies Vaccine (V), giving a total of 23 doses, 1 dose daily for 21 days (or 2 doses daily for 7 days and then 1 dose daily for 7 days). Then for either schedule, give an additional dose 10 and 20 days after the primary series. Give vaccine subcutaneously in the abdomen or thigh, rotating the sites of injection.
   b. For nonbite exposures from escaped dogs or cats in a rabies-endemic area (this is the only indication for using vaccine prophylaxis alone), rabies vaccine should be given daily for 14 days. Injection sites are rotated and given subcutaneously in the abdomen or thigh.

D. Adverse reactions
Human rabies immune globulin (RIG) or Hyperab® is the "biological of choice" for passive immunization of persons exposed to rabies. Local pain and slight febrile response may occur following the administration of RIG. Although not reported after RIG, angioneurotic edema, nephrotic syndrome, and anaphylaxis have been reported very rarely after injection of ordinary human immune serum globulin.

(From The Committee on Trauma: A Guide to Prophylaxis Against Rabies in Exposed Persons. Chicago, American College of Surgeons, 1978.)

be treated as out-patients. Patients with severe burns on the hands, face, and feet, however, should be considered individually.

First-degree burns should not figure into the calculation of burned surface area, since the water barrier of the skin is not disturbed. A first-degree burn is reddened but is not blistered. In terms of water loss, a second-degree burn has the same physiologic significance as a third-degree burn, therefore, second- plus third-degree burns are used to calculate the percentage of surface area involved. The tendency for most physicians is to overestimate the area of the burn. Standard burn charts can be used to calculate the percentage burned, and some attention should be given to detail on the chart to calculate the patient's burn accurately. (See Figure 15-1 in the previous chapter for a burn assessment chart).

Scald Burns

Scald burns are usually second-degree burns, but in the child they may become third-degree burns if infected. Scald burns from soup or other fat-containing cooking liquids can result in third-degree burns. The initial management is the same for all these burns, but the mechanism of the injury that produces a third-degree burn must be borne in mind as therapy progresses. The third-degree burn may require skin grafting at an early or late stage, but that is beyond the scope of this section. Superficial second-degree burns require patience and persistence with sterile dressings and follow-up, but rarely require grafts.

Following recognition of a burn and its classification in terms of degree and percentage, clean cold compresses should be applied and the patient given a narcotic pain reliever. The equipment and dressing supplies will vary from camp to camp, but the basic principle is to dress the wound as aseptically and occlusively as possible. Bulky dressings are preferred because they tend to immobilize and protect better. The interface between the burn and the dressing is best provided by an antibiotic ointment such as bacitracin or, ideally, silver sulfadiazine cream. As an alternative, a topical antibiotic covered with some type of Vaseline gauze may be used. The burn wound should be checked by a health worker every other day for the first week, and then on a schedule determined individually after that.

Healing

A second-degree burn usually requires two to four weeks to epithelialize. The healing process can be seen as individual 1- to 2-mm epithelial buds appear at the periphery of the wound and spread centrally while coalescing. If the periphery of the wound is especially red and tender, blanches, and an exudate apart from the antibiotic ointment is seen, infection is implied, especially when fever is present. Moderate to high fevers are common for the first two to five days following a burn, as is anorexia and some vomiting. For the burn that covers less than 25 percent of the body, plenty of oral rehydration-type fluids should be provided (see Chapter 15). Full fluid resuscitation of major burns is not considered in this section, but salt-rich crystalloid solution should be given in an amount of 4 cc/kg/percentage of body burn in the first 24 hours.

Use of antibiotics is controversial, but they are not recommended unless a definite infection develops. In that case, streptococcal and staphylococcal coverage should be provided. If the patient is not too systemically ill, these can be given orally. Another area of controversy is the unroofing of blisters. In the refugee camp setting, it is better to leave the blister intact and it will separate at the time of dressing changes.

Major Trauma

There are three components in the care of major trauma: initial stabilization; rapid, accurate diagnosis and assessment of injury severity; and management of specific injuries. Aggressive and efficient facilitation of all three phases is crucial to saving lives and decreasing morbidity. This section will be divided in two parts: stabilization, and the handling of specific types of injuries.

The treatment of critically ill patients is a worker-intensive effort. In a refugee camp setting, the director of medical care must take into account the volume of patients, the severity of illness or injury, the skills of the medical staff, the number of physicians and nurses available, and the facilities and supportive services. A triage system must be set up. Some patients will be encountered who would have the potential for survival in a sophisticated tertiary care center with unlimited blood banking, laboratory, and intensive care unit (ICU) facilities. In the refugee camp setting, however, where resources are extremely limited, prolonged treatment of patients who are clearly unsalvageable may not be appropriate. The Western medical and nursing staff will be forced to make treatment priority decisions for which they may have had little emotional preparation.

Stabilization

Management of the airway, control of external hemorrhage, and restoration of intravascular volume are the basic maneuvers required to stabilize the trauma victim.

Airway

The airway of each trauma victim should be inspected immediately and cleared of foreign material, vomitus, blood, and broken teeth. There are four indications for an artificial airway: (1) hypoxia, not responding to mask oxygen; (2) hypoventilation with shock; (3) airway protection in the unconscious patient without a gag reflex; and (4) pulmonary toilet for a patient with copious sputum production and an inadequate cough.

The most common cause of hypoventilation in the trauma victim is upper airway obstruction. The physical signs of upper airway obstruction are inspiratory stridor; paradoxical motion of the chest wall; and supraclavicular and intercostal retractions. Flairing of the *ala nasae* is a nonspecific sign of respiratory distress. If the patient is sweating and has the signs of upper airway obstruction, his PCO_2 is undoubtedly elevated, and rapid correction of the upper airway obstruction is required.

Endotracheal intubation should be considered if the indications for an artificial airway are present. If endotracheal intubation is not possible, a cricothyroidotomy with insertion of a small pediatric endotracheal tube through the cricothyroid membrane will allow resuscitation of the patient. Following resuscitation, a formal tracheostomy or endotracheal intubation can be performed under controlled conditions.

Hemopneumothorax

The patient with war injury or blunt or penetrating trauma must be evaluated for pneumothorax or hemothorax. Tachypnea, cyanosis, tachycardia, and hyperresonant or hyporesonant percussion noted with decreased breath sounds are diagnostic. If in doubt with an unstable patient, rapid thoracentesis (over the fifth rib laterally or second rib anteriorly) with a 20-gauge needle may be helpful. If a gush of air or blood is encountered, a large-bore (32 to 42 F) chest tube should be inserted immediately (see Appendix 16-B). In the absence of a chest tube, sterile rubber tubing or a Foley catheter may be used.

Bleeding

Bleeding is best managed with simple compression, and even severe arterial injuries can usually be managed this way. Tourniquets are generally not indicated when compression is combined with immobilization and elevation. Severe bleeding from the lower extremity is often venous and responds nicely to elevation.

Severe intracavitary bleeding with unstable vital signs requires urgent thoracotomy or laparotomy and is usually controllable only in the operating room. Emergency efforts should be directed toward the replacement and stabilization of circulating blood volume. Type-specific (or type O negative, if available) blood should be given prior to availability of typed and crossmatched blood.

Circulation and Restoration of Blood Volume

Circulation must be maintained and obvious circulatory deficiencies must be addressed immediately. For shock, two large-bore intravenous tubes should be inserted as soon as possible. The femoral or antecubital area and external jugular veins should be considered as the most likely sites. If a clinician has facility in the placement of subclavian or internal jugular catheters, and the patient is not too agitated, this is the method of choice. If there is the least initial difficulty in establishing intravenous access in a patient with circulatory compromise, one should not hesitate to do an antecubital, saphenous, or other venous cutdown (see Appendix 16-A). Either normal saline or, preferably, lactated Ringer's solution should be run wide open until the blood pressure has stabilized. In an adult, 750 cc of blood loss usually stabilizes with 1 to 2 liters of fluid. After that, it is best to administer blood if it is available.

To monitor urine output, a bladder catheter should be inserted. If the patient is male and there is a pelvic fracture, catheterization should be deferred until the patency of the urethra can be established by a spontaneous void. If available, a retrograde urethrogram can rapidly rule out urethral injury. A careful rectal examination may give some indication of injury if the prostate is high or boggy.

For transfer, all intravenous tubing should be secured, the airway reevaluated, and the patient placed on a hard surface [for cardiopulmonary resuscitation (CPR)]. Fractures should be splinted and circulation in extremities ascertained. A nasogastric tube should be inserted (unless there is a basilar skull fracture, in which case the tube is placed orally); vomiting with aspiration is common. Patients transported for surgical care must be given nothing by mouth.

Close monitoring of the hypovolemic patient during resuscitation is essential. A normal blood pressure does not imply full resuscitation; in the young, one quarter to one third of the blood volume may still be deficient. Lips, tongue, conjunctiva, and nail beds are watched for color and capillary filling. The toe and knee temperatures are crucial; if these are cool relative to the thigh, the patient is probably vasoconstricted and needs more intravascular volume. Urine output, neck vein distention, and central venous pressure should be checked continuously to assess the efficacy of fluid resuscitation.

An overly vigorous fluid resuscitation is preferable to protracted shock. The chief error in severe injury is underestimating blood loss and the extent of resuscitation requirements.

Refer to Tables 16-4, 16-5, and 16-6 for the trauma checklists and protocols. Even in major trauma centers, 15 percent of significant injuries may be missed initially. In the heat of resuscitating a severely injured patient, steps are eliminated and important measures are missed. By following a checklist or protocol, the situation can be well organized and errors of omission are minimized.

Handling Specific Types of Injuries

Fractures

Evaluation. Evaluation of the injured patient must begin with assessment of airway, ventilation, and blood pressure. After achieving vascular access, fluid resuscitation, and evaluation of potential central nervous system (CNS), thoracic, and abdominal injuries, attention is turned to evaluation of the skeletal system. The clinical manifestations of fracture include pain, swelling, ecchymosis, deformity in the alignment of the bones, and crepitus. If available, x-ray studies are essential to confirm the diagnosis. Two plain roentgenograms must be taken at right angles to each other. To get the most information about a possible fracture, it is important to include a joint above and below the suspected fracture site on the x-ray plate. By doing so, accurate assessment of the alignment of the fracture can be achieved. The fractures are surgically classified as (1) closed, if there is no laceration of the skin in the region of the fracture site; (2) open, if there is laceration of the skin over the fracture site, thereby causing contamination; (3) pathologic, if the fracture occurs in a diseased area of the bone, that is, tumor, infection, or osteoporosis. The injured extremity must receive a careful vascular and neurologic examination. It is important to assess the pulse status of the extremity distal to the fracture site. In addition, the degree of perfusion and capillary refill of the extremity distal to the fracture must be carefully noted. Neurologic assessment of upper extremity fractures must include assessment of the sensory and motor function of the median, ulnar, and radial nerves. In the lower extremities, the superficial peroneal nerve may be assessed by checking sensation on the dorsum of the foot. The deep peroneal nerve may be assessed by checking sensation between the first and second toe web space. The tibial nerve may be assessed by checking sensation on the plantar aspect of the foot.

Compartment Syndrome. The possibility of a compartment syndrome must be considered. A compartment syndrome occurs when hemorrhage or swelling occurs inside a closed fascial space, thereby leading to myonecrosis, destruction of peripheral nerves, and occlusion of the blood supply. If unrecognized and untreated, a compartment syndrome can progress to complete destruction of the peripheral nerves and muscles, and occasionally progresses to frank gangrene. Check the tenseness of the extremity. It is unusual for a compartment syndrome to occur in the thigh. However, the compartments of the lower leg, forearm, and upper arm are common areas for compartment syndromes to occur. A pulse deficit is usually the last physical sign to occur. More often, the patient will first develop paresthesia or anesthesia in the sensory distribution of the peripheral nerves affected. Check for light touch and pinprick sensory changes distal to the fracture.

Pulse deficits and poorly perfused extremities distal to the fracture site should first be treated by axial traction. If the perfusion and pulse do not return, arteriography, fasciotomy, or vascular reconstruction is indicated. A skilled surgeon and an operating room are then required to achieve limb salvage.

After careful evaluation of the neurovascular status of the extremity and the overlying skin, the fractured extremity is splinted to prevent motion. Movement of fractures increases soft tissue damage and may lead to neurovascular injury and increased blood loss. The fractured extremity should be elevated. Most problems that occur with extremity injuries are due to decreased venous drainage. Early immobilization and elevation of the fracture will minimize this problem. The decision to reduce a closed fracture is based on the clinical and radiologic alignment of the fracture.

Management of Fractures. Anesthesia of some type is usually required. General, regional, or spinal anesthesia may be used. Often, however, a local hematoma block, particularly for distal forearm fractures, yields relatively safe, satisfactory anesthesia. The skin overlaying the fracture is carefully prepared with antiseptic solution. A fine needle is inserted into the hematoma, and some of the hematoma is aspirated. Following this, several cubic centimeters of 2% lidocaine are injected. Satisfactory anesthesia requires a period of 15 to 20 minutes. It is important to use completely sterile lidocaine and to perform this procedure with the utmost sterile technique. Failure to do so may produce osteomyelitis at the fracture site, a devastating complication.

Open fractures also require immobilization, elevation, and antibiotics. Bone ends protruding through the skin should not be placed back in the wound. All open fractures require operative wound care and debridement under anesthesia, as well as antibiotic therapy. The primary goal of therapy is to achieve a healed wound free of infection; the secondary goal is to achieve stable fracture segments.

Therapeutic options in the management of specific open fractures are beyond the scope of this chapter. However, basic principles of operative debridement, wound toilet, immobilization, elevation, and antibiotics are common to all open fractures. As a general principle, the skin should never be closed in the management of open fractures. Rather, the skin should be left open and a delayed primary closure considered. Routine skin closure in the management of open fractures will yield a significant incidence of necrotizing soft tissue infections with gas-forming organisms. This is a limb-threatening and life-threatening complication that is usually avoidable with good wound management.

Penetrating Injuries

Penetrating trauma represents a diverse group of injuries. The characteristics (and treatment) of knife, shotgun, shrapnel, high-velocity, and low-velocity bullet injuries vary significantly. Also, the body region that is wounded dictates management.

In general, most penetrating injuries are cleansed and debrided locally. Tetanus prophylaxis and antibiotics are given. The patient in shock is resuscitated. Beyond this, the considerations related to the injured region prevail. Foreign bodies such as bullets or deep shrapnel are not routinely removed. A patient with a knife or other object protruding from an intracavitary position should not have the wound disturbed. The object should be stabilized in situ and the object removed in the operating room.

Head and Neck. Penetrating intracranial injuries should be handled in a setting where adequate neurosurgical care is available. Dressing the wounds and neurologic stabilization (see Stabilization) are done while transport is arranged. Realistically, such wounds are usually fatal in the best of hands and triage decisions must be made in such cases.

Eye injuries may be repaired or require enucleation, again by specially trained physicians. Untreated penetrating eye injuries may jeopardize the remaining eye.

In penetrating neck injuries, a thorough cranial nerve examination is performed and the wound is carefully inspected. Ideally, subplatysmal neck injuries are explored surgically so, when possible, appropriate arrangements should be made. Exploration of the neck without proper facilities is dangerous and such cases are better observed when transfer is not feasible. The patient should remain in a head-elevated position to decrease venous pressure, and equipment ideally should be available for tracheostomy or cricothyroidotomy or intubation and shock resuscitation.

Chest. Hemopneumothorax is discussed under Stabilization. The most common exsanguinating injury follows knife wounds that sever intercostal vessels. After a large-bore chest tube is inserted, severe blood loss must be replaced unit per unit until a thoracotomy can be arranged.

Criteria for operative intervention vary, but continuous, severe blood loss can be controlled only operatively. Most cases of hemothorax can be managed with a chest tube and water seal drainage alone. The tube may require sterile irrigation to maintain drainage and avoid clot buildup.

Lower chest injuries may penetrate the diaphragm and injure the liver or spleen. Upper chest injuries may injure the trachea or bronchi; a massive air leak through the chest tube may suggest this. All such injuries should be managed operatively. Stabilization may require multiple chest tubes.

Cardiac tamponade is common in penetrating trauma but may not develop immediately. If untreated, it is lethal. Faint, muffled heart sounds, tachycardia, tachypnea, cyanosis, distended external jugular veins, and hypotension are typically seen. So-called paradoxical pulse (varied blood pressure with respiration) is difficult to document and is not important to the diagnosis. Pericardiocentesis, as described in Table 16-6, should be performed emergently and arrangements should be made for surgical intervention where possible. A central venous-type cannula should be left in the pericardium and secured with a suture for transfer. It must be recognized that most cases will not survive without surgery and that long transport will not be tolerated.

Open chest wounds should be covered with occlusive dressings. Vaseline gauze and bulky "fluffed" gauze are ideal if available. Although there are objections because of the possibility of contaminating the wound further, a chest tube may be inserted through the defect and taped in place. If this is not reasonable because the injury is very high, low, or medial, a chest tube should be inserted as described in Appendix 16-B. Intravenous and antibiotic therapy should be given and transport arranged for definitive surgery.

Abdomen. The rule regarding wounds of the abdomen varies with the wounding object. Knife wounds may be carefully explored under local anesthesia. If the peritoneum has been penetrated, laparotomy is indicated. If this is not easily arranged, peritoneal lavage may be done (see Appendix 16-E). If there is no blood, the white count is under 500, and the Gram's stain is negative, the patient may be observed on intravenous therapy and kept from any oral ingestion (NPO). Shrapnel wounds may be managed similarly.

When a large wound or goring injury has occurred, evisceration may result. The patient should be given antibiotics, an IV, nasogastric tube, and be prepared for surgery. Exposed bowel should be covered with saline sponges and covered with a plastic wrap or bag if available. Surgery is obviously required.

Gunshot wounds to the abdomen are managed with laparotomy. Gunshot wounds to the chest or abdomen may cross the diaphragm and injure the other cavity, and this is always a diagnostic consideration. If there is a question of peritoneal penetration in low-velocity missile injuries, the same management as for knife wounds may be considered. X-ray studies may be helpful in locating bullets or fragments.

High-velocity bullet wounds create a shock wave, which may seriously injure tissue far from the actual path of the bullet. Most modern military rifles produce this type of injury. Laparotomy is the only practical option in these cases. Such cases require heroic stabilization, and triage decisions may need to be made.

Extremities. The principle concerns for penetrating extremity injuries are neurovascular injuries and fractures (see above). A careful examination with concern for sensation, range of motion, and pulses is the key to successful management. If neurovascular injury is present, special surgical expertise is required. If not, local debridement, cleansing, and dressing are sufficient if there are no fractures.

If there is a question of fracture, an x-ray film is useful for the diagnosis. If a fracture is present, the wound is treated as an open fracture with generous debridement, irrigation, splinting, or casting of the fracture. Reduction of the fracture and "pins and plaster" fixation is better treatment, if it is available.

Blast Injury

Blast injury (e.g., from land mines) or high-velocity rifle wounds often affect the extremities. Frequently, the soft tissue injury is extensive and part of the extremity is nonviable. Neurovascular injury and fractures must be ruled out, as with other penetrating injuries. Intravenous antibiotics and tetanus prophylaxis are extremely important. Clothing, dirt, and fragments are often propelled deeply into the tissues and debridement should be thorough. After debridement, viability must be assessed again. Often, apparently viable tissue is lost ultimately. Gas gangrene (myonecrosis) may be seen, usually within one to two days after injury (see septic surgery, above). This complication is heralded by tachycardia, mild fever, and crepitation. The wound may exude a thin brownish fluid with a musty odor. When this is recognized, amputation is mandatory emergently. Otherwise, if the extremity is viable, daily dressing with cleansing and debridement should suffice.

THE SURGICAL ABDOMEN

Emergent surgical problems of the abdomen are of three types: obstruction in the gastrointestinal (GI) tract; perforation or inflammation of the hollow visci; and hemorrhage (inside or outside the hollow alimentary tract). Some causes are quite universal; others are more common in underdeveloped countries.

Obstruction

In the United States, most cases of intestinal obstruction are secondary to adhesions (scarring related to previous surgery). In underdeveloped countries, volvulus and intussusception (related to parasitic infestation) are very common, even beyond early childhood. Incarcerated hernia is a common cause of obstruction, and is the most frequent cause in many underdeveloped countries. In fact, bowel obstruction of all types constitutes over half of emergent abdominal operations in parts of Africa.

Historic and physical features of bowel obstruction are similar, regardless of etiology. Symptoms vary as to level of obstruction (proximal versus distal). Table 16-8 shows the principle subjective and objective findings.

If available, plain films (supine and upright) should be obtained. If there is free air (usually seen under the diaphragm on the upright film), perforation has occurred. Paralytic ileus may have scattered air fluid levels but usually there is gas in the colon or rectum. In anatomic obstruction, the gaseous distention of bowel loops is greater, *plicae circularis* are spread or lost, and gas is typically absent in the colon.

Diagnosis

Diagnosis may be aided by a barium enema or barium swallow with delayed films to show small bowel transit. However, contrast studies should definitely not be performed in the presence of fever, generalized tenderness (especially with rebound phenomenon or rigidity), or absent bowel sounds. These findings signify

Table 16-8. Signs and Symptoms of the "Surgical Abdomen"

Subjective	Objective
Obstruction	
Vomiting (more severe with proximal obstruction, may be bilious green or feculent)	Peristaltic waves
	Distention (more pronounced with distal obstruction)
Colicky pain (cramping)	Mild tenderness without peritoneal signs
Stooling (usually decreased or absent; sometimes diarrhea)	"Popping" or tinkling bowel sounds with rushes and rumbles
Thirst	Succussion splash (sound of fluid splashing on movement)
Nausea	
No flatus (late)	Palpable loops
	Empty rectal vault (late sign)
	Fever (not pronounced)
	Shock (very late)
Perforation	
Nausea	Tenderness exquisite[a]
Anorexia	Bowel sounds decreased or absent[a]
Vomiting (not as pronounced as with obstruction)	± Distention
	Rigid or guarded abdomen[a]
Fever, often with chills	Tenderness with movement[a]
Prostration	Rebound phenomenon[a]
Pain with movement	Walking bent over or not at all[a]
Stool pattern ± helpful	Fever, tachycardia
Bloody stools a bad sign	Shock (late)

[a]Peritoneal signs.

compromised bowel viability, with possible perforation, the so-called peritoneal signs. Laparotomy is required when these are definitely present, regardless of diagnosis (except in amebiasis; see below).

Basic laboratory work includes a complete blood count with differential diagnosis. Leukocytosis with a left shift (especially in the presence of fever) suggests compromised bowel with a likelihood of perforation. If available, electrolytes and blood urea nitrogen (BUN) are useful as a guide to proper intravenous therapy. Blood for type and crossmatch should be obtained, if possible. Urine should be checked to rule out diabetes mellitus and obtain a specific gravity, which helps assess overall fluid status. Where applicable, blood should be checked for sickle cell anemia.

Preparation for Surgery

Proper resuscitation prior to surgery is life-saving. D_5 lactated Ringer's solution is given intravenously until adequate urine output is obtained. Because of sequestration of fluid in the bowel and peritoneal cavity (third spacing), heroic amounts of fluid may be required. A nasogastric tube should be inserted and regularly aspirated. Broad-spectrum antibiotics (especially active against gram-negative organisms and gut anaerobes) should be given intravenously. In some parts of Africa, typhoid fever is a major cause of bowel obstruction. If this is suspected, chloramphenicol should be given (initially 100 mg/kg in four doses daily, then reduced gradually to 50 mg/kg/day for a total course of 14 days).

Generally, laparotomy should be arranged as soon as fluid resuscitation can be completed. A surgical maxim is "the sun must not be allowed to rise or set on a bowel obstruction."

Specific Causes of Bowel Obstruction

Volvulus

Volvulus is common in the underdeveloped world and may constitute 15 to 40 percent of cases of bowel obstruction. It may involve any part of the small or large intestine. Volvulus may occur spontaneously due to individual anatomy, or may be secondary to adhesions or ascariasis. The patient is usually extremely distended with "bass drum" percussion note. Cramping pain and bilious or feculent vomiting are common. Classic x-ray findings may be seen, such as a huge bean or U-shaped gas shadow with a "bird beak" pattern for sigmoid or cecal volvulus. Small bowel volvulus may appear as nonspecific obstruction.

Volvulus of the sigmoid may resolve with cautious sigmoidoscopy and passage of a flatus tube through the scope. Other types require laparotomy, usually with resection.

Intussusception

In Europe and America, intussusception of the ileocolic type is typically seen in infants. Overall, intussusception in children and adults constitutes about 20 percent of cases of emergent abdominal surgery in some parts of the underdeveloped world. Infantile intussusception is reducible early in the course of illness by a barium enema with a barium bag height of 1 m. In the underdeveloped world, however, only about 10 percent of cases are of the infantile type. Diagnosis may be difficult because of the prevalence of gastroenteritis, which may be prodromal and an alternative diagnosis from which intussusception must be distinguished. Causes of intussusception in older children and adults include ascariasis, amebiasis, polyps, and, perhaps, dietary factors. Most cases are idiopathic.

Signs and symptoms include colicky pain in nearly 100 percent of cases, vomiting in 80 percent, palpable sausage-shaped mass in 60 to 80 percent, diarrhea in 60 percent, and "current jelly" (bloody mucus) stools in one third to two thirds of cases. Distention is unusual early in the course of the illness. The x-ray films may show an empty right lower quadrant in ileocecal or cecocolic types (Dance's sign). However, the plain abdominal films may be negative early in the course.

Except for the infantile type (when seen early and reduced by barium enema), the treatment is surgical. Preparation for surgery is the same as for other causes of obstruction. The usual approach is reduction or resection, with anastomosis or ostomies.

Ascariasis

Ascaris lumbricoides is a cause of bowel obstruction usually seen in children and young adults. These round worms may cause volvulus or intussusception, but obturator obstruction (plugging the lumen) is the most common finding. See Chapter 35 for a discussion of other aspects of ascaris infection.

Afflicted patients may present with intermittent colic, some vomiting, weight loss, soft or shifting masses, and moderate fever. In the patient's history, a vermifuge may have recently been taken and an obstruction precipitated by dead worms. The patient may also have seen worms in his vomitus or stools. On x-ray examination, worms may actually be seen. If the obstruction is complete, or if volvulus has occurred, the signs and symptoms become more nonspecific.

If obstruction is incomplete, nasogastric suction, intravenous hydration, and antispasmodics may be given. Later, standard antihelminthic treatment may be given. When obstruction is complete, surgical treatment is required.

Incarcerated Hernia

Incarcerated hernia is by far the most common cause of intestinal obstruction worldwide. Inguinal hernia is most prevalent, but several other types are elucidated in surgical texts. In any patient with suspected bowel obstruction, the inguinal and femoral canals, as well as old surgical incisions, should be carefully examined.

Etiologically, a defect in the abdominal wall permits a loop of bowel to herniate. Subsequent edema prevents its return. Both strangulation (resulting in gangrene) and obstruction of the bowel can then occur. During the physical examination, careful attention must be paid to possible peritoneal signs. If they are present, the patient is prepared for surgery without attempted hernia reduction. Forty to 50 percent of strangulated hernias in the underdeveloped world contain dead bowel and therefore should not be reduced.

If the patient has no peritoneal signs, he should be placed in a Trendelenberg (head down) position, given a sedative or narcotic (see Table 16-3), and left alone for about one hour. An ice bag may also be placed on the groin. An intravenous tube may be inserted to begin fluid resuscitation and antibiotics in preparation for surgery, should this method fail.

After one hour, the patient may be resedated, if needed, and reduction may be attempted. Fluid and gas in the hernial content should be squeezed out with slowly increasing pressure beginning at the bottom of the sac. A finger should be placed firmly over the external ring to prevent the sac from overlapping this rigid shelf during attempted reduction. Considerable force may be needed, but not enough to cause an "en mass reduction" (tearing away the ring without reducing the hernia; the entire mass may be forced back into the abdomen). If reduction is successful, surgery to correct the hernia defect should be offered when possible.

If reduction is unsuccessful, another three hours should be allowed for spontaneous reduction, which occurs one half to two thirds of the time. If this, too, fails, the patient should be prepared for operation as an emergency. Mortality is about 10 percent in these cases.

Inflammation-Perforation

Perforation in the GI tract is the main cause of the "acute abdomen." Distinguishing the acutely surgical abdomen from other causes of abdominal pain is a difficult, but invaluable, skill. The history varies with etiology, and some of the more common causes of the acute abdomen are discussed below. The peritoneal signs are recognized only with experience and may be difficult to separate from more nonspecific tenderness and other changes. A reliable physical examination is crucial. The significant findings are given in Table 16-8.

The history is essential to elicit the etiology and obtain information as to the duration of illness. Refer to the Evaluation section of this chapter.

Physical Examination

Inspection classically reveals a patient who lies very still. Writhing suggests colic, such as that seen with a ureteral stone and sometimes with bowel obstruction. The patient's respirations are typically rapid and shallow, with an attempt to splint the abdomen. In the supine position, most normal people breathe with abdominal movement. When "splinting" the abdomen, there is often a paradoxical movement with the abdomen rising during expirations and falling during inspiration. The patient may be more comfortable with the legs flexed at the hips; he or she may have difficulty in a supine position with the legs out straight. The patient is usually not able to walk with a straight back. Hopping is not possible. Sometimes walking or standing is not possible at all. The percussion note usually is tympanitic because of the ileus associated with peritonitis. More typically, percussion produces tenderness, an unusual finding in the absence of peritoneal irritation. Loss of liver dullness suggests free air over the liver from a perforation.

Auscultation can be useful as a palpation technique in addition to its value in assessing bowel sounds. Gentle palpation over the nine areas of the abdomen with the stethoscope head is less threatening to the patient than the examining hand. Rebound can be assessed by gently and slowly pressing in with the stethoscope, then releasing it and observing the patient's face. This also provides a key to the degree of distention and its character.

Bowel sounds are often not entirely absent in the acute abdomen. They are often widely spaced, quiet stacatto notes separated by silence. If this is all that is heard during five minutes of listening, an acute abdomen should be suspected, even if the other signs are equivocal.

Palpation can be done effectively in three stages. The most tender area should be approached last in each stage. First, a scouting palpation with a light touch and a warm hand will help relax the patient and give a clue to specific areas of tenderness. Second, touching each area with a single finger will help localize tenderness, test for guarding and rigidity, and help further assess distention. Finally, full-hand palpation should go deeply to search out masses or distended loops of bowel. If the abdomen is very tender and guarded, this may not be possible and is, itself, an indication of a true surgical abdomen.

The rectal examination is indispensible, and a pelvic examination should be performed in assessing mature females. In all patients, the rectum should be evaluated with the patient supine and the nonrectal hand used to simutaneously palpate the abdomen. Fullness, masses, point tenderness, gas, and qualities of stool should be assessed.

The physical examination of very nervous patients may be facilitated by giving fentanyl or thiopental. Long-acting agents may obscure serial examinations for progression of signs, while shorter-acting agents help eliminate so-called voluntary guarding but do not mask the true peritoneal signs.

Diagnostic Aids

Diagnostic aids for inflammation-perforation are virtually the same ones used for obstruction. The urinalysis should be inspected for increased white blood cells (WBCs), which suggests a nonsurgical urinary tract infection. However, an inflamed viscus or infected peritoneal fluid lying on the bladder can give up to 10 to 15 WBCs per high-power field. A Gram's stain of a spun specimen can help clarify this; if any organisms are seen, a urinary tract infection is likely (see Chapter 36). Typically, the white blood cell count is elevated with a left shift. If the white count is either normal or depressed in the face of very immature polynuclear forms (myelocytes, metamyelocytes), the situation may be grave. Extremely high white counts (20,000 in adults) suggest the possibility of intestinal gangrene.

Abdominal x-ray studies may be nonspecific, but shifts of loops indicate space-occupying masses. Free air and calcifications should also be sought.

Specific Inflammatory Lesions

Appendicitis

The incidence of appendicitis is relatively less common in underdeveloped countries than in Europe and the United States. The natural history of appendicitis has been known for nearly 100 years. Early appendicitis (before perforation) is a fairly minor surgical illness with low morbidity, and nearly no mortality in otherwise healthy patients. When the appendix becomes gangrenous and perforates, a localized abscess or generalized peritonitis occurs. In developed countries, mortality in nonruptured appendicitis is about 0.1 percent and 3 percent in ruptured appendicitis. Morbidity (usually septic complications) is about 5 percent in "simple" appendicitis, and 30 percent in those that rupture.

Appendicitis is a clinical diagnosis that can be difficult because nothing is pathognomonic and most cases are not "classic." The diagnosis is suggested by progressive right lower quadrant abdominal pain and tenderness, fever, nausea, anorexia, and vomiting. Peritoneal signs are progressive with intensifying and spreading tenderness. Rebound tenderness is usually present, as well as referred rebound tenderness (Rovsing's sign). This is a rebound phenomenon tested in the left lower quadrant and experienced as tenderness in the right lower quadrant. Chracteristically, the "appendix shuffle," a gait with the abdomen flexed, is as nearly diagnostic as any other sign.

The rectal examination may reveal a tenderness on the right, with or without a mass. Overall, this is an inconstant sign. The psoas and obturator signs are usually equivocal, but the psoas sign may occasionally be of help in the retrocecal appendix without other compelling signs. The psoas sign is elicited by having the supine patient raise his or her extended leg against resistance. The obturator sign is positive if the patient experiences tenderness when the flexed thigh is rotated externally.

Abdominal films are not particularly helpful in early cases unless a fecolith is seen (calcific density in the right lower quadrant). After perforation, a mass may be appreciated in the right lower quadrant, or an ileus pattern of more generalized peritonitis may be seen.

Although appendicitis cannot be diagnosed on the basis of the white blood cell count, this can be useful. The triad of fever (>38°C), leukocytosis (>10,000/mm^3), and bandemia (bands greater than 5% of the white cells) in the presence of progressive abdominal pain and tenderness, is strongly associated with appendicitis. If the triad is negative, appendicitis will be present less than 10 percent of the time. A urinalysis should be performed to rule out a urinary tract infection, but peritonitis or an inflamed appendix lying on the bladder may give five to ten white blood cells per high-power field. A Gram's stain of the urine may be helpful in such cases.

Treatment is usually removal of the appendix. If the appendix has ruptured with a well walled-off abscess, which the patient is tolerating, antibiotic treatment (usually with metronidazole or chloramphenicol to cover gut anaerobes) may be instituted. A two-week course is recommended. Because recurrent appendicitis occurs in about one third of cases, an interval appendectomy should be performed, usually at about six weeks.

Because rupture may not be appreciated before surgery, antibiotics should be given preoperatively in all cases. Intravenous rehydration must also be considered, especially in advanced cases. If distention and peritonitis are present, a nasogastric tube and intensive resuscitation may be required preoperatively.

Typhoid Fever

Typhoid fever is endemic in many warm climates and presents a common surgical emergency. In 2 to 4 percent of patients, perforation occurs and accounts for 20 to 40 percent of typhoid deaths. Pathologically, ulcerating necrosis of Peyer's patches in the terminal ileum predisposes to perforation. These multiple lesions may necrose translumenally due to typhoid bacilli penetrating the wall.

Clinically, most patients are febrile and

complain of headache and abdominal pain (see Chapter 24). Vomiting and diarrhea or constipation, joint pains, and toxicity may be seen. Dehydration may be severe. Abdominal x-ray films may show distended small bowel loops and fluid levels; blood tests are usually nonspecific except that leukopenia may be observed. When perforation occurs, typical findings are peritonitis and sepsis. This usually occurs during the convalescent phase about one to three weeks after initial onset of symptoms. Late perforation without truly diagnostic prodramata may be difficult to distinguish from other causes of acute abdomen. Laboratory tests and x-ray studies are not particularly useful for specific diagnosis at this stage.

Upon recognition of the disease, oral or intravenous chloramphenicol should be given; if perforation occurs, toxicity with cardiovascular instability may be striking, and aggressive fluid therapy is required. A nasogastric tube should be inserted and the patient prepared for surgery. Patients with significant cardiovascular compromise will usually not tolerate general anesthesia. In such cases, drains may be inserted in the right lower quadrant under local anesthesia using much the same technique as is used in abscess drainage.

At surgery, the perforated ulcers should be excised and the bowel closed in two layers. Occasionally, a small bowel resection may be required. Meticulous peritoneal toilet and irrigation are important. Fascial necrosis, intra-abdominal abscess, and prolonged illness are common sequelae.

Overall, prompt recognition of perforation and aggressive resuscitation offer the best chances for survival.

Amebiasis

Entamoeba histolytica is a common cause of medical illness and has surgical implications in about 2 percent of all cases. The use of metronidazole has decreased the incidence of surgical complications such as perforation and liver abscesses. When these complications occur, making the initial diagnosis of amebiasis is especially important (see Chapter 35).

Amebiasis affects the entire colon, but the cecum and right colon are usually the most severely affected. The presentation of obstruction or perforation is nonspecific to amebiasis, but patients with peritonitis from perforation are particuarly toxic. Massive fluid resuscitation is required. Special attention must be paid to hypokalemia, a frequent finding. Nasogastric suction and broad spectrum intravenous antibiotics (in addition to metronidazole) should be given. Even with perforation, operative intervention should be avoided because of extreme friability of the bowel. After stabilization and medical treatment, however, some organized pericolic abscesses may be surgically drained.

Operative intervention may be required for bowel obstruction secondary to ameboma or intussusception. Strictures may occur later. The mass of an ameboma should decrease in size and the patient should clinically improve after 72 hours on metronidazole. If this does not occur, the diagnosis should be challenged.

Rectal hemorrhage, although rare, may require operation along with massive transfusion and metronidazole.

Amebic liver abscess ("focal necrosis") is secondary to portal spread of *E. histolytica* from the bowel. Most patients have had recent symptoms of amebiasis and most also have tenderness in the right upper quadrant and tender hepatomegaly. The white blood cell count is elevated and the chest x-ray study usually shows an effusion, obliteration of the costophrenic angle with diaphragmatic elevation, and atelectasis. Antiamebic drugs usually produces good results. Open drainage procedures are reserved for secondary infections of the abscess cavity, failure of medical therapy, rupture, or pus too thick to aspirate.

Amebic abscesses of the liver may rupture into the chest across the diaphragm. Intracranial abscesses are rare, but must be considered in an amebiasis patient with focal neurologic signs.

Other Causes of the Surgical Abdomen

There are myriad other causes of the acute abdomen or bowel obstruction. These are well covered in general surgical texts and diagnosis and treatment is usually straightforward.

Gastrointestinal Bleeding

Gastrointestinal bleeding usually requires blood transfusion facilities, as aggressive blood replacement is the key to a successful outcome. Shock must be prevented.

Diagnostically, a nasogastric tube with a bloody return implies bleeding above the ligament of Treitz, and a clear return suggets a colonic cause. Bleeding from the small intestine is unusual.

Unless stigmata of portal hypertension are

present, most upper GI bleeding is from ulcers or gastritis. The medical management is similar in either case.

If available, iced lavage for upper GI bleeding may be done, but its effectiveness is not proven. However, a large-bore (e.g., Ewald) tube with saline lavage is important to prevent large clot formation, which actually perpetuates bleeding.

A large-bore IV is required, and fluids and monitoring are similar to those given in the discussion of circulation in the Major Trauma section of this chapter. The rule of thumb is to intervene surgically after a blood requirement of six units (3 liters, or about half of one blood volume). If available, a surgeon should be informed early in the course of any major GI bleeding.

Colonic bleeding may be secondary to amebic ulceration or arteriovenous malformations but is quite unusual in the underdeveloped countries. The principles of stabilization and surgery for intractible bleeding also apply.

Cancers cause a variety of GI surgical symptoms but are beyond the scope of this chapter. Typically, they are not a source of exsanguinating hemorrhage.

Portal hypertension is common in many countries, and variceal bleeding is a common cause of death in these patients. If a history or stigmata of portal hypertension is present, this should be a suspected cause of upper GI bleeding. Triage decisions may be necessary in that massive variceal hemorrhage is personnel and resource intensive. Massive transfusion requirements and, often, surgery are required, and the results are frequently not gratifying.

Initial management requires shock resuscitation and blood replacement. A nasogastric tube is needed to prevent vomiting and aspiration. The Sengstaken-Blakemore tube, if it is available, provides an intraesophageal balloon tamponade to temporize. Also, if available, vasopressin (or oxytocin) titrated carefully intravenously may dramatically control bleeding.

Bile Stones

Various forms of liver and biliary pathology plague the underdeveloped countries. Specific diseases depend on the population and area under consideration. Details of diagnosis and treatment should be sought in general surgery texts.

Patients with biliary stones are quite prone to sepsis if they are presenting acutely. The patient should be kept NPO, a nasogastric tube should be passed, and intravenous and antibiotic therapies (active against enteric pathogens) should be started as arrangements are made for surgery.

SUMMARY

An array of surgical problems presents in the refugee setting. Depending on local expertise and facilities, most can be managed on site. However, stabilization and transport is more appropriate, when they are possible.

REFERENCES AND SUGGESTED READING

Davey WW: Companion to Surgery in Africa. Edinburgh & London, E&S Livingstone, 1968. Very complete and practical guide with a focus on tropical problems. Weak in trauma. Assumes basic surgical knowledge and skills. Still not dated in approaches to problems.

Hill GJ: Outpatient Surgery, 2nd ed. Philadelphia, WB Saunders, 1980. One of the two "must" books for surgical problems among refugees. The majority of problems encountered in the refugee setting (including major trauma stabilization) are included. The text is not "high tech" and most diagnostic and therapeutic suggestions are practicable in the context of refugee care. This book has an outstanding chapter on "Outpatient Surgery in Developing Countries," which alone is worth the price of the book.

Moore DC: Regional Block, 4th ed. Springfield, IL, Charles C Thomas, 1965. Although old, it includes complete and easy-to-follow descriptions of all principle nerve blocks.

Ramamurti CP: Orthopedics in Primary Care. Baltimore, Williams & Williams, 1981. Good general approach to common orthopedic problems complete with basic anatomic and mechanical background.

Schwartz SI, Adesola AO, Elebute EA, Rob CG: Tropical Surgery. New York, McGraw-Hill, 1971. Well-organized and well-referenced approach to tropical surgical problems. Treatment recommendations are well geared to the environment and are often capable of being implemented by nonsurgeons.

Smith DR: General Urology, 11th ed. Los Altos, CA, Lange, 1984. Excellent and concise approach to common urologic problems. More oriented to problems encountered in developed nations, however.

Way LW: Current Surgical Diagnosis and Treatment, 6th ed. Los Altos, CA, Lange, 1983. One of the two references that will be most useful in managing the surgical problems of refugees. This handbook is concise, well-organized, and amazingly complete. Its major drawback is a Western "high-tech" orientation to diagnosis and treatment. However, its basic approach to most surgical problems, including subspecialty areas, makes it a "must" reference for the nonsurgeon treating refugees.

APPENDIX 16-A

VENOUS ACCESS

Saphenous at Ankle

1. Locate area anterior to medial malleolus.
2. Prepare sterile field and infiltrate with local anesthetic.
3. Make transverse incision (1 cm is adequate).
4. Make three hard spreads with curved hemostat right on the tibia, parallel to the bone (perpendicular to the incision).
5. Scrape hemostat hard against bone from anterior tibia, up across the maleolus. Vein will come up on hemostat.
6. Isolate vein with two ligatures and tie distal one.
7. Cut vein (small scissors or blade) halfway through, 3 to 4 mm proximal to tied ligature.
8. Insert catheter (after flushing). If this is difficult, be sure catheter is beveled and slide catheter in, bevel down, against back wall of vein.
9. Secure proximal tie, close skin, sew in catheter.

Saphenous at groin (easier on adults)

1. One finger breadth below groin fold, and one finger breadth medial to arterial pulse.
2. May use landmarks to attempt percutaneous cannulation.
3. Make transverse 2-cm incision.
4. Dissect perpendicular to incision.
5. Repeat technique from steps 6 to 9 above.

Antecubital (Basilic)

1. Stabilize elbow with thumb pointed out ("hitchhiker" position).
2. One finger breadth proximal to medial epicondyle and one finger breadth lateral (toward radius); in bicipital groove, make transverse incision, 2 to 3 cm.
3. Do standard prep and anesthesia.
4. Make three hard spreads with curved hemostat perpendicular to incision.
5. Curve hemostat in *deep,* spread, close hemostat, bring up to surface. Repeat if vein is missed. Dissect out if unsuccessful.
6. Be sure artery has not been accidentally taken (may check by sticking in No. 22 syringe needle). Isolate and cannulate vein.

Keys to Success

1. Strip excess tissue from vein.
2. Isolate at least 2 to 3 cm of vein between ligatures.
3. Place venotomy properly.
4. Place traction on distal (tied) ligature to open venotomy and straighten vein while doing venotomy and threading catheter.
5. Do not be heavy-handed with catheter once it is out of sight in the vein.

Percutaneous (order of preference in trauma)*

1. Antecubital
2. Femoral
3. Cephalic over bicep (if visible)
4. External jugular vein
5. Saphenous at ankle
6. Hand or forearm vein
7. Dorsal vein of penis

*Subclavian or internal jugular is preferred if the operator is proficient. In a child, a No. 18 steel hypodermic needle may be placed through the femur or the anterior tibia into the marrow space. This will suffice for medications and some fluids. With a "boring" motion, this can be placed fairly easily. This procedure should be performed in emergency situations when other access attempts have failed.

APPENDIX 16–B

CHEST TUBE PLACEMENT

1. Prepare sterile field in midaxillary line with arm over head. Anesthetize the area.
2. Select seventh intercostal space for incision, counting up from the twelfth rib.
3. Make transverse 2-cm incision.
4. Dissect transversely with curved hemostat over sixth rib (one interspace higher than skin incision).
5. Anesthetize interspace and periosteum of top of sixth rib.
6. Poke through with hemostat, turn perpendicular, and spread. Be prepared for gush of air or blood and be ready immediately for next step.
7. Insert chest tube with tip held in needle holder or another hemostat. (It helps to spread intercostal muscles with the hemostat). Attach immediately to suction, Heimlich valve, or glove with fingertips cut off.
8. For hemothorax, angle posteriorly and toward diaphragm. For hemopneumothorax, angle posteriorly and toward head. For pneumothorax, angle anteriorly and toward head.
9. Be sure last hole in tube is within pleural space and tube is not kinked.
10. Close skin with mattress suture and tie tube in.
11. Tape tube and connections securely.

APPENDIX 16-C

SUTURING

Do not close a wound over 12 hours old!

1. Thoroughly irrigate the wound with saline, water, dilute Betadine or dilute soapy water; be sure all debris is out.
2. Prepare a sterile field. Inject local anesthetic into the skin around wound; you may inject into the cut edge itself. Local anesthetic may be injected before irrigation is done if this looks painful.
3. Debride wound.
4. If needed, close in anatomic layers (e.g., fascia of muscle, subcutaneous tissue, and then skin). Use absorbable sutures (gut, chromic, etc.) on deeper layers.
5. Do not leave dead space. If it cannot be closed, insert a drain.
6. Use nonabsorbable suture for skin. Leave tags on knots long enough to facilitate removal later.
7. Approximate skin edges well. Evert edges slightly. Use a vertical mattress suture, if necessary, to take up tension or approximate wound edges. Use an instrument tie; it is quicker and saves suture. Tie square knots, at least three throws. On a straight cut or scalp laceration, a running suture is advisable.
8. Place dressing. If over a joint, immobilize as much as possible.
9. Suture care: Keep dressed and clean; keep dry; observe for signs of infection.
10. Suture removal: Face—3–5 days (and then place tapes across); hand, arm, leg (except pretibial)—one week; feet, trunk, pretibial—10 to 14 days.

APPENDIX 16–D

DRAINAGE OF ABSCESS

1. Wash area and inject anesthetic into dermis only.
2. Prepare sterile field.
3. Use No. 11 blade for opening skin. Go deep enough to get through entire skin. Make cut narrower than the lesion, especially on the face.
4. Cross incision with second incision (cruciate) to allow area free drainage. (Do not use this on the face.)
5. Obtain Gram's stain (and culture if available).
6. Break up loculations with a hemostat. There are frequently septations that need to be thoroughly broken up or the abscess may recur. Do not be afraid of bleeding here.
7. Squeeze abscess to express as much pus as possible. This step is very painful.
8. Pack with strip gauze or insert a drain (and sew to skin).
9. Cover with bulky dressing and keep covered.
10. After packing or drain is out, the patient should bathe or soak the abscessed area (if possible) to keep it open and draining. This will allow healing from the base and will prevent reabscessing from the skin closing over dead space.

APPENDIX 16–E

PERITONEAL LAVAGE

1. Drain bladder and evacuate the stomach with a nasogastric tube.
2. Prepare a sterile field just below the umbilicus. Site of entry is one finger breadth below the umbilicus.
3. Anesthetize the skin, dermis, and then point the needle straight down, injecting lidocaine ahead of the needle. Stay in midline and inject until peritoneal cavity is entered.
4. Make a stab wound with a No. 11 blade.
5. Use a No. 14 needle (an intracath is preferable if available) to enter the peritoneal cavity. Go straight in briskly. A "pop" is felt when the linea alba is pierced.
6. Thread a No. 16 catheter through the needle and into the abdominal cavity. Back out the metal needle.
7. Aspirate for fluid.
8. Instill 1 liter of normal saline.
9. Turn the patient from side to side with the catheter in place.
10. Lower an empty intravenous bottle to the floor and allow the peritoneal lavage fluid to drain. Complete return of all fluid is unusual.
11. Remove the catheter after drainage is complete (5 minutes).
12. Effluent should be tested for the following:
    a. Cell count (significant if the red blood cell count is 60,000, and the white blood cell count is greater than $500/mm^3$).
    b. Gram's stain (positive if organisms or white cells are seen).

17
Maternal Health Care

STEPHEN GLOYD
SANDRA GOVE

The health problems of Third World women and children are rooted in poverty and malnutrition. Poor housing, inadequate drinking water supplies, lack of sewage facilities, early teenage childbirth, short intervals between births, and inadequate hygiene contribute to the high maternal and childhood death rates which are 10 to 100 times higher than the rates in developed countries.

The major causes of maternal death in poor countries today are the same as they were in industrialized countries 50 years ago—hemorrhage, infection, toxemia, obstructed labor, and abortion. The challenge of maternal health services is to create a mix of preventive and therapeutic services to address these major problems and integrate them with child health services.

Good obstetric management of labor and delivery with facilities for obstetrical emergencies reduces maternal and perinatal morbidity and mortality and the risk of anoxic damage to the child. However important the potential benefits, they are frequently less than those achieved with good preventive medical care. In a refugee camp, control of the basic risk factors for diseases—inadequate food, sanitation, water, and shelter—will benefit mothers more than specific antenatal and obstetrical services. Until these factors are addressed, elaborate obstetrical services are out of place. Focused preventive antenatal services (iron and food supplements, chloroquine to prevent malaria, etc.) and basic maternal education programs should precede clinic-based antenatal and obstetrical services.

PLANNING

The development of a maternal health program in a refugee camp requires knowledge of the pattern of childbearing, the local problems associated with the reproductive process, and the attitudes and practices of the local women in pregnancy and childbirth. Moreover, the availability of human and material resources in the camp needs to be assessed.

The Pattern of Childbearing

An estimate of the birth rate in the camp is essential for planning maternity services, family planning, and well-child care. Such an estimate is difficult to obtain if either birth reporting or camp population estimates are unreliable. Therefore, to estimate the birth rate indirectly, a sample household survey is often helpful (see the Appendix and Chapter 2 for methodology). A survey is also useful to gather additional information about the cultural patterns of childbirth, the specific problems one is likely to encounter in the camp, and the effectiveness of existing maternal health programs.

The following is a list of useful subjects to address in the survey:

- Age, parity, level of education of the childbearing population.
- Usual preparation during pregnancy for childbirth.
- Traditional cultural and religious practices regarding childbirth.
- Family and work problems.
- Experiences and attitudes regarding antenatal care.
- Nutritional practices before and during pregnancy and lactation.
- Experience and preferences regarding the place and nature of assistance during delivery.
- Past childbirth experiences: problems and their management.
- Attitudes about the health facilities.
- Attitudes about traditional birth attendants.
- Knowledge and attitudes about family planning.

Available Resources

Trained midwives and traditional birth attendants in the refugee community should be identified and interviewed to assess their training, competence, and potential for further training. Interpreters are essential. Identification of community groups, particularly women's groups within the camp, can be especially helpful to improve the potential credibility and utilization of the maternal health services.

The role of nonrefugee health workers can be determined by their competency and likely length of stay in the camp. Programs based on the presence of highly trained nonrefugee personnel often fail when these workers leave. Training refugees as health workers helps maintain programs and may improve the acceptance of services by the community (see Chapter 4).

Basic equipment considered helpful includes scales, blood pressure cuffs, fetoscopes, stethoscopes, measuring tape, and gloves. A manual pump vacuum extractor is an extremely valuable obstetric tool and should be available where obstetric emergencies are referred for care. Facilities for (or transport to) operative cesarian delivery are desirable, particularly if a system of risk assessment is in place. Instruments for fetal destruction and simple tools for symphysiotomy can reduce the need for cesarian operations. In experienced hands forceps are occasionally useful.

Traditional Birth Attendants versus Midwives

An important early decision in the planning and implementation of obstetric services in refugee camps is whether to use community-based traditional birth attendants (TBAs). TBAs are community members who assist delivery and are often consulted for infant care problems. Their practices vary tremendously depending on local culture and tradition. Some have acquired considerable obstetric skills by apprenticeship. It is estimated that TBAs assist 80 percent of births in underdeveloped countries.

TBAs often serve maternal–child health needs better than trained doctors or midwives. First, they often reach a larger percentage of the women who need them; they provide emotional support and allow delivery in natural and familiar positions; and they usually give valuable advice on nutrition and child care consistent with local customs. Often, TBAs are highly respected in their communities.

TBAs should be considered as part of any strategy to address maternal–child health in refugee camp settings. The decision on whether and how to incorporate TBAs into refugee maternal health services depends on a variety of local factors, including the following:

- Extent and nature of local maternal health problems.
- Status and activities of the local TBAs.
- Willingness of the TBAs to be trained in preventive antenatal care and Western obstetrics.
- Cost-effectiveness of alternative strategies.
- Resources for training and supporting TBAs.
- Quality of the potential referral network.
- Likelihood of trained TBAs remaining in the camp after training.

TBA Training

Among the subjects covered in training programs for TBAs are clean delivery and cord care, management of postpartum hemorrhage, nutrition for the mother, breastfeeding, referral mechanisms, and record keeping. Care must be taken to encourage those practices that are helpful and ignore practices (antepartum massage, external cephalic version) that appear hamless or about which one is uncertain. Proven harmful practices should be discouraged in a tactful manner. Umbilical cord preparations that cause neonatal tetanus (cow dung, soil, etc.) are examples of the latter; however, some traditional cord preparations (spider webs in Central America) have antiseptic properties and may be beneficial.

TBAs benefit from practical demonstrations, discussions in their own language and dialect, and recognition of their strongly held beliefs. Drama is particularly useful in educational programs.

Illiteracy is not necessarily an impediment to good record keeping and referral. A referral system used in Bangladesh is based on different colored vouchers—white vouchers for routine referral of uncomplicated pregnancies, red for complicated pregnancies, blue for infant care referral, and so on. Pictorial representations of both patient care charts and birth registries have been used with good results in many programs (Figure 17-1).

Most TBA programs last from one to six weeks and cost between $20 and $100 (US dollars) per TBA. Successful TBA programs incur substantial support costs after initial training for supervision, resupply, evaluation, and in-service continuing education. UNICEF provides delivery kits; however, kits made from

Figure 17-1. A home visit form for illiterate TBAs in Afghanistan.

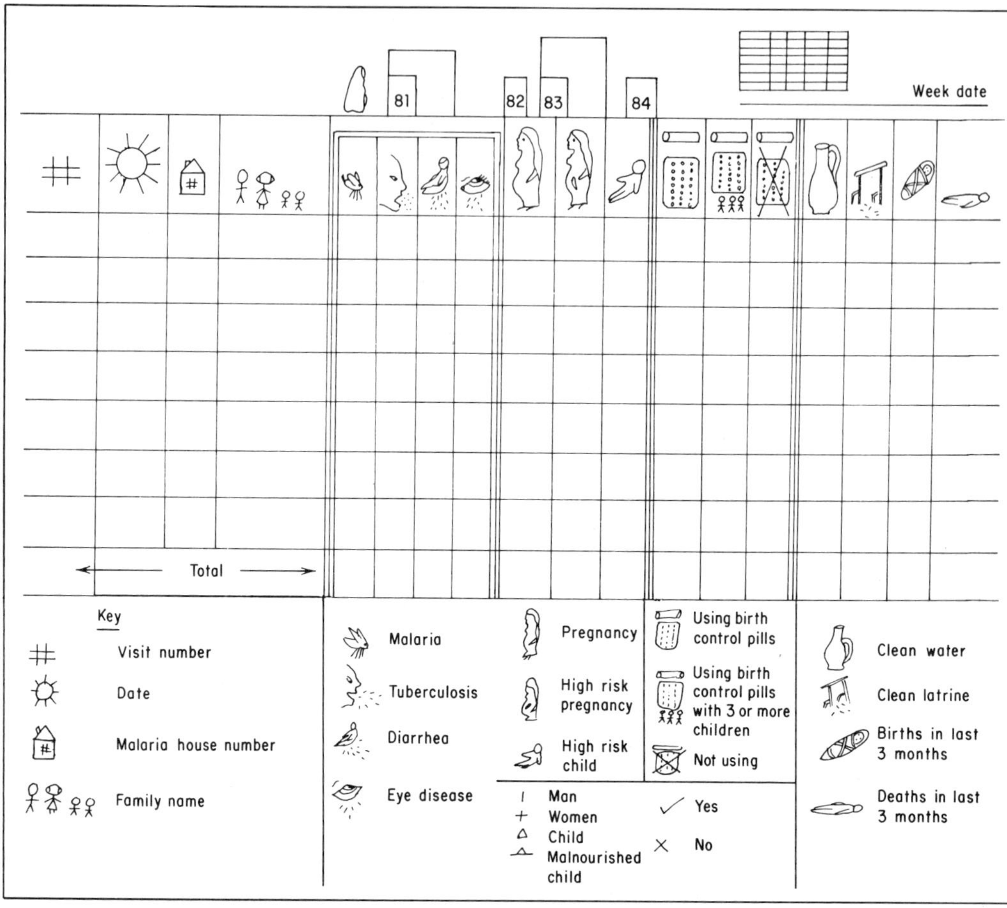

(From Favin, M, et al: Improving maternal health in developing countries. An information for action paper. Geneva, World Federation of Public Health Associations, Aug 1984, p 19.)

locally available materials (sterilized razor blades, cord ties, iodine, cotton balls) are usually easier to resupply. A recently developed TBA trainer's kit is available through UNICEF.

Several factors have been demonstrated as critical to the success of TBA programs (Stinson 1980):

- Teach a limited number of subject areas.
- Build on the existing skills and experience of the TBAs.
- Use a single supervisor, such as a community health nurse.
- Exchange locally available supplies for birth data that can facilitate surveillance and supervision.

Home Versus Hospital Delivery

A number of factors are important in determining whether a delivery system should be home or hospital based. These factors include the appropriateness of using TBAs, maternal preference, availability and reliability of transport, and the potential effectiveness of hospital care. The primary issue is management of delivery; place of birth is secondary.

Hospitals need adequate skilled staff, equipment, and medicines to manage obstructed labor and complicated delivery effectively. Facilities for performing operative delivery should be available or accessible through reliable transportation. If basic standards of institutional care are not met, the disadvantages of a hospital (e.g., nosocomial infection, foreign environment) may outweigh its advantages over home birth.

ANTENATAL CARE

General Preventive Services

General preventive measures such as nutrition programs, health education, immunizations, and prevention of local diseases are the most effective means of reducing maternal and perinatal health problems. Certain preventive services need not be confined to the health sector and may be done more effectively through community action groups.

Nutrition

Maternal malnutrition affects the majority of women in poor areas of the world and leads to a host of maternal problems, including weakness, susceptibility to infections, infertility, amenorrhea, spontaneous abortion, and poor development of the female pelvis during puberty. The most devastating effect of maternal malnutrition is on the fetus and newborn as it causes low birth weight.

Low birth weight (LBW) is common in less developed countries and is an established contributor to excessive perinatal and neonatal morbidity and mortality. Moreover, LBW is associated with mental retardation and impaired immunologic defense throughout infancy. Eighty percent of LBW in many underdeveloped countries is due to intrauterine growth retardation (small-for-gestational-age babies), whereas in developed countries, prematurity is the more common cause. The marked difference in neonatal mortality in developed versus less developed countries is, in large part, due to the higher incidence of LBW. Therefore, a major impact on infant survival can be expected when LBW is prevented.

The principal factors that lead to maternal malnutrition are poverty and unavailability of food. Refugee women are often subjected to extremely poor nutrition while seeking asylum. Other factors include overwork, the added nutritional demands of pregnancy and lactation (an estimated 300 to 800 additional calories per day), lack of general education and specific knowledge about foods, and cultural practices. In some West African cultures, consumption of fish by pregnant women is thought to make their babies liars, and eggs are thought to make them bald. Women in many cultures are often the last in families to receive food and get the least food in times of shortage. It is also a widespread belief that women should limit weight gain during pregnancy to avoid a difficult delivery.

Many women in poor countries become progressively depleted nutritionally with successive, closely spaced pregnancies. The result is what is called the maternal depletion syndrome—thin, prematurely aged, and often severly anemic multiparas who are at high risk for poor pregnancy outcomes.

Nutritional Interventions

The first and foremost step in nutritional intervention is to ensure the availability of adequate calories, proteins, and vitamins to women in their daily ration. Where the general ration is not adequate for maternal nutrition during pregnancy and lactation, a supplementary feeding program should be instituted. The addition of iron and vitamins C and D is considered appropriate to meet special needs of pregnancy, particularly when women have little access to meat or other high-protein and iron sources.

Nutritional education is essential during pregnancy. Demonstration of the choice and preparation of available food is preferable to a lecture on nutrition. Cultural beliefs that affect maternal nutrition should be investigated. Vegetable gardens and other food projects can be helpful. Community kitchens are a useful and efficient way of providing nutritious food combinations for the whole family. Assisting women to create income-generating projects that will enable them to buy more food is also helpful. Also see Chapter 13 on nutritional interventions.

Immunizations

In the underdeveloped world, neonatal tetanus is the second most important cause of neonatal mortality (LBW is the first). Neonatal tetanus can be prevented by proper cord care and prenatal immunization against tetanus. Administration of at least two doses of tetanus toxoid during pregnancy reduces the incidence of neonatal tetanus by more than 80 percent. Another strategy that yields similar results is the immunization of all women of childbearing age on two or more occasions. If the second of these immunizations is during pregnancy, the protection against neonatal tetanus exceeds 90 percent (Lancet 1983). (See Chapter 6.)

Iron Supplementation

Anemia is a major problem of pregnancy, which contributes to low birth weight and depleted infant iron stores. Anemic women have less reserve and therefore a higher risk of morbidity and mortality from hemorrhage during labor and delivery. Severely anemic women are also at risk for congestive heart failure during and immediately after pregnancy.

Oral iron and folate supplements are essential for all pregnant women in most refugee settings. The usual supplemental dose is ferrous sulfate (or equivalent), 400 mg per day (200 mg for iron consumption plus 200 mg for probable depletion of iron stores). Folate 0.5 mg per day is also considered advisable for prophylaxis. For women who do not take tablets regularly, oral supplementation should be pursued with health education and assitance by health workers from the community. Parenteral iron and transfusions are a last resort.

It is often useful to determine the local prevalence of anemia in the camp's pregnant population using hemoglobin, hematocrit, or qualitative measurements such as the "anemiometer" and "anemia recognition card" (Favin 1984). If the prevalence of anemia is high, consideration should be given to mass treatment with therapeutic levels of oral iron. Underlying infectious causes of anemia such as hookworm and malaria should be investigated to assess the value of mass preventive or therapeutic measures. Routine hemoglobin and hematocrit values are of limited value in camps where most women are anemic and would be treated with supplementary iron anyway.

Iodine Supplementation

Iodine-deficient goiter is a common condition in certain highland regions or where foodstuffs (e.g., cassava) interfere with the absorption or utilization of iodine. Goiter in pregnant women may result in their bearing deaf, mentally retarded, or small-for-gestational-age babies. Where there is organized commercial distribution of salt, goiter can be prevented easily through the consumption of iodized salt. Iodine-supplemented flour and bread are also available. Intramuscular injections of iodized oil can be used as a one-time-only prevention and treatment of goiter.

Malaria Prophylaxis

Pregnant women are at considerable risk for malarial infection and its complications. Malaria increases the risk of spontaneous abortion and is considered a major cause of intrauterine growth retardation.

The effects of malarial infection on the fetus depend on the endemicity of malaria: in unstable malaria areas or where migrants without immunity enter an endemic area, malaria can cause first-trimester abortion, premature labor, and intrauterine fetal death.

In communities where malaria is holoendemic and transmission is stable, maternal immunity is better and there is no clear association between malaria and stillbirths. Even with substantial maternal immunity, however, malaria does reduce birthweight. A study in Gambia recorded that 20 percent of all placentas were infected with malaria and associated with an average birth weight reduction of 170 g (McGregor 1983).

See Chapter 25 for more on malaria prophylaxis.

Antenatal Health Education

A good time to educate pregnant women and mothers on a variety of important issues is during antenatal care. Some issues that should be addressed are the following:

- Nutrition
- Sanitation and safe water use.
- Sexually transmitted diseases.
- Family planning.
- Danger signs during pregnancy (bleeding, swelling, membrane rupture, etc.).
- Management of common conditions of pregnancy (heartburn, nausea, backache, etc.).
- Working during pregnancy.
- Smoking and alcohol consumption.
- Importance of wearing shoes.

Prior to delivery is an ideal time to discuss issues of child rearing. The mother plays the key role in her child's survival in the first five years and she should be considered an important health worker. Preparation for the promotion of breastfeeding should be stressed. The timing and practices of weaning need to be discussed. Mothers should be taught how to manage diarrhea with oral rehydration solution (see Chapter 15) and to recognize and treat other common childhood illnesses.

Discussion of harmful traditional health practices is appropriate in some circumstances. Examples include female circumcision, umbilical cord treatment with home remedies, and harmful infant feeding practices. Some of these issues and their implications are extremely sensitive and often not well understood by the expatriate health worker. Open-ended, nonjudgmental community discussions are helpful to explore these issues. Often, the presence of local midwives, elder women, husbands, and male community leaders can give the discussions a wider scope and can help facilitate change of harmful customs and reinforcement of good ones.

HIGH-RISK SCREENING

The risk approach is an epidemiologic and management tool intended to enable health workers to concentrate attention on the individuals with the greatest need. Screening implies that the capacity to manage certain patients adequately in referral hospitals or clinics exists. If this is not the case, then specific screening should be reevaluated. Furthermore, a prime requirement for high-risk screening is maximum prenatal coverage of the population. If the users of health services are a selected group, the majority of community women in high-risk categories may not benefit from such identification.

Risk factors vary from community to community. For intervention to be specific, there is a need to mount small-scale investigations of local risk factors and pregnancy outcomes. Table 17-1 shows a simple scoring system for risk allocation and family planning priorities developed from a WHO system for a north African country; it is applicable to both pregnant and nonpregnant women. Many refugee camps might elect to develop scoring systems with scores based on their own use of services and their capacity to handle high-risk situations.

Early identification of the pregnant woman is important to facilitate measures against anemia, malnutrition, and parasite infection in the critical first trimester of gestational growth. Even with intensive community education, first-trimester prenatal attendance is often unsuccessful, particularly where the local culture encourages concealing early pregnancy. House-to-house visits by community women and health personnel is one way of identifying early pregnancies.

Although many prenatal programs recommend that pregnant women be examined several times (even monthly) during pregnancy, each program must set realistic goals for itself. In rural areas of the Third World, the goal is often one visit in early pregnancy and once in the third trimester unless problems or high-risk situations develop. Most refugee camps have the resources for more frequent attendance, but the benefits accrue less from the number of visits than from the quality of health education and other preventive interventions.

Table 17-1. Pregnancy Risk Scoring Scheme (PAHO/WHO)[a]

	Characteristics	Points
Age	under 19, over 40	4
	Between 30 and 39	2
	Between 20 and 29	0
No. of children	10 or more	4
	0–1	2
	2–9	0
Interval between deliveries	Less than 24 months	1
	More than 24 months since last delivery	0
Medical history	Previous obstetric complications, deaths	3
	Diabetes, heart or renal disease, psychoses, etc.	5
Maternal education	Illiterate	1
	Can read/write	0

[a]The points are added up to give a total score and decisions taken as follows:

Points	*Recommendation*
5 or more	highest risk, referral obligatory
3–4	high risk, referral recommended
0–2	usual risk, usual local care

(From Risk Approach for Maternal and Child Health Care. WHO Offset Publication No 39, Geneva, World Health Organization, 1978.)

Antenatal cards are available that combine risk factors associated with history and prenatal course. Experience has shown that, with encouragement, most women given their own cards reliably bring them to antenatal clinic. This practice obviates the need for time-consuming and difficult-to-manage filing systems.

The use of Western pregnancy weight and height standards may be misleading. Weight for height and arm circumference standards, however, tend to remain relatively stable in different populations, as does weight gain in pregnancy.

Infectious Diseases in Pregnancy

Screening for common infectious diseases can be productive when the disease under consideration is sufficiently prevalent (over 5%) to justify screening but not so common that universal treatment is more cost-effective than identifying individual cases (e.g., malaria, intestinal parasites). Such screening can often be done with a careful history alone. The use of laboratory tests is generally necessary only for definitive diagnosis and management.

Tuberculosis is a prevalent disease in refugee camps (see Chapter 33) and is particularly dangerous during pregnancy. Pregnant women are at greater risk of rapidly progressive and life-threatening tuberculous disease; infants born to tuberculous mothers risk congenital infection, dissemination, and miliary or meningeal disease. Thus, diagnostic measures and treatment for tuberculosis should not be delayed in pregnancy.

Pregnant women with prolonged cough or unexplained weight loss should be evaluated for tuberculosis, and sputum should be obtained if indicated. Treatment should begin as soon as possible after definitive diagnosis is made. INH, ethambutol, thiacetazone, and rifampin are considered safe in pregnancy. Streptomycin, ethionamide, and pyrizinamide should be avoided during pregnancy and lactation.

Urinary Tract Infections. Routine urinalyses are not commonly performed on pregnant women in underdeveloped countries because the cost of screening is usually not worth the benefits. However, in symptomatic patients a significant infection should be identified and treated (see Chapter 36).

Intestinal parasites. Screening for parasites such as hookworm, ameba, ascaris, and *Schistosoma* species is costly and a positive result is not necessarily indicative of a clinically significant infection. With a high prevalence of hookworm or ascaris, mass treatment may be cheaper and more effective than individual case finding. Mebendazole, thiabendazole, praziquantel, oxamniquine, metriphonate, and trichloroethylene (TCE) should not be given in pregnancy. Pyrantel pamoate and piperazine should be used only after the first trimester.

Hepatitis. An epidemic form of non-A, non-B hepatitis has been noted in Somali refugee camps and has resulted in fulminant hepatitis during the third trimester of pregnancy with high maternal mortality and fetal loss. Unlike posttransfusion non-A, non-B hepatitis transmission, which resembles hepatitis B, epidemic non-A, non-B transmission appears to be by fecal–oral spread (Deinhardt 1982). Thus, prevention must emphasize proper human waste disposal, clean water, and good handwashing technique.

Hypertensive Diseases of Pregnancy

Pregnancy-associated hypertension (preeclampsia) and eclampsia are common in the Third World. Reported preeclampsia varies between 1 and 20 percent of all pregnancies worldwide, and eclampsia is a leading cause of maternal mortality (Davies 1979).

Health workers should screen for the signs and symptoms of preeclampsia (edema, sudden large weight gain, blood pressure greater than 140/90, or rapid, sustained rise in blood pressure). Blood pressure screening is suggested for the first antenatal visit, for all third-trimester visits, during labor, and for several hours after delivery. A urine dipstick showing more than 2+ protein can be helpful to diagnose suggestive cases, but it is of limited use in areas where *Schistosoma hematobium* is prevalent, since this commonly causes proteinuria.

Treatment of preeclampsia by complete bed rest at home is the only option in many refugee camps, but this may be difficult to achieve. Women often perform the bulk of their family's work. Unless a concrete plan is made to relieve her of cooking, childcare, and the fetching of water and firewood, conservative management is likely to fail. Education of the husband is therefore equally important to education of the woman. Sedatives such as diazepam (only after the first trimester) or phenobarbital are often useful to ensure rest and better define the woman's illness for her family. The woman with preeclampsia must be carefully monitored; warning signs that convulsions may be imminent include acceleration of hypertension, right upper quadrant or epigastric pain, blurred vision, tremulousness, and increasing headache. The prompt administration of magnesium sulfate and transfer for delivery as soon as possible are important.

Diabetes Mellitus

Unless local studies indicate an unusually high prevalence of diabetes, routine screening by urine or blood glucose is marginally important in poor countries. Screening should be considered in refugees from urban populations where the incidence of diabetes may be higher.

EXTERNAL CEPHALIC VERSION (ECV)

Antenatal version of breech presentations is not commonly used in developed countries because most primiparous breech presentations are delivered by cesarean section. In poor countries, the risk of cesarean section to the mother is much greater because anesthesia, equipment, sterile conditions, postoperative care, and blood transfusion capability are suboptimal. The postoperative infection rate is very high throughout the developing world. While ECV carries its own inherent risk due to placental abruption, cord knotting, and induction of premature labor, most observers feel that ECV reduces the overall maternal and perinatal mortality by reducing vaginal breech deliveries and cesarean sections (Thornton 1985). In experienced hands, a trial of carefully monitored (by fetoscope) external version of breech presentations at 32 to 34 weeks gestation seems appropriate.

INTRAPARTUM CARE

Whether delivery is planned for home or hospital, the key to a good outcome is preventive management and limited intervention. Adequate nutrition, fluids, and hygienic management of labor and delivery are particularly important. Practices used for delivery should not conflict with the customs and practices of the refugee population; otherwise, women may avoid seeking care even when they have problems. Local practices may sometimes be preferable to common Western medical practice. Some traditional delivery positions, including squatting or kneeling, have been shown to preserve adequate maternal–placental blood flow and facilitate fetal descent and delivery better than the standard hospital lithotomy position.

Frequent handwashing and simple techniques for clean delivery and sterile umbilical cord care can significantly reduce the incidence of maternal and newborn infections. Vaginal examinations are best performed only when necessary. Where deliveries are in hospitals or maternity units, early discharge of the mother and infant reduces nosocomial infection. In some camps, mothers leave the hospital a few hours after delivery.

Dehydration and weakness commonly occurs with continuous expenditure of energy accompanied by profuse sweating and respiratory fluid loss from prolonged or obstructed labors. Fluids are best administered orally, with added carbohydrates; this can prevent servere dehydration and acidosis (see Chapter 15). Intravenous fluids are expensive and inhibit the natural maternal movement which can facilitate descent of the fetus.

Ambulation and frequent urination during labor should be encouraged. Bladder distention frequently inhibits labor, and the descending head may impede urination; sitting in warm water often facilitates urination. In persistent cases, in–out catheterization may be helpful. Amniotomy is discouraged as a routine procedure. It may be helpful in occasional cases of delayed, late first stage of labor and when it is essential to know if the amniotic fluid is meconium stained. Analgesic use during labor may interfere with optimal uterine contractions and should be discouraged except under unusual circumstances.

Auscultation of fetal heart tones by fetoscope is probably the optimal manner of detecting fetal distress in refugee settings. Inexpensive conical fetoscopes are widely available.

Specific standards for the three stages of labor are helpful to enable early identification by birth attendants of problems that may require intervention. Guidelines for intervention in the developed world may be inappropriate for refugee camp settings where the complications of cesarean section are frequent. Each program must balance the risk of problems, such as prolonged labor, or ruptured fetal membranes, with the estimated local risk of intervention (e.g., cesarean section), to establish local standards for birth attendants. In general, the balance will be shifted toward acceptance of longer labors in all stages and a longer interval between fetal membrane rupture and delivery.

Management should include clearly defined referral mechanisms that can be established for each type of provider. Attention must be given to realistic transport possibilities, capabilities of the referral destination, and effective communication up and down the referral ladder.

Induction and augmentation of labor are dangerous in settings where accurate control of oxytocin infusion is not available. The use of oxytocin should be restricted to cases of ineffective uterine contractions when the pelvis is considered of adequate size for fetal passage and the fetal head presentation is normal. Augmented labor is relatively contraindicated in grand multiparas because of the high risk of uterine rupture. Intramuscular oxytocin during labor is not considered safe in any setting.

Back-up care for obstructed labor should include the use of the hand-pump vacuum extractor. Vacuum extractors are easy to use and are available from international health agencies (e.g., UNICEF) for $75 to $100 (US). They require no external power source and only a fraction of the skill to operate that forceps require. Furthermore, knowledge of the position of the fetal head is not crucial. The vacuum extractor can be placed on the fetal head on occiput anterior or posterior positions; when the head is engaged, the extractor may be used with a less than fully dilated cervix. The fetal head can spontaneously rotate while the provider is slowly assisting its delivery. Maternal anesthetic is not required, and the mother can bear down and push when the vacuum cup is applied.

A referral facility for cesarean section delivery should be identified. Performing cesarean sections with local anesthesia may be safer than using spinal anesthetic block (SAB) anesthesia, particularly in cases of maternal hypotension from hemorrhage (Lawson & Stewart 1977). Cesarean delivery should not be attempted unless the anesthesia and operating room conditions meet mimimal standards. Operative mortality and postpartum infection rates for cesarean operations are much higher in poor areas than in the developed world.

Symphysiotomy is a recognized alternative to cesarean section in the management of obstructed labor (Gebbie 1984). Some consider this procedure preferable to cesarean section in areas where equipment, conditions, and skills for major operative procedures are not optimal. Furthermore, cesarean operation capability requires considerable staff time and equipment, and in many areas these resources may be more usefully devoted to the cost-effective tasks of prevention.

Fetal craniotomies can be life-saving procedures for the mother in cases of fetal death from obstructed labor. Cesarean section is rarely necessary for evacuation of the dead fetus in cephalic position and, in poor areas of the world, is much more risky to the mother than fetal-destructive procedures. Skills and equipment for these operations are easily acquired (Lawson & Stewart 1977).

POSTPARTUM CARE

The most common puerperal problems likely to be encountered in refugee camps are postpartum hemorrhage, infection, mastitis, and thromboembolic disease. Both hemorrhage and infection are likely to be more prevalent and severe in refugee camps as a consequence of the common underlying anemia and malnutrition.

TBAs and midwives have been taught to handle most cases of postpartum hemorrhage sucessfully. Immediate postdelivery hemorrhage can be managed by uterine compression, ice, oral or intramuscular ergot, or manual removal of the placenta. Rudimentary shock management (supine position, legs elevated) and ready access to oral or parenteral fluids can be life-saving in hemorrhage with significant volume loss. Birth attendants should be able to determine significant blood loss by postural blood pressure and gross anemia measurements.

Hemorrhage occurring 24 or more hours after birth is common and is usually caused by retained placental fragments. Oxytocics are the first-line conservative treatment, followed by gentle curettage and antibiotic therapy. Oral iron therapy (ferrous sulfate, 400 mg per day) is indicated for all women up to six months postpartum, with higher therapeutic doses (ferrous sulfate, 600–900 mg per day) given to anemic women. Transfusion is indicated, if available, for hemoglobins less than 6 g/dl or for anemia-associated heart failure.

Puerperal infections usually occur between the third and seventh days postpartum and are commonly caused by endometritis and mastitis. Endometritis is usually associated with lower abdominal/uterine tenderness, foul-smelling discharge, high temperatures, and a rapid pulse. Untreated, it is frequently fatal. Predisposing factors for endometritis include prolonged rupture of fetal membranes, long labor, multiple vaginal examinations, trauma (e.g., from forceps), and cesarean section. Its pathogenic spectrum is polymicrobial; gram-negative enteric, gram-positive, and anaerobic bacteria are all common. Numerous antibiotic regimens are used, one of which is ampicillin combined with an aminoglycoside and clindamycin in severe infections. Chloramphenicol and antistaphylococcal antibiotics are also helpful. Isolation of women with postpartum infections is important in a hospital setting. Blood transfusion can be helpful when severe anemia is associated with septic infections.

Mastitis can often be prevented by drainage of obstructed mammary ducts through continued nursing or breast pumping and hot packs. Nursing should be temporarily discontinued only in the case of gross pus drainage or an actual abscess. Antibiotics (cloxacillin or cotrimoxazole) are indicated with local inflammation or generalized symptoms including fever.

Thrombophlebitis, which is not uncommon in the postpartum period, is best treated in the refugee camp by local heat, elevation, and anti-inflammatory medications such as aspirin. Anticoagulation is not usually indicated in refugee camps.

Most postpartum care will necessarily be home based since, even in those camps with institutional deliveries, few allow extensive postpartum hospital stays. Thus, the home visit becomes an important tool in the identification and management of postpartum conditions as well as in health education. Home visits also facilitate the assessment of the hygienic conditions of the household and allow the visitor to give concrete suggestions regarding sanitation issues. Refugee camps are well suited for home-based care because of the proximity of residences.

The home visit is an ideal time to discuss the possibilities of child spacing (family planning) when both the mother and father are present. The home visitor should be well versed in the methods of family planning available in the camp and keep records of users (see Chapter 7).

NEWBORN CARE

Birth attendants often care for newborns and should be trained in newborn resuscitation, management of feeding problems, and treatment of common infant diseases. The birth attendant should encourage the mother to enroll the child in well-child preventive care programs. Some maternal–child health programs train midwives to be primary providers in the under-five clinics to preserve continuity of care and emphasize the interdependence of maternal and child health.

Newborn Resuscitation

Immediately after delivery, the oropharynx should be cleaned with a mucus trap (if available) or a clean cloth. Stimulation of the extremities usually initiates respiration. If breathing is absent or weak, mouth-to-mouth resuscitation is effective and easy to learn. If oxygen is available, ambu bags may be preferred. External cardiac massage is indicated if the newborn remains unresponsive with a heart rate less than 70. Maintenance of newborn body temperature is important even in warm climates; it can be done most easily by maximizing skin contact with the mother and drying and covering the newborn with a clean cloth. (See Chapter 12 for more details on pediatric resuscitation.)

Birth attendants should have specific instructions in umbilical cord management. Placing the newborn below the level of the mother's uterus for at least 30 seconds before the cord is interrupted gives the child an early red blood cell boost. The cord should be cut approximately 5 cm from its abdominal base, treated with an antiseptic, and covered with a sterile or clean dressing. Thereafter, the cord should be kept dry until it falls off in seven to ten days.

Ophthalmia neonatorum prophylaxis can be done with erythromycin, neosporin, or 1 percent silver nitrate ointment. Vitamin K (1 mg IM or 5mg PO) may reduce the incidence of neonatal bleeding but is not essential.

The birth attendant should perform a standard, simple newborn physical examination, including birthweight determination. A delay of 24 hours can significantly change the weight of the newborn. Hanging scales are available to facilitate weighing in the home. Color-coded scales are available for illiterate TBAs for less than $2 (US) per scale (Program for Appropriate Technology in Health, Seattle, WA).

INFANT CARE

Mothers should be instructed to begin nursing in the first few hours after birth to give the newborn the benefit of the antibody-rich colostrum and to stimulate uterine contraction in the mother. Water is not necessary. Breastfeeding alone, without any food or fluid additives, is appropriate for the first four months.

The birth attendant should examine the baby on the second or early on the third day for neonatal jaundice. An "icterometer" (Thos Ingram and Co., Birmingham, UK) is available to measure the depth of jaundice in newborns without taking a blood specimen. Exposure to daylight is a highly effective means of treating moderate levels of hyperbilirubinemia. Breastfeeding should be continued in newborns with jaundice.

Health education regarding the treatment of infant diarrhea with oral rehydration solution and continued nursing is essential. Management of infant fevers and upper respiratory infections should also be taught. Awareness of local customs is important. In some Asian communities babies are not given breast milk for the first three days; they are given a sticky rice instead. Clearly harmful practices should be discussed with local midwives so that appropriate behavior can be encouraged.

EVALUATION AND SURVEILLANCE

The birth attendant should register birth information in the mother's own antenatal/intrapartum chart and in a cumulative birth register. The mother's chart includes birth weight, complications of the mother and newborn, assistance in labor, and medications administered. The cumulative registry should include for each pregnancy the date of birth, the mother's parity, multiple gestation, birth weight, fetal or newborn deaths (including the age, in days, at death), and other complications.

The information in the mother's chart is primarily useful in the child's care and in subsequent pregnancies. The birth register can be quite useful in planning services. The rate of low-birth-weigth newborns is an excellent indicator of maternal malnutrition, and the perinatal death rate is a good measure of the performance of the maternal health services. The total number of attended births can be compared with the estimated total number of births in the camp to estimate the utilization of maternity care.

When reporting is reliable, computations can be made of a number of other useful indicators:

- Total birth rate (number of births per 1000 population per year).
- Stillbirth rate (fetal deaths from 28 weeks until birth).
- Neonatal mortality rate (deaths of live newborns from 1 to 28 days).
- Perinatal mortality rate (stillbirth plus neonatal death rates).
- Infant mortality rate (deaths of infants up to one year of age per 1000 live births).

It is particularly important to share the information with the birth attendants. This valuable feedback about their work encourages active participation in the health data collection and thus improves the reliability of the surveillance system.

REFERENCES

Davies AM: Epidemiology of hypertensive disorders of pregnancy. Bull WHO 1979;57:373–86.
Deinhardt ID: Viral hepatitis. Bull WHO 1982;60(5):661–91.
Favin M et al: Improving Maternal Health in Developing Countries. An Information for Action Paper. Geneva, World Federation of Public Health Associations, Aug 1984, p 19.
Gebbie DAM: Symphysiotomy. Clin Obstet Gynaecol 1982;9:663–83.
Lancet (editorial): Prevention of neonatal tetanus. Lancet 1983; 1:1253–54.
Lawson JB, Stewart DB (eds): Obstetrics and Gynecology in the Tropics and Developing Countries, London, pp 193–97, 237–38. Edward Arnold, Ltd, 1977.
McGregor IA: Malaria infection of the placenta in the Gambia, West Africa. Trans Roy Soc Trop Med Hyg 1983;77:232–44.
Stinson W: Aid for International Development (AID) Seminar on TBAs. Washington DC, American Public Health Association, March 4, 1980.
Thornton JG: External cephalic version, is it still justified in developing countries? Tropical Doctor 1985;15:173–74.

APPENDIX 17-A

BIRTH RATE DETERMINATION

Information should be gathered from a sample household survey using methods of random selection (see Chapter 2). From the sample, estimate the proportion of women of childbearing age in the camp population. This is usually about 25 percent in most Third World countries, but this percentage is often skewed in refugee camps where few men are present. This proportion multiplied by the estimate of the total camp population gives an estimate of the total number of women of childbearing age in the camp. Also from the sample, one can determine the proportions of women of this age group who are pregnant, nursing, or menstruating (generally 20, 30, and 50%, respectively). One then can estimate the number of pregnant women in the camp. This number multiplied by 1.3 will give a gross estimate of the annual number of expected births in the camp.

18
Ophthalmologic Diseases

ETIENNE OTT
RUDOLF BOCK
WILLIAM HAWKS

This chapter outlines a basic approach for the common eye diseases encountered in refugee camps. Both vitamin A deficiency and trachoma (the leading causes of blindness, after trauma and cataract, in these settings) are preventable and treatable. Other common eye problems include easily removable corneal foreign bodies and conjunctivitis. Simple standard lenses can be supplied to provide clear vision.

THE PATIENT EXAMINATION

Before examining the patient, take a patient history. Note any symptoms that may indicate eye disease, such as blurred vision, pain, headaches, tearing, discharge, burning sensation, sensitivity to light (photophobia), foreign body sensation, itching, or double vision.

For a basic eye examination, the following tools are needed:

- A Snellen illiterate E chart for far vision or tumbling E card.
- A Jaeger chart for near vision testing.
- A good flashlight for focal illumination.
- A hand-held magnifying loupe (4× or 6× magnification).
- Fluorescein strips for examination of the cornea (e.g., foreign bodies, erosions, ulcers).
- A Schiotz tonometer and topical anesthesia drops (e.g., 0.5% tetracaine) for measuring intraocular pressure.
- An ophthalmoscope for evaluating cornea, lens, and vitreous transparency.

Vision testing should be done on all patients. The procedure is as follows: A Snellen chart is placed in a well-lit location (avoiding glare) 20 feet (6 meters) from the patient. Showing the chart to the patient, explain the concept of indicating the direction of the Es by rotating the patient's hand so that his or her fingers point in the direction of the various Es. Then move the patient back to the testing distance. To avoid peeking, have a helper cover one of the patient's eyes securely with a hand or cover, being careful not to press on the eye, while the other eye is being tested. Always test the right eye first and start by pointing to the large Es (20/200 or 6/600), then proceeding to the smaller Es as the patient answers correctly. Record the smallest line the patient can read correctly. If the patient cannot see the largest letter, hold up your hand against a contrasting background to check if the number of fingers held up can be counted correctly (recorded, for example, as CF at 20 feet). If the patient cannot count fingers at 20 feet, gradually shorten the distance until he can do so. If he cannot count fingers even close up, check if he can perceive hand movement (HM). If he is unable to see hand movement, take him to a dark room to test if he can perceive light (LP). Always be sure that the eye that is not being tested is securely covered. Distance vision can be tested outdoors, but it is much better to test near vision and conduct all other eye examinations in a partially darkened room with focal illumination. Near vision is tested with the Jaeger chart at 35 to 45 cm in good illumination, again testing each eye separately and recording the J number.

Physical Examination of the Eye

Start with the eyelids and proceed step by step as follows.

Eyelids and Lacrimal (Tear) Sac Area

Begin by examining the eyelids and lacrimal (tear) sac area (see Figure 18-1). Note any swelling, redness, or tenderness (e.g., sty, lid abscess, chalazion, tear sac infection, eczema). Check the position of the lid border—it may be turned out (ectropion) or turned in (entro-

Figure 18-1. Eyelid and lacrimal (tear) sac anatomy.

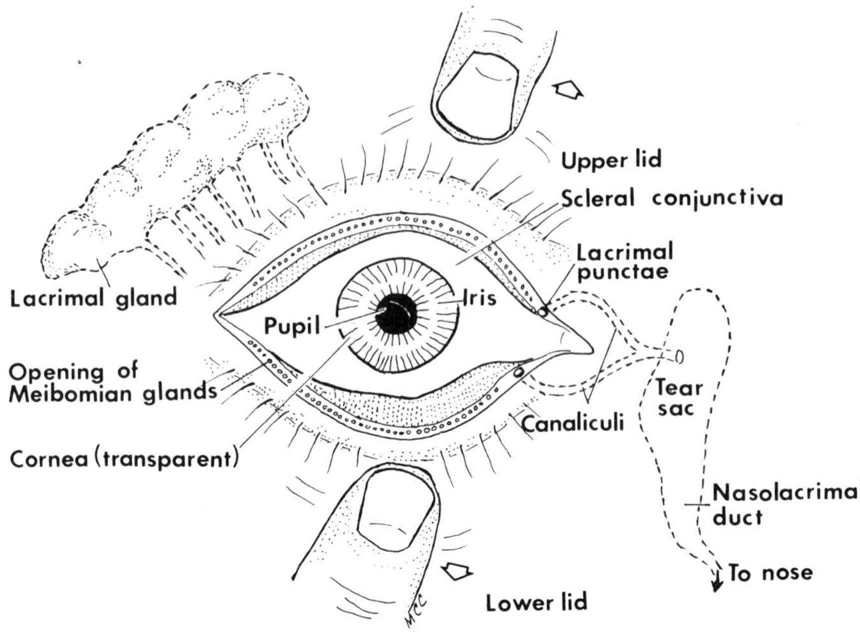

pion). In the latter case, the eyelashes may be rubbing against the cornea (trichiasis, common in trachoma).

Conjunctiva

Next examine the conjunctiva. This is the thin mucous membrane that covers the white of the eyeball (bulbar conjunctiva) and lines the inside of the lids. To see the upper lid conjunctiva, it is necessary to flip that lid around. To do this, ask the patient to look down, and then pull down on the upper eyelashes. Apply a cotton swab about 1 cm above the lid border as a fulcrum around which the lid may then be turned upward. It is important to practice this on normal eyes. Inspection of the upper middle half of the upper lid conjunctiva is essential for making the diagnosis of various infections, especially trachoma. Foreign bodies also often lodge there and may be gently wiped off with a cotton swab.

In examining the conjunctiva, look for redness, swelling, pigmentation, and dryness.

Redness of the bulbar conjunctiva is the most common and obvious sign of eye disease. In making a diagnosis and assessing the severity of the disease, close attention must be paid to the color pattern and distribution of this redness, and to accompanying symptoms. It is not uncommon to see a localized, irregular, blood-red area after minor injuries, coughing, or heavy lifting. This is called subconjunctival hemorrhage (see Figure 18-2) and is due to circumscribed bleeding beneath the conjunctiva. It may look frightening but is almost always harmless, disappearing spontaneously in a few days. If the redness is diffuse (all over the bulbar conjunctiva), one must try to distinguish whether it is more intense in the periphery (conjunctival injection) (Figure 18-3) or around the cornea (ciliary or pericorneal injection) (Figure 18-4). The former indicates a harmless condition (usually conjunctivitis), the latter a serious one (inflammation of the iris or cornea, or acute glaucoma).

Swelling is found in patients with allergies (to insect bites, animal hair, plants, chemicals, etc.).

Figure 18-2. Subconjunctivial hemmorhage.

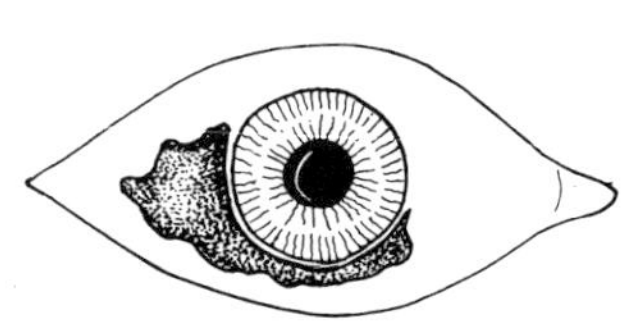

Figure 18-3. Conjunctival injection.

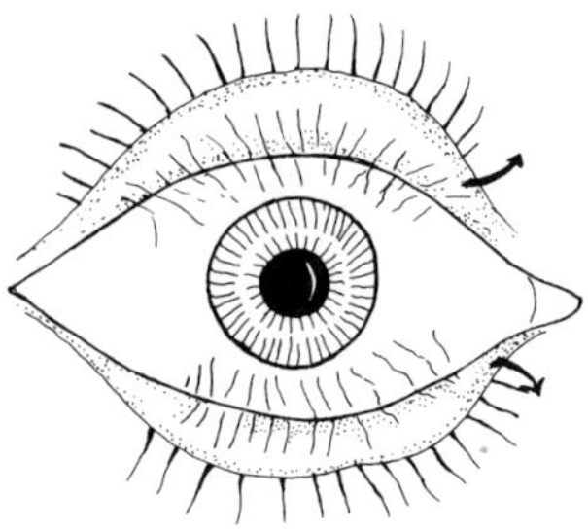

Figure 18-4. Ciliary injection.

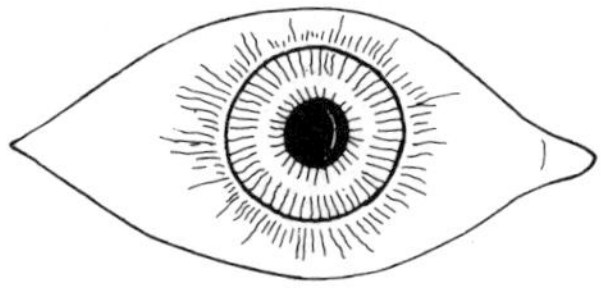

Yellowness is seen with jaundice; brown-black discoloration is seen with a nevus, usually occuring as a birthmark in black children.

Xerosis (dryness) is found in vitamin A deficiency. This is best seen just medial and/or lateral to the cornea.

Cornea

In examining the cornea, look for grayish white areas and new blood vessels. Insert a fluorescein strip for a moment behind the lower lid for staining. Then, in a darkened room, use a flashlight and magnifying loupe for close inspection. A gray area may be either an ulcer or corneal scar. Ulcers appear dull and take up the fluorescein as a bright yellow-green color; scars have a smooth surface and do not stain. It is important to look for newly formed blood vessels in this otherwise avascular and completely transparent tissue. For example, with trachoma, the cornea is invaded by fine blood vessels coming from above (pannus) (Figure 18-5), and in phlyctenular ulcers (Figure 18-6) the vessels may come from any direction.

Anterior Chamber

The anterior chamber (AC) is normally filled with clear fluid (aqueous) and is therefore transparent. However, if blood fills the chamber after trauma (hyphema) or pus is present as in severe corneal ulcer or iritis (hypopyon), a fluid level can be seen while the patient is sitting (Figure 18-7). The depth of the AC varies from person to person and may be evaluated by directing the beam of a flashlight at an oblique angle. If the chamber is shallow because of a forward bulging of the iris, as with acute glaucoma, a shadow will appear on the opposite side of the iris (Figure 18-8).

Pupil

Examination of the pupil is of great diagnostic significance. Look at the size (comparing the

Figure 18-5. (*A*) Trachoma follicles; (*B*) trachoma pannus.

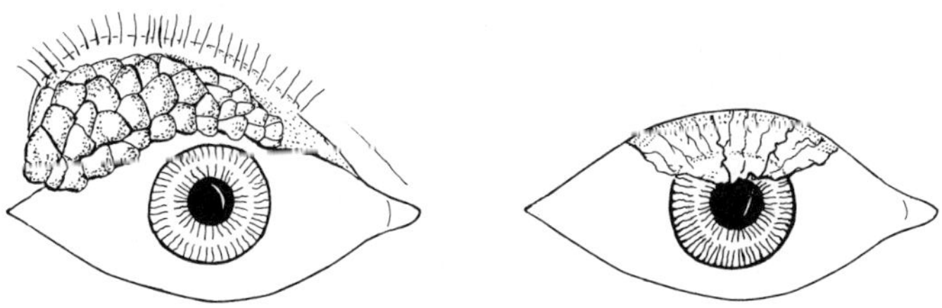

Figure 18-6. Phlyctenular disease: (*A*) corneal and (*B*) limbic.

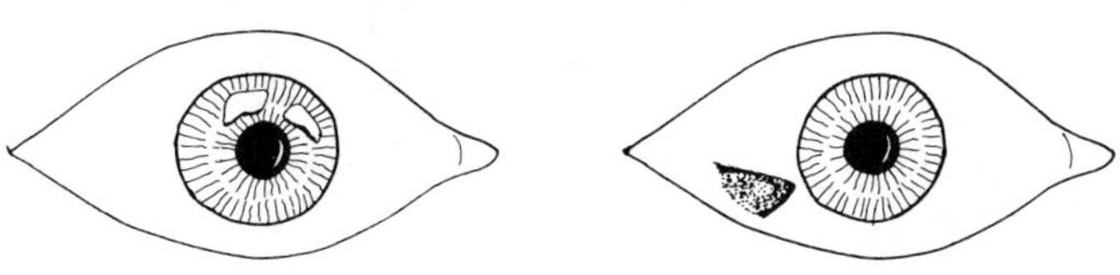

two sides), shape, and reaction to bright light (tested in a darkened room). The normal pupils are round, equal in size, and react (constrict) promptly to light. A large nonreactive pupil on one side may be a sign of a brain hemorrhage after head injury or, if the eye is inflamed and painful, of acute glaucoma. A small nonreactive pupil may be seen in late syphilis, or the patient may be on morphine. If the pupil is irregular in shape (Figure 18-9), it is usually attached to the lens due to inflammation of the iris (iritis). Normally, the color of the pupil is black. If it appears partially or totally gray, suspect a cataract (a clouding of the lens, which is located just behind the pupil).

Measuring Intraocular Pressure

An important examination in glaucoma (see below) is measurement of intraocular pressure (IOP—the pressure inside the eyeball). When IOP is high, it is usually possible to estimate the pressure by palpating the eyeball with two fingers. This is done by asking the patient to look down while placing your two index fingers on the upper lid, exerting pressure with one finger while feeling the increasing hardness of the eyeball with the other finger. If the pressure is very high, the eye may feel stony hard. Compare the two sides.

The Schiotz tonometer is a relatively simple instrument that is indispensable in obtaining accurate measurements of IOP in the lower ranges. The method of Schiotz tonometry is easy to learn (Figure 18-10). One or two drops of a topical anesthetic (e.g., 0.5% tetracaine) is instilled while the patient is lying on his back. He is asked to hold both eyes open and steady while looking straight at a fixed point on the ceiling or at the finger or thumbnail of his outstretched hand. Hold the lids open without pressing on the eyeball while placing the footplate of the tonometer gently on the cornea. There should be no pressure of the vertically held instrument except for its own weight. A normal pressure is a scale reading above 3. The instrument is calibrated in such a way that the higher the reading, the lower the pressure in millimeters of mercury interpolated on a chart. It is very important to clean and dry the instrument (remove the plunger) after each use to prevent the smooth plunger surface from

Figure 18-7. Hyphema.

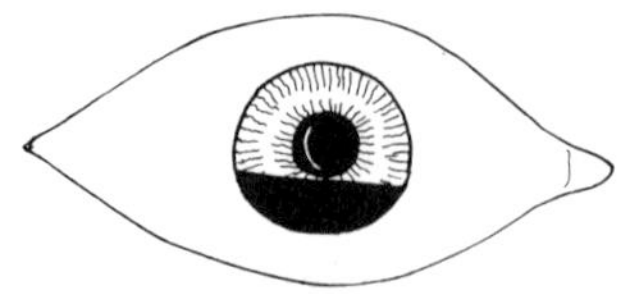

Figure 18-8. Detection of a shallow anterior chamber.

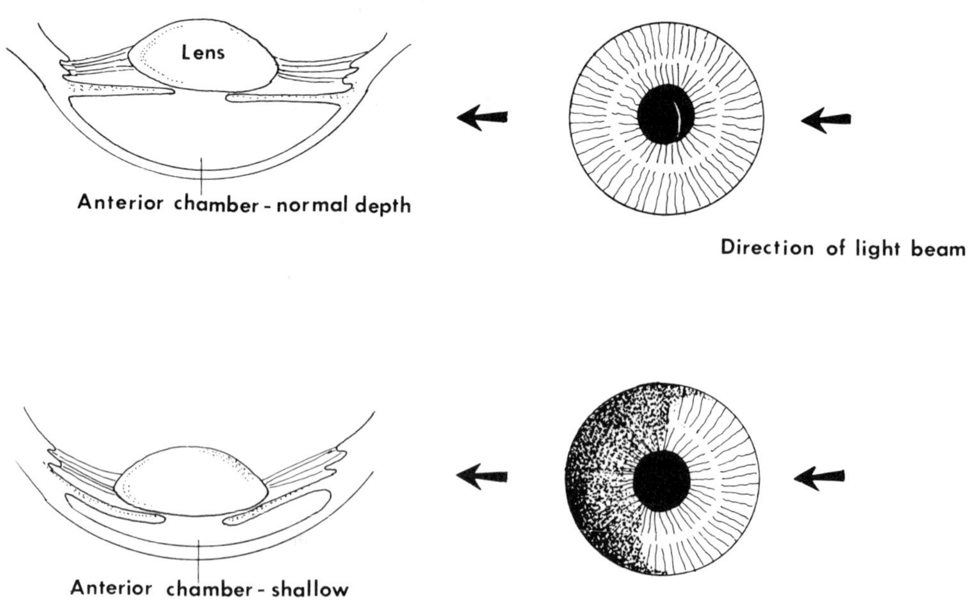

Figure 18-9. Irregular pupil (iritis).

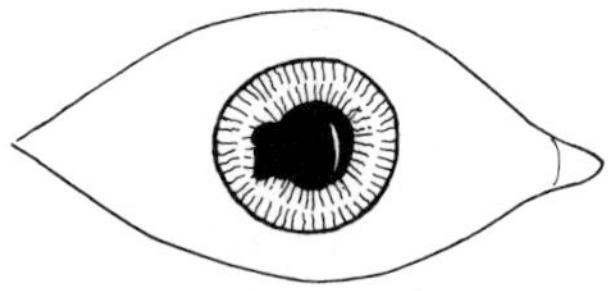

corroding. If this happens, the readings become unreliable and the instrument is useless. Cleaning is also important to prevent spread of infectious diseases.

Examination of the Visual Field by Confrontation

Examination of the visual field by confrontation is done to test the patient's side vision and can be useful for diagnosing retinal detachment, brain tumors, and advancing glaucoma. The method is as follows: have the patient sit at about an arm's length away, covering his left eye. Ask him to fixate steadily on your left eye with his right eye. Bring your left hand in from the far left side while slightly wiggling two fingers. Ask the patient when he first notices these fingers moving. Repeat the same procedure, bringing your hand from above and below, and finally from the right side using your right hand as the target. You may also test the oblique meridians. Always watch the patient's eye to make sure it is not moving to find your moving fingers. If the patient's field is normal, he should notice the moving fingers at about the same moment that the examiner notices them. Repeat the procedure in the same manner with the patient's right eye covered and his left eye fixing on your right eye.

Figure 18-10. Schiotz tonometry.

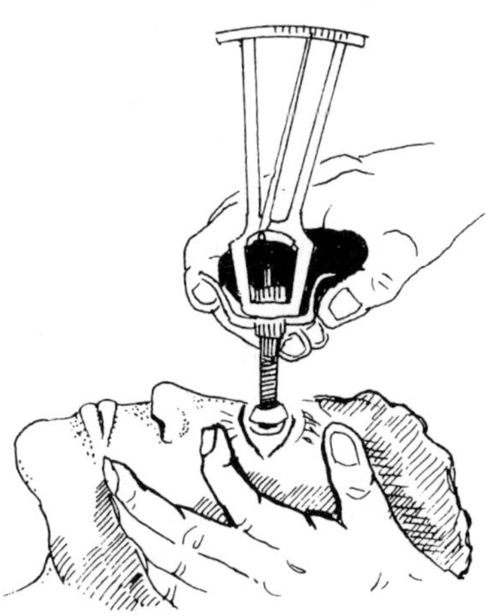

SYMPTOMS, SIGNS, AND MANAGEMENT OF VARIOUS EYE CONDITIONS

Conditions of the Eyelids

Hordeolum (sty) is an acute inflammation of the meibomian lid glands. There is localized redness, pain and tenderness, and swelling of the lid. It usually clears in a week to ten days but may develop into a lid abscess—a larger lesion. Treatment with antibiotic ointments and hot compresses several times a day is helpful. If lid abscesses progress, antibiotics have to be given systemically (by mouth or injection).

Acute tear sac infection may give rise to similar symptoms, but the center of the inflammation is localized nasally in the area of the tear sac. Pain can be intense and there may be fever. The patient usually gives a history of tearing for a long time in that eye, which may be a sign of a chronic tear sac infection. At that stage, because of obstruction of the nasolacrimal duct (see Figure 18-1), mucopurulent fluid can often be expressed from the tear sac by gently pushing upward with a finger in the inner corner of the eye. Acute tear sac infection must be treated with systemic antibiotics. Hot compresses relieve the pain somewhat. If treatment is started in time, a perforation (pus breaking through the skin) can usually be avoided. Chronic tear sac infection may respond to antibiotic ointments or drops, but usually a surgical repair (making a new opening from the tear sac to the nose) is necessary.

Chalazion is a painless, slowly developing lump deep in the lid. It may be a residue of a sty or become secondarily infected and then present as a sty. Treatment with hot compresses may help, but usually excision is necessary. A variety of tumors can occur in the lids. Most papillomas look like warts, change very little, and are harmless. Malignant tumors show definite enlargement and should be treated as soon as possible.

Conditions of the Conjunctiva

Conjunctivitis

Conjunctivitis is usually caused by bacteria or viruses. It is often very contagious, particularly the common types caused by bacteria (*Staphylococcus* sp.). Transmission is through direct or indirect contact (e.g., dirty hands, rags, flies). It is common where poor hygienic conditions exist (such as those often found in refugee camps or settlements). In acute bacterial conjunctivitis, the peripheral bulbar conjunctiva and the lid conjunctiva are markedly inflamed, and there is a burning sensation, discomfort, and purulent discharge. There is minimal pain, and vision is not impaired, except momentarily by a film or discharge. Usually treatment with antibiotic ointments will clear up the disease quickly. Cold compresses often relieve the symptoms and stop the growth of bacteria. With severe infection that is not treated, a dangerous ulcer of the cornea may develop. In cases of profuse discharge, gonorrhea must be suspected. Rapidly spreading corneal ulcers are common with gonococcal infections and can lead to blindness. Newborn babies can become infected during birth. One percent silver nitrate drops or antibiotic ointment should be instilled into the eyes of all babies right after birth to prevent this blinding disease.

Trachoma

Trachoma is a chronic infection of the conjunctiva caused by chlamydia, a small, intracellular bacteria. Initially, because a staphylococcal or pneumococcal conjunctivitis is often superimposed, the picture may be that of an acute infection. When treated with antibiotics, staphylococcal conjunctivitis subsides quickly without leaving any permanent damage to the eye; however, trachoma infection scars the conjunctiva and cornea, leading to visual impairment. Infection usually occurs in early childhood from close family contacts, and is often passed on in the acute phase to other family members (most often the mother). It is difficult to break this vicious circle unless the poor hygienic conditions can be improved.

In the early stages of trachoma, the conjunctiva of the lids (mostly upper eyelids) have a red velvety appearance, interspersed with tiny, bubblelike structures called follicles (see Figure 18-5). Much later, scars form that will curl the lid margins inward as they start to shrink (entropion), until finally the eyelashes rub against the cornea (trichiasis). The trachomatous process invades the superficial cornea with new blood vessles (pannus) like a thick curtain (see Figure 18-5). Ulcers in the pannus may develop, and eventually the patient loses vision from clouding of the cornea. Prolonged treatment with tetracycline antibiotic eye ointment (three times daily for six weeks) is effective. In the early stages of the disease, daily washing of the eyes with clean water may affect a cure. In severe cases, tetracycline may be supplemented with PO sulfa or other antibiotics. Surgical correction of the entropion and trichiasis is often necessary. In a refugee camp setting, a screening of all patients (especially children) and treatment of those with trachoma is mandatory. If an entire community is being treated, then tetracycline ointment can be applied twice daily for one week each month for six months, or once a day for two weeks each month for six months. Teaching about hygiene and the contagious nature of the disease is important. The availability of water for washing may be a problem.

Xerophthalmia

Any person (particularly a child) whose diet lacks vitamin A, or who cannot absorb vitamin A because of chronic or acute intestinal disease, may develop night blindness. Conversely, any person (particularly a child) who complains of night blindness should be suspected of having vitamin A deficiency. Any condition that interferes with the delivery of retinol to the distal retina cells can create clinical disease. Dryness of the skin and conjunctiva (xerosis), and/or white foamy spots (Bitot's spots) in the exposed area of the bulbar conjunctiva may be secondary to vitamin A deficiency (Figure 18-11). Often the whole conjunctiva appears dry, wrinkled, and almost leathery. The greatest danger is the sudden development of a rapidly extending corneal ulcer from a breakdown of the tissue (keratomalacia). This may occur during an acute attack of diarrhea.

Prompt treatment with vitamin A may arrest the process of corneal melting, which can

Table 18-1. Classification of Active Xerophthalmia

xN	Night blindness
x1A	Conjunctiva xerosis
x1B	Conjunctiva xerosis with Bitot's spots
x2	Corneal xerosis
x3A	Corneal ulceration, i.e., keratomalacia involving less than one third of the corneal surface
x3B	Corneal ulceration, i.e., keratomalacia involving more than one third of the corneal surface

Figure 18-11. Xerophthalmia.

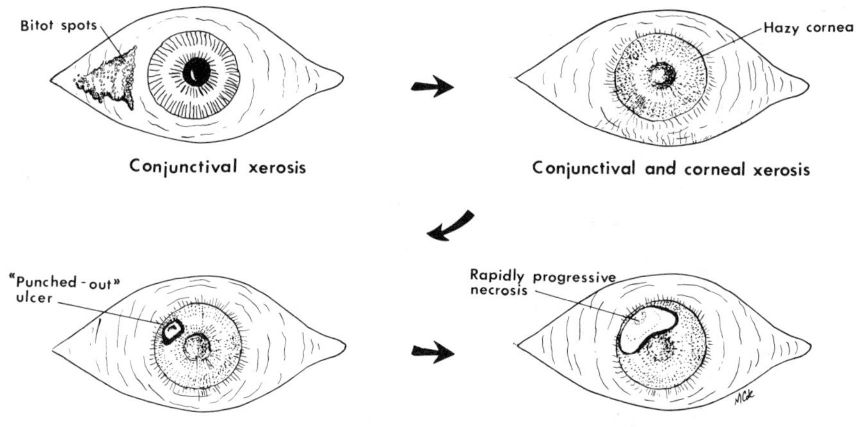

occur within hours. In addition to treating all patients with signs of xerophthalmia (including night blindness), the WHO (1981) recommends that all severely malnourished children and all children with measles should be treated for vitamin A deficiency whether or not symptoms are apparent. The recommended dose is 200,000 IU orally (well absorbed) on days 1, 2, and 8. Alternatively, 100,000 IU can be given intramuscularly for the first dose. For prophylaxis of older children and adults 200,000 IU is given every four to six months. Each of the above doses should be halved for children under one year of age. The WHO also recommends that all women receive 200,000 IU of Vitamin A orally within one month of delivery.

The corneal ulcers of xerophthalmia should be treated prophylactically with broad-spectrum antibiotic ointment. One risk of these ulcers is corneal rupture, so care should be taken not to put pressure on the globe.

Allergic Conjunctivitis

In patients who are hypersensitive (allergic) to certain substances such as insect bites, animal hair, pollen, shampoos, and detergents, the conjunctiva may become edematous and pruritic. Tearing is seen. The conjunctiva may be somewhat red and may also balloon up as a pale blister. Treatment consists of cold compresses and cortisone drops, if available. However, cortisone should not be used if there is any suspicion of herpes virus infection (see below, under viral infections). Patients should avoid future contact with the allergen if it can be identified.

Pterygium

Pterygium is a winglike vascularized extension of the conjunctiva into the cornea in the lid fissure area. It is much more common on the inner (nasal) side of the cornea and invades it very slowly (see Figure 18-12). Eventually, after many years, it may reach the pupillary area and interfere with vision. It should therefore be surgically removed before it grows that large. The lesion is believed to be due to prolonged exposure to excessive sun (ultraviolet light), wind, and dust.

Corneal Diseases

Corneal Ulcer

The most common lesion of the cornea is a corneal ulcer (Figure 18-13), a circumscribed, gray, depressed area that is always dangerous if it is located anywhere near the pupil, because it heals with a scar that interferes with vision.

Figure 18-12. Pterygium.

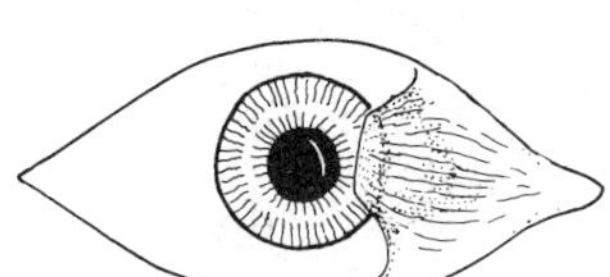

Figure 18-13. Corneal ulcer.

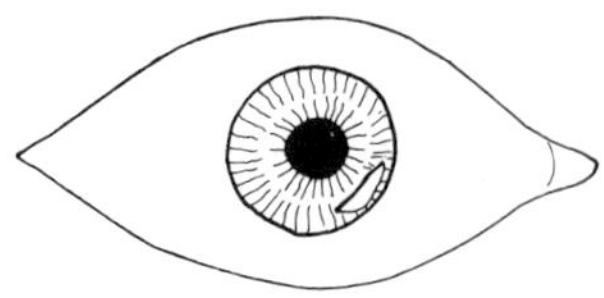

Ulcers are inflammatory lesions of the cornea with marked redness around their borders (pericorneal injection). These are accompanied by pain, tearing, and photophobia. Vision is also impaired. If none of these signs of inflammation is present, a gray spot in the cornea is a scar (or healed ulcer). Most of these ulcers are caused by common bacteria and will respond well to most antibiotics. *Pseudomonas,* a bacterium that can destroy the cornea in two to three days, should be suspected if the ulcer appears somewhat greenish. It can spread in a few hours, sometimes from a very small scratch. Gentamicin and tobramycin are the only drugs to which it may respond. Severe ulcers may show a hypopyon, more common with pneumococcal infectious ulcers (usually with chronic tear sac infection) and *Pseudomonas.* The patient complains of pain, tearing, and photophobia. A corneal scar, the end product of a healed ulcer, also appears as a gray area, but the surface of the gray area is smooth and shining. There is no redness around the cornea, and the patient is asymptomatic except for impaired vision. Some viral infections can also cause corneal ulcers (see below).

Phlyctenular Keratoconjunctivitis

Phlyctenular keratoconjunctivitis is believed to be an allergic reaction of the cornea and conjunctiva to the toxin of tubercle bacilli. It is therefore often seen in populations in which tuberculosis is common. Its active phase is usually in childhood. These patients are extremely sensitive to light and there is much tearing. The typical lesion is either a white spot at the limbus, with adjacent sector-shaped redness of the conjunctiva, or small corneal ulcers that stain with fluorescein and have small vessels extending from the limbus toward them with pericorneal redness (see Figure 18-6). Eczema of the skin around the eyes and elsewhere on the face is also often present. As the ulcers recur, vision may eventually be impaired. Antibiotics with steroids are effective treatment, after ascertaining that herpetic infection of the cornea is not present. The patient's nutritional state should be improved. Hot compresses relieve the irritation, and dark glasses are helpful against the photophobia.

Viral Infections

Epidemic keratoconjunctivitis (EKC) is a contagious, chronic viral disease afflicting the cornea with multiple, tiny gray spots just beneath the surface. The corneal lesions are more clearly seen with fluorescein staining. Discomfort and pericorneal redness sometimes lasts for many months. There is no specific treatment for EKC and it does not respond to antibiotics. Sunglasses help to relieve the photophobia.

Another important viral infection is dendritic ulcer of the cornea or herpetic keratitis caused by the herpes simplex virus. Symptoms are photophobia, moderate pain, and irritation. On fluorescein staining, the diagnosis can be made with a slit lamp or powerful magnifying loupe if the typical branchlike (dendritic) corneal ulcer is seen (Figure 18-14). Pericorneal redness is present. Steroid drops are absolutely contraindicated in this disease. Antibiotics are ineffective, but topical acyclovir may be of value (Maudgel et al 1985; Nicholson 1984).

Figure 18-14. Herpetic keratitis.

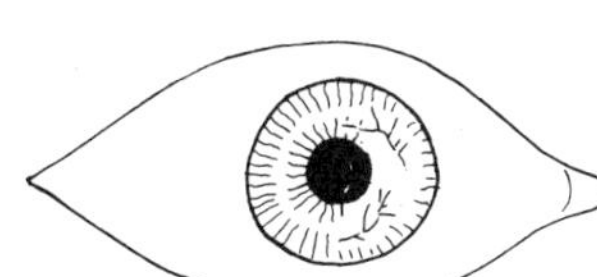

Iritis

The cause of iritis (inflammation of the iris) is often obscure. It may be associated with rheumatic disease in children, tuberculosis, syphilis, leprosy, trauma, or corneal infections. There is much pain deep in the eye, tearing, or photophobia. The eye has pericorneal redness, and vision is somewhat blurred. Pupil size is decreased, compared with that of the normal eye, and reacts more sluggishly to light. If adhesions of the pupillary border to the lens have formed, the pupil has an irregular shape, making the diagnosis easy (see Figure 18-9). The eyeball is tender to the touch and the intraocular pressure may be slightly lower than normal. Treatment for acute iritis is with atropine drops (one drop, two to four times a day, until tenderness is gone); first make sure that acute glaucoma is not present because this is made worse by atropine. Frequent application of steroid drops (one drop every one to two hours) and hot compresses is also helpful.

Glaucoma

Acute Glaucoma

Acute glaucoma is a relatively rare condition but requires immediate treatment. If possible, an ophthalmologist should be consulted. Correct diagnosis is essential for proper handling. It must not be confused with acute iritis. In both diseases there is often severe pain and redness. The distinguishing features are the size and reaction of the pupil (large and nonreactive in glaucoma, small with sluggish reaction in iritis) (Figure 18-15), and most important, the intraocular pressure (very high to palpation in glaucoma soft in iritis). Close observation may reveal the anterior chamber to be shallow in glaucoma (see Figure 18-8). If the pressure cannot be brought down, an attack of acute glaucoma may lead to blindness in two or three days.

Treatment consists of glycerol (1 cc/kg PO) mixed 1:1 with water, which osmotically decreases the intraocular pressure. Lemon juice is added to the solution to make it more palatable. Pilocarpine (4%) is placed on the affected eye every 15 minutes for several hours to constrict the pupil. Acetozolamide (Diamox) (500 mg PO or IM) can be added to the regimen. If the pressure cannot be brought down quickly, surgery (iridectomy) has to be done by an ophthalmologist (who, as noted earlier, should handle such cases in any event).

Figure 18-15. The "steamy" cornea of glaucoma.

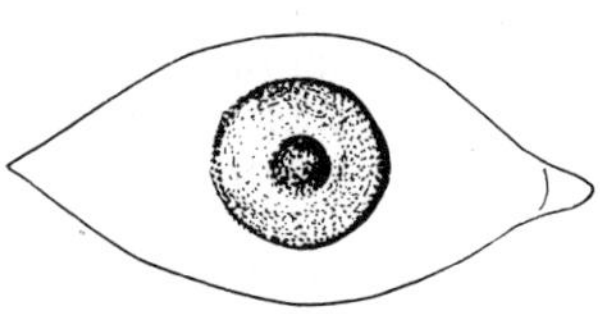

Chronic (Open-Angle) Glaucoma

Chronic (open-angle) glaucoma is much more common than acute glaucoma. Here, the intraocular pressure is moderately elevated, slowly and insidiously leading to blindness. The peripheral vision is lost, first, leading to tunnel vision, while central reading vision remains good for a relatively long time. Despite obvious symptoms, the patient may seek treatment only after one eye is blind and the other has far-advanced disease. The diagnosis can be made in the early stages by Schiotz tonometry. These patients should also be under the care of an ophthalmologist if possible.

Ophthalmologists can often see the effect of increased intraocular pressure by looking at the optic nerve with the ophthalmoscope. It appears pushed back (cupping). The disease is uncommon before the age of 40. Since it begins painlessly, it is a good idea to do tonometry when in doubt about the diagnosis.

Treatment consist of 4 percent pilocarpine (one drop in the affected eye every 6 hours) with or without 0.5 percent timolol eye drops (Timoptic) (one drop every 12 hours). Acetazolamide (Diamox) is sometimes added (250 mg PO every 6 hours). Operative relief of the intraocular pressure (trabeculectomy) is sometimes required.

There is also a congenital form of glaucoma, a serious disease in which the whole eye becomes enlarged. Sight is usually lost because treatment (surgery) is often unsuccessful.

Cataract

Cataract is a clouding of the lens and appears as a whitish or gray discoloration of the pupil. It is common in older people and may impair vision severely. If the pupil reacts promptly to light, and if the patient can perceive color (red, green, and blue) and can indicate, in a darkened room, from which side the flashlight beam enter his or her eye (has "good light projection"), surgical removal of the cloudy lens has an excellent chance of restoring good vision. After the operation, however, glasses or contact lenses have to be worn to replace the focusing power of the removed lens. Cataracts may also occur in children, usually beginning at birth. These should be treated surgically as early as possible to minimize the danger of amblyopia (lazy eye, see below).

Onchocerciasis (River Blindness)

Onchocerciasis (river blindness) is a chronic disease caused by a parasitic filaria *(Onchocerca volvulus)* that is transmitted by a fly. It is the main cause of blindness in equatorial Africa. The infection occurs in childhood through the transmission of the larva of the filaria during the bite of a river-breeding fly. It matures over the years in nodules under the skin and produces millions of microfilariae that spread all over the body, frequently settling in the eyes. There it produces a chronic optic neuritis, uveitis (iritis), corneal inflammation with scarring, and secondary glaucoma, all of which combine to destroy vision. The excision of the subcutaneous nodules containing the adult worms is sometimes helpful. Eradication of the disease-carrying flies has not been successful. Removal of infected persons from endemic areas (who act as intermediary hosts) has not been practicable so far. A single oral dose of ivermectin (150 to 200 mg/kg) has resulted in a rapid decrease in the density of the skin microfilariae (Coulaud et al 1984).

Tumors

Tumors of the eye are uncommon. Skin cancers can occur on the lids. The most dreaded ocular malignancy is retinoblastoma in children. This arises from the retina, filling the inside of the eye and eventually invading the brain. It may first be noticeable as a white reflex in the pupil. The eye is blind and even its removal will often be too late to save the child's life.

INJURIES TO THE EYE

Minor cuts of the eyelids with good apposition of the wound borders can be allowed to heal with just antibiotic ointment and a sterile dressing. Larger cuts (lacerations), particularly if they go through the lid border, need careful primary suturing by a doctor trained in this work to prevent ugly deformities.

Corneal abrasion (a superficial scratch) is very painful. The patient has much tearing and photophobia, and a drop of tetracaine is usually necessary to allow inspection of the cornea. Staining with fluorescein will show the extent of the erosion. Antibiotic ointment and patching tight enough to keep the lid shut may be helpful because blinking is painful and delays healing. The stratch usually heals in 24 to 48 hours.

Corneal foreign body symptoms may be the same as for an erosion. Tiny foreign bodies can be seen more easily after fluorescein staining. A magnifying loupe and good light are essential for seeing and removing foreign bodies. Pericorneal redness is most marked near the site of the foreign body. A brown rust ring quickly develops around metallic foreign bodies. The cornea must be well anesthetized with several drops of tetracaine before removal of the foreign body is attempted. A sterile cotton swab (moistened with a few drops of an antibiotic solution) is often successful. If not, a sterile needle mounted on a syringe as handle dislodges the foreign body using a loupe and light. Rust rings should be scraped out with a needle to avoid prolonged irritation. An antibiotic ointment and a patch are applied. Thorns stuck in the cornea may break off at or underneath the corneal surface. They often penetrate the cornea, occasionally causing uveitis. Antibiotic ointments and patching should be applied and the patient referred to an ophthalmologist, if possible.

Lacerations of the globe from penetrating injuries should be treated by topical antibiotics, patching, and referral. Systemic antibiotics should be given prophylactically and tetanus immunization status updated as needed (see Chapter 31). These are serious injuries that can easily lead to blindness.

Blunt injuries to the eye may cause bleeding in the skin of the lids (harmless) or in the anterior chamber. The blood cells settle down to the bottom of the chamber, forming a hyphema (see Figure 18-7). The whole anterior chamber is sometimes filled with blood, causing the cornea to appear black ("black ball hemorrhage"). Usually the blood is absorbed readily within a few days, but if it does not, the pressure inside the eye may rise, causing severe pain and secondary glaucoma. Surgical intervention may be necessary. After such an injury the patient should be kept quiet; some doctors still feel such patients should be kept in bed with both eyes patched for four to five days to avoid a spontaneous recurrence of the bleeding that is often more severe than the original bleed. Aspirin must be avoided. There may also be bleeding in the vitreous after blunt eye trauma. With an ophthalmoscope, one cannot see the normal red reflex in the pupil. The blood interferes with vision and takes a long time to be absorbed.

Chemical injuries such as those caused by alkali solutions (lye burns) are the most destructive to the cornea, and usually lead to blindness. Acid solutions are less dangerous. Whatever the agent, the eye should be washed out immediately with a lot of clean water. A few drops of tetracaine will make it easier for the patient to keep the eye open during this prolonged rinsing procedure. Dress the eye with antibiotic ointment.

STRABISMUS AND AMBLYOPIA

Strabismus (a turning in, out, up, or down of one eye in relation to the other) is of minor significance in refugee camps. However, amblyopia in one eye (lazy eye, which may be associated with strabismus) needs mention. A lazy eye appears anatomically normal but has not learned to see clearly during the first six years of life. This is often a result of strabismus or an unequal focusing in the two eyes. Treatment for amblyopia is to force the lazy eye to see by continuous patching of the good eye. This is most successful before one year of life, and has little effect after the age of eight. The earlier it is done, the better.

Early detection is therefore crucial. This is done by testing vision in small children (each eye separately—see the section on vision testing above) with the illiterate E chart. Most children can do this test reliably after the age of three and a half. Make sure the patient is not peeking with the other eye during testing; children with amblyopia are clever at doing this by turning their heads. The test is meaningless if they peek.

REFRACTIVE ERRORS AND PRESBYOPIA

The pinhole test can be used to easily detect refractive errors. Poke a hole with a medium-sized safety pin (less than 1 mm) through a piece of cardboard, or better still, through the bottom of an aluminum can, the top of which has been cut off (a "beer can telescope"). Test the patient's vision by letting him look at the vision chart through the tiny hole held close to his eye. If his sight improves significantly, one can assume that he has a refractive error and not some eye disease that blurs his vision. Errors of refraction blur vision because the optical system of the eye does not focus a seen object sharply on the retina. Usually this is because the axial length (cornea to retina) is either too long (myopia or nearsightedness) or too short (hyperopia or farsightedness) for the focusing system (cornea and lens).

Astigmatism blurs vision because the cornea has a slight distortion and fails to focus in a point on the retina (*stigma* means "point"). The far vision of nearsighted people is blurred and usually gets progressively worse during the teen years. Farsighted people can see both far and near objects well while they are young, but need glasses for reading well before the age of 45 when normal eyes require them. Eventually, farsighted individuals also need glasses for far vision.

Presbyopia (aging sight) is the normal decrease in ability to focus on near objects (e.g., reading) that ordinarily starts at about the age of 45 (earlier in tropical climates). Older farsighted patients may need corrective lenses to help their far vision.

To examine and fit refugee patients for correction of their exact refractive error would not be feasible because of the lack of trained personnel, but it may be helpful to dispense simple standard "dime store" reading glasses. These can be obtained cheaply and may be a source of tremendous comfort to those who like to read or work with their hands. The following standard dioptric lenses should be stocked: +1.0, +1.5, +2.0, +2.5, +3.0, +3.5, and +4.0. It is also helpful to keep some +10.0 and +12.0 dioptric lenses on hand for cataract patients if surgery is performed.

REFERENCES AND SELECTED READING

Coulaud JP, Lariviere M, Azia MA et al (letter): Ivermectin in onchocerciasis. Lancet 1984;2:526–7.

Dawson CR: Pathogenesis and control of blinding trachoma. In Duane TD, Jaeger EA: Clinical ophthomology, Vol 5, Chapter 60, pp 1–11. Philadelphia, Harper & Row, 1984.

Duane TD, Jaeger EA: Clinical Ophthomology. Philadelphia, Harper & Row, 1984.

Dawson CR, Schachter J: Strategies for treatment and control of blinding trachoma: Cost-effectiveness of topical or systemic antibiotics. Rev Infect Dis 1985;7:768–73.

Greene BM: Selective primary health care: strategies for control of disease in the developing world. VI. Onchocerciasis. Rev Infect Dis 1983;5:781–89.

Lumicao GG, Heggie AD: Chlamydial infections. Pediatr Clin North Am 1979;26:269–82.
Maudgal PC, Vrijghem JC, Molemans M et al: Effect of topical acyclovir therapy on experimental herpes simplex keratouveitis. Arch Ophthalmol 1985;103:1389–92.
Newell: FW: Ophthomology: Principles and Concepts. New York, CV Mosby, 1982.
Nicholson KG: Antiviral therapy. Respiratory infections, genital herpes, and herpetic keratitis. Lancet 1984;2:617–21.
Sanford-Smith J: Ophthalmology in developing countries. Br Med J (Clin Res) 1984;289:811–13.
Schachter J: Chlamydial infections. N Engl J Med 1978;298:428–35,540–49.
Schwab L, Taylor HR: Cataract and delivery of surgical services in developing nations. In Duane TD, Jaeger EA: Clinical Ophthomology, Chapter 57, pp 1–9. Philadelphia, Harper & Row, 1984.
Sommer A: Field Guide to the Detection and Control of Xerophthalmia. Geneva, World Health Organization, 1982.
Sommer A: Introduction to geographic and preventive ophthomology. In Duane TD, Jaeger EA: Clinical Ophthomology, Vol 5, Chapter 50, pp 1–2. Philadelphia, Harper & Row, 1984.
Taylor HR: Onchoceriasis. In Duane TD, Jaeger EA: Clinical Ophthomology, Vol 5, Chapter 62, pp 1–12. Philadelphia, Harper & Row, 1984.
Taylor J: Appropriate methods and resources for third world ophthomology. In Duane TD, Jaeger EA: Clinical Ophthomology, Chapter 58, pp 1–7. Vol 5. Philadelphia, Harper & Row, 1984.
Tielsch JM, Sommer A: The epidemiology of vitamin A deficiency and xerophthalmia. Annu Rev Nutr 1984;4:183–205.
Vaughan D, Asbury T: General Ophthalmology. Los Altos, CA, Lange, 1980.
WHO: Xerophthalmia Treatment and Prevention Schedule. New York, Hellen Keller Institute, 1981.

19
Dental Care

KYLE L. COBLE

This chapter provides a brief introduction to simple dental problems. With the help of this chapter, a health worker who is already familiar with basic aspects of medicine and surgery should be able to perform rudimentary dental procedures such as cleaning, temporary fillings, and extractions with adequate anesthesia.

Oral disease, besides being painful, may contribute to malnutrition, general malaise, and infection. Although there may be pressure to create sophisticated dental clinics replete with compressors and high-speed drills, there are more appropriate uses for scarce dental resources, such as provision of preventive educational services and the training of auxiliary dental health workers (see Chapters 4 and 9). Treatment of dental pain is an important health service, but the teaching of such simple dental self-care techniques as toothbrushing and the training of dental health workers are more important for overall benefit to community dental health. Once trained, an organized staff of dental assistants can function with minimal supervision and make dental services more available to the community while helping to ensure continuity.

TOOTH DEVELOPMENT AND ANATOMY

A child usually has a full set of 20 primary or baby teeth by 2 years of age. By the age of 21, all 32 of the permanent or adult teeth have usually erupted. The primary teeth are labeled from A to T, and the permanent teeth from 1 to 32 (Figure 19-1).

Figure 19-2 displays the basic tooth anatomy. Maxillary and palatine nerves innervate the maxillary teeth, while mandibular, buccal, and lingual nerves innervate the mandibular teeth. It is important to know the number of roots a tooth has when performing extractions (see the section on extractions). For maxillary teeth, the first, second, and third molars usually have three roots, the first premolars have two, and the second premolars, canines, and incisors usually have one. For mandibular teeth, the first, second, and third molars have two roots, and the remaining teeth have one.

DENTAL PATHOPHYSIOLOGY

Plaque is a densely packed layer of bacteria attached to the tooth surface. Calculus (tartar) is calcified bacterial matter, usually covered by a softer layer of plaque.

Gingivitis, a general term referring to inflammation of the gums (gingiva), can usually be prevented by proper toothbrushing. Although it is most often due to plaque and infection, malnutrition may also cause red, swollen, and painful gums. When gingivitis extends to involve the nearby bone and supporting tissues, it is called periodontitis.

Tooth decay (cavities) results from bacterial manufacture of acids, which cause erosion of the tooth enamel. A tooth abscess is a painful infection of the tooth pulp. Abscesses that begin in the space between the teeth and gums (gingival sulci) are called periodontal abscesses. Food, especially sugar, provides nutrients for bacterial growth. Brushing, flossing, and scaling help remove both bacteria and food debris.

Prevention of Tooth Decay

Preventing tooth decay is better than curing it. Brushing regularly is the key. If toothbrushes are not available, a stick can be chewed at one end to make a brush. Salt or baking soda can be used instead of toothpaste. Brushing should be done after each meal, especially in the evening so that food is not resting in tooth crevices overnight. A circular, scrubbing motion should be used for brushing. Each tooth surface needs to be brushed, including both sides and the crown, followed by thorough rinsing of the mouth.

Figure 19-1. Tooth development chart: (*A*) primary teeth; (*B*) permanent teeth.

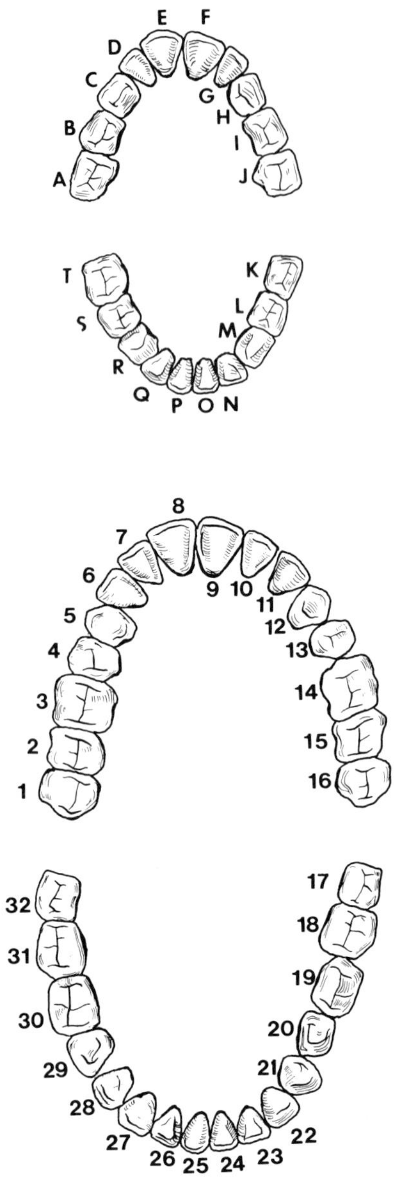

Diet is also important for prevention of tooth decay. Vegetables, fruits, and other firm, fibrous foods help to "scrub" the teeth, and should be eaten at the end of each meal when possible. Concentrated sweets should be avoided and, if eaten, should be done so with meals, again being careful to brush the teeth after eating. Fluoride, although helpful in preventing tooth decay, is usually impractical to supply to refugee populations.

DENTAL EXAMINATION AND DIAGNOSIS

The case history is obtained first; this should include the present illness and relevant past history. It is important to keep in mind systemic conditions that could cause postoperative complications, such as bleeding disorders, heart disease, diabetes, or malnutrition. Patients with cardiac disease may have tachycardia, dizziness, or chest pain if anesthetic with epinephrine is used, whereas diabetic and malnourished patients are more prone to infection and slow wound healing.

For an oral examination, a light source (flashlight, sportsman's headlamp, or lamp), a mouth mirror, and an explorer (pointed probe) are needed. Observe the patient's face, noting asymmetry or swelling. Palpate the glands under the mandible and along the neck for swelling and tenderness. Check inside and outside the mouth for abnormalities of the lips, tongue, sublingual area, floor of the mouth, inside of the cheeks, palate, and throat. Is the patient able to open and close his or her mouth normally? Is halitosis (bad breath) present (suggestive of an infection)? Are cavities present? Are there partially erupted, mobile, or broken teeth? Are there teeth with a blackish internal discoloration (suggestive of nonvital, or dead, teeth)?

Ask the patient to open his or her mouth and point to the source of pain. Apply pressure to the affected tooth or gum area. Tap lightly on the suspect tooth with the mirror handle. Check for tenderness, bleeding, pus, or tooth mobility.

Complaint of tooth pain alone is not adequate reason for tooth extraction. Clear signs of caries should be seen on examination. Most often in relief settings, those who seek attention for oral pathology have advanced disease. A grossly decayed tooth with a large cavity poses little diagnostic difficulty, and extraction is the treatment of choice. If there is only a small hole in the tooth without abscess formation, then a temporary filling can be provided if facilities permit.

An abscess is commonly present around a carious tooth and is recognized by swelling, pus, and mobility of the affected tooth. If satisfactory analgesia can be obtained, then the

Figure 19-2. Anatomy of the tooth.

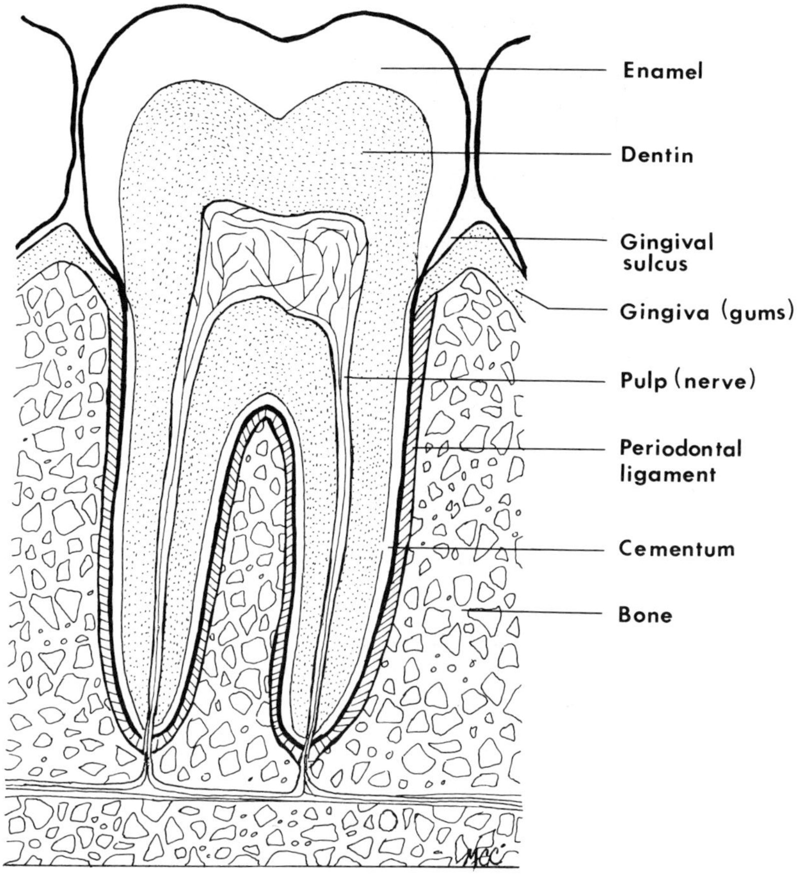

tooth can be extracted right away. If the pus and swelling prevent adequate anesthesia, or if the abscess is associated with facial swelling, antibiotics (usually oral penicillin) can be used for two to five days to quiet the infection, after which the offending tooth is extracted. The importance of returning for extraction should be explained to the patient because symptoms will recur if the extraction is not performed. Incompletely erupted, diseased teeth are difficult to extract and should be referred to experienced personnel.

ESSENTIALS OF TREATMENT

Treatment begins with seating the patient to take maximum advantage of the light source. A low chair is ideal for extraction of lower teeth, and a higher chair for extraction of upper teeth. A head rest should be provided (Figure 19-3), or a wall can be used. Hands are scrubbed and protective gloves used when available. (Health workers with cuts or abrasions on their hands should either wear gloves or not operate, for the protection of the patient and themselves.) Previously sterilized instruments and supplies are neatly organized within easy reach. A waste receptable is necessary for disposables and for expectorate (spit).

Scaling

Tartar or calculus harbors bacteria and promotes gum disease, with loss of periodontal attachment, supporting bone, and eventually the teeth. Although prophylactic tooth cleaning is ideal, resource limitations in refugee camps

Figure 19-3. A head rest that allows adaptation of an upright chair for use as a dental chair.

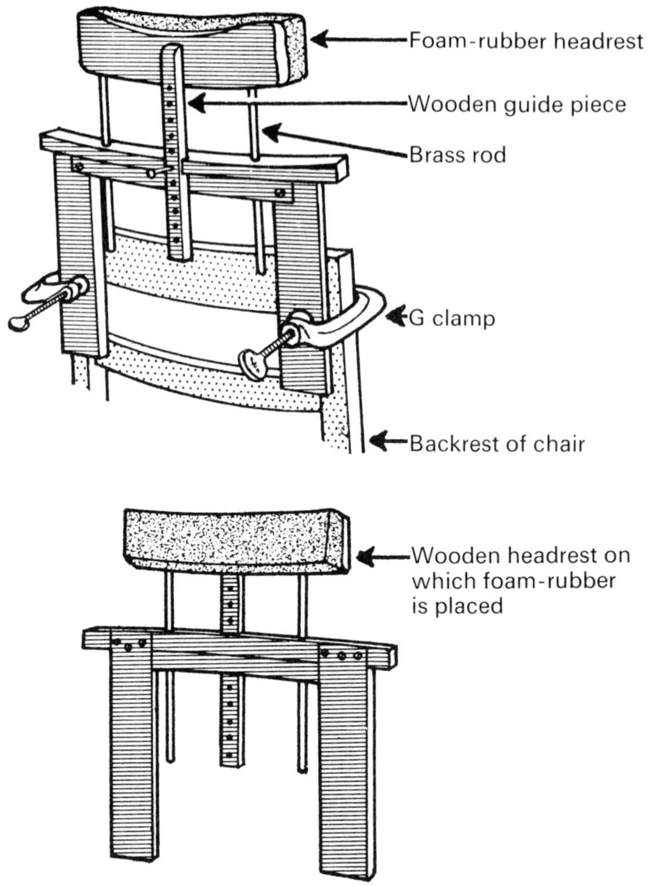

(Reproduced with permission from Halestrap DJ: Simple Dental Care for Rural Hospitals. London, Medical Missionary Association, 1981, p 26.)

often dictate that treatment be confined to removal of calculus causing pain, periodontal abscess, and gingivitis.

The Jacquette U 15-30 is recommended for general scaling procedures. Use the scaler on each surface of the tooth, beginning by using the tip of the scaler below the gingiva under the calculus and pulling against the tooth toward the crown. The scaler point should be sharpened regularly, being sure to maintain the proper cutting angles.

Extractions

Injection of Anesthetic

The most commonly used anesthetic is 2 percent lidocaine with 1:100,000 epinephrine supplied in 1.8-cc carpules mounted into an aspiration-type cartridge syringe. Although it provides shorter anesthesia, lidocaine without epinephrine is sometimes used for patients with cardiac disease. The minimum amount of anesthetic should be used to do the job properly. The maximum dose is six cartridges for adults and two for children, although usually just one carpule or less is needed. Twenty-seven-gauge needles are used. Ideally these should be disposed of after a single use, although in refugee camps they may need to be sterilized for reuse.

Before injection, the cartridge and needle should be cleared of air (try not to terrify the patients by waving the needle in front of them). Injecting anesthetic into areas of inflammation or abscess is relatively ineffective and should be avoided. If fainting occurs after injection, place the patient in a supine or head-down, feet-up position and maintain an airway. Remember to advise patients that they should not chew anything until the numbness wears off, for they might unwittingly bite their anesthetized lip.

Three major methods of local anesthesia are used in dentistry. These are superficial injection to anesthetize superficial nerves, local infiltration near the root of the tooth, and nerve block near the nerve trunk before the nerve branches reach the teeth.

Anesthesia for the Upper and Anterior Lower Teeth

The infiltration method is effective for the upper teeth. Although somewhat less effective, the infiltration method can also be used for the lower front teeth (canines and incisors). This method requires two injections to anesthetize each tooth, one inside (palatal) and one outside (facial) (Figure 19-4*A* and -4*B*). The cheek is retracted, and the needle aligned with the bevel toward the tooth. For the injection on the facial side, the needle is advanced through

Figure 19-4. Anesthesia techniques for upper (*A*) and anterior lower (*B*) teeth.

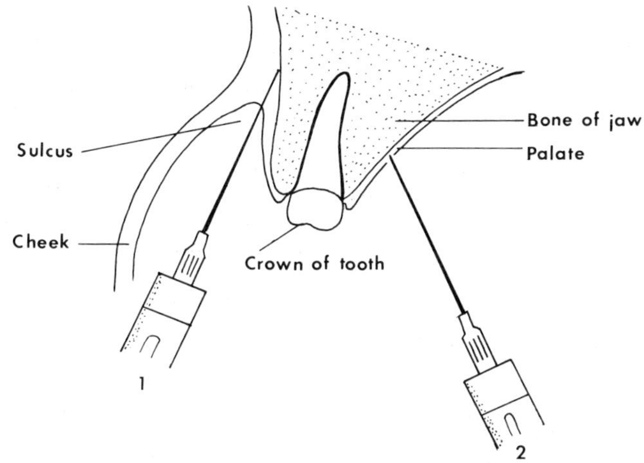

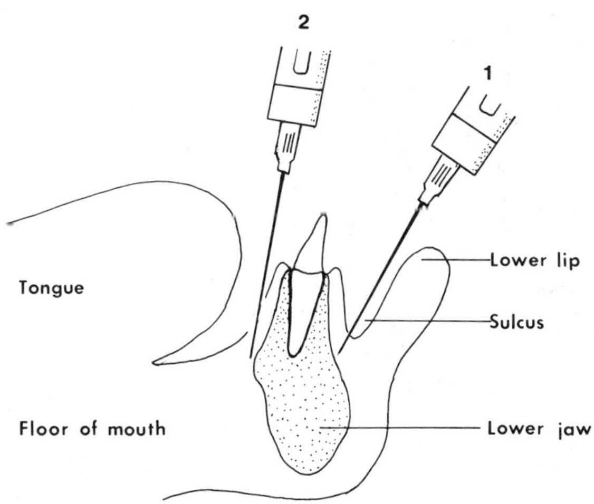

(Adapted with permission from Halestrap DJ: Simple Dental Care for Rural Hospitals. London, Medical Missionary Association, 1981, pp 12 and 14.)

the mucobuccal fold (between the jaw and the cheek). Estimate the needle angle and depth of penetration required to place the point of the needle near the apex (root end) of the tooth (maxillary teeth are about 20 to 25 mm long). The needle should be aligned parallel to the anterior teeth, and angled posteriorly for the premolars and molars. About 1.5 cc of anesthetic is injected on the facial side. Only a shallow injection, with enough anesthetic to blanch the tissue, is given on the palatal side since only a thin layer of mucosa covers the bone in this region. Wait about five minutes for the anesthetic to take effect, testing the area with a sharp probe before proceeding.

Anesthesia for the Lower Molars and Premolars

Three nerve blocks (using a total of two injections) are required to achieve adequate anesthesia for extraction of the lower molars and premolars. The first injection blocks the inferior alveolar nerve, anesthetizing half of the mandible from the molars to the central incisor, along with half of the lower lip. The lingual nerve lies near the inferior alveolar nerve and can be blocked with the same injection, thereby numbing half of the tongue. A second injection blocks the buccal nerve, numbing the buccal gingiva (gums).

To perform these nerve blocks, the patient must open his or her mouth as widely as possible. Visualize the bilateral fibrous bands (pterygomandibular raphe) that connect the upper and lower jaw, located anterior to the mandibular rami, just posterior to the molars (Figure 19-5). Holding the syringe in the dominant hand, use the index finger of the nondominant hand to locate the raphi, and then slide the finger laterally into a deep sulcus (the coronoid notch). Aim the anesthetic needle toward the center of this notch, at the level of the center of the fingernail. The needle should lie just above the mandibular teeth, with the barrel of the syringe lying between the premolars on the opposite side of the mouth. This places the axis of the syringe at about 45 degrees to the midline of the mandible (Figure 19-6). The inferior alveolar nerve is anesthetized by advancing the needle about 1 cm until the mandible is met. The needle is withdrawn slightly, and about 1 cc of anesthetic is injected. Withdrawing the needle about halfway will bring it near the lingual nerve, where about 0.5 cc should be injected.

Figure 19-5. Anesthesia for the lower molars and premolars. The first injection blocks the inferior alveolar nerve.

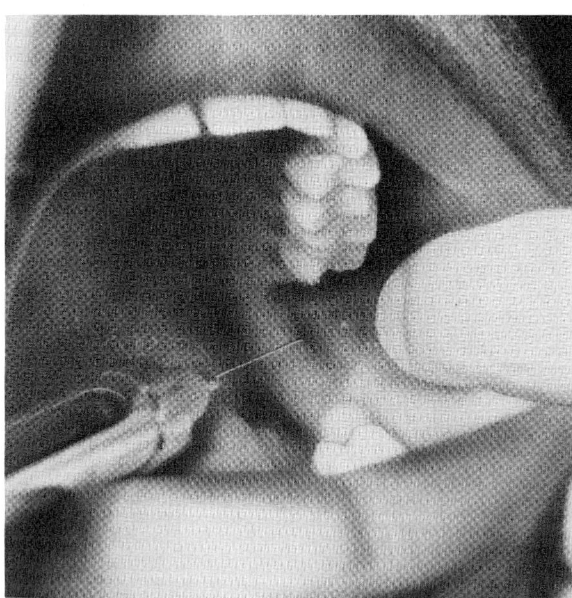

(Reproduced with permission from Halestrap DJ: Simple Dental Care for Rural Hospitals. London, Medical Missionary Association, 1981, p 16.)

Figure 19-6. Anesthesia for the lower molars and premolars. The second injection blocks the buccal nerve.

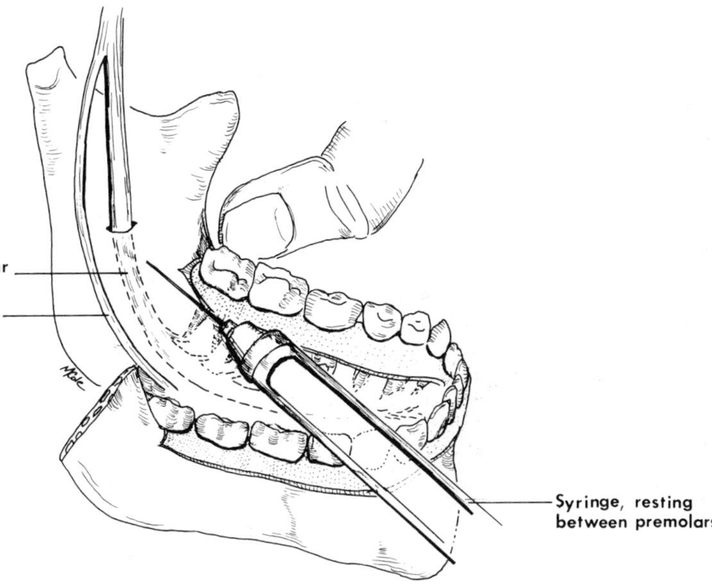

(Adapted with permission from Halestrap DJ: Simple Dental Care for Rural Hospitals. London, Medical Missionary Association, 1981, p 15.)

A final injection is needed to block the buccal nerve. This need be done only on the facial side of the teeth to be extracted, using the infiltration technique described above.

Extraction Techniques

Teeth should be extracted only when necessary. Be certain of the diagnosis and that the correct tooth has been identified. Right-handed health workers should stand in front of the patient for extraction of all but the lower right teeth. Minimum equipment for performing extractions includes a mouth mirror, an explorer or probe, a straight elevator, and an upper (No. 150) and a lower (No. 151) universal forceps (Figure 19-7).

Briefly explain the procedure to the patient. Next, anesthetize the tooth as described above. The first operative step is to loosen the tooth from its supportive tissue using the straight elevator. The tool should be held with the index finger extended along its length, with the finger pad resting near the tip. This is done both for better control and for the patient's safety in case the instrument slips. Guide the tip around the neck of the tooth to a depth of about 0.5 cm below the gum line, separating the gingival attachment from the tooth without tearing the gums. Next, placing the tip of the elevator against the tooth or root to be extracted, use the adjacent tooth as a fulcrum and pry the tooth or root fragment while rotating the elevator handle to provide a lifting motion. Do this on all sides of the tooth or root, if necessary, to loosen it.

One cautionary note about use of the elevator to remove the upper premolar and molar roots—since there is only a thin rim of bone between these roots and the maxillary sinuses, very little upward force should be exerted in these regions.

The tooth should now be ready for extraction using the forceps. The beaks of the forceps should be aligned with the long axis of the tooth, as far toward the root as possible. Full arm motion is used rather than hand-wrist force. The final motion in extraction is a pulling away from the tooth's insertion toward the facial surface. However, while trying to loosen the tooth before extraction, always initially apply firm upward force for the upper teeth, and firm downward force for the lower teeth. It may seem counterintuitive to apply force in

Figure 19-7. Basic equipment for extractions.

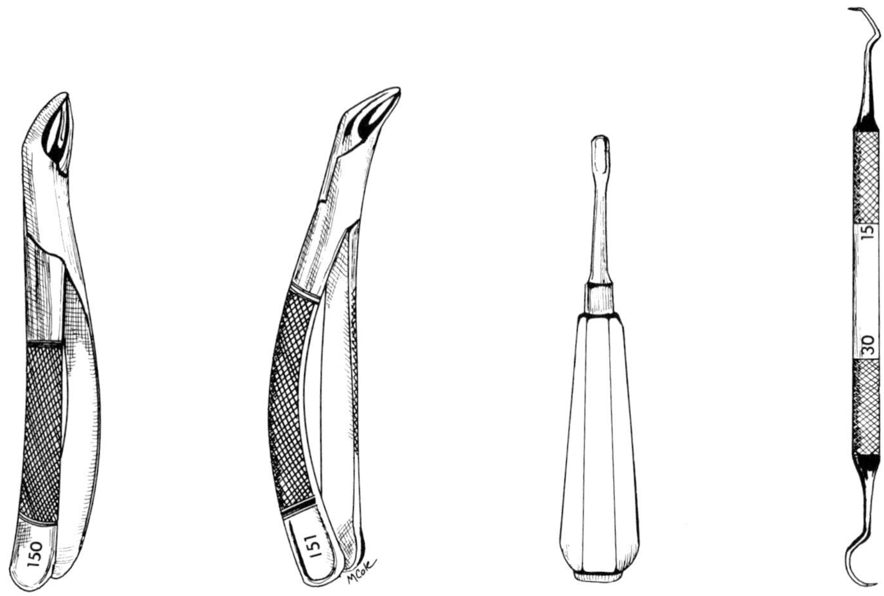

Maxillary Universal Forceps #150 | Mandibular Universal Forceps #151 | Straight Elevator #34 | Jacquette U-15-30 Scaler

the opposite direction of the final extraction, but if force is not exerted in this manner root fracture is likely. Beware, however, of excessive force, which may also fracture roots or alveolar bone.

When loosening lower teeth, remember to support the patient's mandible with the nondominant hand to avoid dislocating the jaw. When loosening upper teeth, place the index finger and thumb of the nondominant hand on either side of the tooth. If two or more teeth are extracted, it is a good idea to place one or more sutures to close the wound (see Chapter 16). Finally, examine each tooth after extraction to check for broken roots. Further specifics of extraction technique vary according to the tooth to be extracted:

- Primary teeth. Since these are similar in shape to their permanent counterparts, the same techniques are used except that greater care is exercised to avoid fracture of the more fragile roots, or damage to the underlying permanent teeth.
- Upper incisors and canines. Because of the conical shape of the root, a rocking movement toward the lip and palate is used, along with upward force. This is followed by back-and-forth rotational movements. Repeat the side-to-side and rotational motions until the tooth is loosened. Extraction is finally achieved by a downward force toward the lip.
- Upper premolars. These teeth have thin roots necessitating a combined upward force with careful side-to-side and rotating movements. When the tooth is loose, it is extracted toward the cheek with a downward and outward force.
- Upper molars. These teeth normally have three roots, two toward the facial and one toward the palatal side. The tooth will loosen with a combined upward pressure and a rocking movement between the cheek and palate. After the tooth is loose, use downward force to remove the tooth toward the cheek.
- Lower incisors and canines. Rotational movement should be avoided with these teeth because they usually have a flattened, ribbon-shaped root. While supporting the mandible, apply side-to-side pressure along with a downward force. The tooth is extracted toward the cheek with an upward force after loosening.
- Lower premolars. Because these teeth have a single conical-shaped root, side-to-side and rotational movements can be used along with a steady downward force. Support the mandi-

ble while pushing downward. After the tooth is loosened, it is extracted toward the cheek with an upward force.

- Lower molars. These teeth usually have two broad roots. Along with a downward force, the initial movement is toward the lingual side, followed by force toward the facial side. Support the mandible while exerting downward force. When the tooth is loose, it is extracted with upward force toward the cheek.

After extraction, the patient should rinse the mouth out once and then bite on gauze for 30 minutes. To avoid dislodgement of the extraction site blood clot, the patient should be told not to rinse the mouth or spit until the next morning. Then they should start rinsing their mouth with salt water (one-quarter teaspoon of salt per cup) after each meal and at bedtime for three to five days. Soft foods may be eaten two hours after extraction but should be chewed on the side opposite the extraction. Routine follow-up is not required, but the patient should be told to return if the swelling, bleeding, or pain is not clearly improved in 24 hours, is getting worse, or fails to resolve after four to five days.

Complications of Tooth Extraction

The five most common extraction complications besides discomfort are broken roots, bleeding, infection, "dry socket," and occasionally jaw dislocation. Broken roots may be a source of infection and, in general, should be removed. The elevator is used, as noted above, to loosen the roots by pushing the tip of the instrument between the roots and the socket wall, after which the fragments are removed with forceps or a hemostat. However, if the fragments cannot be located or dislodged, or if the roots are very small, then the patient should be sent home with analgesia and instructed to use frequent saltwater rinses. After one to five days, healing may occur despite the fragments and, if not, they may be easier to remove.

The use of pressure and sutures to help control bleeding have already been mentioned. Antibiotics (usually oral penicillin) may be needed to treat infection, along with saltwater rinses.

Dry socket is a painful condition that may occur several days after extraction. It is due to failed healing of the extraction site which, instead of containing a resolving blood clot, is dry or packed with food. Treatment consists of sterile saline irrigation and iodoform or other antiseptic packing placed into the extraction site every two to four days as needed, along with frequent saltwater rinsing and analgesics.

Jaw dislocation can be prevented by using the nondominant hand to stabilize the mandible when downward force is exerted during extraction. If the jaw does dislocate, analgesia and muscle relaxants such as meperidine and diazepam are given, followed by steady downward pressure using both thumbs against the patient's lower molars and premolars. After the mastication muscles have stretched enough to allow the mandibular condyle to reach the level of the joint socket, then the mandible can be eased into place posteiorly while maintaining the downward force.

Temporary Fillings

Temporary fillings are placed in teeth with small cavities as a short-term alternative to extraction. Their use is contraindicated in painful teeth. Temporary fillings may be appropriate in camps with adequate dental resources for refugees who will be transferred in weeks to months to a location where permanent fillings are available.

The procedure is straightforward. Debris is removed from the cavity with a spoon excavator. The tooth is then thoroughly dried and isolated with cotton gauze. The cement (usually eugenol or oil of cloves with powdered zinc oxide) is mixed into a stiff, puttylike paste and pressed into the dry cavity using any small-bladed tool. The patient bites down and excess cement is removed. A good filling can last for weeks to months.

STERILIZATION

Recent studies demonstrating the risks of blood-borne diseases such as hepatitis and AIDS, emphasize the importance of using sterile instruments and supplies. When possible, disposable items such as gloves, needles, and gauze should be used. If there is a surgical team in camp, they can be consulted about sterilization techniques and materials.

The autoclave is the best alternative for instrument sterilization. If an autoclave is not available, instruments exposed to blood can be placed in boiling water for 30 minutes with 20 ml of light machine or olive oil added for each liter to prevent rusting. If a pressure cooker is used, boiling time can be reduced to 15 minutes. Alternatively, instruments can be heated (red-hot) with an alcohol burner flame, but this method is less effective than boiling and can ruin the instruments. Liquid sterilizing solutions with antirust tablets are another option, although six or more hours of soaking is required.

Instruments not exposed to blood can be cleaned by soaking for 30 minutes in a bleach solution. To mix, add nine parts water with one part sodium hypochlorite, being sure to change the solution daily. Thorough rinsing of metal instruments after soaking is important to avoid corrosion.

REFERENCES AND SUGGESTED READING

Clark J: Clinical Dentistry, New York, Harper & Row, 1976.
Dickson M: Where There Is No Dentist, Palo Alto, CA. Hesperian Foundation, 1983.
Halestrap DJ: Simple Dental Care for Rural Hospitals. London, Medical Missionary Association, 1981.
Kruger G: Textbook of Oral Surgery, St. Louis, CV Mosby, 1974.

20
Psychiatric Care of Refugees

JOSEPH WESTERMEYER

EXTENT AND SEVERITY OF THE PROBLEM

Numerous studies of refugees over the last few decades have demonstrated high rates of psychiatric disorder. These rates have been higher than comparable rates in the sociey-of-origin for all disorders studied, including depression, anxiety, paranoia, substance abuse, schizophreniform psychosis and schizophrenia, somatoform disorder, and other disorders. Social disruptions with potentially deleterious effects on mental health are also increased among refugees. These include marital and family dysfunction, divorce, intrafamily violence, and juvenile delinquency. Compared with psychiatric rates of the society into which the refugees migrate, the refugees' psychiatric morbidity is often higher, depending on the particular diagnostic category (Eitenger 1959; Murphy 1955; Williams & Westermeyer 1986).

During the early months and years of flight, disruption, and readjustment, almost all adult refugees experience high and sustained levels of psychophysiologic, emotional, and cognitive symptoms (Lin et al 1979; Westermeyer et al. 1983a). Depending on social policies and clinical resources available for refugees, symptoms may persist at high levels or may gradually resolve over several years. The presence of psychiatric symptoms per se does not necessarily warrant a diagnosis of psychiatric disorder, since many grieving, hypochondriacal, fearful, or suspicious refugees may remain productive and optimistic. Some psychiatric symptoms, if within the limits of functioning and coping, may be necessary to motivate adjustment and change. The risk of major psychiatric disorder requiring clinical attention is highest in the first few years, and gradually decreases thereafter. Psychiatric syndromes are so prevalent among refugees that some clinicians have given self-rating scales (e.g., translations of the 90-item Symptom Checklist or the Zung Depression Scale) to adult patients in general medical clinics (Westermeyer et al 1983b).

Several factors affect the prevalence of psychiatric disorder among the refugee population. Those elements that favor lower overall rates of psychiatric disability include remaining in one's own country or culture, brief flight with limited risks, absence of malnutrition and infectious diseases, remaining within an intact social network, continued employment (or education), maintenance of social roles, and promise for an early return to place-of-origin. On the other hand, malnutrition and infectious diseases, considerable loss of life and property, disruption of the refugee's social and political organization, prolonged residence in camps, loss of occupation and social roles, or relocation to a markedly different cultural milieu can be expected to increase rates of psychiatric disorder. Personal characteristics of the refugee population may affect psychiatric morbidity. For example, among those who fled Cuba in the late 1970s were many individuals with a history of mental disorder, criminality, or social deviance. Finally, the policies adopted and implemented by program administrators, relocation agencies and workers, and health officials can ameliorate or exacerbate the rate of psychiatric disorder, and the transience or permanence of psychiatric morbidity (Mezey 1960a).

ETIOLOGIC CONSIDERATIONS

Conditions experienced during flight and characteristics of the refugees themselves can provide clues to the types of problems likely to be encountered. Extensive malnutrition is apt to result in impaired brain development and mental retardation in younger children and those newborns whose mothers were malnourished while pregnant. Pellagra from niacin deficiency can produce dementia, dermatitis (typically a butterfly-type rash of the face), and diarrhea in adults. Despite frequent cardiovascular beriberi, the complete syndrome of cerebral beriberi (or Wernicke's syndrome) has rarely been observed. Malnutrition may mimic depression, with resultant apathy, physical immobility, social withdrawal, anhedonia, weakness, and anergy (Helwig-Larsen et al 1952).

Infectious diseases can also produce organic brain syndromes. Cerebral malaria, measles, and encephalitides can produce temporary impairment or result in permanent damage. Systemic infections, such as typhus and typhoid, and toxic conditions affecting other systems, such as lobar pneumonia or urinary tract infections, can similarly precipitate bizarre behavior, hallucinations, delusions, and disorientation. Such complications are especially likely to occur in the elderly, or in those with anemias or with borderline nutrition.

Acute brain syndromes from closed head trauma may produce personality change, irritability, emotional lability, paranoia, or hyperactivity. These may persist for a few weeks to several months. Blast injuries, falls in rough terrain, or direct blows to the head can produce this picture. The diagnosis of head trauma may be difficult to make because a reliable history is not available and external evidence of trauma is minimal or absent; absence of localizing findings and a gradual resolution of symptoms suggest the diagnosis.

The refugee experience involves numerous life experiences often associated with reactive depression or mania, acute paranoia, anxiety states, phobic disorders, panic attacks, schizophreniform psychosis, and other conditions that may be stress related. Disruption of one's social network by separation or death of family, friends, relatives, co-workers, and neighbors can undermine security and a sense of social connectedness. Loss of home, vocation, and material belongings often creates an acute grief reaction with resultant disengagement, impoverished thought content, and immobilization. If the move involves relocation outside of the country of origin, the new language and customs can produce a culture shock phenomenon with concomitant threat to one's own social and cultural identity. The ordinary loci for control or influence over life events composed of clan, community, regional and national government are replaced by unfamiliar institutions controlled by others (Scheuty 1944).

Extensive life change has been associated with nonpsychotic psychiatric syndromes and a large number of other medical conditions (Holmes & Masuda 1973). These include depression, fractures, hypertension, congestive heart failure, endocrine abnormalities, and even pregnancy. Because refugee movements inevitably produce massive life changes, refugees are at increased risk for stress-related medical disorders.

Psychiatric patients with chronic disorders are at special risk in the refugee setting. Although they may have achieved a level of adjustment and partial function in their home environment, relocation to a new and stressful environment often disrupts this former stability. Regressive behavior and an exacerbation of the clinical condition can be expected. This is most likely to occur with mental retardation, schizophrenia, paranoid disorders, affective illness, and organic brain syndromes (Mezey 1960b).

DIAGNOSIS

Methods of psychiatric diagnosis in the refugee setting do not differ greatly from the standard procedures employed in out-patient, emergency room, and in-patient facilities of general acute care hospitals. The essentials include establishing rapport, taking a thorough present and past history, obtaining a detailed social and developmental history, inquiring about familial psychiatric disorders, and conducting a formal mental status examination (i.e., orientation, recent and remote memory, cognition including abstraction, mood, presence of hallucinations or delusions, and suicidal or assaultive ideation). With this information in hand, the well-trained clinician can make a working psychiatric diagnosis.

There are some special aspects to psychiatric diagnosis in the refugee setting. If the clinician does not speak the patient's language, the nuances of working with a translator must be learned (described in Westermeyer, 1985). The clinician must become familiar with the refugees' traditions involving birth, illness, death, notions about health and illness, nonmedical curing, relationships between older and younger persons and between men and women, and local customs for dealing with crisis and change. This information can be acquired through anthropological ethnographies, orientation from clinicians with experience in the culture, and immersion in the refugees' community, music, literature, and art.

Psychometric evaluation can be useful in ascertaining organic impairment, intelligence level, learning problems, personality characteristics, and certain psychopathologic symptoms. At the simplest level, even the draw-a-person test can be accomplished if the patient is familiar with the use of pencil and paper. Certain tests are nonverbal and relatively culture-fair (e.g., Porteus maze). Even seemingly culture-bound tests (e.g., Minnesota Multiphasic Personality Inventory) and self-rating scales (e.g., Zung Depression Scale) have been widely translated and renormed in other languages and cultures.

Two psychiatric symptom complexes that tend to be overdetermined in refugee populations are paranoia and somatization symptoms. These often accompany, and may even appear to dominate, the clinical picture of major depression, anxiety, phobia, or panic. The reasons for the exaggeration of these symptoms are not clear. Somatization may result from blocking of feelings, from attribution of dysphoric affect to somatic illness (rather than the reverse), or from the patient's unwillingness to relate personal feelings to an outsider. Somatic delusions may spread in epidemic form and present as a *foile á famille* (madness of the family). Paranoia may be stimulated from the danger and distrust that accompany refugee migration, or from the projection of hostility (felt as a result of recent losses) onto others. Paranoid symptoms are fairly frequent and include delusions regarding the fidelity of a spouse, or paranoia toward social and health workers (Pedersen 1949; Kino 1951; Prange 1959; Kendler 1982).

TREATMENT

Early recognition and timely treatment of malnutrition, infectious diseases, and head trauma reduce both acute psychiatric crises and long-term psychiatric disability. During the early provision of medical services, psychiatric consultation is probably less critical as a clinical service than as an organizational service for future administrative planning.

During the acute phase of refugee medical care, the basic skills of crisis intervention can be very useful. These involve the following:

- Facilitation—helping the patient and family to tell their stories and express their feelings about the problem.
- Clarification—asking questions that help define the problem.
- Consideration of alternatives—determining what actions, if any, might be feasible to address the problem.
- Determination of priorities—assessing the relative importance and sequence of appropriate interventions.
- Decision making—negotiating who will do what, when and where. Final or irrevocable decisions should be avoided during a crisis.

Grief work is another critical aspect of work with refugees. For months or years following flight, they may need to grieve the loss of home, country, material belongings, role, status, and occupation. It may be necessary to grieve for relatives or friends who died, especially when funerals were not conducted or when there was no time for a period of grieving. Survivor guilt is a widespread problem in refugee groups. Refugees often need help in thinking about the deceased person, expressing their feelings, conducting appropriate rituals, finding personal meaning in suffering and death, internalizing and emulating valued aspects of the deceased, and sublimating losses through altruistic or creative expressions.

Brief or time-limited psychotherapy, consisting of one to several sessions, can be valuable in helping refugees to identify unresolved emotional problems, deal with them, and get on with their lives. To conduct psychotherapy across cultural boundaries, the therapist must have previous experience in this type of treatment (ideally under supervision of an experienced cross-cultural therapist) and know the symbols and values of the refugees' culture well. Naive attempts are useless, at best, and alienating or detrimental, at worst. If translators are necessary, they should receive appropriate training relevant to this specialized work.

Involvement of family members or friends can be valuable in the therapeutic process. These ancillary persons can help the therapist to understand the problem within the family and cultural context. They can also support and guide the patient between therapeutic sessions, functioning as auxiliary therapists. It is also crucial in brief therapy to bridge conflicts between the patient and the immediate social network of family and friends. Healers of various kinds from the refugees' indigenous culture may sometimes be of value in establishing communication links between patients and their families, the social structure, and other health care workers.

Medications can be valuable, but should not be administered in a reflex or merely supportive fashion. Indications are essentially the same as for psychiatric care in other settings. Sedatives impede grief work and facilitate hostile and uncontrolled outbursts. They should be used only for the treatment of alcohol or sedative withdrawal. Tricyclics and other antidepressants can help many patients whose major depressive symptoms continue and exacerbate, rather than resolve, over several weeks, but they require close medical supervision and frequent reassessment to ensure their judicious use. Neuroleptics in small doses may aid in the management of brain syndromes, while large doses may be required for exacerbations of mania or schizophrenia. Lithium treatment for mania is feasible even in remote locations lacking laboratory backup for blood levels, but should be prescribed only by those familiar with its potentially toxic effects.

PREVENTION

Several important primary measures should be taken to reduce the incidence of psychiatric disorders. Adequate nutrition must be maintained and daily vitamin supplements provided if adequate food supplies cannot be arranged. Such nutritional support can prevent pellagra and beriberi and their permanently damaging effects on children and fetuses in utero. Infectious diseases should be controlled through immunization programs, eradication of disease vectors such as mosquitoes and rats, early recognition and treatment of potentially epidemic disorders, quarantine of infectious cases, and a clean water supply. These steps are critical to maintain an optimal level of adjustment within the community and to prevent chronic brain syndromes.

In addition, the refugees need assistance in their transition from the past to the future. If they are to step into the unknown future, they must have a firm and secure foot planted in the past. Focusing on continuity with the past helps to maintain self-esteem, a positive identity, and a sense of personal integrity. This can be accomplished by maintaining daily routines, occupational and family roles, avocations and hobbies, recreation, and religious practice. Families should persist in their daily, weekly, seasonal, and annual rituals to the extent possible by eating meals together and observing religious and national holidays. Activities that require community participation (such as festivals, celebrations, and cultural activities) should be encouraged. Producing and selling indigenous crafts may be a vehicle for creativity and economic gain (Westermeyer et al 1983c).

Foreign aid and the activities of religious missions and international organizations can stifle the refugees' own social reorganization. This pitfall must be carefully avoided. If refugees have migrated as an entire clan, village, town, or district, then morale, self-identity, and a sense of control over present and future events are more easily maintained. If fragmented groups have arrived at an already established relocation site, administrative personnel may assist them in developing a social organization appropriate to the needs of the residents. Committees can be established to promote health and disease prevention, education and vocational training for adults and children, daily work assignments, weekend recreation and social activities, and care of the sick and elderly and to arrange distribution of food, clothing, information, and available resources. A goal of resettlement to a permanent site should be to locate a setting appropriate for the social needs of the refugees. A village of farmers might be relocated to a rural area where they are able to maintain contact with one another. An extended family of artisans or skilled workers would do best in a town or city in need of their particular skills. Professional or executive families with previous experience abroad might be able to relocate as a nuclear family, although isolated family placement should be avoided. Local needs and the likelihood of acceptance should be taken into account lest the refugees suffer further rejection and insecurity in their new community.

Orphans, widowed persons, solitary soldiers, and others without family should be integrated into an existing family of their cultural peers. This can best be accomplished if some previous tie exists such as clan membership or origin in the same village or district. Childless adults may take a parentless child, or a couple with children may be able to take an older woman who can provide child care.

Orientation to the new setting must begin as soon as practical. This may entail clearing new farmland and building houses, learning the new language, and acquiring new job skills. Such efforts raise morale and involve the refugee in an ongoing process of readjustment and commitment to a new life and future.

SPECIAL PROBLEMS

Culture-bound syndromes may occur among refugee populations. Some of the best known examples are latah, koro, and amok. These syndromes involve psychiatric symptoms such as ticlike movements, social withdrawal, assault, fear, and panic. None of these syndromes necessarily conveys a psychiatric entity in and of itself. For example, koro symptoms may occur as a manifestation of reactive group hysteria, or an individual adjustment reaction, panic disorder, or psychotic depression, each of which has a different course and treatment. Thorough psychiatric assessment is needed in the case of culture-bound syndromes, as in any nonspecific presenting symptom such as a suicide attempt or social withdrawal.

Psychiatric disorder may occur as an epidemic phenomenon, especially among groups exposed to frustrating or stressful situations, or to poor administration or leadership. These syndromes usually involve shared somatoform, psychophysiologic, emotional, or behavioral symptoms such as weakness, pain, trouble with sensory organs, complaints relative to sexual function, fears, memory problems, and anxiety. Interventions consist of addressing the environmental problem, along with providing support and reassurance of eventual recovery for sufferers.

Children and adolescents usually adjust well to refugee situations, especially if nutrition is adequate and the family remains intact (Pattison 1984). Children and adolescents with severe malnutrition or prior psychiatric conditions, those unaccompanied by family, those who have lived as street children, or those placed with families of a different culture and language are at high risk for developing a psychiatric disorder (Williams & Westermeyer 1983).

Foreign relief workers themselves are at risk for psychiatric disorders. Typically, like the refugees, they have left their homes and social networks for a new environment with a different language and culture. Often, the opportunity for relocation to a refugee setting has followed a recent major life change such as the completion of professional training, termination of previous employment, divorce, children leaving home, retirement, or the death of a spouse or parent. The work often involves dealing with man's inhumanity to man on a massive scale, sometimes in the context of risk to one's own health and life. Living conditions are often primitive, and recreational outlets are few. To maintain a positive mental state, work schedules should include regular weekly or biweekly recreational or "time out" trips away from the camp. Medical care should be readily available to the relief workers, and program administrators must attend to the adjustment and well-being of their staff. In rare instances, some workers will require evacuation back home in the event of major psychiatric disorder, but timely on-site care enables most psychiatric casualties to complete their tours of duty (Talbott 1969). The espirit de corps that develops among relief workers under stressful conditions is probably critical to maintaining good mental health.

REFERENCES AND SUGGESTED READING

Eitinger L: The incidence of mental disease among refugees in Norway. J Ment Sci 1959;105:326–38.

Friedmann CTH, Faguet RA: Extraordinary Disorders of Human Behavior. New York, Plenum Press, 1982.

Helwig-Larsen P, Hoffmeyer H, Kieler J et al: Famine disease in German concentration camps, complications and sequels, with special reference to tuberculosis, mental disorders, and social consequences. Acta Psychol Neurolog Scand (Suppl) 1952;83:1–441.

Holmes TH, Masuda M: Life change and illness susceptibility. In Scott JP Senay EC (Eds): Separation and Depression: Clinical and Research Aspects. Washington DC, American Association for the Advancement of Science, 1973.

Kendler KD: Demography of paranoid psychosis (delusional disorder): A review and comparison with schizophrenia and affective illness. Arch Gen Psychiatr 1982;38:890–92.

Kino FF: Alien's paranoid reaction. J Ment Sci 1951;97:589–94.

Lin KM, Tazuma L, Masuda M: Adaptational problems of Vietnamese refugees: I. Health and mental health status. Arch Gen Psychiatr 1979;36:955–61.

Mezey AG: Personal background, emigration and mental disorder in Hungarian refugees. J Ment Sci 1960a;106:618–27.

Mezey AG: Psychiatric illness in Hungarian refugees. J Ment Sci 1960b;106: 628–37.

Murphy HBM: Flight and Resettlement. Geneva, UNESCO, 1955.

Pattison EM: War and mental health in Lebanon. J Operational Psychiatr 1984;15:31–38.

Pedersen S: Psychopathological reactions to extreme social displacements (refugee neurosis). Psychoanal Rev 1949;36:344–54.

Prange AJ: An interpretation of cultural isolation and alien's paranoid reaction. Int J Soc Psychiatr 1959;4:254–63.

Scheuty A: The stranger: An essay in social psychology. Am J Soc 1944;49:499–507.

Talbott JA: The American expatriate in South Viet Nam. Am J Psychiatr 1969;126:555–60.

Tseng WS, McDermott JF: Culture, Mind and Therapy: An Introduction to Cultural Psychiatry. New York, Brunner Mazel, 1981.

Westermeyer, J: Clinical considerations in cross cultural diagnosis. Hosp Comm Psych, in press.

Westermeyer J, Vang TF, Neider J: Migration and mental health: Association of pre- and post-migration factors with self-rating scales. J Nervous Ment Dis 1983a;171:92–96.

Westermeyer J, Vang TF, Neider J: A comparison of refugees using and not using a psychiatric service: An analysis of DSM-III criteria and self-rating scales in cross-cultural context. J Operational Psychiatr 1983b;14:36–41.

Westermeyer J, Vang TF, Neider J: Refugees who do and do not seek psychiatric care: An analysis of premigratory and postmigratory characteristics. J Nervous Ment Dis 1983c;171:86–91.

Williams CL, Westermeyer J: Psychiatric problems among adolescent Southeast Asian refugees: A descriptive study. J Nervous Ment Dis 1983;171:79–85.

Williams C, Westermeyer J: Refugees and Mental Health. New York, Hemisphere, 1986.

21
Rehabilitation Medicine in Refugee Camps

JEAN BAPTISTE RICHARDIER
DAVID WERNER

There is no simple answer to the problem of helping physically disabled people in a refugee or disaster setting. Refugee camps are often situated in inhospitable areas near borders close to guerilla or war activities, and in host countries where refugees are often unwelcome and the health system is barely capable of meeting the most urgent and basic needs of the indigenous population.

Disabled individuals are the most vulnerable and often the earliest victims of war or famine. The services that were provided in their country of origin, if any, were probably the first to be discontinued during a crisis and will be the last services restored. Within this context, it is essential to determine the most appropriate means to provide durable assistance to the disabled. While striving to provide the best possible solution for the patient's immediate needs, it is necessary that the patient be prepared for a situation in which support services may be totally absent. This is a difficult task which is complicated by the imposed inertia of refugees that may induce indifference and lack of motivation.

It is difficult to claim that one technical solution perfectly suits a specific situation. Only continous research, a critical evaluation of achievement, progressive application of the experiences of the situation, and repeated adjustment based on the experience of others in similar situations will allow success. Each new situation will require a genuine experimental approach with the inherent right to be mistaken but not to be obstinate or unrealistic.

With a commitment to this philosophical approach, the founders of Operation Handicap International created a voluntary agency devoted to the rehabilitation of the physically disabled in underdeveloped countries and, particularly, in the refugee setting. Because locomotor disabilities account for the majority of handicaps among refugees, this chapter is devoted primarily to the management and rehabilitation of these patients.

The World Health Organization (WHO) has defined impairments, disabilities, and handicaps (WHO 1980b). Impairment may be caused by various diseases or disorders including malnutrition, communicable diseases, insufficient quality of prenatal and postnatal care, accidents, or a variety of traumas including battle injuries. An impairment is any loss or abnormality of psychological, physiologic, or anatomic structure or function. This definition includes any anomaly, defect, or loss of limb, organ, tissue, or other body structure, or a defect in a functional system, including the mental functions, either temporary or permanent. A disability is any restriction (resulting from an impairment) or lack of ability to perform an activity in the manner or within the range considered normal. A handicap is a disadvantage resulting from an impairment or disability that limits or prevents the fulfillment of a role that is normal relative to age, sex, and cultural factors.

The WHO classification emphasizes the importance of timely preventive measures aimed at either prevention or reversal of the progressive process. The role of rehabilitation is to reverse the disabling effect of an impairment. Rehabilitation includes all measures aimed at reducing the impact of disabling or handicapping conditions and at allowing disabled and handicapped individuals to achieve social integration (WHO 1980b).

The level of rehabilitative services will be influenced by numerous features of the refugee setting. Rehabilitation programs for disabled refugees should not be based on standards higher than those available to the disabled within the host country or region, as this would inevitably create discontent among local authorities and the local population. Refugee situations should be regarded as temporary.

Eventually, the disabled are likely to face a more difficult environment in which meeting even the most basic needs will be more difficult.

Even with a large, highly motivated staff, the future of some patients is bleak. Therapy for tetraplegic patients, for example, will fail in most refugee situations. Confronted with an impressive disability (such as poliomyelitis complications), the rehabilitation team should cautiously question the decision to intervene. For example, the rehabilitation team should not try to fit a hip disarticulation or a double above-knee amputee with very short stumps with prostheses since such attempts are doomed to failure. The rehabilitation team should give first priority to the disabled who will benefit the most from therapy as well as those with the most common disabilities. Patients requiring a lot of attention and long-term treatment for minimal improvement should be considered second priority.

Rehabilitation programs in the refugee setting require difficult choices. It is not helpful to raise false hopes, especially for disabled refugees facing an uncertain future.

SURVEY AND ASSESSMENT OF REHABILITATION NEEDS

Although a comprehensive survey of the disabled people in a refugee setting is not a precondition to practical action, it is important to initiate a method of identifying the disabled and assessing their needs. In an established refugee settlement, such a survey can be accomplished through home visits by locally trained staff or regular clinic consultations, or by relying on information from refugee leaders. If a large number of refugees arrive together, a screening system to identify disabled individuals who will need immediate assistance and those to be treated later should be established.

To facilitate the screening process and the identification of the disabled and their needs, the UNHCR Social Services division has set guidelines to train refugee workers and has created an assessment form to be used by all health workers. Although this form must be abbreviated when used as a mass screening tool, it provides an excellent framework (see Appendix 21-A).

General principles of prevention and assessment of disabilities should be followed, but implementation procedures require flexibility. Each refugee setting poses new problems, and priorities and solutions will differ according to the country of asylum, the culture of the refugees, the geographical environment of the settlement, the presence of comprehensive medical and surgical facilities, and the types of disability. While the program is being implemented, methods of training rehabilitation workers should be developed. It is important to evaluate the previous technical level of trainees as well as their ability to learn new, and sometimes abstract, principles.

SETTING UP A BASIC REHABILITATION PROGRAM IN A REFUGEE SETTING

Even when the WHO and UNHCR recommendations and guidelines are carefully adapted for a specific refugee setting, implementation is often complicated by difficulties that limit or delay their development and application.

In the refugee setting, first priority is usually given to emergency programs; thus, agencies concerned with rehabilitation of the disabled are often inadequately funded and poorly organized. Because social integration is the ultimate goal of rehabilitation, close cooperation is required among surgeons, general medical staff, physical therapists, orthotic and prosthetic technicians, social workers, and the disabled and their families. Often, each component of the rehabilitation process is handled by a different agency, each with a different philosophy regarding the required level of care, priorities, and methods. Coordination among these agencies is essential for the successful implementation of a rehabilitation program.

SETTING UP SYSTEMS FOR COORDINATION AND REFERRAL

Coordination with Various Medical Care and Surgical Programs

The rehabilitation and surgical teams should establish close collaboration to define and carry out the most appropriate surgical techniques for amputation, surgical stump correction, elective surgery, postoperative follow-up, and rehabilitation. In addition, the physical therapists should set up an intensive program in the postsurgery ward.

Coordination with Adult Medicine Programs

Hospitalized patients in general, and particularly those whose illness can induce a temporary or permanent disability, benefit from simple physical therapy techniques, walking aid devices, and the availability of orthotic and prosthetic manufacturing. In case of suspected impairment of the neuromuscular system, as in poliomyelitis, expertise in rehabilitation medicine can prove to be very helpful. Tuberculosis and leprosy patients usually benefit from special care in separate wards, with rehabilitation techniques being an important component of their treatment. Obstetric and pediatric facilities should also be included, as timely preventive measures are essential for congenital deformities and delivery complications. Early identification of a clubfoot, for instance, will allow a simple but spectacularly effective treatment that can reverse an otherwise poor prognosis. Regular visits by the rehabilitation staff to the obstetric and pediatric facilities will encourage referals of newly discovered anomalies.

Coordination with the Out-Patient Clinics

The out-patient clinic staff will constitute a permanent referral network if they are sensitized to the possibilities of rehabilitation treatments. The staff should be instructed to identify disabled patients and refer them for consultation.

Coordination with the Feeding Center

Supplementary feeding may be necessary for those undergoing rehabilitation since this process may be particularly demanding for the patient. It is also necessary to check the disabled individual's access to the food and water distribution system inside the refugee camp because they may experience special limitations to the acquisition process.

Coordination with Agencies in Charge of Construction and Sanitation

To improve the living conditions of the disabled in a refugee settlement, it is important to coordinate activities with those agencies responsible for construction and sanitation. Several additional toilets should be built that are large enough to accommodate a disabled individual and a wheelchair. Minor modifications will also permit easier access to the houses and communal buildings.

Coordination with Social Services, Schools, and Vocational Training

The rehabilitation team should ensure that disabled children have access to the schools in the camp or settlement. Agencies in charge of vocational training should be convinced of the need to welcome a minimum quota of disabled individuals. These same agencies should also be encouraged to create training adapted to the needs of the disabled such as secretarial and handicraft skills, and production of items that assist self-reliance. In the same spirit, as many positions as possible should be made available to the disabled. One task of the refugee social workers should be to maintain close contact with the disabled through regular home visits, as well as visits to school and vocational training programs. Such visits will allow follow-up on the progress of each disabled patient and timely intervention in case of difficulty.

REQUIREMENTS FOR PROPER REHABILITATION

Construction of the Facility

Construction materials used in building rehabilitation facilities are not as important as a spacious design. Ideally, several departments for the various disabilities should be able to work within the same facility.

Hospital Ward

A hospital ward is important if there are many patients suffering battle wounds, or if the number of severely disabled patients, including paraplegics, is significant. This ward can help to free surgery beds needed for new patients and it will facilitate more dynamic rehabilitation. Ideally, the hospital ward should include the following facilities: (1) nursing and examination rooms with simple and easily accessible, specially adapted toilet and bathing facilities; (2) a physical therapy department; (3) an orthotics and prosthetics workshop (constructed with large windows for proper light and ventilation, a molding room, an examination room, a storage room, parallel bars, a strong table, wooden work benches, water, and, if possible, electricity); (4) a lecture room with a blackboard; (5) an out-patient department with adequate space for family members to accompany the patient during consultations; (6) an optional specialized consultation room for clubfoot consultation, amputee consultation, and so on; (7) an infant play area and activities room; and (8) a sports field or playground area.

TRAINING REHABILITATION HEALTH WORKERS

Basic Training Principles

Training health workers in the theories of the mechanics of motion must be done in progressive stages of increasing difficulty. Those teaching the courses should set aside much of the complex and abstract terminology and look for simple images to make the information comprehensible. This requires a dynamic, inventive, and patient approach to the health worker trainees and frequent self-evaluation by the trainer. The most efficient and practical training method is the immediate transfer of newly acquired information from one health worker to another under the guidance of a supervisor. The trainees should be encouraged to arrive at their own technical solutions and initiatives, thus building self-confidence and allowing more complete integration into the rehabilitation staff.

MANUFACTURE OF PROSTHETIC DEVICES

The equipment for the prosthetic workshop should include standard carpentry and metal working tools. The workshop should not rely on imported materials. Leather, wood or bamboo, iron bars, iron rods, and different qualities of rubber, including used tires, are usually available locally and are adequate to manufacture fair-quality prosthetics and orthotics. Trainees will progress more quickly because they are accustomed to using these materials. Figures 21-1 and 21-2 show examples of prosthetic devices used in the rehabilitation of Cambodian refugees.

Although the technology used must be functionally accurate and efficient, it is better to rely on materials that can withstand the unavoidable errors and lack of precision in the trainees' work. In this respect, leather is an ideal material for the molded sockets for prostheses, orthopedic shoes, and orthotic devices. In hot and humid climes, leather is more

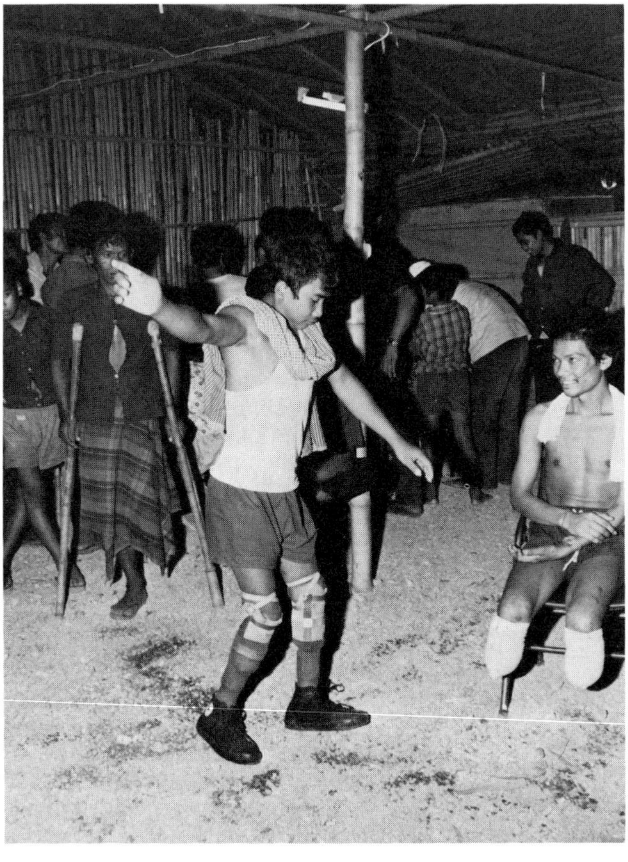

Figure 21-1. Two below-knee amputees. One watches as his friend takes his first steps without crutches.

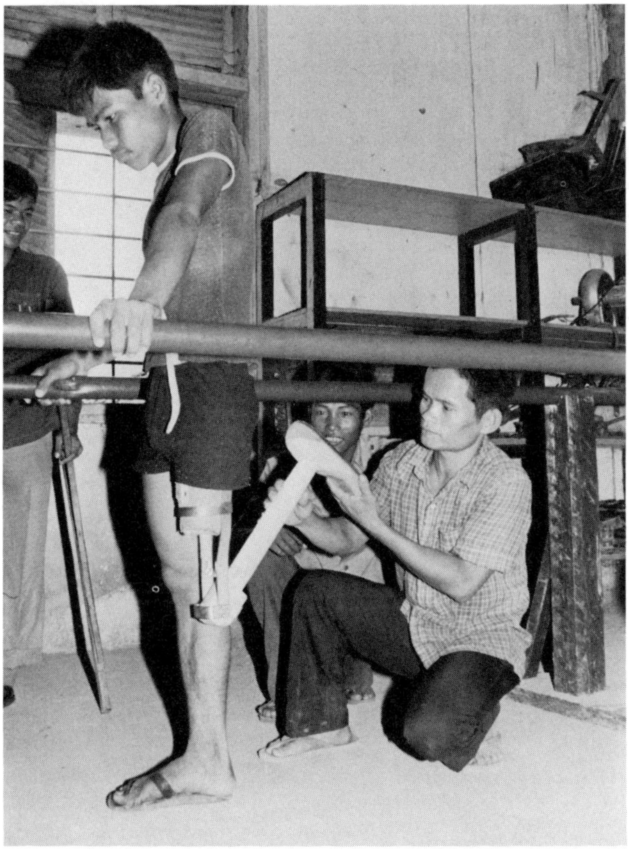

Figure 21-2. Left leg prosthesis being checked at Mairuth camp in Thailand.

comfortable than most man-made materials. Leather also permits the fitting of badly shaped stumps, whereas more rigid materials would require stump surgery. The use of locally available materials will allow the manufacture of adjustable and mendable artificial devices and aids. Needed adjustments can usually be made by the trainees or by the patients.

The following illustrations, adapted with permission from an upcoming book by David Werner, provide examples of aids for rehabilitation including aids to prevent contractures (Figure 21-3) and exercise and walking aids (Figures 21-4 and 21-5).

Figure 21-3. Examples of aids for rehabilitation and prevention of foot contractures.

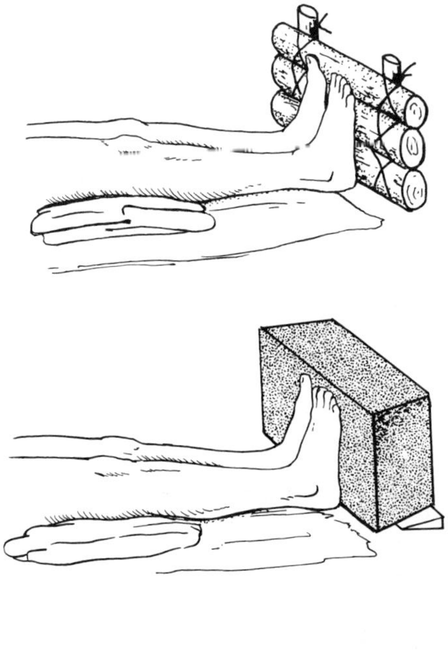

Artificial Legs (Lower Limb Prostheses)

Below the Knee

The most common leg amputation is below the knee. A leg that is amputated in the middle part of the lower leg is also the easiest to adapt to an artificial limb. There are a number of al-

Figure 21-4. Strengthening and straightening exercises.

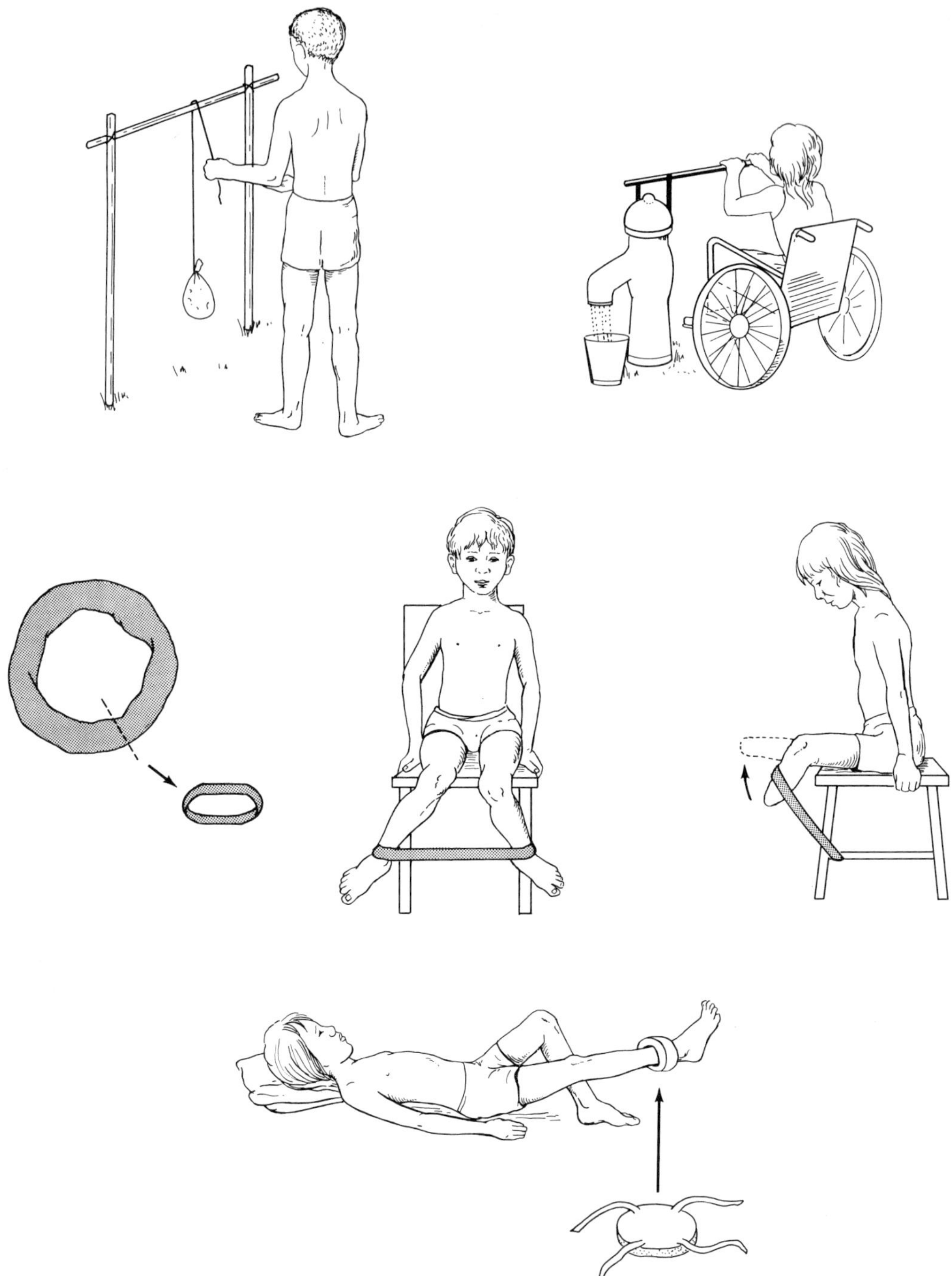

(Figures 21-3 through 21-11 adapted from Werner D, Richardier JP: Disabled Village Children. A Guide for Health Workers and Families. Palo Alto, CA, Hesperian Foundation, and Sinaloa, Mexico, Proyecto PRO-JIMO, 1987.)

ernatives for the construction of a below-the-knee prosthesis, including hand-held pole legs, a "sawed-off crutch" leg, bamboo and plaster legs, and plastic pipe legs with a foot attached (Figure 21-6).

It is important to note that artificial limbs on which the patient walks with the knee bent are easy to make, but run the risk of causing knee contractures. The contractured knee cannot easily be straightened to fit a better, more useful limb. Bent knee limbs should be for temporary or emergency use only. Knee straightening and strengthening exercises should be done every day.

With limbs adapted for use with a straight knee, the knee has a full range of motion. Walking is easier and more natural. However, great care must be taken that weight bearing is evenly distributed over the entire stump, not only at the end of the stump.

Preparing the Stump

In the first weeks or months after an amputation, the stump tends to swell. The swelling may, in time, lead to a knobbed, deformed stump, which is difficult to fit with an artificial limb. For this reason, it is important to wrap the stump with elastic bandage from the time the leg is amputated until a limb is fitted, or until there is no more swelling. When the person is not wearing the prosthesis, an elastic bandage should be worn to control the stump size.

Study the Leg

Before starting to make an artificial limb, study the leg (Figure 21-7). A good fit of the socket on the stump and at the knee is one of the most important, and difficult, parts of limb-making. It is helpful to have an understanding of the bones and muscles in the leg. Study the knee and stump carefully. Note the positions of the kneecap, the bony bumps on the sides of the knee, and the shin bone. Pressure on bony bumps and over the shin bone should be avoided. Instead, pressure should be placed over muscle masses.

A good prosthetic socket does not press on the bony lumps just under the skin but against the muscle masses. It should press in firmly just below the kneecap, where the main weight should be borne. Enough space should be left at the stump tip so that the tip will not be injured if the stump settles a little deeper into the socket.

Measurements for a Below-Knee Limb

A number of measurements should be accurately recorded before a limb is made (Figure

Figure 21-6. Artificial legs (below-knee).

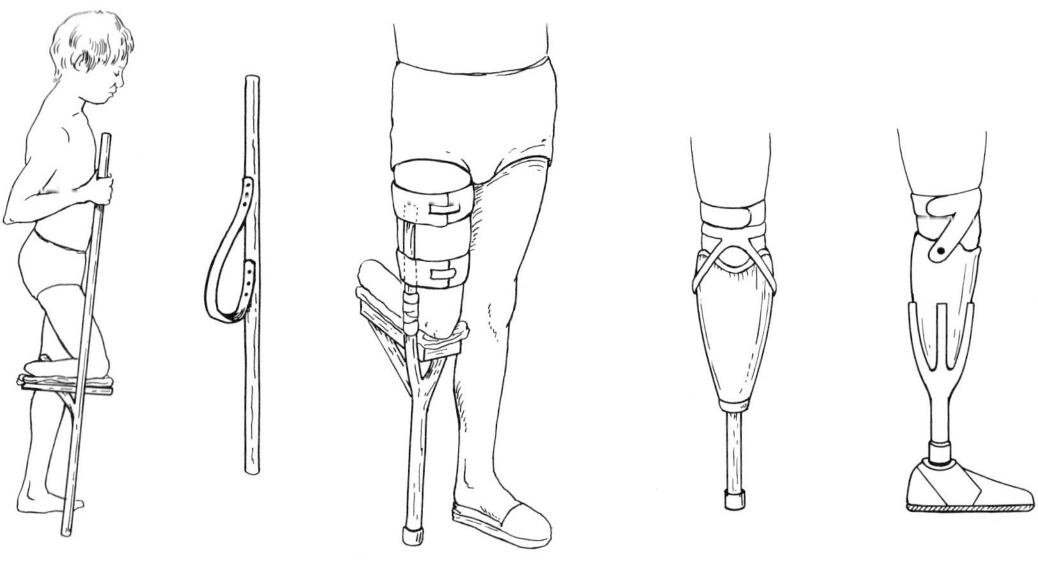

Figure 21-5. Aids for walking: (*A*) parallel bars; (*B*) crutches modified to form a walker; (*C*) wh
(*D*) underarm crutches; (*E*) below-elbow crutches; (*F*) cane with a wide base; and (*G*) walking sti

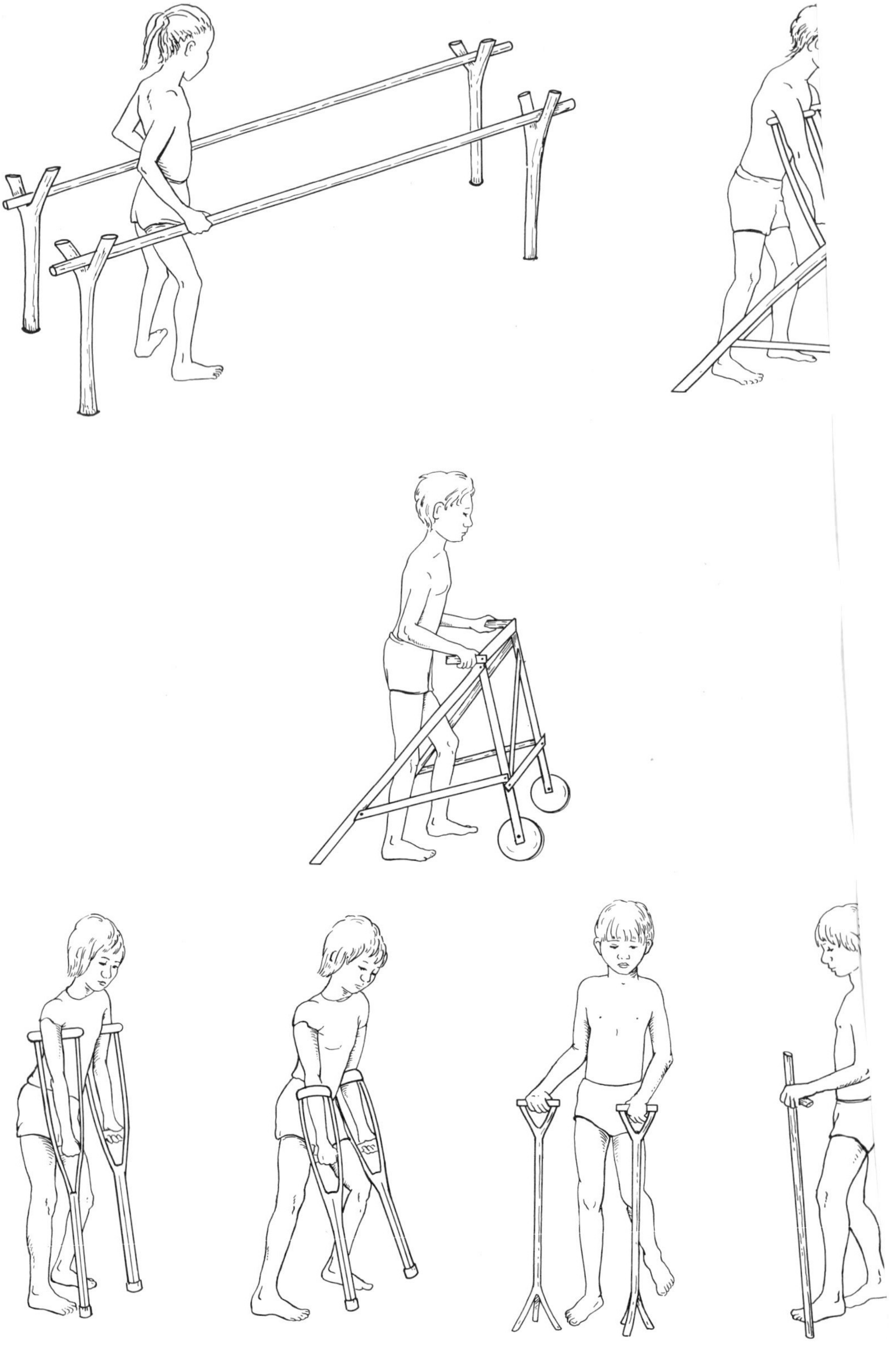

Figure 21-7. Study of the leg.

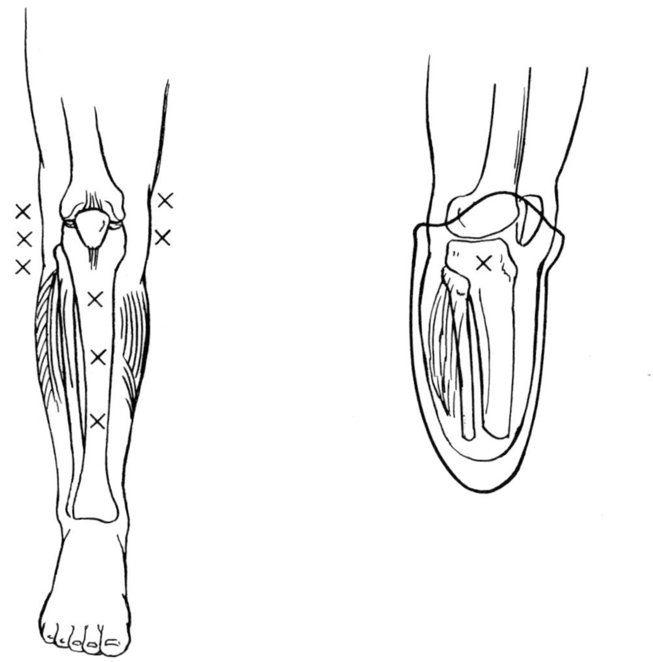

21-8). The distance around the knee, just below the knee, and every two inches around the leg above the knee should be measured. The distance from the front to the back of the knee just below the cap; from side to side; from midknee to bone end; from the knee to the end of the stump; from midknee to the heel; around the thickest part of the good leg; around the ankle; and around the front of the ankle to the back bottom of the heel should be measured as well as the foot length. The artificial limb should be the same length as, or a little shorter than, the other leg.

Above-the-Knee Prosthesis

Children who are growing quickly need a low-cost limb that can be easily replaced or lengthened. Small children usually learn to walk well with a straight leg limb without a knee joint.

A bamboo or polyvinyl chloride (PCV) plastic tube above-the-knee limb can be made in much the same way as one for the below-the-knee limb (Figure 21-9). The top edge of the socket should be rounded out to form a high lip on the back, on which the butt can sit. Weight bearing should be on the buttock and over the entire stump, not mainly on the end of the stump.

For older children and adults, an above-the-knee limb with a knee joint can be made. Figure 21-10 illustrates the construction of such a limb. The socket piece can be made of plaster with glue, resin, or wood with support strips of metal. To help keep the knee from bending when weight is on it, a piece of rubber can be stretched across the front of the knee (see the front view).

Putting feet on artificial legs makes them look better because shoes, sandals, or boots can be worn. The wide base helps prevent the leg from sinking into mud or sand, and a well-made foot can make walking easier. Two types of foot attachment are illustrated in Figure 21-11.

OCCUPATIONAL THERAPY

Occupational therapy plays an important role in the rehabilitation process. Any physical activity is desirable as long as it stimulates gait-training, recuperation of limited function, compensation, coordination, and balance, and

Figure 21-8. Measurements for a below-the-knee limb.

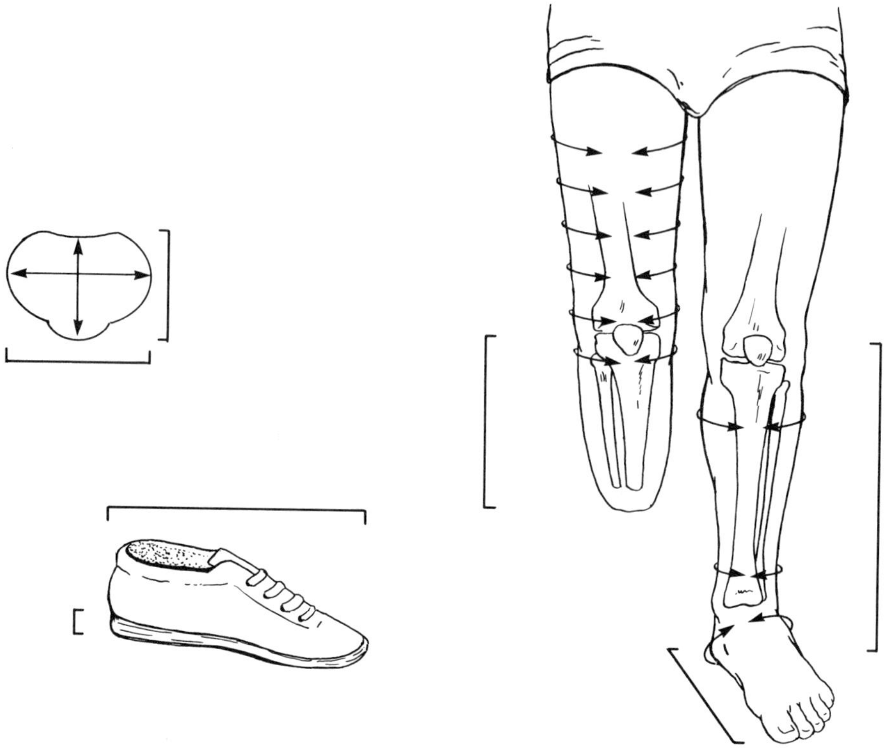

Figure 21-9. Above-the-knee limb without a knee joint: back view; front view; and socket shape.

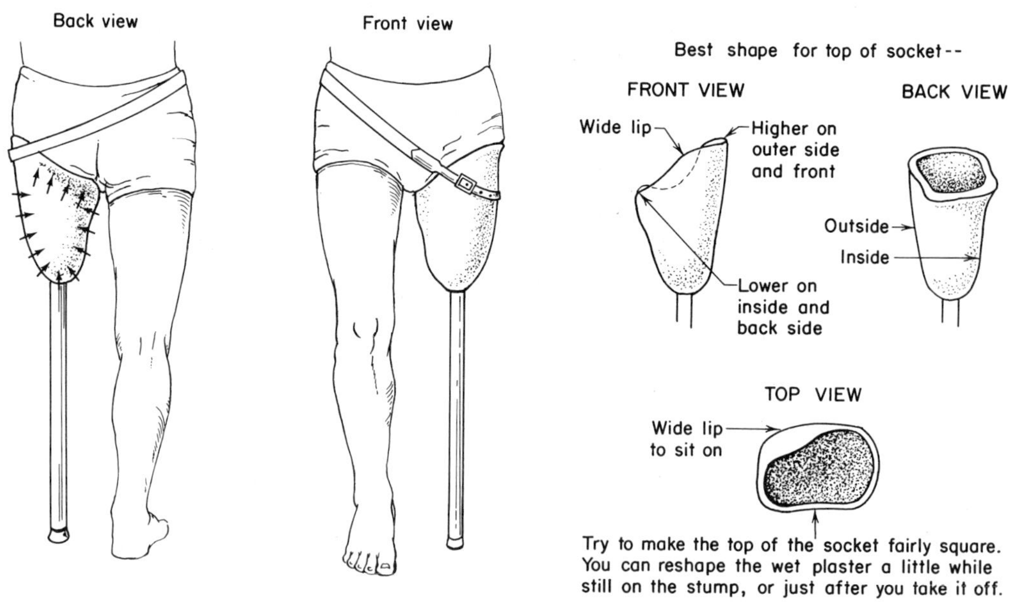

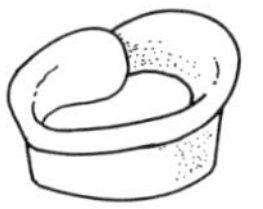

Note: In some countries, thin plastic cuffs the right shape for socket tops can be purchased in different sizes from orthopedic supply distributors. They can be placed around the leg before casting and can be reused. Ask for 'prefabricated ischial weight bearing cuffs'.

Figure 21-10. Above-the-knee limb with knee joint: (*A*) side and front views; (*B*) making the knee joint.

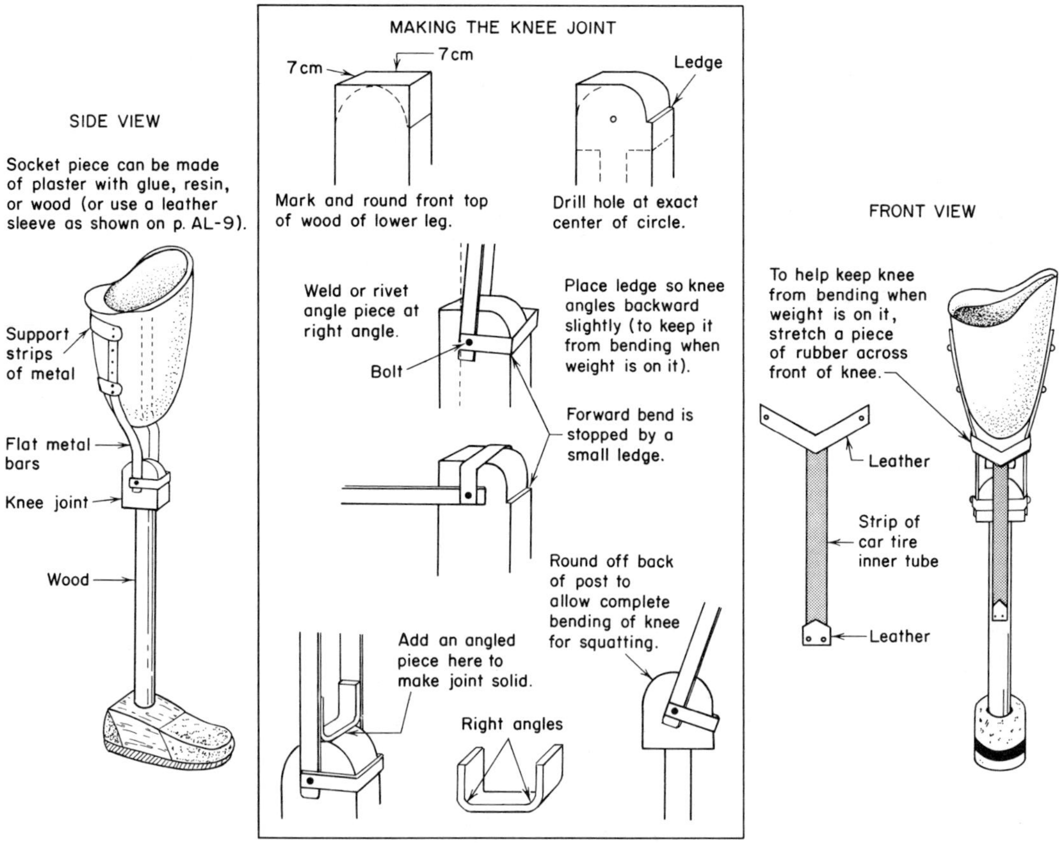

as long as it creates a sense of joy and optimism among the patients. Games, sports, and competition must be organized with enthusiasm and energy from the staff to encourage active participation by the disabled patients. In addition, the occupational therapists should teach the disabled and their families how to carry out the basic activities of daily life, to prepare the patient for future independent living. Simple adaptations that allow the patient to integrate into the school and work environment should be devised as well.

SPECIAL PROBLEMS IN REHABILITATION

Programs for Patients in a Scattered Refugee Setting

The disabled may be scattered among numerous, and sometimes distant, camps, and their number will not justify setting up a comprehensive rehabilitation program in each camp. Rehabilitation efforts in this setting should be focused primarily on the training of family members in accordance with WHO recommendations described in the manual, *Training Disabled People in the Community* (1983). The manual presents details and illustrations on how to organize and conduct a community-based rehabilitation program.

When the geographical environment and distances permit, the rehabilitation team should organize one or more mobile units. Each unit, ideally, should include one technician, one physical therapist, and the basic equipment needed to manufacture artificial devices and aids. Local technicians and therapists will differ in their level of training according to the specific situation. When necessary, patients should be precisely measured and the devices made in a well-equipped, established workshop.

Figure 21-11. Two types of feet.

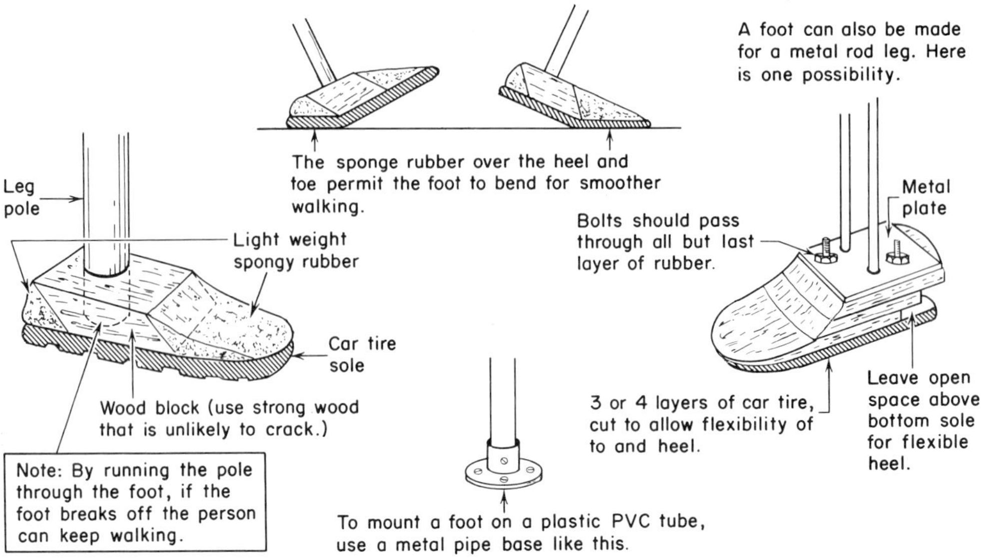

Programs That Are Part of a Permanent Health Care System

Refugees are more welcome in some countries than in others, and they may be granted a permanent status in order to be integrated with the local population. In such situations, the best way to establish appropriate and lasting assistance for the disabled is to assist in developing the existing health system in the country of asylum. This approach benefits both the refugees and the local population and encourages a smooth integration of the disabled into the local population.

Resettlement in Other Countries

As a matter of principle, the rehabilitation team does its best to guarantee the disabled an equal chance of being resettled in another country. However, resettlement is not necessarily the most desirable future for refugees in general, and disabled refugees in particular, despite the expectation of better health care.

When resettlement is available to disabled refugees, the rehabilitation team should work closely with the screening agency on a case-by-case basis to identify the disabled for whom resettlement is either urgent or the most reasonable solution. For those who are considered for resettlement, the social and medical benefits in another country should clearly surpass the difficulties of adaptation to another country. For those who do not fit this criteria, health workers should remember that disabled people in underdeveloped countries are often accepted and cared for by family members to a greater extent than the disabled in many of the developed countries.

REFRENCES AND SELECTED READING

AHRTAG: Aids for Living: The Newsletter on Low-Cost Technologies for Prevention of Disability and the Rehabilitation of Disabled People. London, AHRTAG, 1985a.

AHRTAG: Low Cost Aids, Low Cost Physiotherapy, Low Cost Walking Aids, Personal Transport for Disabled People, Primary Health Care in Developing Countries. London, AHRTAG, 1985b.

Dartnell C: Simple Orthopaedic Aids. Appropriate Designs for a Developing Country. London, Leonard Cheshire Foundation International, 1983.

Helander E, Mendis P, Nelson G: Training Disabled People in the Community. A Manual on Community-Based Rehabilitation for Developing Countries. Geneva, World Health Organization, 1983.

Huckstep RL: Poliomyelitis: A Guide for Developing Countries. London, English Language Book Society, 1979.

Jaccard P, Jaccard R: Un Homme Nouveau. Le lépreux handicappé, opéré et appareillé. Paris, Association Francaise Raoul Follereau, 1983.
Operation Handicap International: Simple Above-Knee Prosthesis. Simple Below-Knee Prosthesis. Simple Orthopaedic Shoes and Calipers. Simple Wooden Wheelchairs. Lyon, Operation Handicap International, 1983.
Shirley O (ed): A Cry for Health. Poverty and Disability in the Third World. Somerset, Third World Group for Disabled People, 1983.
Taussig G: Guide pratique du traitement de la poliomyélite. Paris, Recontre de l'Enfant Handicapé, 1983.
UNESCO: Constructive Education for Special Groups: Handicapped and Deviant Children. Paris, UNESCO, 1980.
United Nations High Commissioner on Refugees: Handbook for Social Services. Geneva, United Nations High Commissioner on Refuges, 1984.
Werner D: Where There Is No Doctor. A Village Health Care Handbook. Palo Alto, CA, Hesperian Foundation, 1977.
Werner D, Richardier JP: Disabled Village Children. A Guide for Health Workers and Families. Palo Alto, CA, Hesperian Foundation, and Sinaloa, Mexico, Proyecto PROJIMO, 1987.
World Health Organization: The Primary Health Worker (rev ed). Geneva, World Health Organization, 1980a.
World Health organization: International Classification of Impairments, Disabilities, and Handicaps. Geneva, World Health Organization, 1980b.

APPENDIX 21-A

ASSESSMENT FORM FOR A PERSON WHO IS DISABLED OR CHRONICALLY ILL

Principal Applicant's
Name: ______________________________
(Underline family name)

Case No. ______________________________

> Complete a separate form for each member of a family who is disabled or chronically ill.

1. Name of person who is disabled or chronically ill ______________________________
(Underline family name)
Sex: ☐ male ☐ female Year of birth: ____________________
2. Has lived ☐ with family ☐ with relative(s) ☐ with friend(s) ☐ alone
since ☐ months ☐ years
3. If the disabled or chronically ill person lives with someone who is registered separately, provide the full name of the head of that family: ______________________________
(Underline family name)
4. Does this person have an *illness* that has lasted more than three months?
☐ yes ☐ no
If "yes," give the name of the illness and explain how it affects this person. ____________
____
____
____
____
5. This person has difficulty (mark any boxes that apply):
☐ using his/her legs ☐ speaking
☐ using his/her hands or arms ☐ learning
☐ seeing ☐ because of sometimes acting in a strange way
☐ hearing ☐ with fits
☐ other (specify): ______________________________
6. Describe this disability: ______________________________
____
____
____

7. Explain *how* and *when* the disability began:

____

____

____

____

8. The list below includes activities required for normal daily living.

Mark the *"Immediate Assistance"* box for any activities that the person is not now able to do and does not have someone to help with.	Mark the *"Training"* box beside any activity the person cannot do without assistance. This will show areas where rehabilitation training may be helpful.

Immediate Assistance	*Training*	
☐	☐	Obtaining food, water, fuel (cross out any that do not apply)
☐	☐	Preparing food
☐	☐	Eating food
☐	☐	Washing himself/herself
☐	☐	Dressing
☐	☐	Washing clothes
☐	☐	Cleaning his/her house
☐	☐	Preventing injuries to parts of his/her body that have no feeling
☐	☐	Moving around *inside* his/her house and immediate living area
☐	☐	Going to the toilet or latrine
☐	☐	Working
☐	☐	Going to school
	☐	Understanding what is said to him/her
	☐	Expressing thoughts, needs, and feelings
	☐	Taking part in family activities
	☐	Taking part in community activities
☐	☐	Other (Describe): ____________________

____

____

____

____

9. Explain how the person previously has been able to accomplish any of the tasks for which immediate assistance is needed:

____

____

____

____

10. If a change in the location where the person is living or any special adaptations in or around the house (such are hand rails or a ramp) would help in meeting daily needs, please explain:

____

____

____

____

11. If the person is an adult, indicate any:
previous occupation ________________________________
current occupation ________________________________

12. Describe any assistance this person needs to establish or improve an occupation: __________

____

____

____

13. Has the person ever regularly taken medicine to cure or control illness or disability?

☐ yes ☐ no

If "yes," explain *who* told the person to take this medicine, *where* it was obtained, *when* the person started taking it, *whether* the person is still taking it, and *what* the medicine and its dose were:

____
____
____
____

14. Describe any other rehabilitation training or medical treatment the person has had for the illness or disability. Explain *who* provided this treatment, *where* it was provided, *when* it began, and *whether* it is still being provided:

____
____
____
____

15. Add any further details that may be useful to those arranging assistance for this person:

____
____
____
____

16. ____________________ ____________________ ____________________

Name of Interviewer	Organization of Interviewer	Date of Interview

Plan for Immediate Action

The space below is to be used by medical, rehabilitation, and social services staff to indicate what action should be taken in regard to this case.

Action Required	*To Be Carried Out By*	*Recommended By*	*Date*
☐ Immediate assistance with ____________ ____________ ____________ ____________			
☐ Further assessment of ____________ ____________ ____________ ____________			
☐ General medical examination			
☐ Specialized medical examination (specify type), ____________ ____________ ____________ ____________			

Additional comments: ______________________________
____
____
____
____
____

(Adapted from UNHCR, Handbook for Social Services. Geneva, UNHCR, 1984.)

III

DIAGNOSIS AND MANAGEMENT OF INFECTIOUS DISEASES

22

Approach to Infectious Diseases in Refugee Camps and Field Laboratory Techniques

THOMAS C. JONES
JOHN DYKE

The most common medical problems facing refugees are malnutrition, trauma, and infectious diseases. This section focuses on how to approach the diagnosis and treatment of infectious diseases in the absence of sophisticated diagnostic testing. During management of the patient's illness, health workers may have to take into account the complications of poor nutritional status and/or trauma, a limited spectrum of available therapy, and complications posed by cultural or language barriers.

It is most important to constantly remind oneself that the *most* compulsive, comprehensive approach within the constraints of the environment must be used—not the least; that is, if a microscope is available, it must be used; if a translator is available, he or she must be trained in the subtleties of history-taking; if time is available, a careful history and physical must replace a superficial triage examination. Unfortunately, too often a pattern of rapid diagnosis, unconfirmed by available testing, followed by shotgun therapy becomes the norm of treatment, even when facilities allow a more logical approach to patient care. This temptation, often due to overwork, frustration, and fatigue, must be resisted. This chapter is designed to provide a framework for a rational approach to diagnosis and treatment of infectious diseases in a low-technology setting.

The standard methods of diagnosis, in the setting of a solid understanding of pathogenesis of the diseases under consideration, must be relied on. These include careful history of the illness, a focused physical examination, and use of limited laboratory testing. To these standard methods is added the important use of the epidemiologic setting as a diagnostic tool. In addition, one may focus diagnosis on similar treatment approaches rather than on a specific microbial genus or species diagnosis. For example, finding fecal leukocytes does not identify an infecting agent but usually indicates a need for the use of antibiotics. Unexplained fever with an eschar and a rash may place the patient's illness in a group with one of the tetracycline-responsive illnesses such as scrub typhus.

As described in Chapter 24, one important step in diagnosis of infectious diseases is to determine whether the process is confined predominantly to one organ system. This is accomplished primarily through the history and physical examination and is the reason why these steps must be done with care. As is noted in the following chapters, once focus on a specific organ system is possible, the differential diagnosis and use of the laboratory become manageable.

The following sections describe in detail the techniques that are useful during history-taking, physical examination, and use of the laboratory. One should be aware that the laboratory techniques available are never static; that is, as the refugee situation changes (which it often does), the use of laboratory support must change. The laboratory must be viewed as a dynamic part of the health care process, not a legislated limitation. When an available microscope is not used because "these people never had this as part of their health care before and probably never will in the future," we see an excuse for further reducing the already deplorable status of the refugee. One should recall such statements as they were applied to the Cambodian refugees in Thailand each time one sees a resettled Cambodian enter a sophisticated medical unit in New York or Paris.

Fortunately, the refugees' status is often not permanent; they deserve the best care available, including appropriate laboratory support for diagnosis. Decisions about distribution of limited resources may affect the availability of laboratory supplies, but this should not affect their use when available nor exclude the possibility of a change in this resource allocation in the future. Our task is to constantly provide the best care possible, not to be bound to the past or to predict the future.

SPECIAL USES OF THE HISTORY AND PHYSICAL EXAMINATION

Patient History

Patient history is traditionally divided into the categories "present illness" and "past medical history." This separation of events based on time is often unavailable or not useful in the refugee camp setting. There are two reasons for this: time is an abstract concept requiring milestones for definition (e.g., a watch, calendar, or event orientation), and time is subject to different interpretations due to language and culture differences. Physicians often become discouraged by the difficulties of grasping the time problem in history-taking and quickly resort to a form of veterinary medicine. This is unnecessary if the problems in time orientation are considered, if translators are carefully prepared regarding the information desired from patients, and if questions are constructed in a manner likely to yield a helpful response.

In addition, the level of understanding of the patient (or family member) regarding the signs or symptoms under investigation must be considered. For example, to gain an adequate response to the question "How long have you been sick?" a clear separation between sickness and health in the mind of the patient is required, even if time has been properly defined. A more accurate answer may be obtained by referring to some functional activity such as walking, working, or deep breathing, rather than using the general concepts of sickness and health. The rule, therefore, is to be as specific as possible about the activity that might be affected and that can lead to dating the onset of a specific organ dysfunction. Pulmonary symptoms of a gradual, progressive, disabling type are more likely due to tuberculosis, whereas an illness of rapid onset and short duration suggests pneumococcus or *Hemophilus* infection.

The information that is of critical importance if the history of the present illness is to be of value includes the following: date of onset, character of the progression of symptoms (progressive, intermittent); location (limited to one organ system, migratory), and relationship of a major symptom to secondary symptoms.

The past history is often of little benefit for the various time, cultural, and language reasons already indicated. Attention should be directed primarily to the patient or the patient's family concerning the following: previous attacks similar to the present illness; history of medication taken and possible allergies; and obvious environmental issues that might aid in diagnosis, such as duration in the camp, nutritional status, and social situation. The history should also be directed toward a review of organ systems not included in the present illness to ensure that major symptoms have not been omitted by the patient.

Physical Examination

The approach to physical examination can be divided into three general areas: triage for infectious diseases, identification of organ system dysfunction, and complete evaluation.

Triage for Infectious Diseases

The rapid evaluation of patients regarding infectious diseases focuses attention on emergency conditions which affect the following: the central nervous system and meninges, respiratory function, and fluid balance and gastrointestinal function.

Rapid evaluation of the central nervous system (CNS) is done by determining the level of consciousness, and evaluating meningeal signs by flexing the neck and, in infants, by checking the fontanels for bulging.

Respiratory function is evaluated by determining the rate of respiration and by checking for the presence of intercostal retraction (indicative of airway obstruction), wheezing, and cyanosis of the mucosa or skin.

Fluid balance is determined by examining for skin turgor and depressed fontanels in infants and by blood pressure readings.

This rapid evaluation of the central nervous system, meninges, lungs, and fluid status can be accomplished within one to two minutes. In addition, the feel of the skin will yield an estimate of the level of fever, and a check for the ecchymotic skin lesions of meningococcus can complete a triage examination. This evaluation will permit an immediate decision concerning hydration, airway assistance, CNS evaluation (lumbar puncture), or cooling.

Identification of Organ System Dysfunction

The tools needed to identify the source of fever rapidly and efficiently include a stethoscope, an otoscope, and tools for clearing wax from the ear canals. The order of examination varies depending on the age of the patient (see Chapter 12 for more specifics on the physical examination of infants and children), but it must include the following:

- Mental status and vital signs (pulse, blood pressure, and temperature).
- Careful examination of the eardrums for signs of inflammation.
- Examination of the pharynx.
- Auscultation and palpation of the lungs.
- Cardiac examination for murmurs or arrhythmias.
- Palpation of the abdomen for areas of tenderness, distention, and liver and spleen size, as well as auscultation for bowel activity.
- Evaluation of extremities for asymmetry or altered function.
- Examination of the skin.

The data obtained by these points of focus will allow the best determination of whether or not fever is rising from one organ system. The following chapters indicate the diseases to be considered when abnormalities in one of the organ systems appear to predominate.

Complete Evaluation

When time is available and the patient's condition requires a full evaluation, the standard approach for complete physical examination should be taken. This evaluation should be recorded carefully in a place that allows easy reference, because repeated evaluation, perhaps by a different clinician, may be necessary.

When a complete evaluation is augmented by routine screening laboratory tests, these tests should include the following:

- Complete blood count (hematocrit, white blood cell count, and differential).
- Malaria smear.
- Gram's stain and TB stain of sputum or drainage material.
- Stool examination for leukocytes and ova and parasites.
- Urinalysis.
- Serologic tests.
- Cultures.

FIELD LABORATORY TECHNIQUES

Complete Blood Count

The most important screening tests for infection or blood loss are white cell count, red cell count, and white cell differential smear. These can be done in any refugee setting in which a microscope, glass slides, cell counting chambers, simple diluting fluids, and stains are available.

Manual Pipet Methods of Red and White Cell Counting

Cell counting requires diluting fluids to prepare the anticoagulated whole blood for addition to the counting chamber.

Procedure for Red Blood Cell Counts

Anticoagulated whole blood is diluted with an isotonic diluting fluid to facilitate counting and to prevent lysis of the red blood cells. The cells are counted in a standard hemocytometer. The normal range is as follows:

- Males: 4.0 to 5.5×10^6 mm^3
- Females: 3.5 to 5.0×10^6 mm^3

Reagents Needed. Any one of the following diluting fluids may be used:

- Hayem's solution:

Sodium sulfate	2.50 g
Sodium chloride	0.50 g
Mercuric chloride	0.25 g
Distilled water	100.00 ml

- Gower's solution:

Sodium sulfate	12.5 g
Glacial acetic acid	33.3 ml
Distilled water	200.0 ml

(Gower's solution is superior to Hayem's solution because it prevents rouleaux and clumping of red cells.)

- Sodium chloride, 0.85 percent (weight/volume):

Sodium chloride	0.85 g
Distilled water	100.0 ml

Equipment Needed. The following equipment will be needed:

- Tri-Lyne blood-diluting pipets (for red blood cells) and aspirator tubing.
- Improved Neubauer hemocytometer with nondisposable cover glass (see below).
- Clean gauze or microwipe.
- Microscope.

Procedure

1. Dilute the blood as follows:
   a. Using the aspirator and red blood cell (RBC) pipet (see Figure 22-1), draw the blood up to the 0.5 mark in the pipet.
   b. Remove blood from outside the pipet with clean gauze or a microwipe. Be careful that the gauze does not withdraw any blood from the stem of the pipet. Place a nonabsorbent material at the end of the pipet, bringing the blood down to exactly the 0.5 mark.
   c. Holding the pipet almost vertically, place its tip into a small vial of red cell count diluting fluid. Draw the diluting fluid into the pipet slowly while gently rotating the pipet with your hand to ensure the proper amount of mixing. Aspirate the diluting fluid until the mixture reaches the 101 mark. If the blood falls below the 0.5 mark at any time during this step, repeat the entire procedure using a clean pipet. If any blood has dripped into the bottle of diluting fluid, the solution is contaminated and fresh diluting fluid must be used. If the pipet is not held in a vertical position while aspirating the diluting fluid, air bubbles will tend to form in the bulb. If this occurs, the dilution will be inaccurate and the procedure must be repeated using a clean pipet.
   d. Place the pipet in a horizontal position and firmly hold the index finger over the tip of the pipet. Detach the aspirator tubing from the other end of the pipet.
   e. The dilution of blood is now complete. The fluid in the pipet bulb is at a dilution of 1:200.
2. Clean the counting chamber and cover glass with a clean, lint-free microwipe. Alcohol will facilitate the cleaning process. Carefully replace the coverglass on top of the ruled area of the counting chamber.
3. Mix the diluted red cell counts for approximately three minutes to ensure adequate mixing. This is done by placing the thumb over the tip of the pipet and the middle finger over the other end. Moving only the hand, shake the pipet back and forth.
4. Fill the counting chamber with two samples of the pipet dilution (one on each side of the hemocytometer) after expelling the first five drops onto a piece of gauze. Once the chamber is filled, place the hemocytometer in a moist chamber (a Petri dish lined with moistened filter paper), label it, and allow the cells to settle for a few minutes. The moist chamber should prevent evaporation of the solution from under the cover glass. Evaporation of the solution can be identified by fluid retreating from the edges of the plated area. Evaporation causes the concentration of cells in the remaining fluid on the ruled area and an erroneously high count.
5. Count the red cells as follows:
   a. Place the hemocytometer on the microscope stage. using low power (10× objective), place the large center square in the middle of the field of vision. Examine the entire large square for even distribution of red cells.
   b. Change to the high-dry objective (45×). Move the counting chamber so that the small upper left corner square (R) is completely within the field of vision. This square is subdivided into 16 smaller squares to facilitate cell counting.
   c. Count all of the cells in the square. Count the cells on two of the outer margins but exclude those lying on the other two outside margin lines. If any white cells are in the area being counted, do not include them in your count. (The white cells will be larger than the red cells and will not have as smooth an appearance.) Count the five red cell squares (the four corners and one center square) on each side of the chamber. The two counts should agree to within 10 percent.
   d. Add the counts from the two samples on each side of the chamber to get the total number of cells counted. The volume of the red cell portion of both sides of the hemocytometer used in this calculation is 10 squares $\times (0.2 \times 0.2 \times 0.1) = 0.04\ mm^3$.

$$\text{Total number of RBCs/mm}^3 = \frac{\text{Total No. RBCs counted} \times 200}{0.04\ \text{mm}^3}$$

Procedure for White Blood Cell (WBC) Counts

Anticoagulated whole blood is diluted in acetic acid, which hemolyzes the erythrocytes and preserves the leukocytes. The cells are counted in a standard hemocytometer. The leukocytes remain intact for at least 24 hours at room temperature (18 to 27°C) after dilution. The standard normal range is 4000 to 12,000/mm^3.

Reagent Needed. The following diluting fluid should be used: glacial acetic acid, 2 percent. This is prepared by diluting 2 ml of gla-

Figure 22-1. Blood cell diluting pipet.

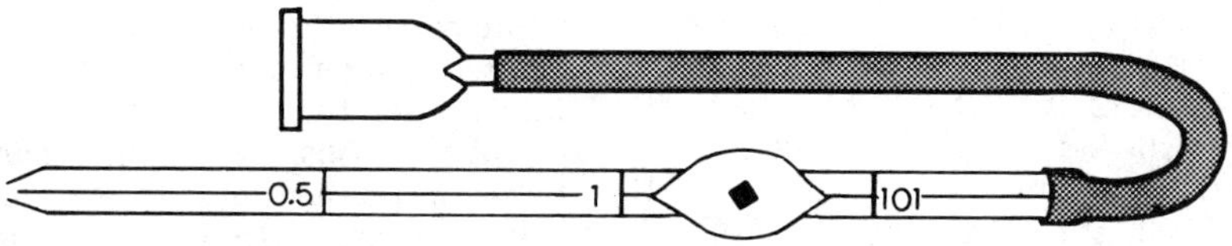

cial acetic acid in 100 ml distilled water. The solution is stable for 60 days.

Equipment Needed. The equipment required for the white blood cell count procedure is the same as that for red cell counting except for the diluting pipet, which is larger for WBC counting.

Procedure

1. Dilute the blood as follows:
   a. Use the pipet and aspirator to draw blood to the 0.5 mark following the same techniques used for RBC counting.
   b. Holding the pipet vertically, place the tip of the pipet into a small vial of the white count diluting fluid. Draw the diluting fluid into the pipet slowly, while gently rotating the pipet with your hand to ensure the proper amount of mixing. Aspirate the diluting fluid until the mixture reaches the 11 mark. The dilution of blood is now complete with 0.5 in 10 or 1:20 dilution.
2. Clean the counting chamber. Follow the mixing procedures described for RBCs and fill the counting chambers.
3. Count the white blood cells as follows:
   a. Using low power only (10× objective), make certain that the microscope light is adjusted properly. In proper focus, the white cells should look like small dark, or black, dots. The red cells will have been lysed; red cell stroma may be present. Scan the four large corner squares marked "W" on the counting chamber (see Figure 22-2). For accurate white counts, there should be an even distribution of cells in all four large squares.
   b. Beginning with the upper left square (W), count all the white cells in the four large corner squares and add the results together to obtain the total number of cells

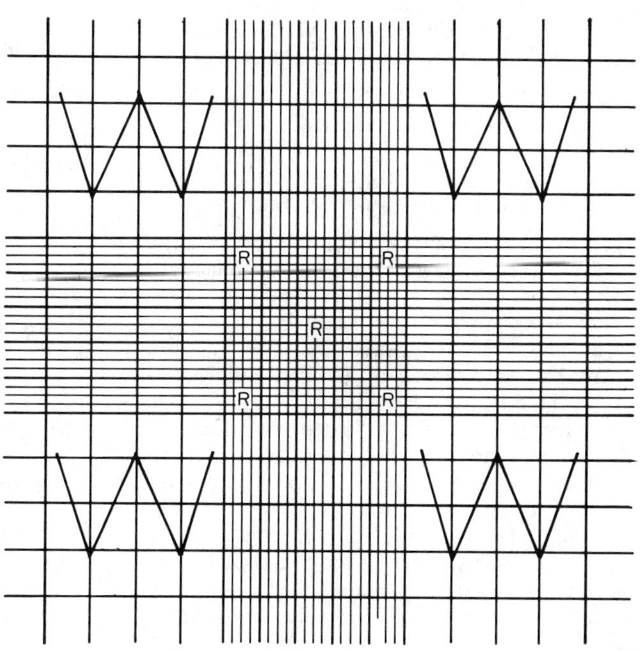

Figure 22-2. Magnified appearance of Neubauer hemocytometer markings.

counted. If the chamber has triple lines, count those cells that touch the middle of the three outside lines on two sides and disregard those touching the corresponding lines on the other two sides. Count the cells on the opposite side of the counting chamber and record the number of cells counted in these four large squares.

c. Add the counts from each side of the chamber to get the total number of cells counted. The volume of the white cell portion of both sides of the hemocytometer used in this calculation is 8 squares × (1.0 × 1.0 × 0.1mm) = 0.8 mm^3.

$$\text{Total number of WBCs/mm}^3 = \frac{\text{Total No. WBCs counted} \times 20\ \text{(dilution)}}{0.8\ \text{mm}^3}$$

Peripheral Blood Smears

Making the Smear

The information gathered from the examination of a blood smear is extremely important in diagnosing hematopoietic disorders as well as aiding in the diagnosis of some infectious diseases such as malaria. The reliability of the information obtained depends to a considerable extent on the quality of the smears. Fresh EDTA anticoagulated whole blood or venous blood obtained by capillary puncture (finger or heel stick) is used.

Reagent and Equipment Needed. The reagent and equipment required are as follows:

- Wright's stain
- Precleaned microscope slides with frosted ends
- Precleaned 22 × 30 mm coverslips
- Microscope with oil immersion lens

Procedure. Touch one small drop of capillary or fresh venous blood to the edge of a clean slide (see Figure 22-3). Then bring this edge to the surface of a second, scrupulously clean slide that is supported by a flat, firm horizontal surface. Wait until the blood spreads along the edge while holding the two slides at a 45 degree angle. Then, just before the blood has spread to the outer edges, push the spreader slide ahead of the drop of blood with a rapid, but not too brisk, movement. Label the slide, for example, by writing the slide number on the smear with a pencil. Allow the slide to air dry, stain it, and if indicated, place a coverslip over it with an available mounting fluid.

Blood films of the proper thickness will dry quickly and will appear yellow when placed on white paper. The smaller the angle between the slides and the more slowly the blood is spread, the thinner the film will be. The well-made blood film consists of a thick band (at the application point) that is drawn out into a thin, feathery portion. In the thick portion, the cells are too closely placed and overlapping to be studied, while in the thin portion they exhibit artifacts because of their wide separation. Cell morphology is best in the intermediate zone where the cells just touch each other. The blood smear is about 2 cm wide and 3 cm long, and its sides do not extend to the edges of the glass slide.

Among the causes of a poor blood smear are the following:

- Drop of blood too large or too small.
- Spreader slide pushed across the slide in a jerky manner.
- Failure to keep the entire edge of the spreader slide against the slide while making the smear.
- Failure to keep the spreader slide at a 30 degree angle with the slide (increasing the angle results in a thicker smear, whereas a smaller angle gives a thin smear).
- Failure to push the spreader slide completely across the slide.

Staining Blood Smears

The Romanovsky formula is the combination of acidic and basic components that allows the use of one stain to produce a variety of predictable color reactions. Basic dyes stain acid tissue components such as nuclear DNA and cytoplasmic RNA blue, whereas acid dyes stain hemoglobin and eosinophilic granules pink. Other structures show affinity for the neutral dye.

Reagents and Equipment Needed. The reagents and equipment required include Wright's stain, a methyl alcohol solution of eosin and a complex mixture of thiazines, including methylene blue, azure B, and other derivatives; and potassium–sodium phosphate buffer, pH 6.4.

Procedure

1. Place fresh air-dried blood smear, film side up, on a staining rack. For best results films should be fixed in 70% methanol before staining. If the films are air dried without

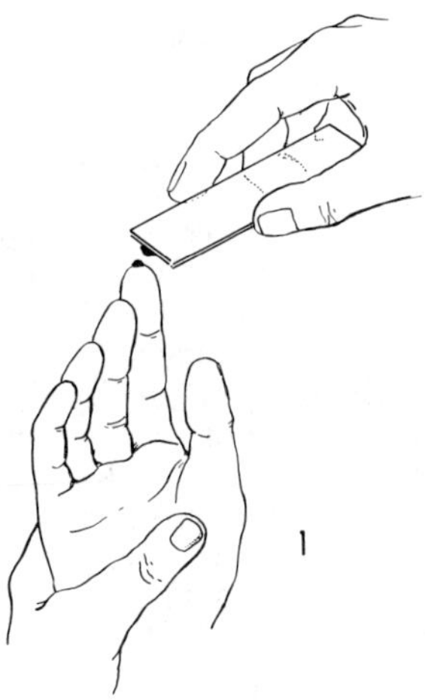

Figure 22-3. Method of preparing a peripheral blood smear: (1) Touch a drop of blood to the edge of a clean slide; (2) bring this edge to the surface of another slide. Wait until the blood spreads along the whole edge; (3) holding the two slides at a 45 degree angle, push the top slide with a rapid, but not too brisk, movement; (4) write the slide number on the smear with a pencil.

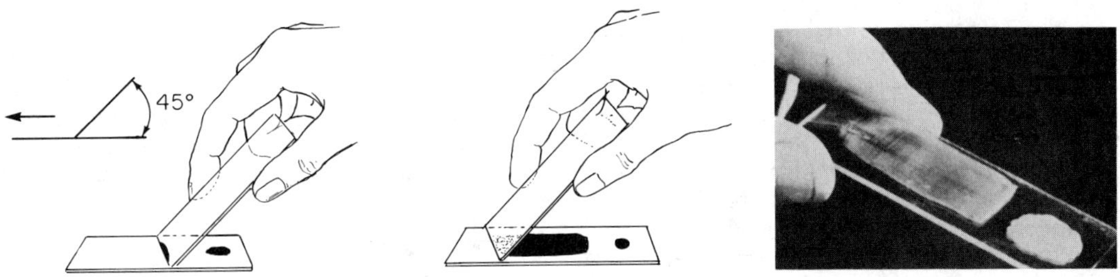

fixing, then they should be examined within a few hours.

2. Cover the blood smear completely with Wright's stain. Allow the stain to react for two minutes (the time may vary slightly depending on the quality of the stain used). This fixes the blood film to the slide.
3. Add to the stain on the blood smear an equal quantity of buffer solution. Add the buffer slowly, taking care that the solution does not run over the edge of the slide. To mix the stain with the buffer, blow gently on the diluted stain on several portions of the slide to set up gentle currents and to make an even distribution. Look for a green metallic sheen to appear, then allow the stain and buffer to react for approximately four minutes (the time may vary slightly depending on the pH of the buffer solution).
4. Wash the stain-buffer solution from the slides with a gentle flow of distilled water. The stain should be "floated" off the slide by adding water slowly at first and then more briskly while the slide is in a horizontal position. It is important to complete the washing while the slide is still horizontal; otherwise a film tends to settle on the smear (precipitate), which may be difficult to remove by subsequent washings. The stain remaining on the back of the dried slide can be removed with gauze moistened in alcohol.
5. Allow the slide to dry by evaporation by leaving it in a tilted position.
6. When the slide is thoroughly dry, it is ready to be coverslipped or observed under the microscope.

Problems. Common problems in staining include the following:

1. Excessively blue stain. Thick films, prolonged staining time, inadequate washing, or too high an alkalinity of stain or diluent tends to cause excessive basophilia. In such smears, the erythrocytes appear blue or green, the nuclear chromatin is deep blue to black, and the granules of the neutrophils

are deeply overstained and appear large and prominent. The granules of the eosinophils are blue or gray. Such a stain may be corrected by staining for a shorter time or by using less stain and more diluent. If these steps are ineffective, the buffer may be too alkaline, and a new buffer with a lower pH should be prepared.

2. Excessively pink stain. Insufficient staining, prolonged washing time, mounting the coverslips before they are dry, or a stain or buffer that is too acidic may cause excessive acidophilia. In such films, the erythrocytes are bright red or orange and not pink, the nuclear chromatin is pale blue, and the granules of the eosinophils are sparkling, brilliant red. One of the causes of the increased acidity is exposure of the stain or buffer to acid fumes. The problem may be a low pH buffer, or it may be the methyl alcohol, which is prone to develop formic acid as a result of oxidation on standing. A given powder may afford perfect results when dissolved in fresh methanol, but poor results when dissolved in the same lot of methanol after some months of exposure to air. After these steps have been checked, one might suspect that the dye does not have the proper polychrome components and should try another lot.
3. Inadequate stain. Inadequately stained red cells, nuclei, or eosinophilic granules may be due to understaining or excessive washing. Prolonging the staining or reducing the washing may solve the problem.
4. Precipitate on the film. Precipitate on the film may be due to unclean slides, drying during the period of staining, inadequate washing of the slide at the end of the staining period (especially common if one fails to hold the slide horizontally during the initial washing), inadequate filtration of the stain, or dust settling on the slide or smear.

Interpretation. Blood smears stained well with Wright's stain are pink when viewed with the naked eye. The red cells are pink, not lemon yellow or red. There should be only a minimum of precipitate. The areas between the cells are clear. The color of the film should be uniform without pale or dark green areas, which are indicative of excessive staining of thick portions of film. The blood cells should be free of artifacts, such as vacuoles. The nuclei of leukocytes are blue to purple, the basichromatin and oxychromatin (chromatin and parachromatin) are clearly differentiated, and the cytoplasmic neutrophilic granules are tan. The eosinophilic granules are red-orange and each is distinctly discernible so that one can count the individual granules.

The basophil has dark blue to purple granules. Platelets have dark lilac granules. Bacteria (if present) are blue. The cytoplasm of lymphocytes is generally robin's egg blue; that of the monocytes has a faint bluish tinge. These colors are variable and two films stained from the same bottle sometimes differ greatly. In general, a preparation is satisfactory when both the nuclei and the neutrophilic granules are distinct, regardless of their color and when the film is free from precipitated dye. The colors are prone to fading if the preparation is mounted in poor-quality balsam or if it is exposed to light.

Morphology of Peripheral Cells

The differential blood smear analysis involves classifying and enumerating the white blood cells present on a peripheral smear, examining the smear for RBC and WBC morphology, and estimating platelet adequacy.

Procedure for Examining the Stained Smear

1. Examine the blood smear using the low power (10X) objective.
   a. The white cells should be evenly distributed over the smear.
   b. Estimate the white cell count by noting the number of white cells in relation to the number of red blood cells. The result should agree with the WBC count obtained. If it does not, the white count should be repeated.
   c. Examine the thin peripheral edge of the smear. If there is an increased number of white cells in this area, the differential cell count is inaccurate. Most of the cells at the edge of the smear are the larger white cells, namely, neutrophils and monocytes. Therefore, this shows poor distribution of white cell types in the smear. If there are clumps of platelets in this area, the smear then shows a decrease in platelets. In such situations, the blood smear should be discarded and another made.
   d. In scanning the blood smear, it is important to note anything unusual or irregular, such as large, abnormal-looking cells, or rouleaux formation of the red cells.
   e. Choose that portion of the blood smear

where there is only slight overlapping of the red cells. Place a drop of oil on the slide and carefully change to the oil immersion objective (100×).

2. Perform the differential cell count and examination of the white cell morphology.
   a. Begin in the thin area of the slide where the red cells are slightly overlapping. Gradually move the slide as shown in Figure 22-4. Count each white cell seen and record them on a differential cell counter until 100 white cells have been counted. If any nucleated red cells are seen during the differential count, enumerate them on a separate counter. These cells are not to be included in the 100-cell differential count. Record the percentage of neutrophils, band forms, eosinophils, monocytes, basophils, and lymphocytes.
   b. While counting the white cells, make a note of any abnormalities present in the cells, such as very immature forms or atypical lymphocytes.
3. Examine the red cell morphology in a thin area of the slide where the red cells either do not overlap or overlap slightly. Note any variations from normal, such as anisocytosis, poikilocytosis, microcytosis, macrocytosis, hypochromia, or the presence of unusual cells such as target or sickle cells, basophilic cells, stippling cells, spherocytes, or parasite-containing cells. Six to eight fields should be reviewed before morphology is graded.
4. Examine the platelets on the smear for morphology and number present. Using the same fields on various parts of the smear as in step 3 for the red cell morphology, determine the approximate number of platelets per field.

Malaria Blood Smears

The advantages and disadvantages of thick and thin smears are discussed in Chapter 25. The Giemsa stain used below is available commercially or can be mixed from 0.175 g of Giemsa stain powder, 65 ml of pure methyl alcohol, plus 35 ml of pure glycerol. Phosphate buffer should be used to bring the solution to the correct pH. Improper pH of the Giemsa stain may result in parasites being unrecognizable. (See Table 22-1 and Figure 22-6 for malaria parasite morphology.)

Thick Smears

1. Place one drop of blood from a finger stick on a thoroughly clean slide labeled with the patient's name, the date, and the time.
2. Using the tip of a broken wooden applicator stick or pointed edge of a glass slide, evenly spread out the blood with a circular motion to a diameter of 1 to 2 cm. (See Chapter 25 for further details of making thick and thin malaria smears.)
3. Air dry for at least 30 minutes in an environment protected from flies, since the blood can be removed from the slide during the drying period.
4. Immerse in distilled water until all hemoglobin is removed.
5. Flood with properly diluted (usually 1:20) and buffered (pH 6.4) Giemsa stain for 20 to 30 minutes.
6. Wash with buffered water (pH 7.0).
7. Air dry.
8. Examine under high-dry magnification for gametocytes (observing for other diseases in addition, such as evidence of microfilaria), and then with the oil immersion objective.

Figure 22-4. Pattern for moving the slide to examine cells.

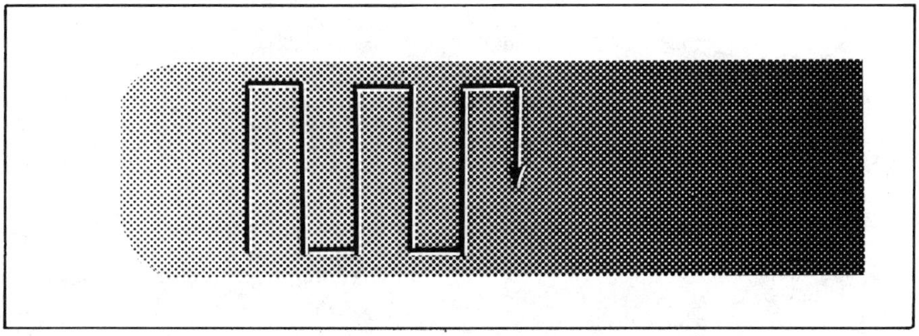

Thin Smears

1. Place one drop of blood from a finger stick toward the end of a clean glass slide. Using the edge of a second slide, smear the blood over a 2 to 3 cm^2 area, obtaining a "feathered edge" as when preparing a slide for routine hematologic examination.
2. Air dry.
3. Fix in absolute methanol for one minute.
4. Air dry.
5. Flood with diluted (1:20) Giemsa stain buffered to pH 6.4 for 20 to 30 minutes.
6. Rinse with buffered water (pH 7.0).
7. Air dry.
8. Examine under high-dry and then oil immersion objectives.

Staining Material for Bacteria

Gram's Stain

The Gram's stain technique is the same regardless of the consistency of the specimen. A thin smear should be made of samples that contain large amounts of debris such as sputum or feces. If a specimen is very thin, inscribing a circle on the slide with a diamond marker or wax pencil helps to locate the specimen after staining. Sputum samples should be examined before placement on the slide for the best areas of purulence (globular gray-green). Sputum specimens with greater than 25 squamous epithelial cells per low-power field generally indicate significant contamination with oral–pharyngeal secretions.

Solutions Required

The Gram's stain requires the following solutions:

- Crystal (gentian) violet.
- Gram's iodine stain (This can be made either by diluting 60 ml Lugol's solution [3.0 g of iodine crystals, 6.0 g of potassium iodide, 60 ml of distilled water] with 840 ml of distilled water, or by mixing directly 1.0 g of iodine and 2.0 g of potassium iodide in 300 ml of distilled water. The solution is stable for about two weeks.
- Decolorizing mixture. (Although plain 95% ethanol can be used alone, a 50/50 mix of this with acetone generally works better.)
- Safranin solution.

Gram's Stain Procedure

1. Apply the specimen to a clean microscope slide.
2. Air dry and gently heat fix.
3. Flood the slide with crystal (gentian) violet for one minute.
4. Wash with water.
5. Cover the slide for one minute with Gram's iodine.
6. Wash with water.
7. With the slide at a 45° angle, apply the 50/50 mixture of 95 percent ethanol and ace-

Table 22-1. Important Morphologic Characteristics Useful for Species Diagnosis in Human Malaria as Seen on Giemsa Smears

Species	Infected RBCs	Trophozoite	Schizont	Gametocyte
P. falciparum	Normal size; multiply infected RBCs seen more often than with other species	Small rings with beadlike cytoplasm (blue) and double chromatin dots (red)	Seldom seen in peripheral blood smear	Diagnostic banana-shaped gametocyte
P. vivax	Enlarged in size; Schuffner's dots (red) present	Ameboid cytoplasm	Can be seen on smear	Round
P. malariae	Somewhat enlarged	Compact cytoplasm	Merozoites arranged in rosette around central pigment clump	Round

tone until the crystal violet is no longer coming off the slide. This takes about five to ten seconds and is the most critical step of the Gram's stain procedure. If the decolorizing solution is applied for too long, gram-positive organisms may become decolorized and will falsely appear as gram-negative organisms after the safranin counterstain is applied.
8. Wash with water.
9. Counterstain with safranin for 30 seconds.
10. Wash with water.
11. Air dry, or gently blot dry with a clean paper towel.

Acid-Fast Bacillus (AFB) Staining

Presented here is the modified Kinyoun's acid-fast stain. It is used to detect *Mycobacterium* organisms such as tuberculosis. *Mycobacterium leprae* can also be seen using the same technique but only for sputum, urine, tissue pulp, and similar samples. This is not the proper technique for staining leprosy biopsy specimens. A positive red-staining bacillus is usually a mycobacterium, but *Nocardia* species may also appear partially acid fast.

AFB staining requires the following solutions:

- Kinyoun carbol-fuchsin solution. (This is made by dissolving 4.0 g of basic fuchsin in 20 ml of 95% alcohol. Then 8 ml of liquefied phenol and 100 ml of distilled water are added.)
- Fifty percent ethanol. (Dilute 52.5 ml of 95% ethanol with 47.5 ml of distilled water.)
- One percent sulfuric acid decolorizer. (Add 1.0 ml of concentrated sulfuric acid to 99 ml of distilled water.)
- Methylene blue counterstain. (Dissolve 2.5 g of methylene blue in 100 ml of 95% ethanol.)

Procedure for Staining

1. Ideally, since the staining can be variable and difficult to interpret, simultaneous known positive and negative controls should be included.
2. Air dry and gently heat fix the smears.
3. Flood the slide with Kinyoun carbol-fuchsin stain, and let stand for two minutes.
4. Pour off excess stain and rinse with water.
5. Drop by drop, decolorize with acid-alcohol until the decolorizer flows colorless.
6. Rinse with water.
7. Counterstain with methylene blue for 30 seconds.
8. Rinse with water.
9. Air dry. Do not blot.

Stool Analysis

Examination for Fecal Leukocytes

There appears to be a good correlation between the presence of leukocytes in diarrheal stools and certain invasive bacterial enteric pathogens, especially *Salmonella* and *Shigella.* Viral and parasitic diarrheas are rarely associated with the finding of significantly increased leukocytes in the stool.

The procedure is simple. A small fleck of stool is placed on a clean glass slide. Although adding two drops of methylene blue makes it easier to distinguish the leukocytes, staining is not required. A coverslip is placed on the slide, and the specimen is examined with the high-dry lens. Findings are positive if there are greater than ten leukocytes per high-power field in more than five fields.

Stool Concentration Technique

Although stool concentration is not necessary for identification of moderate to heavy numbers of parasites in stool, a method for concentrating the stool is helpful if a diagnosis is needed on patients with light parasite burdens in the stool. One useful technique is as follows:

1. Place approximately 0.5 g of fecal material into a centrifuge tube.
2. Add 1 ml of formol-saline (50 ml of formalin in 450 ml of normal saline) until a uniform suspension is obtained.
3. Add 8 ml of formol-saline, mixing thoroughly with a wooden applicator stick.
4. Centrifuge at 800 rpm for five minutes or allow to separate by gravity for one to two hours.
5. Gently pour off the fluid, leaving the sediment in the tube.
6. Add 8 ml formol-saline and mix to obtain a uniform suspension.
7. Add 2 ml of ethyl acetate to the fecal suspension.
8. Cap the tube and mix by inversion.
9. Centrifuge at 800 rpm for five minutes or allow to separate by gravity for one to two hours.

10. Pour off the top layer. Occasionally, the fat plug may have to be reamed with an applicator stick.
11. The remaining sediment contains concentrated ova, parasties, and bacteria with vegetable matter removed.

Stool Examination for Ova and Parasites

A simple wet prep is the most useful examination for ova and parasites. This is done by mixing a small specimen of stool with one drop of normal saline on the slide. Examine under low power to locate the parasite and under high-dry power to identify the organism.

For further identification of protozoa, it is helpful to stain a portion of the slide with an iodine solution, such as a 1:14 dilution of Logol's stock solution (10 g of potassium iodine, 5 g of iodine crystals, with 100 ml of distilled water). The same working solution can be mixed directly without an intermediate stock solution (e.g., 1 g of potassium iodine, 0.5 g of iodine crystals, plus 140 ml of distilled water). The disadvantage of the latter technique is that the working solution must be mixed fresh daily, while the stock solution can be stored for about four weeks.

Stool samples should be examined microscopically within a few hours after collection. Cysts will remain intact for a few days, but trophozoites can be seen only for about one to three hours before they deteriorate. If longer periods of delay are anticipated, freshly passed stool specimens should be placed in formalin or another appropriate preservative. (See Figure 22-5 for relative sizes of protozoa and helminths in stool.)

Urinalysis

Examination of urine in the diagnosis of infectious diseases is done by determining the presence of glucose, protein, red blood cells, white blood cells, casts, and bacteria. In addition, management of acute illness can be monitored by measuring urine volume and specific gravity. The first step in urine examination is to collect urine uncontaminated by vaginal or urethral discharge material. This is best done by using a midstream "clean catch" of the urine. Urine should be examined soon after collection so that cells are not allowed to disappear by lysis and bacteria are not able to grow.

Testing of urine for glucose and protein is done by use of "dipstick" kits and recording the shade or color of reagents impregnated in the cardboard stick. The presence of large amounts of glucose will indicate diabetes and the kinds of bacterial infection associated with diabetes will be more likely. Excessive amounts of protein will indicate glomerular damage, which is common in streptococcal infections as well as numerous other microbial diseases including malaria, schistosomiasis, and leprosy. The specific gravity of urine at room temperature is measured with a hydrometer.

Examination of the urine sediment is done by centrifugation of 10 ml of urine at 2000 rpm for five minutes, removal of 9 ml of the supernate, and resuspension of the sediment in the remaining 1 ml. Thus, a tenfold concentration of cellular elements and bacteria is achieved. A drop of the urine is placed on a slide and a 22-mm coverslip is placed over it. This is examined using the low-power microscope objective (10×) and indirect lighting. The casts (clumps of cells in the shape of collecting tubules) are counted under low power and the number per ten fields recorded. Under high-power magnification (40 to 45× objective) the number of erythrocytes and white blood cells per high-power field is determined. Increased numbers of white cells indicates bladder infection. Increased numbers of erythrocytes may indicate infection or urinary tract trauma or tumor.

Recording the presence of bacteria, fungi, protozoa, or helminth ova in the urine may be of diagnostic value. Bacteria seen by oil immersion microscopy in uncentrifuged, unstained fresh urine indicates more than 100,000 organisms per milliliter; urinary tract infection is very likely. Sedimented urine samples may be Gram stained to distinguish urinary tract infection due to gram-negative rods from the occasional infection with gram-positive cocci (see Chapter 36). Occasionally, helminths (schistosome ova), protozoa (trichomonads), or fungi *(Candida)* may be seen in the urine and can cause hematuria or pyuria. Urine culture and antibiotic sensitivities are of use in recurrent, complicated urinary tract infections, but in a refugee setting they are of limited value (see Chapter 36).

Serologic Testing

In a refugee setting, serologic testing may be unavailable but, if they are accessible, kits or reagents may be very useful for diagnosis of syphilis, typhoid fever, and meningococcal meningitis. Common methods include latex agglutination for bacterial antibodies, and the card test for syphilis.

Agglutination Test

Agglutination tests are done using organisms or other particles, such as latex, bentonite, or red blood cells coated with the appropriate antigen, which are mixed with the patient's serum in various dilutions to determine the presence of antibody to the specific microbial antigens. Serial twofold dilutions of serum are used and the highest dilution of serum that yields visible agglutination is recorded as the antibody titer. These tests are potentially useful in the refugee setting because they usually require only test tubes for making dilutions of serum with sodium chloride, clean slides or multiwell plates for mixing the serum and antigen, and a quality control system including known positive and negative sera. The exact steps for the agglutination will vary depending on the antigen, the particle, and the quality control procedures. These steps should be included in the instructions provided with the antigen-control sera kit. The slide agglutination test is the assay most easily done in the field. A drop of antigen-coated latex or bentonite particles is mixed thoroughly with a drop of serum. The degree of flocculation of the white particles is read visually by holding the slide in indirect light against a black background.

The diseases most likely to be evaluated with agglutination tests include salmonellosis (typhoid), brucellosis, and amebiasis. Another use of agglutination tests is for identification of bacteria grown on blood agar, chocolate agar, or MacConkey's agar plates. A colony of bacteria is mixed with the known antisera for identification of the organism. These tests depend on the availability of antisera, but are most likely helpful in identifying *Salmonella, Shigella,* meningococcus, pneumococcus, and *Hemophilus* infections (see the section on cultures).

Rapid Plasma Reagin Card Test

The rapid plasma reagin (RPR) card test is a nontreponemal testing procedure for the serologic detection of syphilis. RPR card antigen suspension is a carbon-containing cardiolipin antigen that detects "reagin," an antibodylike substance present in sera of syphilitic patients and occasionally in sera of others with acute or chronic conditions unrelated to *Treponema pallidum.* When a specimen contains reagin, flocculation occurs with a coagglutination of the carbon particles of the RPR card antigen, which appear as black clumps against the white background of the card. This coagglutination can be read macroscopically. By contrast, nonreactive specimens appear to have an even, light gray color.

Materials Needed

The agglutination test requires the following materials:

- RPR card antigen (store at 2 to 8°C). Allow the antigen to warm to room temperature—23 to 29°C—before use. Shake ampule vigorously for 10 to 15 seconds before opening.
- Brewer diagnostic cards.
- Dispenstirs.
- Dispensing bottle and needle. [The 20-gauge needle is calibrated to deliver 30 drops (±1 drop) per 0.5 ml of antigen.]
- Control sera, including reactive, weakly reactive, and nonreactive human serum.
- Rotator—95 to 110 rpm.
- Moisture chamber cover.

Procedure

1. Using a clean Dispenstir for each specimen, add control and patient sera to individual wells of the card.
2. Gently shake the antigen-dispensing bottle before use. Holding it in a vertical position, dispense one or two drops to make sure the needle passage is clear. Place one drop of antigen onto each test area. *Do not restir* because mixing of the antigen and specimen is accomplished during rotation.
3. Place the card on the rotator with a moisture cover. Rotate for eight minutes at 100 rpm.
4. Following rotations, to help differentiate nonreactive from minimal reactive results, the card must be briefly rotated and tilted by hand (three or four times). Immediately read the card macroscopically under a high-intensity lamp; do not read under fluorescent lighting.
5. If the control results are satisfactory, record control and patient results on the worksheet. If control results are unsatisfactory, the test must be repeated using new controls and/or antigen.

Technical Notes

Lipemia will not interfere with the RPR card test unless it is at such a high level that it obscures the state of the antigen particles.

Slight hemolysis will not interfere. However, a specimen should be rejected if it is so hemolyzed that printed matter cannot be read through it.

RPR antigen suspension must be stored at 2 to 8°C and brought to room temperature (23 to 29°C) before use. Storage in sunlight or at temperatures above 30°C may cause the antigen to appear rough with nonreactive sera. If the ampule of antigen is frozen during shipment, it can be reconstituted once by warming to room temperature. Repeated freezing and thawing should be avoided. Immediate use of a refrigerated antigen may decrease the sensitivity of the test.

Interpretation

- Reactive—shows characteristic clumping ranging from slight but definite (minimal reactive) to marked and intense (reactive).
- Nonreactive—shows slight roughness or no clumping.

There are only two possible reports with the card test—reactive or nonreactive—regardless of the degree of reactivity. Minimal or moderate reactive (showing slight but definite clumping) is always reported as reactive.

Bacterial Culture

Bacterial culture facilities are usually not available in a refugee setting. One should be aware that if agglutination testing of sera for identifying bacteria is available, systems for growing colonies of bacteria to be tested can be organized easily. One needs the following equipment: 37°C incubator, culture dishes, appropriate agar media, and wire loops for streaking and selecting colonies of bacteria.

At a minimum, if culturing is to be done, three kinds of medium should be used: blood agar, chocolate agar, and an enteric bacterial differential medium such as MacConkey's. With these culture dishes, specimens of sputum, spinal fluid, exudative fluid, and feces can be tested for the most common bacteria. In addition, disks impregnated with various antibiotics may be available. These make it possible to detect resistance or sensitivity of the organism to antibiotics, even in the absence of genus and species taxonomic classification of the organism.

Blood agar is useful for culturing exudates and sputum in order to identify important causes of disease such as staphylococci or streptococci. Chocolate agar is useful for culturing spinal fluid, sputum, and exudates for the growth of *Hemophilus* and *Neisseria,* and MacConkey's differential media will allow culture of feces and identification of the colorless colonies of organisms such as *Salmonella* and *Shigella,* which do not ferment lactose.

MORPHOLOGY OF IMPORTANT BLOOD AND STOOL PARASITES

Figure 22-5 shows the major morphologic features and sizes of protozoa and helminths found in stool specimens. The diseases associated with these organisms are described in Chapter 35. When examining stool specimens, the low-power objective is used (10× objective and a 10× eyepiece). Under this magnification, the eggs 50 to 60 μ in length will fill 1/20 of the field, while those 100 to 120 μm in length will fill 1/10 of the field. With the high-power objective (40×) the 50-μ eggs will fill 1/5 of the microscopic field. Under the high-power objective, a protozoan, such as a *Giardia* cyst, will fill only 1/25 of the field. For protozoa, the oil immersion lens should be used (100× objective) to examine details of the organism. The *Giardia* cyst will fill 1/10 of an oil immersion microscopic field. *Entamoeba coli* trophozoites and cysts are not pathogens, but they are included in the figure because they are commonly confused with *E. histolytica.* Red blood cells and white blood cells in stool may be used to judge relative sizes of parasites (RBC = 6 to 8 μ ; WBC = 15 to 20 μ).

Figure 22-6 shows photomicrographs of two important blood protozoa (malaria, trypanosomes) of one bacterium, *Borrelia,* and of one helminth (microfilaria). The malaria smears (Figure 22-6*A* to *C*) are evaluated using the oil immersion objective. Figure 22-6*A* shows the typical delicate ring with double chromatin dots of *P. falciparum.* Figure 22-6*B* shows a heavy *P. falciparum* infection with numerous ring-form nuclei and one gametocyte. Figure 22-6*C* shows a trophozoite and segmented form of *P. vivax.* Figure 22-6*D* shows the characteristic picture of an extracellular flagellate,

Figure 22-5. Major morphologic features and size of protozoa and helminths found in stool specimens.

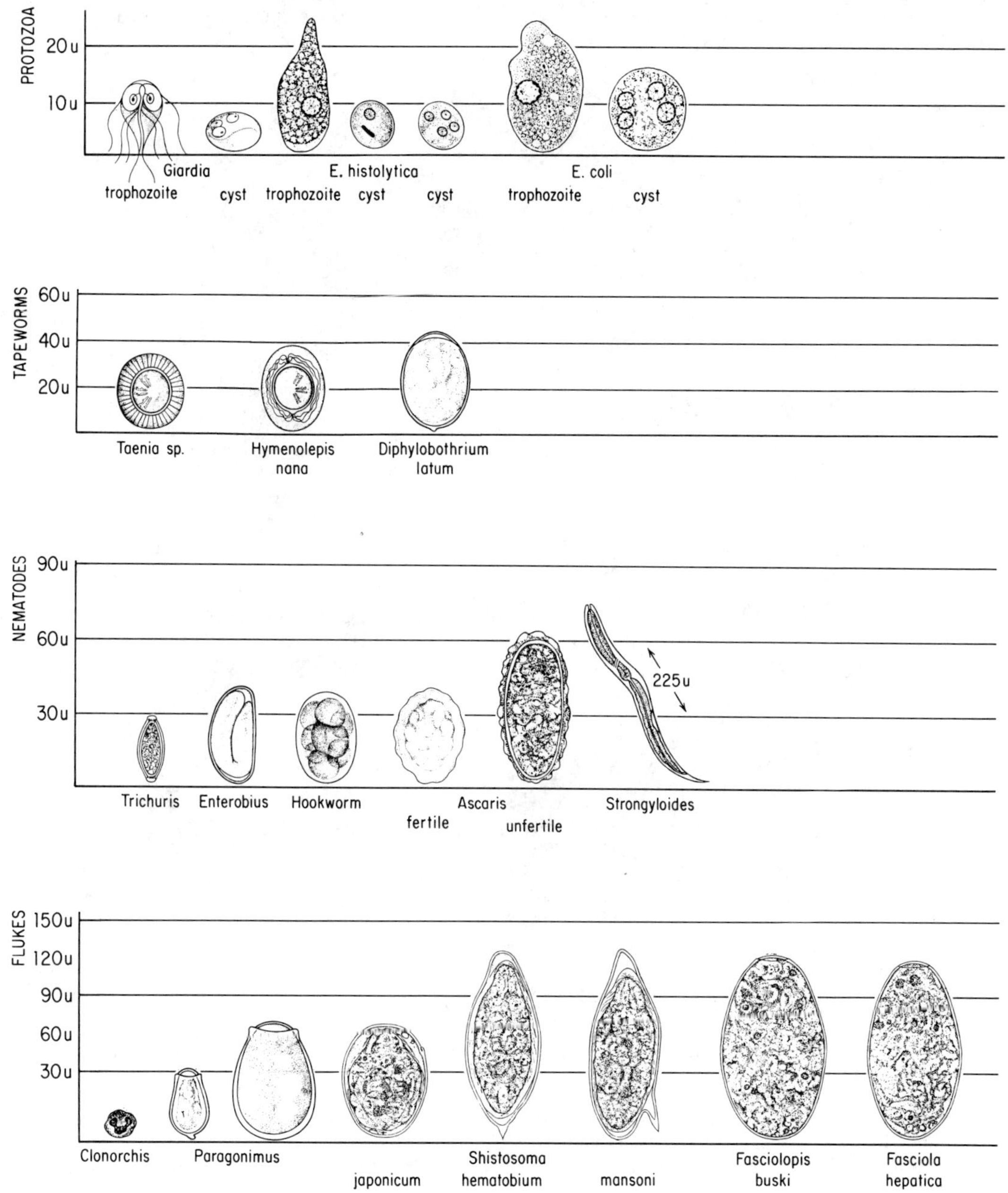

Tryanosoma rhodesiense. Figure 22-6*E* shows the threadlike extracellular bacteria *Borrelia recurrentis.* Figure 22-6*F* is a low-power microphotograph of the microfilaria of *W. bancrofti,* the cause of filariasis. Note the size of the microfilaria in relation to the leukocyte nuclei and compared with the leukocyte in Figure 22-6*D.*

Figure 22-6. Photomicrographs of three blood protozoa and one helminth. *A*, *B*, *C* are malaria smears using oil immersion objective: (*A*) ring with double chromatin dots of *P. falciparum;* (*B*) a heavy *P. falciparum* infection with numerous ring-form nuclei and one gametocyte; and (*C*) trophozoite and segmented form of *P. vivax;* (*D*) *trypanosoma rhodesiense;* (*E*) *Borrelia recurrentis;* (*F*) high-power view of *W. bancrofti.*

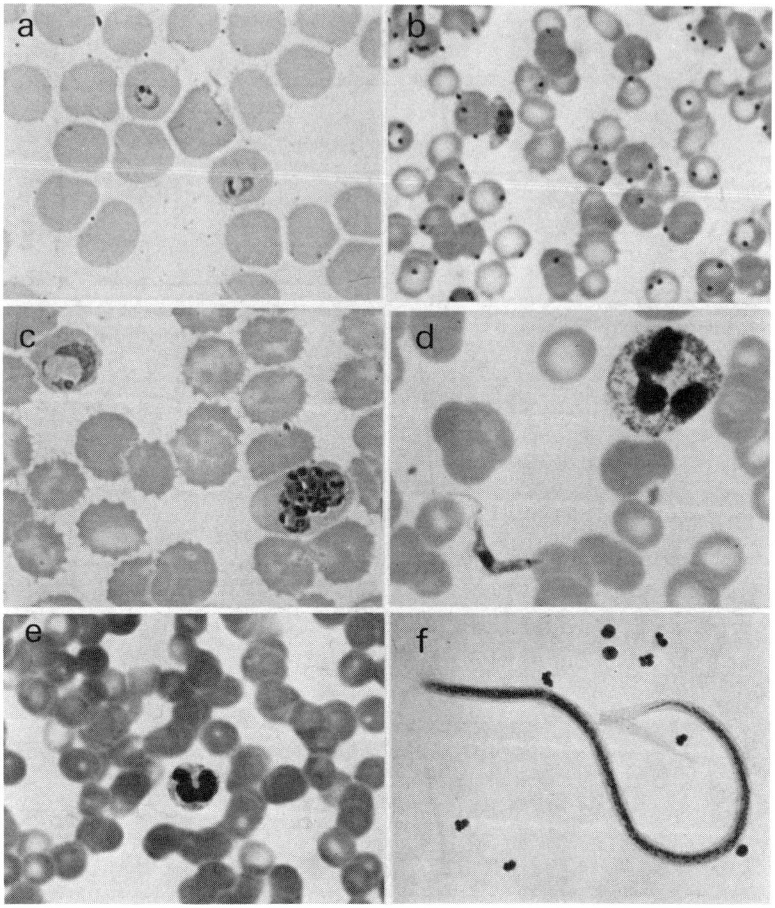

REFERENCES AND SELECTED READING

Bradley GM, Benson ES: Examination of the urine. In Davidson I, Henry JB (eds): Clinical Diagnosis by Laboratory Methods, 15th ed, pp 15–83. Philadelphia, Saunders, 1974.

Brown BA: Hematology: Principles and Procedures, 3rd ed, pp 75–81. Philadelphia, Lea & Febizer, 1980.

Cheesbrough M: Medical Laboratory Manual for Tropical Countries. Vol. 2. Microbiology. Cambridgeshire, England, Tropical Health Technology, 1984.

Henry JB: Clinical Diagnosis and Management by Laboratory Methods, 16th ed, pp. 892–93. Philadelphia, Saunders, 1979.

Shaffer JD, Goldin M: Medical microbiology. In Davidson I, Henry JB (eds): Clinical Diagnosis by Laboratory Methods, 15 ed, pp 921–1019. Philadelphia, Saunders, 1974.

Sonnenwirth AC, Jarrett L (eds): Gradwohl's Clinical Laboratory Methods and Diagnosis, 8th ed, pp 640–43; 763–64. St. Louis, Mosby, 1980.

U.S. Department of HEW: Manual of Tests for Syphilis. Atlanta, Centers for Disease Control, 1969.

23
Drug Choice and Usage

THEODORE C. M. LI
THOMAS C. JONES

This chapter provides a rapid guide to drug choice and usage with special emphasis on infectious diseases. Antimicrobial drug choice is organized by organ system rather than by infectious agent, since it is the differential diagnosis of organ dysfunction that the clinician is facing. The treatment of *S. haematobium* is therefore found in the genitourinary section, whereas *S. mansoni* is in the gastrointestinal section. The organization parallels the review of systems used in history taking: general (including undifferentiated fever), skin, ears, eyes, nose, and throat, lymphatics, lung, gastrointestinal tract, genitourinary tract, extremities, and central nervous system. Each section is subdivided according to common clinical entities, the usual causitive organisms, and the antimicrobial agents of choice.

After locating the drug(s) of choice, the reader should refer to Appendix 23-A for specific dosage schedules and adverse drug reactions. It would be best to consult this book's index for further references on the disease or drug of interest, since many are discussed in detail elsewhere. Specifically, Chapters 25, 29, 33, and 37, should be consulted for more detailed treatment schedules for malaria, leprosy, tuberculosis, and sexually transmitted diseases, respectively.

The antimicrobials listed have been limited to those most likely to be available in a refugee setting. For example, second- and third-generation cephalosporins are not included even though they might be preferable. An exception is ceftriaxone. Since its long half-life permits twice-daily dosing, ceftriaxone might occasionally be a cost-effective alternative in the treatment of meningitis.

Cost and efficacy are critical in refugee care. Table 23-1 provides a list of common antimicrobial drugs and their direct purchase cost from pharmaceutical companies in the United States. Prices in other countries may differ. The list demonstrates that although one agent, such as doxycycline, might have better bioavailability and ease of administration, tetracycline is only one sixth the cost. It is also clear that parenteral drugs are more costly than oral agents. One gram of oral chloramphenicol costs one dollar while the intravenous form is almost five times more expensive.

Another important consideration for drug use in refugee camps is the stability of these agents when exposed to heat, sunlight, and humidity. Table 23-2 is a list of the major drugs suggested by the WHO for emergency settings, organized by their temperature stability. Finally, Appendix 23-B lists the dosages for non-antibiotic medications selected from the WHO emergency drug list (WHO 1983).

There are a few special considerations for antibiotic usage in children. Dosages should be calculated in milligrams per kilogram (Appendix 23-A). In general, neonates require a lower dose than older infants and children because of their slower renal and hepatic elimination and metabolism. Three classes of drugs deserve special mention for use in children.

- The use of chloramphenicol should be avoided in premature infants and normal newborns since it causes an often-fatal "gray syndrome." Chloramphenicol can cause bone marrow suppression in all patients, and consideration should be given to obtaining hematocrits and reticulocyte counts every few days while patients are taking this drug.
- The tetracycline drugs can lead to permanent staining of teeth and growth retardation. These drugs should be avoided in growing children when possible (especially for those under eight years of age), and for pregnant women.

• The use of drugs such as sulfonamides, anticonvulsants, and penicillins, and infections with a few organisms such as *Mycoplasma pneumoniae,* have been associated with an increased risk of developing Stevens–Johnson syndrome. This presents as erythema multiforme with rapidly advancing erythematous and vesiculobullous skin and mucosal lesions. Mortality may be as high at 10 percent.

Every effort has been made to ensure the accuracy of the drug dosage information con-

Table 23-1. Representative Examples of Antimicrobial Cost

Drug	Route	Dose	Cost (US$)
Antibacterials			
INH	po	300 mg	0.02
Sulfisoxazole	po	500 mg	0.04
Penicillin VK	po	500 mg	0.05
Tetracycline	po	500 mg	0.05
Ampicillin	po	500 mg	0.11
Erythromycin	po	500 mg	0.15
Ethambutol	po	100 mg	0.15
Amoxicillin	po	500 mg	0.23
Chloramphenicol	po	250 mg	0.25
Pyrazinamide	po	500 mg	0.42
Sulfa/trimethoprim	po	1 tablet	0.45
Doxycycline	po	100 mg	0.61
Rifampin	po	300 mg	0.89
Penicillin G	IM,IV	1 million U	0.94
Cephalexin	po	500 mg	1.14
Streptomycin	IM	1 g	1.21
Gentamicin	IM,IV	80 mg	1.77
Chloramphenicol	IV	1 g	4.72
Cefazolin	IV	1 g	5.73
Nafcillin	IV	1 g	5.95
Cefoxitin	IV	1 g	6.82
Vancomycin	IV	500 mg	17.91
Antiparasitic			
Quinine	po	300 mg	0.08
Quinacrine	po	100 mg	0.12
Thiabendazole	po	500 mg	0.35
Metronidazole	po	500 mg	0.53
Chloroquine	po	500 mg	0.98
Sulfa/ pyrimethamine	po	1 tablet	1.19
Niclosamide	po	500 mg	1.49
Mebendazole	po	100 mg	2.37
Praziquantel	po	600 mg	5.50
Pyrantel pamoate	po	60 ml	15.25

Table 23-2. WHO Drug List Organized by Temperature Stability

A. Refrigerate at 2 to 8°C (35 to 46°F)
   - Procaine benzylpenicillin injection

B. Store at or below 30°C (86°F)
   - All creams and ointments
   - Aspirin
   - Benzylpenicillin and phenoxymethylpenicillin (dry forms for reconstitution)
   - Phenoxymethylpenicillin tablets
   - Glyceryl trinitrate (nitroglycerin)
   - Sulfadimidine tablets
   - Tetracycline tablets

C. If facilities permit, store at or below 30°C (86°F)
   - Chloramphenicol caps
   - Chlorihexidine
   - Cloxacillin caps
   - Codeine tabs
   - Dextran (structural changes if temperature exceeds 100°F)
   - Diazepam tabs and injectable
   - Digoxin tabs and injectable
   - Ergometrine (ergonavine) tabs and injectable
   - Furosemide injectable
   - Hydrocortisone injectable
   - Iodine solution (temperature not to exceed 35°C, 95°F)
   - Isoprenaline (isoproterenol) injectable
   - Mebendazole caps
   - Metronidazole tabs
   - Niclosamide tabs
   - Promethazine tabs, syrup
   - Quinine injectable
   - Retinol
   - Sulfadoxine pryimethamine tabs
   - Sulfamethoxazole trimethoprim tabs

D. Medications unlikely to lose significant potency when stored for 3 to 6 months at over 30°C (86°F)
   - Aluminum hydroxide tabs
   - Beclomethasone for inhalation
   - Benzyl benzoate lotion
   - Chloroquine tabs, syrup
   - Chlorphenamine tabs
   - Ferrous salt-folic acid
   - Furosemide tabs
   - Gentian violet crystals
   - Oral rehydrations solution (dry for mixing)
   - Lidocaine injectable
   - Paracetamol (acetaminophen)
   - Pethidine (meperidine)
   - Piperazine tabs, syrup
   - Propranolol tabs

Table 23-2. WHO Drug List Organized by Temperature Stability (*Continued*)

D. Medications unlikely to lose significant potency when stored for 3 to 6 months at over 30°C (86°F)
- Salbutamol for inhalation
- Senna (vegetable product—protects from insects and rodents)
- Sodium chloride injectable
- Thiabendazole tabs
- Water for injection

[a]This is a complete list of the drugs recommended for use in refugee camps by the World Health Organization (WHO 1983), arranged according to their temperature stability by Barry Bunting, BS Pharm. To minimize drug degradation it is also important to protect pharmaceuticals from moisture and sunlight. Medications that are photosensitive are usually supplied in light-resistant containers, and these should be used when possible.

tained here, but the clinician should check with product inserts, the Centers for Disease Control, and other sources for recent changes.

DISEASES PRESENTING WITH FEVER, WITH OR WITHOUT ORGAN SYSTEM LOCALIZATION

Fever or other signs of sepsis, such as tachypnea or hypotension, will be the only manifestations in several bacterial, rickettsial, and protozoal diseases. Treatments for the most common or important of these are listed below. Clinical and laboratory clues that may aid in distinguishing these diseases are described in Chapters 22, 24, and 25. The most important antibiotics for use in these conditions are chloramphenicol, penicillin, tetracycline, quinine, and metronidazole.

Diseases	*Organism(s)*	*Primary Choice*	*Alternatives*
Typhoid fever	*Salmonella typhi*	Chloramphenicol × 2 weeks	Ampicillin; SMX/TMP
Neonatal sepsis	Group B streptococcus, *E. coli, Listeria,* etc.	Gentamicin and ampicillin × 1–2 weeks	
Leptospirosis	*L. icterohemorrhagiae, L. pomona,* etc.	Penicillin G	Tetracycline; ampicillin
Brucellosis	*B. melitensis, B. suis*	Tetracycline × 3 weeks and Streptomycin × 2 weeks	SMX/TMP × 4 weeks
Louse, murine or scrub typhus	*R. prowazekii, R. typhi, R. tsutsugamushi*	Tetracycline	Doxycycline; chloramphenicol
Amebiasis	*E. histolytica*	Metronidazole × 10 days plus iodoquinol × 20 days	Emetine or dihydroemetine × 10 days, then chloroquine × 2 weeks plus iodoquinol × 20 days
Visceral leishmaniasis	*L. donovani*	Stibogluconate sodium × 10–30 days	Pentamidine × 2–3 weeks
Malaria		See Chapter 25	
Trypanosomiasis	*T. gambiense* (early)	Pentamidine isethionate × 10 days	Suramin
	T. rhodesiense (early)	Suramin	Pentamidine isethionate
	T. gambiense or *T. rhodesiense* (late)	Suramin and melarsoprol	Suramin and tryparsamide

SKIN INFECTIONS

Skin infections are caused by external injuries, such as bruises, animal bites, trauma, and ectoparasites, often with secondary bacterial infection; or the skin may be one manifestation of systemic disease, such as scrub typhus, leprosy, meningococcemia (see Brain and Meninges section); or the skin may be the primary site of microbial-induced inflammation such as dermatomycoses, cutaneous leishmaniasis, cutaneous treponemes, scabies, or impetigo. Treatments for various skin disorders are listed below.

Diseases	*Organism(s)*	*Primary Choice*	*Alternatives*
Cellulitis			
Abscess (−)	Group A *Streptococcus*	Penicillin	Erythromycin
Abscess (+)	*S. aureus* or Group A *Streptococcus*	PCNase-resistant penicillin	Cephalosporin; erythromycin
Erysipelas	Group A *Streptococcus*	Penicillin	Erythromycin
Impetigo (bullous)	*S. aureus*	PCNase-resistant penicillin	Cephalosporin
Impetigo	Group A *Streptococcus*	Penicillin	Erythromycin
Specific skin diseases			
Anthrax	*B. anthracis*	Penicillin G, 2 million units IV q 6 h until edema subsides, then penicillin VK for 7–10 days	Erythromycin × 5–7 days; tetracycline × 5–7 days
Scrub typhus	*R. tsutsugamushi*	Tetracycline × 3–7 days	Chloramphenicol × 3–7 days; doxycycline once
Dermatomycosis	*Candida, Microsporium Trichophyton*	Clotrimazole	Nystatin
Hanson's disease (leprosy)	M. leprae	See Chapter 29	
Treponemes			
Syphilis, bejel, pinta, yaws	*T. pallidum, T. pallidum* (var), *T. carateum, T. pertenue*	Benzathine penicillin once	*Tetracycline × 10 days, erythromycin × 10 days*
Parasites			
Cutaneous leishmaniasis	*L. tropica, L. braziliensis*	Stibogluconate sodium × 20–30 days	Pentamidine × 3 weeks
Loiasis	*Loa loa*	Diethylcarbamazine × 2–3 weeks	
Onchocerciasis	*O. volvulus*	Ivermectin once	Diethylcarbamazine followed by suramin (add steroids, e.g., dexamethasone 2 mg/dose bid with heavy infection); mebendazole
Bites			
Dog	*P. multocida, S. aureus,* anaerobes	Penicillin or ampicillin	Tetracycline
Human	Group A *Streptococcus,* Non-Group A *Streptococcus,*	Penicillin	Add PCNase-resistant penicillin if *Staphylococcus* is suspected

Diseases	*Organism(s)*	*Primary Choice*	*Alternatives*
	S. aureus, anaerobes, gram-negative bacteria		
Ectoparasites			
Lice		Pyrethrins to affected areas × 10 minutes, repeat in 1 week.	Benzobenzoate to affected areas × 8–12 hours
Scabies	Mites	Gamma-benzene hexachloride, apply from neck down for 8–12 hours × 1	Crotamiton 10 percent, apply from neck down for 12 hours × 3 days; benzyl benzoate, apply from neck down for 8-12 hours
Burns			
Clean	———	Silver sulfadiazine	Silver nitrate
Infected	Gram-negative bacteria	Sulfamylon	

EYE, EAR, SINUS, MOUTH, AND THROAT INFECTIONS

Bacterial infections localized to the orifices of the head are very common in refugee populations and they can become serious in malnourished patients or in those immunosuppressed by systemic disease. Otitis media is a major cause of illness among children. Poor dentition leads to oral cavity abscesses. Treatments for the most common of these conditions are listed below.

Diseases	*Organism(s)*	*Primary Choice*	*Alternatives*
Conjunctivitis			
Bacterial	*S. pneumoniae, S. aureus, H. influenza*	Erythromycin ointment every 2 hours × 7 days	Bacitracin ointment every 2 hours × 7 days; chloramphenicol ointment every 2 hours × 7 days
Trachoma	*C. trachomatis*	Tetracycline po × 3–4 weeks	Erythromycin po × 3–4 weeks; SMX/TMP po × 3–4 weeks; sulfonamide, tetracycline, erythromycin, or rifampin ointment four times a day, × 6 weeks
Viral	Adenoviruses	None	
Keratitis			
Bacterial	*S. aureus*	PCNase-resistant penicillin by subconjunctival injection, and erythromycin ointment every 2 hours	
	Pseudomonas	Colistin or gentamicin, subconjunctival	

Diseases	*Organism(s)*	*Primary Choice*	*Alternatives*
		injection, and polymyxin ointment	
	S. pneumoniae, N. gonorrheae	Penicillin G, subconjunctival injection, and penicillin G (high dose) IV every 6 hours and tetracycline ointment	
Parasitic	*O. volvulus*	Surgical excision of primary nodule and ivermectin once or diethylcarbamazine × 19 days followed by suramin × 5 weeks	
Orbital cellulitis			
Children under five years	*H. influenza, S. pneumoniae*	Ampicillin[a]	Chloramphenicol[a]
	Group A *Streptococcus*		
	S. aureus	PCNase-resistant penicillin	
Adults	*S. aureus*	PCNase-resistant penicillin	Cephalosporin
	Group A *Streptococcus, S. pneumoniae*	Penicillin	
External ear infections (otitis externa)			
Uncomplicated otitis externa	*Pseudomonas*	Corticosteroids topically and colistin or polymyxin	Acetic acid (2%) or half-strength Burow solution (aluminum acetate 1:20) topically
Malignant otitis externa	*Pseudomonas*	Carbenicillin and gentamicin	
Furuncle with cellulitis	*S. aureus*	PCNase-resistant penicillin	Erythromycin
Fungal	*Aspergillus*	Acetic acid (2%) or vinegar topically	Tolnaftate solution
Middle ear infections (otitis media)			
Neonate	*S. pneumonia, H. influenazae,* gram-negative rods	Ampicillin and gentamicin	
Children	*S. pneumoniae, H. influenzae*	Ampicillin[a]	SMX/TMP × 7 days
Adults	S. pneumoniae	Penicillin VK Ampicillin	Erythromycin
Mastoiditis	*S. pneumoniae, S. aureus*	PCNase-resistant penicillin	Cephalosporin
Sinusitis			
Acute	*S. pneumoniae, S. aureus,* Group A *Streptococcus,*	Ampicillin (may use phenylephrine drops as adjunct therapy)	SMX/TMP

[a]See footnotes[a–c] on page 263 for important information on treatment of resistant strains of *H. influenzae.*

Diseases	*Organism(s)*	*Primary Choice*	*Alternatives*
	anaerobes (often with dental infections)		
Chronic	Anaerobes	Ampicillin	Clindamycin; penicillin VK
Dental abscess	Mouth flora, anaerobes	Penicillin VK	Tetracycline
Epiglottitis	*H. influenzae*	Chloramphenicol[a]	Ampicillin[a]
Parotitis	*S. aureus*, anaerobes in chronic disease	PCNase-resistant penicillin	
Pharyngitis			
Febrile, exudative	Group A *Streptococcus*	Benzathine penicillin once, or penicillin VK × 7–10 days, bid[b] or tid	Erythromycin
Viral		None	
Membraneous	*C. diphtheriae*	Penicillin VK and diphtheria antitoxin	Erythromycin; tetracycline
Submandibular abscess (Ludwig's angina)	Anaerobes, spirochetes	Clindamycin and drainage	Penicillin VK or chloramphenicol and drainage

DISEASES OF LYMPHATIC TISSUE

Lymphatic inflammation may be divided into inflammation of the groin lymph nodes, which results from genital infection, and more generalized lymphadenopathy from several bacterial or parasitic organisms. Nongenital localized lymphadenitis may arise from cellulitis of the extremities or subtle pharyngitis due to streptococci. In children, tuberculosis may be an important cuase of cervical lymphadenitis. The common causes of lymphadenopathy in a refugee setting and their treatments are listed below.

Diseases	*Organism(s)*	*Primary Choice*	*Alternatives*
Streptococcal lymphadenitis	*Streptococcus*	Penicillin	
Tuberculous lymphadenitis	*M. tuberculosis*	(See Chapter 33)	
Bubonic plague	*Y. pestis*	Streptomycin × 10 days	Tetracycline × 10 days; chloramphenicol × 10 days
Filariasis	*W. bancrofti, W. malayi, W. timori*	Diethylcarbamazine × 3 weeks	
Lymphogranuloma venereum (LGV)	*C. trachomatis*	Tetracycline × 2–3 weeks	Erythromycin × 2–3 weeks; SMX/TMP × 2–3 weeks
Granuloma inguinale	*C. granulomatis*	Tetracycline × 10–14 days	SMX/TMP × 10 days Ampicillin × 10 days
Chancroid	*H. ducreyi*	SMX/TMP 2 tablets/dose × 5 days	Erythromycin × 1–2 weeks; ceftriaxone once
Primary syphilis	*T. pallidum*	Benzathine penicillin 2.4 million U	Tetracycline × 15 days
Sporotrichosis	S. schenckii	Potassium iodide	

[a]See footnotes [a–c] on page 263 for important information on treatment of resistant strains of *H. influenzae.*

[b]Twice daily (bid) dosing is probably as effective for the treatment of streptococcal pharyngitis as tid or qid dosing (Gerber and Markowitz 1985).

LUNG INFECTIONS

The most important lung infections in the refugee setting are bacterial pneumonia, abscess, and tuberculosis. The management of these illnesses are described in Chapters 32 and 33. The most commonly used antibacterial drugs are penicillin and chloramphenicol. The treatments for pulmonary infections are listed below.

Diseases	*Organism(s)*	*Primary Choice*	*Alternatives*
Bacterial pneumonia	*S. pneumonia*	Penicillin[a]	Erythromycin
	H. influenzae	Chloramphenicol[b]	Ampicillin[b]
	S. aureus	PCNase-resistant penicillin	Cephalosporin; erythromycin
	P. pseudomallei	Tetracycline × 60–150 days	Chloramphenicol × 60–150 days; SMX/TMP
Lung abscess	Anaerobes	Clindamycin	Penicillin; chloramphenicol
Aspiration pneumonia	Anaerobes	Penicillin	Clindamycin; chloramphenicol
Cavitary pneumonia			
Tuberculosis	*M. tuberculosis*	See Chapter 33	
Paragonimiasis	*P. westermani*	Praziquantel × 1–2 days	Bithional × 10–15 doses

GASTROINTESTINAL AND HEPATIC DISEASES

Most gastrointestinal infections are associated with diarrhea; their treatment is primarily directed at replacing fluid loss, as described in Chapters 15 and 34. The presence or absence of fecal leukocytes may aid in determining whether erythromycin, SXM/TMP, or tetracycline may be used. Specific stool protozoa or helminths may be treated as the clinical situation dictates, as described in Chapter 35. Hepatic disease consistent with cholangitis or abscess will require both antibacterial and antiamebic therapy.

Diseases	*Organism(s)*	*Primary Choice*	*Alternatives*
Gastroenteritis with stool leukocytes			
Campylobacter enteritis	*Campylobacter* sp.	Erythromycin × 5–7 days	Tetracycline × 5–7 days
Salmonellosis	*Salmonella* sp.	None in uncomplicated diarrhea; with bleeding or sepsis, use ampicillin × 5–6 days	SMX/TMP × 5–6 days
Shigellosis	*Shigella* sp.	SMX/TMP × 5–6 days	Tetracycline 2.5 g once
Intestinal amebiasis	*E. histolytica*	Metronidazole × 5–6 days and iodoquinol × 20 days	Emetine × 5 days and tetracycline × 10 days
Without stool leukocytes			
Viral enteritis		None	
Giardiasis	*G. lamblia*	Quinicrine × 7 days	Metronidazole × 7–10 days or furazolidone × 7 days

[a]Since drug levels obtained with benzathine penicillin alone are too low, full courses of penicillin G or penicillin VK should be used for *S. pneumonia* infections. Penicillin remains the drug of choice for pneumococcal pneumonia throughout most of

Diseases	*Organism(s)*	*Primary Choice*	*Alternatives*
Cholera	*V. cholera*	Tetracycline × 3–4 days	Furazolidone × 3–4 days; SMX/TMP × 3–4 days
Specific intestinal parasites			
Flukes			
Fasciolopsiasis	*F. buski*	Praziquantel × 1 day	
Schistosomiasis	*S. mansoni, S. japonicum*	Praziquantel × 1 day	Oxamniquine once; or niridazole × 2 wk
Roundworms			
Ascariasis	*A. lumbricoides*	Pyrantel pamoate once	Mebendazole × 3 days
Hookworm	*A. duodenale, N. americanus*	Pyrantel pamoate once	Mebendazole × 3 days
Trichuriasis	*T. trichuris*	Mebendazole × 3 days	
Strongyloides	*S. stercoralis*	Thiabendazole × 2 days	Pyrantel pamoate once
Tapeworms			
Fish tapeworm	*D. latum*	Niclosamide once	Praziquantel once
Dwarf tapeworm	*H. nana*	Praziquantel once	Niclosamide × 5–7 days; paramomycin × 5–7 days
Beef tapeworm	*T. saginata*	Niclosamide once	Praziquantel once
Pork tapeworm	*T. solium*	Niclosamide once	Praziquantel once
Cysticercosis	*T. solium* (larval)	Praziquantel (use with high-dose steroids in neurocysticercosis) × 10 days	
Echinococcosis	*E. granulosus*	Surgical removal of cysts	Mebendazole × 3 months (high dose)
Hepatitis	Hepatitis A, B, and non-A, non-B viruses	None	
Hepatic abscess			
Amebic	*E. histolytica*	Metronidazole × 10 days and iodoquinol × 20 days	Emetine × 5 days followed by chloroquine phosphate 600 mg base × 2 days, then 300 mg base QD × 2–3 weeks and iodoquinol × 20 days.
Pyogenic	Anaerobes, gram-negative bacteria	Metronidazole and gentamicin	Chloramphenicol or clindamycin, and gentamicin
Cholangitis and cholecystitis			
Bacterial	Gram-negative bacteria, anaerobes, enterococci	Chloramphenicol or clindamycin, and gentamicin	Metronidazole and gentamicin
Clonorchiasis	*C. sinensis*	Praziquantel × 1 day	
Fasciolasis	F. hepatica	Praziquantel × 1 day	

---

the world. However, a few locals have reported strains of *S. pneumonia* relatively insensitive to the pencillins (Berman and McIntosh 1985).

[b]See footnotes[a−c] on page 263 for important information on treatment of resistant strains of *H. influenzae.*

GENITOURINARY TRACT INFECTIONS

Urinary tract infections are most easily treated with sulfa, SMX/TMP, ampicillin, or Tetracycline. Careful clarification of the cause of the infection, as outlined in Chapter 36, will allow the best therapeutic success. Treatments for genital infections are outlined in Chapter 37 and in this chapter under management of lymphatic infections.

Diseases	*Organism(s)*	*Primary Choice*	*Alternatives*
Cystitis			
Adults			
Initial, nonfebrile	Gram-negative rods	Sulfisoxazole 2 g once	SMX/TMP once; ampicillin 3.5 g once
Recurrent or febrile	Gram-negative rods	SMX/TMP × 1 week	Ampicillin × 1 week; tetracycline × 1 week
	Gram-negative cocci	Ampicillin × 1 week	
Children	Gram-negative rods	Ampicillin × 1 week	Cephalosporin (first generation) × 1 week
Pyelonephritis	Gram-negative rods	Gentamicin	SMX/TMP × 1 week, ampicillin
	Gram-negative cocci	Ampicillin × 1 week	
Schistosomiasis	*S. haematobium*	Praziquantel × 1 day	Metriphonate
Genital infections	See Chapter 37 and this Chapter under Diseases of Lymphatic Tissue		

DISEASES OF JOINT, BONE, AND MUSCLE

Bacterial infections of the joints, bones (osteomyelitis), or muscles require vigorous, often prolonged therapy, sometimes in conjunction with surgical drainage (arthritis) or extensive debridement (gas gangrene).

Diseases	*Organism(s)*	*Primary Choice*	*Alternatives*
Septic arthritis			
Infants and young children	*S. aureus*	PCNase-resistant penicillin × 3 weeks	Cephalosporin × 3 weeks
	H. influenzae[a]	Ampicillin or chloramphenicol × 3 weeks	
Adults	*S. pneumoniae*[b]	Penicillin G (high dose) × 3 weeks	Erythromycin × 3 weeks
	N. gonorrhea	Penicillin G (high dose) × 3 days	Erythromycin; ampicillin and probenecid 1 g once, then 500 mg/dose every 6 hours or tetracycline 1.5 mg once, then 500 mg/dose every 6 hours × 10 days
Osteomyelitis	*S. aureus*	PCNase-resistant penicillin	Cephalosporin; clindamycin
Myositis			
Gas gangrene	*C. perfringens*	Penicillin G (high dose)	Tetracycline; metronidazole
Pyomyositis	*S. aureus*	PCNase-resistant penicillin	Cephalosporin

[a]See footnote[a−c], next page.
[b]See footnote[a] on page 260.

DISEASES OF THE BRAIN AND MENINGES

Treatment of meningitis should be prompt and may precede lumbar puncture. The selection of antibiotics for patients with fever and meningismus is usually based on age and local epidemiology. Therapy may be amended subsequently based on Gram-stain analysis of the CSF.

Diseases	*Organism(s)*	*Primary Choice*	*Alternatives*
Meningitis	Neonatal or infant, organism unknown	Ampicillin and gentamicin	
	Child, organism unknown	Ampicillin[a] or chloramphenicol[a]	Ceftriaxone[a,b], gentimicin plus carbenicillin[a,c]
	Adult organism unknown	Penicillin G	Chloramphenicol or ceftriaxone
	N. meningitis	Penicillin G	Chloramphenicol
	S. pneumoniae[d]	Penicillin G	Chloramphenicol
	Streptococcus	Penicillin G	Chloramphenicol
	H. influenzae	Ampicillin[a] or chloramphenicol[a]	Ceftriaxone[a,b], gentimicin plus carbenicillin[a,c]
	L. monocytogenes	Ampicillin	
	Gram-negative rods	Gentamicin	
Brain abscess	Anaerobes	Chloramphenicol	Metronidazole
	S. aureus	PCNase-resistant penicillin	
	P. falciparum	See Chapter 25	
Malaria			
Trypanosomiasis	*T. gambiense, T. Rhodesiense*	See section on diseases presenting with fevers, in this chapter	

[a]As many as 60% of *H. influenzae* organisms in certain parts of the world may be resistant to ampicillin. These strains are usually sensitive to chloramphenicol. If sensitivity testing is available, both drugs can be started initially, discontinuing one after sensitivities are known. In certain areas of the world where *H. influenzae* is known to be occasionally sensitive to ampicillin but resistant to chloramphenicol, the use of both concomitantly may be considered. Finally, Campos and coworkers (1986) have reported multiply resistant *H. influenzae* type b organisms causing meningitis in Spain. Sixty percent of their 35 cases were resistant to ampicillin, 66% to chloramphenicol, and 57% to both antibiotics. All *H. influenzae* organisms were sensitive to cefotaxime.

[b]Alternatives include other appropriate second- or third- (not first-) generation cephalosporins such as cefuroxime, cefotaxime, or moxalactam.

[c]The combination of gentamicin and carbenicillin has been shown to be effective against multiply resistant *H. Influenzae* organisms (Mathies et al 1986; Uchiyama et al 1980).

[d]See footnote [a] on page 260.

REFERENCES

Abramawicz M (ed): Drugs for parasitic infections. The Medical Letter 1986;28:9–18.

Abramawicz M (ed): Handbook of Antimicrobial Therapy. New Rochelle, NY, The Medical Letter, 1984.

Behrman RE, Vaughan VC: Nelson Textbook of Pediatrics. Philadelphia, WB Saunders, 1983.

Berman S, McIntosh K: Selective primary health care: strategies for control of disease in the developing world. XXI. Acute respiratory infections. Rev Infect Dis 1985;7:674–91.

Campbell WC, Fisher MH, Stapley EO et al: Invermectin: A potent new antiparasitic agent. Science 1983;21: 823–27.

Campos J, Garcia-Tornel S, Gairi JM et al: Multiply resistant *H. influenzae* type b causing meningitis: Comparative clinical and laboratory study. J Pediatr 1986;108:897–902.

Cole CH: The Harriet Lane Handbook. Chicago, Year Book Medical Publishers, 1984.

Conn HF: 1985 Current Therapy. Philadelphia, WB Saunders, 1985.

Drug Information 85. Bethesda, MD, American Society of Hospital Pharmacists, 1985.

Gerber MA, Markowitz M: Management of streptococcal pharyngitis reconsidered. Pediatr Infect Dis 1985;4:518–26.

Goodman LS, Gilman A: The Pharmacological Basis of Therapeutics. New York, Macmillan, 1985.
Mathies AW Jr, Leedom JM, Ivler D et al: Antibiotic antagonism in bacterial meningitis. Antimicrob Agents Chemother 1967;7:218–24.
Peter G, Giebink GS, Hall CB, Plotkin SA (eds): Report of the Committee on Infectious Diseases. 12th ed. Elk Grove Village, IL, American Academy of Pediatrics, 1986.
Physicians' Desk Reference. Oradell, NJ, Medical Economics, 1986.
Sanford JP: Guide to Antimicrobial Therapy. San Antonio, Texas, 1986.
Uchiyama N, Greene GR, Kitts DB et al: Meningitis due to *H. influenzae* type b resistant to ampicillin and chloramphenicol. J Pediatr 1980;97:421–24.
Vaughan D, Asbury T: General Ophthalmology. Los Altos, CA, Lange, 1985.
WHO: WHO Emergency Health Kit: Standard Drugs and Clinic Equipment for 10,000 Persons for 3 Months. Geneva, World Health Organization, 1983.

Appendix 23-A. Antimicrobial Dosages and Adverse Reactions

Drug	Route	Adult Dosage	Pediatric Dosage	Adverse Reactions
Amodiaquine	po	25 mg base/kg/dose qd	Same as adult	Insomnia, fatigue, fever
Ampicillin				
	po	250–500 mg/dose qid	15–25 mg/kg/dose q6h	Diarrhea, rash, fever, urticaria, hemolysis
Meningitis or sepsis	IV or IM	1–2 g/dose q4–6h	Newborns, and infants less than 7 days old: If birth weight < 2.0 kg give 50 mg/kg/dose q12h. For birth weight > 2.0 kg give 50 mg/kg/dose q8h. Infants over 7 days old: If birth weight <2.0 kg give 50 mg/kg/dose q8h. If birth weight > 2.0 kg give 50 mg/kg/dose q6h. Children: 75 mg/kg/dose q6h.	
Bithionol	po	1 g/dose tid every other day over 30 days	10–15 mg/kg/dose tid every other day over 30 days	GI upset, urticaria
Carbenicillin	IV or IM	50–80 mg/kg/dose q4h	17 mg/kg/dose q4h	Rash, urticaria, fever, hemolysis, fluid retention, sodium excess
Ceftriaxone				
H. ducreyi	IM	250 mg/dose once	———	Rash, fever, diarrhea
Severe illness	IV or IM	1–2 g/dose q12–24h	25–35 mg/kg/dose q12h	
Meningitis	IV or IM	50 mg/kg/dose q12h	Same as adult	
Cephalothin	IV	1–2 g/dose q12h	20–40 mg/kg/dose q6h	Diarrhea, rash, fever, phlebitis
Cephazolin	IV or IM	1–2 g/dose q8h	10–30 mg/kg/dose q8h	
Chloramphenicol				
Mild infection	———	Not recommended	Not recommended	Aplastic anemia. GI upset, fever, rash, headache, neuritis, urticaria, "gray syndrome" in infants
Moderate infection	IV, po	250–500 mg/dose q6h	Infant: not recommended	
Severe infection	IV, po after initial IV therapy; very well	12–25 mg/kg/dose q6h	Premature infant under 7 days: contraindicated	

Appendix 23-A. Antimicrobial Dosages and Adverse Reactions (*Continued*)

Drug	Route	Adult Dosage	Pediatric Dosage	Adverse Reactions
Chloramphenicol	absorbed po, poorly absorbed IM		Premature infant over 7 days: not recommended, but 6 mg/kg/dose q6h can be used Term newborns less than 7 days: 6 mg/kg/dose q6h Term newborns 7–28 days: 12 mg/kg/dose q6h Infants and children: 15 mg/kg/dose q6h	
Chloroquine	po	600 mg base (1 g salt), then 300 mg in 6 h, then 300 mg qd × 2 days	10 mg base/kg once, then 5 mg/kg once in 6 h, then 5 mg/kg/dose qd × 2 days	GI upset, ocular damage, headache, rash, hemolysis, leukopenia
Clindamycin				
Serious infection	po	150–300 mg/dose q6h	4 mg/kg/dose q8h	Diarrhea, colitis, rash, urticaria, hepatitis, sterile abscess
Severe infection	IV	400–1000 mg/dose q8h	Infants under 1 month: 5–7 mg/kg/dose q8h Children over 1 month: 7–13 mg/kg/dose q8h	
Diethylcarbamazine				
Filariasis/ *Loa loa*	po	Day 1: 50 mg/dose once Day 2: 50 mg/dose tid Day 3: 100 mg/dose tid Days 4–21: 2 mg/kg/dose tid	Day 1: 25–50 mg/dose once Day 2: 25–50 mg/dose tid Day 3: 50–100 mg/dose tid Days 4–21: 2 mg/kg/dose tid	Fever, vertigo, urticaria, headache, vomiting, Herxheimer reaction
O. volvulus	po	25 mg/dose qd × 3 days, then 50 mg/dose qd × 3 days, then 100 mg/dose qd × 3 days, then 150 mg/dose qd × 12 days	0.5 mg/kg/dose tid × 3 days, then 1.0 mg/kg/dose tid × 3 days, then 1.5 mg/kg/dose tid × 3 days, then 2 mg/kg/dose tid × 2–3 week	
Doxycycline	po	100 mg/dose bid Pregnancy: not recommended	2.5 mg/kg/dose bid Children under 8 years: not recommended	GI upset, rash, fever, hepatitis, candidiasis, photosensitivity
Emetine	IM	1 mg/kg/dose (up to 60 mg/day) qd × 5 days	0.5 mg/kg/dose bid (up to 60 mg/day) × 5 days	Local pain at injection site
Erythromycin	po	500 mg/dose qid	20–50 mg/kg/dose qid	GI upset, rash
Ethambutol	po	15–25 mg/kg/dose qd	Same as adult	Optic neuritis, rash, GI upset, fever, gout, CNS changes
Eurazolidone				
G. lamblia	po	100mg/dose qid × 7 days	1.25 mg/kg/dose qid × 7 days	GI upset, malaise, headache, fever,

Appendix 23-A. Antimicrobial Dosages and Adverse Reactions (*Continued*)

Drug	Route	Adult Dosage	Pediatric Dosage	Adverse Reactions
Eurazolidone				
G. lamblia			Infants under 1 month: contraindicated	rash, hypotension
V. cholera	po	100 mg/dose qid × 3–4 days	1.25 mg/kg/dose qid × 3–4 days Infants under 1 month: contraindicated	
Gentamicin	IV or IM	1–1.7 mg/kg/dose q8h × 7 days	Newborns under 7 days: 2.5 mg/kg/dose q12h Infants and children: 2 mg/kg/dose q8h	Renal toxicity, rash, vertigo, ototoxicity
INH (isoniazid)	po	5 mg/kg/dose (maximum 300 mg) qd	10–20 mg/kg (maximum 300 mg) qd	Neuropathy, vitamin B^6 deficiency, GI upset, hepatitis, agranulocytosis, hemolysis
Iodoquinol	po	650 mg/dose tid × 20 days	10–13 mg/kg/dose tid × 20 days	Rash, acne, GI upset
Ivermectin	po	150–200 μg/kg/ dose once	Unknown	Hypotension, fever
Mebendazole				
E. granulosis	po	40 mg/kg/dose qd	Unknown	GI upset, rash, neutropenia in high doses
O. volvulus	po	1g/dose bid × 28 days	Unknown	
Roundworms	po	100 mg/dose bid × 5 days Pregnancy: contraindicated	Same as adult	
Mefloquine	po	1.5 g/dose once	Unknown	GI upset, vertigo
Melarsoprol	IV	2–3.6 mg/kg/dose qd × 3 days, stop for 1 week, then 3.6 mg/kg/ dose qd × 3 days; repeat after 10–21 days.	0.36 mg/kg/dose qd increasing slowly to 3.6 mg/kg/dose qd over 1–5-day intervals for a total of 18–25 mg/kg in 1 month	Myocardial damage, proteinuria, GI upset, encephalopathy, neuropathy, Herxheimer reaction
Metriphonate	po	10 mg/kg/dose alternate weeks × 3 doses	Same as adult	GI distress, weakness
Metronidazole				
E. histolytica	po	750 mg/dose tid × 8 days	15 mg/kg/dose tid × 10 days	Seizures, neuropathy, metallic taste, candidiasis, Antabuse reaction
G. lamblia	po	250 mg/dose tid × 5 days	5 mg/kg/dose tid × 5 days	
Anaerobes	po	500mg/dose tid	10 mg/kg/dose tid	
	IV	15 mg/kg/dose once, then 7.5 mg/kg/dose q6h	Same as adult	
Niclosamide	po	2 g once	11–34 kg: 1 g once Over 34 kg: 1.5 g once	GI upset, pruritus
Oxamniquine	po	15 mg/kg/dose once	15–20 mg/kg/dose once	Fever, dizziness, GI upset, drowsiness, seizures
Paromomycin				
E. histolytica	po	8–10 mg/kg/dose tid with meals × 7 days	Same as adult	GI upset

Appendix 23-A. Antimicrobial Dosages and Adverse Reactions (*Continued*)

Drug	Route	Adult Dosage	Pediatric Dosage	Adverse Reactions
Paromomycin				
H. nana	po	45 mg/kg/dose qd × 5–7 days	Same as adult	
Penicillin, benzathine	IM	1.2 million units/ dose	Under 68 kg: 300–600,000 IU Over 68 kg: 900,000 IU	Anaphylaxis, rash, urticaria, hemolysis
Penicillin G				
Usual dose	IV or IM	300–600,000 IU/ dose q6h	6–12,000 IU/kg/dose q6h	Anaphylaxis, rash, urticaria, hemolysis
High dose	IV	1–2 million units/ dose q4–6h	25,000 IU/kg/dose q6h	Anaphylaxis, rash, urticaria, hemolysis
Meningitis	IV	1–2 million U/dose q2h	20,000 IU/kg/dose q2h	Anaphylaxis, rash, urticaria, hemolysis
Penicillin VK	po	250–500 mg/dose qid, tid, or bid[a]	6.2-12.5 mg/kg/dose qid or tid	Anaphylaxis, rash, urticaria, hemolysis
Penicillin, PCNase resistant				
Cloxacillin/ dicloxacillin	po	250–500 mg/dose qid	12.5–25 mg/kg/dose qid	Anaphylaxis, rash, urticaria, hemolysis
Nafcillin/ oxacillin	IV or IM	1–2 g/dose q4–6h	40–50 mg/kg/dose q6h	Anaphylaxis, rash, urticaria, hemolysis
Pentamidine				
L. donovani	Slow IV/IM	2–4 mg/kg/dose qd for up to 15 doses	Same as adult	Hypotension, sterile abscess, vomiting, neutropenia, hypocalcemia
T. gambiense	Slow IV/IM	4 mg/kg/dose qd × 10 days	Same as adult	
Potassium Iodide	po	10 drops/dose tid after meals, increasing to 40 drops/dose tid	1–10 drops/dose tid, increase 1 drop each dose to 10–40 drops/ dose tid	GI upset, metallic taste
Praziquantel				
D. latum, T. saginata, T. solium	po	10–20 mg/kg/dose once	Same as adult	GI upset, fever, headache, malaise
H. nana	po	25 mg/kg/dose once	Same as adult	
F. buski, C. sinensis	po	25 mg/kg/dose tid × 1 day	Same as adult	
P. westermani	po	25 mg/kg/dose tid × 1–2 days	Same as adult	
S. hematobium, S. mansoni	po	40 mg/kg/dose once	Same as adult	
Pyrantel pamoate	po	11 mg/kg/dose (up to 1 g) once	Same as adult	Dizziness, GI upset
Quinacrine	po	100 mg/dose tid × 5 days	2 mg/kg/dose tid × 5 days	Yellowish skin discoloration, psychosis, rash, hemolysis, fever, blood dyscrasias

[a]For streptococcal pharyngitis, bid dosing is probably as effective as tid or qid dosing (Gerber and Markowitz 1985).

Drug	Route	Adult Dosage	Pediatric Dosage	Adverse Reactions
Quinine (may substitute quinidine)	po	650 mg/dose tid × 3 days	8 mg/kg/dose tid × 3 days	Visual disturbances, vertigo, fever, rash,
	IV	600 mg in 300 cc normal saline/dose over 8 h, continue until po can be started	12.5 mg/kg in normal saline/dose over 2 h, repeat in 6–8 h if unable to tolerate po; continue until po can be started	Tinnitus, headache, confusion, GI upset, hemolysis, hypotension
Rifampin	po	600 mg/dose qd	10–20 mg/kg/dose qd	Hepatitis, GI upset, mild CNS changes
Silver sulfadiazine	Topical	Apply to 1–3 mm thickness qd or bid	Same as adult	Rash, rare interstitial nephritis
Stibogluconate	IV or IM	10 mg/kg/dose (up to 600 mg) qd × 10 days, course may be repeated	Same as adult	Vomiting, GI upset, muscle stiffness
Streptomycin				
Moderate illness	IM	1–2 g/dose qd	20 mg/kg/dose bid	Ototoxicity, vertigo, rash, fever, muscle weakness, urticaria
Severe illness	IM	1–2 g/dose bid	40 mg/kg/dose bid	
Sulfamylon	Topical	Apply to 1–3 mm thickness qd to bid	Same as adult	Local reactions, rash, urticaria
Suramin				
O. volvulus	IV	100 mg test dose, then 1 g/dose weekly × 5 doses	10 mg test dose, then 20 mg/kg/dose weekly × 5 doses	Vomiting, shock, urticaria, neuropathy, proteinuria, nephropathy
Trypanosomiasis				
Early	IV	100 mg test dose, then 20 mg/kg/dose (up to 1 g) every other day × 5 doses	Same as adult	
Late	IV	10 mg/kg/dose every 5 days × 12 doses	Unknown	
Tetracycline	po	500 mg/dose qid Pregnancy: not recommended	12.5 mg/kg/dose qid Children under 8 years: contraindicated	GI upset, hepatitis, photosensitivity, candidiasis, fever, rash; do not mix with food, milk, antacids
Thiabendazole	po	25 mg/kg/dose bid (up to 3 g/day) × 5 days	Same as adult	GI upset, rash, CNS changes, tinnitus, hypotension
TMP/SMX (trimethoprim/sulfamethoxazole)	po	TMP 160 mg/SMX 800 mg/dose bid	TMP 4 mg/kg/SMX 20 mg/kg/dose bid	Rash, fever, erythema multiforme, Stevens–Johnson, urticaria, colitis, blood dyscrasias
Tryparsamide	IV	1-g test dose, then 30 mg/kg/dose weekly × 15 doses	Unknown	CNS changes, rash, hypotension, visual changes, tinnitus, vomiting

Appendix 23-B. Dosages for Nonantibiotic Medications

Drug	Adult Dosage	Pediatric Dosage
Aluminum hydroxide tabs	1–2 tab po pc, hs, and prn	½–1 po pc, hs, and prn
Aspirin		
Fever or pain	1–2 tab po q4–6h prn	10–15 mg/kg/dose q4–6h prn
Arthritis	3–5 tab po q 6 h	25 mg/kg/dose qid
Atropine	Usual dose is 0.5 mg/dose q4–6h prn po, IV, or SC. For cardiac arrest give 0.5 mg/dose q 5 minutes IV or via an endotracheal tube (maximum total dose 2.0 mg).	Usual dose is 0.01 mg/kg/dose (up to a maximum of 0.4 mg) q4–6h prn po, IV or SC. For cardiac arrest give 0.01–0.03 mg/kg/dose IV or via an endotracheal tube, q 5 minutes × 3, with a minimum dose of 0.4 mg/dose.
Beclomethasone for inhalation	2–3 puffs q6–8h and prn (maximum of 20 puffs/day)	1–2 puffs q6–8h and prn (maximum of 10 puffs/day)
Chlorpheniramine tabs	1 tab po q6h	Children over 6 years: ½ tab po q6h
Codeine tabs		
Pain	30–60 mg/dose q4–6h	0.5–1.0 mg/kg/dose q4–6h
Cough	10–20 mg/dose q4–6h prn	1–1.5 mg/kg/dose q4h (maximum 30 mg/day)
Diazepam tabs and injectable		
Sedative/muscle relaxant		
po	2–10 mg/dose q6–8h prn	0.03–0.2 mg/kg/dose q6h
IM or IV	2–10 mg/dose q3–4h prn	0.04–0.2 mg/kg/dose q2–4h (maximum 0.6 mg/kg/8 h)
Status epilepticus (seizures)	5 mg/dose q 5–10 minutes (maximum total dose = 20–30 mg)	1 month–5 years: 0.2–0.5 mg/kg/dose q 15–30 minutes (maximum total dose = 5 mg) 5–12 years: 1 mg/kg/dose q 15–30 minutes (maximum total dose = 10 mg)
Digoxin		
Digitalization (½ total dose STAT, then ¼ of the digitalizing dose q8h × 2)	1.0 mg	Premature: 0.020mg/kg Term newborn: 0.040 mg/kg Child: 0.050 mg/kg
Maintenance dose	0.125–0.250 mg po q day	Premature: 0.0025 mg (2.5 μg/kg/dose po q12h Term newborn or child: 0.005 mg (5.0 μg)/kg/dose po q12h
Epinephrine (adrenalin)	0.5–1.0 mg/dose SC q 15 minutes × 3, or q4h prn. For cardiac arrest give 0.5–1.0 mg/dose IV or via an endotracheal tube q 5–10 minutes.	0.01 mg/kg/dose SC q 15 minutes × 3, or q4h prn. For cardiac arrest, give 0.01 mg/kg/dose IV or via an endotracheal tube q 5–10 minutes.

Appendix 23-B. Dosages for Nonantibiotic Medications (*Continued*)

Drug	Adult Dosage	Pediatric Dosage
Ergometrine (ergonavine)		
po	1 mg/dose	0.5–1.0 mg/dose
IM or sc	0.3–1.0 mg/dose	0.25–0.5 mg/dose
Furosemide		
po	20–80 mg/day as qd or bid may increase 20–40 mg/day to maximum of 600 mg/day	2 mg/kg/dose q6–8h
IV or IM	20–80 mg/dose (maximum 6 mg/kg)	1 mg/kg/dose q 12 or prn
Hydrocortisone		
Shock	3 gm IV STAT, then 1 g IV q6h	50 mg/kg STAT, then 15 mg/kg/dose q6h
Status asthmaticus	350 mg IM or IV STAT, then 150 mg IV or IM q6h	6 mg/kg IM or IV STAT, then 3 mg/kg IM or IV q6h
Isoprenaline (isoproterenol) (To mix, add 1 mg to 100 ml D5W. Then 0.6 cc/kg/h = 0.1 μg/kg/h)	0.1–1.5 μg/kg/minute Titrate to desired affect, or heart rate > 150 or arrhythmia	0.1–1.5 μg/kg/minute Titrate to desired effect and heart rate > 180 or arrhythmia
Paracetamol (acetaminophen)	1–2 tabs po q4–6h prn	10 mg/kg/dose po q4–6h prn
Pethidine (meperidine)	50–100 mg po, IM or IV q3–4h	1–1.5 mg/kg/dose po, IM or IV q3–4h
Promethazine		
Antihistaminic	12.5–25 mg po tid	0.1–0.5 mg/kg/dose po tid
Nausea	12.5–25 mg po or IM q4–6h	0.25–0.5 mg/kg/dose q4–6h po or IM
Sedation	25–50 mg/dose po or IM	0.5–1.0 mg/kg/dose po or IM
Propranolol		
Arrhythmias	1 mg/dose q 5 minutes IV (maximum 5 mg)	0.01–0.10 mg/kg/dose IV q6–8h (maximum single dose = 1.0 mg IV), or 0.1–0.35 mg/kg/dose po q6h
Hypertension	10 mg/dose po qid May increase 10–20 mg/dose every 3–7 days to maximum dose of 320–480 mg/day po	0.5–1.0 mg/kg/day divided q6–12h, up to a maximum dose of 2 mg/kg/day
Retinol		
Treatment of vitamin A deficiency	200,000 IU po (or 100,000 IU IM) STAT, and on days 2 and 8 for a total of 3 doses	Less than 1 year: 100,000 IU po (or 50,000 IU IM) STAT, and on days 2 and 8 for a total of 3 doses
Prophylaxis	200,000 IU po q 3–4 months	Less than 1 year; 100,000 IU po q 3–4 months
Salbutamol for inhalation	1–2 puffs q4–6h or 15 minutes before exercise	1 puff q4–6h or 15 minutes before exercise
Senna	1–3 tab po q day	½–1 tab po q day

(These drugs, except for atropine and epinephrine, are selected from the WHO Emergency Health Kit: Standard Drugs and Clinic Equipment for 10,000 Persons for 3 Months, Geneva, World Health Organization, 1983.)

24
Systemic Febrile Illnesses

THOMAS C. JONES

One of the most difficult diagnostic problems facing health care personnel in a low-technology setting is that posed by the patient presenting with fever without localized signs or symptoms. A challenge arises because the physical examination is often negative for a source of the fever and the history of the febrile illness does not often provide specific clues. One must rely on epidemiologic data; that is, awareness of the predominant febrile illnesses in the environment, a few diagnostic tests such as blood count and malaria smears, and the course of the illness after initiating presumptive therapy. This chapter focuses on the most common diseases and management methods in caring for such patients.

When a patient develops fever, the clinician first carries out a careful history and physical examination by organ system to identify localized processes as a cause of the fever. A number of febrile illnesses should be considered. For example, subtle pneumonia, otitis media, or enteritis commonly present with fever as the first sign of the infectious process. Once the search is completed and no localized process is identified, the term undifferentiated febrile illness is applied (Deller & Russell 1967; Rowland 1970). For purposes of diagnostic efficiency, the clinician must then consider common infections in the region for which diagnostic tests are readily available; common infections that are usually diagnosed by exclusion; and rare infections that must be considered as diagnostic and therapeutic setting dictates.

The most important cause of undifferentiated febrile illness in the tropics is malaria. This is so important that in many regions endemic for malaria, the definition of undifferentiated febrile illness is applied only after the patient has not responded to treatment for malaria. A malaria smear should be done on every febrile patient when possible (see Chapter 25). The second most important diagnostic consideration is typhoid fever. This, too, is so common in the tropics that many clinicians initiate a therapeutic trial with chloramphenicol before considering other diagnostic possibilities. Another important febrile disease to consider is amebiasis, which can also present with fever alone. All three of these diseases can be confirmed within a few days by appropriate diagnostic testing and/or response to therapy.

Some febrile illnesses are not easily diagnosed and must be defined by the course of the illness and by exclusion. Febrile syndromes caused by viruses are very common, examples being such mosquito-borne viruses as dengue fever, and enteroviruses such as ECHO virus. Although clinical clues during the course of the illness may support a presumptive diagnosis, specific diagnostic tests or response to therapy are usually not helpful. Some rickettsial diseases, such as African tick fever or scrub typhus, fall into the same category but differ in that, occasionally, response to antibiotics may be informative. As in diseases in temperate climates, tropical infectious diseases may move from the initial diagnosis of undifferentiated febrile illness to organ system diagnosis during the period of observation. Thus, the course of the illness will aid in the diagnosis if fever was an early sign preceding specific organ dysfunction. Viral hepatitis is a common example of an illness presenting with fever. The appearance of jaundice after several days provides the clue. Leptospirosis may also begin as a febrile illness and then demonstrate inflammation of the meninges, liver, or kidneys characteristic of that infection. Tuberculosis is a common infectious disease for which diagnostic support may not be available and its clinical course yields the diagnosis.

Uncommon infectious diseases may also present with fever, and, in the absence of diagnostic tests, the clinician must rely heavily on his or her knowledge of the environment from which the patient came. The following diseases, although uncommon, would be placed near the top of a differential diagnosis of fever if the environmental setting dictates.

Acute Chagas' disease (recent residence in a mud and stick hut in South or Central America); schistosomiasis (exposure to fresh water in areas known to be endemic for the disease; the presence of eosinophilia, a characteristic of helminth infections, lends further support to this diagnosis); visceral leishmaniasis (residence in an area endemic for the disease and having experienced sandfly bites; the presence of enlarged spleen or bone marrow dysfunction will further increase the probability of this diagnosis); and brucellosis (travel to cattle-raising areas and ingestion of unprocessed milk products).

Very specific regional histories would lead to consideration of coccidiomycosis, African tick fever, African trypanosomiasis, relapsing fever, bartonellosis, and Colorado tick fever. These special environmental diagnostic considerations are added to the diagnostic list that would be developed for a febrile patient from any place in the world: meningococcemia, endocarditis, gram-negative sepsis, hidden abscess, and malignancies.

MANAGEMENT OF FEBRILE PATIENTS

A logical approach to diagnosis and management of febrile patients will lead to the earliest diagnosis and therapy. After careful history and physical examination, and initiation of supportive therapy, the laboratory tests to be done immediately include (1) malaria smear; (2) stool for protozoa and helminth ova; (3) complete blood count; and when possible (4) blood culture, stool culture, and liver function tests. The malaria smear will detect malaria parasites but, in addition, may aid in the diagnosis of relapsing fever, trypanosomiasis, bartonellosis, and filariasis. A stool for helminth ova and protozoa will detect *Entamoeba histolytica* or *Strongyloides* larvae. If the fever is due to schistosomiasis, the stool may not be helpful, as fever usually antedates the appearance of schistosome eggs in the stool. A complete blood count will detect eosinophilia associated with schistosomiasis, filariasis, and strongyloidiasis; the leukopenia and anemia associated with leishmaniasis; the leukopenia of typhoid; or the leukocytosis of amebic abscess. Blood cultures detect typhoid and other causes of bacteremia, and stool cultures identify salmonella and shigella intestinal infections. Abnormal liver function tests may be an early sign of hepatitis or leptospirosis. Subsequent diagnostic testing will be dictated largely by the history but may include serologic testing for typhoid, leptospirosis, rickettsia, brucellosis, and amebiasis.

For the patient who presents with hepatic dysfunction and fever, the most important diagnostic considerations are malaria, hepatitis, leptospirosis, and typhoid fever. When faced with the need to distinguish among these four causes of fever and jaundice, the order of evaluation is apparent. The most emergent diagnostic test is a malaria smear, since malaria is the most likely to progress rapidly to death and is easily diagnosed and treated. After appropriate blood cultures are obtained for typhoid fever (if available), and the blood count or serologic tests have been examined for supportive evidence of that diagnosis, antibacterial therapy directed against *Salmonella typhi* may be initiated. Leptospirosis and hepatitis are diagnosed during the subsequent days of observation in the absence of specific therapy because of the appearance of jaundice. During this time, unusual causes of jaundice such as cholangitis secondary to common duct obstruction from *Ascaris lumbricoides* or *Clonorchis,* will be evaluated by stool examination for helminth ova. In addition, amebic abscess of the liver, which does not usually cause jaundice, may become clear because of the appearance of tenderness over the liver, right shoulder pain, and/or leukocytosis. Amebic abscess of the liver is difficult to distinguish from pyogenic liver abscess and cholangitis; the clinician must often rely on the therapeutic response to antiamebicides rather than antibacterial drugs.

Therapeutic trial with antimicrobial agents, though not encouraged, may be the only available course under some conditions. Chloroquine, quinine, or pyrimethamine sulfa are frequently used in areas endemic for malaria. There is no doubt that this procedure leads to confusion in some cases and microscopic diagnosis is preferred whenever possible. Health workers frequently resort to initiation of chloramphenicol or co-trimoxazole for typhoid fever. This is often done concurrent with obtaining blood cultures because firm diagnosis may require four to six days. One must be aware, however, that these are broad-spectrum antibiotics and may influence the course of a number of infections. One of the most specific therapeutic trials is the use of emetine or metronidazole in the diagnosis or extraintestinal amebiasis. Since the alternative is laparotomy for exploration of the intestine or the liver, 24 to 48 hours of observation following antiamebic therapy may avoid a major surgical procedure. The use of tetracycline for presumed rickettsial diseases may also provide further information regarding therapeutic response while one awaits the serologic test results. The same may apply to the initiation of antituberculosis therapy while awaiting results of skin testing and cultures. There are few indications for therapeutic antimicrobial trial other than these in the practice of infectious diseases in the refugee setting.

SPECIFIC FEBRILE DISEASES

Specific diseases that present with fever as the primary sign are discussed in the following pages. They include typhoid fever, leptospirosis, dengue fever and other arbor virus infections, amebiasis, leishmaniasis, trypanosomiasis, and brucellosis. Other important diseases that may present with fever are discussed in other chapters of this book, including malaria, pneumonia, tuberculosis, and meningococcemia.

Typhoid fever

Typhoid fever is caused by the bacterium *Salmonella typhi* after it is ingested in adequate numbers in contaminated food or water. In addition to *S. typhi,* eight to ten other species of salmonella have been associated with bacteremia as a common manifestation (Parker 1984). The tendency to bacteremia separates these salmonella from those that primarily cause gastroenteritis (see Chapter 34 on Intestinal Illness).

After ingesting *Salmonella,* the patient typically experiences a few days of diarrhea and vomiting followed by fever associated with severe prostration (endotoxemia), hypotension, abdominal pain, and constipation. Depending on the infecting dose of organisms, the incubation period is one to three weeks.

After malaria, typhoid fever should be at the top of the differential diagnosis list for any patient with fever. Clues to the presence of *Salmonella typhi* include "rose spots" on the abdomen, an enlarged, soft spleen, temperature–pulse dissociation (inappropriately low pulse), leukopenia, and slight changes in liver function tests. Diagnosis may be confirmed by culturing *S. typhi* from the blood or stool. In some cases, the serologic responses to the H and O antigens of *Salmonella* suggest the diagnosis. This is useful primarily when blood cultures are unavailable. The main problems are that antibody titers may indicate previous infection, rather than the cause of the present illness, and high titers may not appear until after resolution of the febrile illness. In patients who have received typhoid vaccine, use of serologic tests for diagnosis is unreliable.

The treatment of *S. typhi* infection requires attention to where the typhoid fever was acquired because of the variation in drug susceptibility in different areas. In general, chloramphenicol is the drug of choice for treatment of typhoid fever, although ampicillin can be used instead. It is important to realize that the temperature may not begin to return to normal for five or six days after initiation of therapy; therefore, the absence of a response during the first few days should not be taken as evidence of inappropriate diagnosis or ineffective antibiotic therapy.

Leptospirosis

Leptospirosis is another bacterial infection that causes fever, hepatitis, and meningitis. This is caused by various species of the spirochete *Leptospira.* It is primarily transmitted to humans who come into contact with water contaminated by the urine of infected animals. Leptospirosis should be suspected in a patient with progressive fever, liver dysfunction, meningitis, conjunctivitis, and renal impairment. The diagnosis is confirmed by serologic testing. Penicillin may be helpful early in the course of illness, however, primary care of the patient with leptospirosis includes management of the complications of hepatitis, coagulation disorders, and renal failure.

Septicemia with Unknown Microbe

Some patients will present with fever due to bacteremia originating from a localized infection that cannot be identified. The clinical pattern of the illness is dominated by the fever and evidence of a "septic" state because of the patient's weakness, prostration, confusion, hyperventilation without pneumonia, and/or hypotension. The most common causes of this illness are gram-negative bacteria such as *Escherichia coli, Klebsiella,* or *Pseudomonas;* neonatal sepsis caused by *E. coli* or *Listeria monocytogenes;* and *Staphylococcus aureus* arising from a hidden abscess or heart valve infection.

Gram-negative sepsis most often arises from a urinary tract or bowel source but, particularly in a hospitalized patient on antibiotics, it may arise from lung, skin, or intravenous line infections, which then develop into bacteremia. Therapy includes gentamicin and ampicillin, plus chloramphenicol or metronidazole if anaerobic bacteria are suspected. Identification of the source of the bacteremia is done by follow-up examination during therapy.

Neonatal sepsis is discussed in Chapter 12. It is also treated with gentamicin and ampicillin. Fever may not be a part of the clinical picture of neonatal sepsis.

Sepsis due to gram-positive bacteria such as *Staphylococcus* or *Streptococcus* requires use of a penicillinase-resistant penicillin such as nafcillin or cephalosporin. If an abscess is suspected as the source, its presence should be checked for daily and surgically drained when identified.

Dengue and Other Systemic Viral Illnesses

Many febrile illnesses are associated with viral infections (see Chapter 26). In some parts of the world, as in Africa, viral exanthems such as measles are still a common cause of fever. Some of the enteroviruses transmitted by contaminated water or food are also common sources of fever. For example, ECHO viruses and coxsackieviruses can be identified with increased frequency in those in the tropics and subtropics. In some regions, insect-borne viral infections are very common. For example, in Central America and Southeast Asia, the mosquito-borne infection dengue fever is a common cause of illness. Dengue fever is often diagnosed after other diseases that cause fever and muscle pain are excluded such as malaria, leptospirosis, and typhoid fever. The typical pattern is one of fever lasting five to ten days occasionally associated with rash. After the illness has subsided, testing for arbovirus antibodies may confirm the diagnosis.

Other febrile viral infections must be considered on the basis of epidemiologic data on viruses present in the region. Management is supportive because specific antiviral drugs are not available.

Amebiasis

Amebiasis is an illness with two main clinical presentations: intestinal amebiasis and extraintestinal amebiasis. The disease is caused by the protozoa *Entamoeba histolytica,* which is transferred to humans when they ingest raw vegetables or water contaminated with *E. histolytica* cysts. Intestinal amebiasis is characterized by the invasion of the *E. histolytica* trophozoite between the epithelial cells of the colon, and initiation of necrotic submucosal ulcers in the wall of the large bowel. This illness presents with signs of colitis including abdominal pain, diarrhea with mucus and blood, and fever. Extraintestinal amebiasis is due to invasion of the blood vessels of the bowel and transfer of trophozoites to the liver and, rarely, to other organs. If this process occurs with limited colonic irritation, the patient may present only with fever. Patients with extraintestinal amebiasis, particularly amebic abscess of the liver, will present with fever, weight loss, malaise, and right upper quadrant pain (Peters 1981). Diagnosis of the intestinal phase of amebic infection rests on identifying the ameba in the stool of a symptomatic patient. Liver abscess caused by ameba is suspected when the liver is found to be tender to palpation and when there is severe, localized, so-called point tenderness at one area over the liver, determined by exerting pressure between the ribs overlying the liver. Right shoulder pain and signs of fluid in the right lung may indicate diaphragmatic irritation due to the abscess. Amebic abscess of the liver is diagnosed by aspiration of the abscess and identification of motile ameba in the aspirate, by leukocytosis in the peripheral blood count and, if available, by high titers of antibody against ameba in the circulation.

Amebiasis is treated with metronidazole for the tissue infection and with diiodohydroxyquin or diloxanide furoate for the luminal phase of the infection. In serious disease, emetine or chloroquine are often added for treatment of extraintestinal amebiasis.

Leishmaniasis

Leishmaniasis is the general name applied to three different clinical illnesses caused by obligate intracellular protozoa that replicate in histiocytes. These are cutaneous leishmaniasis, and visceral leishmaniasis caused by the organisms *Leishmania tropica, L. brasiliensis mexicana* complex, and *L. donovani* or *L. chagasi,* respectively. Cutaneous leishmaniasis and mucocutaneous leishmaniasis are skin and mucosal infections that do not cause fever; they are considered in Chapter 28.

Visceral leishmaniasis presents a different clinical pattern because the amastigotes of *L. donovani* replicate in histiocytes in the reticuloendothelial system and, therefore, affect the size and function of the liver, spleen, lymph nodes, and bone marrow (Geraci et al 1980). Patients present with fever and complications of the functions of these organs, particularly the bone marrow. For this reason, presentation is often similar to that of acute leukemia since anemia, thrombocytopenia, and leukopenia may be common. The complications leading to death in this illness include bleeding or sepsis associated with bone marrow dysfunction. All forms of leishmaniasis are treated with pentavalent antimony. If this drug fails, amphotericin B has been shown to be effective (Medical Letter 1984).

Trypanosomiasis (African)

African trypanosomiasis is an unusual disease in humans who have been in the central regions of the African continent. It presents with symptoms of fever, malaise, weakness, irritability, and progressive central nervous system dysfunction (Foulkes 1981). The disease is caused by *Trypanosoma gambiense* on the west coast of Africa, and *T. rhodesiense* in southeastern parts of Africa. A pathologic response in African trypanosomiasis includes lymph node enlargement followed by signs of generalized vasculitis. This phase of the illness may be confused with malaria or other causes of vasculitis. Myocarditis, with or without congestive heart failure, is an important part of this phase. Following this, the picture of progressive encephalitis becomes the dominant clinical feature, heralded by irritability and sleeplessness, followed by somnolence and coma. The diagnosis of African trypanosomiasis in the febrile patient is made by identifying flagellated protozoa in the peripheral blood. These organisms are not intracellular but live and divide freely in the circulation. On examination of spinal fluid, a finding of elevated cell count and protein and, occasionally, identification of the flagellate will confirm central nervous system infection.

The type of treatment depends on whether or not the central nervous system has been invaded. If the diagnosis is made early, before central nervous system infection occurs, the drug suramin is sufficient; after central nervous system infection, the arsenical Mel-B is necessary.

Chagas' Disease (American Trypanosomiasis)

American trypanosomiasis is an illness characterized by two different clinical patterns: acute Chagas' disease and chronic Chagas' disease (Brener 1982). The illness is caused by the protozoan *Trypanosoma cruzi,* which is transmitted to humans by the bite, and subsequent defecation, of a reduviid bug. The protozoa replicates at the site of inoculation and invades the bloodstream. The acute illness is rarely seen, except in highly endemic areas, and presents as fever and unilateral conjunctivitis or a trypanosomal chancre. Myocarditis may be a complication of this febrile illness. Acute Chagas' disease may be a severe, fatal illness, or it may go unnoticed by the infected patient. The illness may resolve spontaneously but does appear to respond to antiprotozoal drugs such as nifurtimox or benzidazole. Following the initial period, the patient will demonstrate continued infection by serum antibodies against the protozoa. Identification of the organism in the bloodstream can sometimes be made using xenodiagnosis.

Years later, the signs and symptoms of chronic Chagas' disease appear. Progressive myocardial enlargement, myocardial failure, rhythm disturbances, and pulmonary emboli are characteristic of chronic Chagas' disease. In addition, autonomic dysfunction of the esophagus and colon result in megacolon and megaesophagus. There is no effective therapy for this stage of Chagas' disease except supportive care for the heart failure, rhythm disturbances, and emboli.

Helminthic Infections

Worm infections may present with fever during the period of larval migration. Two of the most important of these are *Schistosoma* sp., the cause of schistosomiasis (Nash 1982), and *Strongyloides stercoralis,* the cause of strongyloidiasis (Purtilo 1974). These are discussed in Chapter 35. Both of these causes of fever should be considered if eosinophilia is present in the peripheral blood smear. In addition, strongyloides larvae can be identified in a fresh stool sample. Schistosome eggs may not be seen in the stool at the time the patient presents with fever and eosinophilia, but subsequent stool examinations over a period of several weeks will confirm the diagnosis. Therapy is with praziquantel for schistosomiasis (Pearson & Guerrant 1983) and thiabendazole for strongyloidiasis (Medical Letter 1984).

Patients being treated with immune suppressives such as corticosteroids are at risk for developing the severe form of strongyloidiasis. In these patients, eosinophilia may not be associated with the fever. Stool examination for strongyloides is the only diagnostic test available. Because hyperinfection strongyloidiasis is often caused by medical treatment of allergic conditions such as asthma, stools should be checked for strongyloides before such therapy.

Other conditions presenting with fever and eosinophilia include filariasis, diagnosed by peripheral blood smear stain for microfilaria; cysticercosis, often associated with seizures; and tropical pulmonary eosinophilia, associated with cough and shortness of breath. These illnesses are treated with antihelminthic drugs, such as diethylcarbamazine for filaria and tropical eosinophilia, and praziquantel for cysticercosis (Medical Letter 1984).

REFERENCES

Brener Z: Recent developments in the field of Chagas' disease. Bull WHO 1982;60:463–73.

Deller JJ, Russell PK: An analysis of fevers of unknown origin in American soldiers in Vietnam. Ann Intern Med 1967;66:1129–43.

Foulkes JR: Human trypanosomiasis in Africa. Br Med J 1981;283:1172–74.

Geraci JE, Wilson WR, Thompson JH: Visceral leishmaniasis (kala-azar) as a cause of fever of unknown origin. Mayo Clinic Proc 1980;55:455–58.

Hornick RB: Selective primary health care: strategies for control of disease in the developing world. XX. Typhoid fever. Rev Infect Dis 1985;7:536–46.

Marsden PD: Selective primary health care: strategies for control of disease in the developing world. XVI. Chagas' disease. Rev Infect Dis 1984;6:855–65.

Medical Letter. Drugs for parasitic diseases. Med Lett 1984;26:27.

Nash TE et al: Schistosome infections in humans: Perspectives and recent findings. Ann Intern Med 1982;97:740–54.

Parker MT: Enteric infections: Typhoid and paratyphoid fever. In Smith GR (ed): Topley and Wilson's Principles and Practice of Bacteriology, Virology and Immunity, 7th ed, vol 3. New York, Edward Arnold Publishers, 1984.

Pearson RD, Guerrant RL: Praziquantel: A major advance in antihelminthic therapy. Ann Intern Med 1983;99:195–98, 574.

Peters RS, Girlin N, Libke RD: Amebic liver abscess. Annu Rev Med 1981;32:161–74.

Purtilo DT, Meyers WM, Connor DH: Fatal strongyloidiasis in immunosuppressed patients. Am J Med 1974;56:488–93.

Rowland HAK: Management of patients recently arrived from the tropics. Br Med J 1970;3:447–49.

Warren KS, Mahmoud AAF: Tropical and geographical medicine. New York, McGraw-Hill, 1984.

25
Malaria

IRA K. SCHWARTZ

With few geographic exceptions, refugees in Latin America, Asia, and Africa must contend with malaria, an infectious disease that is a leading cause of morbidity and mortality among displaced persons throughout the tropics. Malaria also poses profound risks to the personal health of relief workers who live and work in these areas. More than 100 million cases of malaria occur worldwide each year. Depending on the refugee setting and diagnostic facilities, 1 to 10 percent of visits to an emergency health care station arc due to malaria. The most important problems in refugee camps regarding control of malaria include (1) prevention of fatal disease due to falciparum malaria including that due to chloroquine-resistant strains; (2) prevention of the spread of the disease in the refugee settlement; (3) availability of blood smear examination to enable an accurate diagnosis; (4) control of malaria relapses; and (5) protection of nonimmune health workers. This chapter reviews issues of pathogenesis, clinical symptoms and signs, diagnosis, and treatment of malaria in an effort to confront these problems

ETIOLOGY AND PATHOGENESIS

Malaria is caused by a unicellular protozoan parasite that belongs to the genus *Plasmodium.* Humans are infected by four species: *Plasmodium falciparum, P. vivax, P. malariae,* and *P. ovale* (Table 25-1). *Plasmodium vivax* has the widest geographic range, extending throughout the malarious world with the exception of sub-Saharan Africa and Haiti. *Plasmodium falciparum* is the most common human malaria parasite and is the species responsible for the greatest threat to life. Certain inherited hemoglobinopathies (e.g., HbS, thalassemia, and G6PD) are associated with some protection from *P. falciparum* infection. *Plasmodium malariae* is usually found in the same areas as *P. falciparum,* but is always less common. The prevalence of *P. ovale* is low and geographically restricted to tropical Africa and some western Pacific islands.

Malaria is a vector-borne disease that humans acquire after being bitten by an infected female *Anopheles* mosquito. It is important to note that, in most parts of the world, malaria-transmitting anophelines are nocturnal in their blood-seeking habits. Therefore, humans are exposed to the disease primarily from dusk through dawn. Human behavior during this time can substantially alter the risk of acquiring the disease.

As an infected anopheline mosquito feeds on a human host, she inoculates malaria sporozoites from her salivary glands into the human peripheral circulation. Within an hour, these parasites are carried to the liver, where they invade hepatic parenchymal cells. Most of these parasites undergo a spectacular transformation and, within one to two weeks, multiply into large multinucleate bodies (preerythrocytic schizogony). These hepatic schizonts may contain as many as 40,000 merozoites, each of which is capable of invading a red blood cell after bursting from a hepatocyte.

After entering the erythrocyte, parasites continue to multiply asexually (erythrocytic schizogony), metabolizing hemoglobin, and growing from young trophozoites to schizonts. This process continues until the host cell is lysed, liberating 6 to 24 new merozoites, each of which reinvades a red blood cell to continue this intravascular cycle. This periodic rupture of parasites from red cells is responsible for the paroxysmal fever and chills of acute attacks of malaria.

For reasons that remain unclear, some merozoites do not develop in this manner, but rather, invade erythrocytes, begin sexual development, and differentiate into male or female gametocytes—the sexual forms of the malaria parasite. When a susceptible anopheline mosquito ingests both male (micro-) and female (macro-) gametocytes during a blood meal, sexual union (fertilization) occurs in the gut of the insect. The resultant zygote trans-

Table 25-1. Some Characteristics of Human Malarias

Species	Plasmodium Vivax	Plasmodium Falciparum	Plasmodium Malariae	Plasmodium Ovale
Incubation period (days)	12–17	9–14	18–40	16–18
Secondary exoerythrocytic cycle	Present	Absent	Absent	Present
Merozoites per tissue schizont	10,000	40,000	2,000	15,000
Erythrocytic cycle (hours)	42–48	48	72	49–50
Parasitemia (average) (per mm^3)	20,000	20,000–500,000	6,000	9,000
Severity of attack	Mild to moderate	Severe	Mild	Mild

forms into an ookinete and, subsequently, penetrates the wall of the mosquito midgut where it forms an oocyst. The oocyst matures over several days and releases many thousands of sporozoites, which are harbored in the mosquito's salivary glands. This entire sexual process is called sporogony.

Plasmodium falciparum is the most virulent parasite and causes the greatest morbidity and mortality. Parasitized red cells lose their oxygen-carrying capacity and deformability, which causes functional anemia and ischemia. In general, the higher the number of *P. falciparum* parasites in the peripheral blood, the greater the risk of complications or death from the infection. As a rule, individuals with parasitemia of 10 percent or greater and a hematocrit of less than 30 percent carry a grave prognosis unless aggressive treatment is started immediately. At this level of parasitemia, acute renal failure associated with hemolytic anemia is common. Respiratory failure, with or without pulmonary edema, may be seen and requires careful fluid management. A true bleeding diathesis is uncommon, but functional hypersplenism with sequestration of platelets in the spleen will cause peripheral thrombocytopenia. Disseminated intravascular coagulopathy rarely occurs.

Disturbances in mentation, from disorientation to psychoticlike states, and focal or global neurologic changes associated with cerebral hypoxia occur with *P. falciparum* infections. This syndrome is referred to as cerebral malaria if the patient becomes comatose or experiences major motor seizures. Lumbar puncture for examination of the cerebrospinal fluid (CSF) may be indicated to rule out pyogenic meningitis or other causes of encephalitis. Increased CSF pressure may be present, but the fluid should be clear, with a normal glucose and, rarely, with elevated protein. CSF pleocytosis is uncommon.

Blackwater fever is a syndrome of rapid and severe acute hemolysis, massive hemoglobinuria (dark brown urine), and renal failure. The pathogenesis of this uncommon, but serious, syndrome is unclear. Individuals with blackwater fever often give a history of intermittent quinine use in the past, and an autoimmune mechanism associated with quinine is postulated. Treatment consists of supportive fluid therapy, transfusions as needed, and appropriate antimalarial chemotherapy.

Infections with the three other species of malaria are usually not fatal. Splenomegaly from *P. vivax* will occasionally lead to splenic rupture and intraabdominal hemorrhage. Chronic infection in children with *P. malariae* has been implicated as a cause of an immune complex–induced nephrotic syndrome, a nephropathy that responds poorly to steroids but may respond to azathioprine.

DIAGNOSIS

Health care workers trained in nonmalarious areas of the world must develop a high level of suspicion of malaria infection. Malaria may be the cause of any febrile illness in individuals living in, or coming from, malaria endemic regions. The disease can be reliably diagnosed only through careful microscopic examination of properly prepared peripheral blood films. Both thick and thin blood smears should be made on a clean, grease-free, glass slide. Blood is most easily obtained from the lateral aspect of the third or fourth finger of the hand or, in infants, the heel or big toe (earlobes are not recommended). The skin should be cleansed with alcohol and allowed to dry prior to puncture with a sterile lancet or needle. Squeezing the extremity gently will allow a drop of blood to well up and permit adequate smears to be made (Figure 25-1). Take time to ensure that all smears are accurately labeled with the patient's name and/or number, and the date. The simplest method is to write directly on the thin film with an ordinary lead pencil. The blood films should be allowed to dry completely; in hot and humid climes, this process may be accelerated through the use of a fan or hair dryer. (Be careful not to heat and, thereby inadvertently, fix the thick smear.) During the drying process, flies and other insects are attracted to the blood smears; if laboratory workers are not attentive, these vermin may destroy the preparations before they are stained. Once dry, *only* the thin smear should be dipped in methanol and then air-dried for fixation. It is crucial that the thick smear not be fixed, in order to allow red blood cell (RBC) lysis to occur. The entire slide—both thick and thin smears—is then stained with Giemsa stain (see Chapter 22).

The microscopic examination of blood films for *Plasmodium* forms requires both practice and an understanding of the differential staining characteristics of infected erythrocytes. In general, the thick smear is 20 to 40 times more sensitive than the thin smear for determining the presence of parasites in the blood. However, the correct speciation of parasites is more easily accomplished from a thin smear.

Correct identification of the species of the infecting parasite is always desirable to make

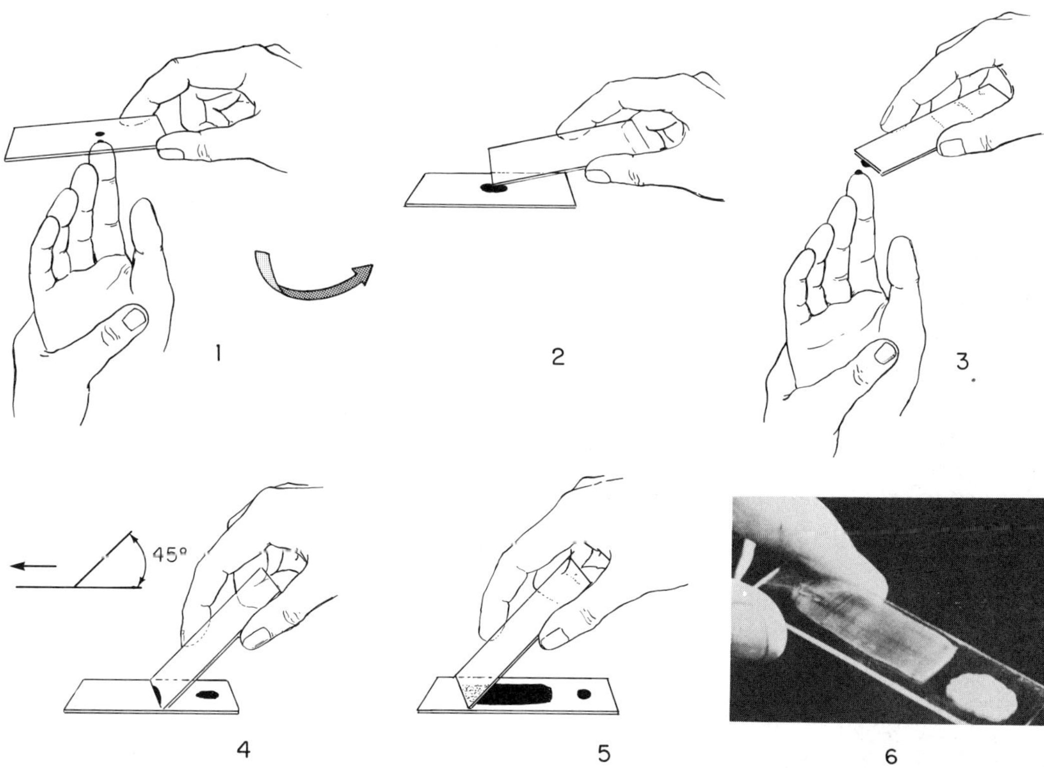

Figure 25-1. Preparation of a thin and thick blood film on the same slide: (1) Touch the drop of blood with a clean slide; (2) spread the drop of blood with the corner of another slide to make a circle or a square about 1 cm^2; (3) touch a new drop of blood with the edge of a clean slide; (4) bring the edge of the slide carrying a drop of blood to the surface of the first slide and wait until the blood spreads along the whole edge; (5) holding it at an angle of about 45 degrees, push it forward with a rapid, but not too brisk, movement; (6) write the slide number on the thin film with a pencil. Wait until the thick film is quite dry.

appropriate therapeutic decisions. The major clinical question posed in the diagnosis of acute malaria is always to distinguish *P. falciparum* malaria from malaria caused by nonfalciparum species. With practice, this skill can be acquired.

Under the microscope, *P. falciparum* appears as uniform, small, intraerythrocytic ring forms (young trophozoites) which stain as a dark red chromatin body (nucleus) attached to a thin crescent of bluish cytoplasm—a "signet ring"-like shape. On thin smears, some cells may have more than one parasite and may appear to have more than one chromatin body. The falciparum gametocyte (in itself, nonpathogenic to humans) has a characteristic sickle shape and, when seen, is an aid in the microscopic identification of infection with this species. *Plasmodium falciparum* parasites mature asexually while attached to endothelial surfaces in deep viscera. Therefore, it is very unusual to see any asexual parasite stage other than ring forms in the peripheral smear.

Species of malaria other than *P. falciparum* rarely infect more than 2 to 3 percent of circulating erythrocytes. Therefore, microscopic thin fields with more than 2 to 3 percent of red blood cells infected, with only ring forms present, are almost always diagnostic of *P. falciparum*.

Infections with other species of malaria are diagnosed in the peripheral smear by the typical appearance of the stages of the asexual life cycle of the parasites. *Plasmodium malariae* rings are large and coarse in shape. The older trophozoite of this species may look like a rectangular band extending across the cytoplasm of the red blood cell. Circulating schizonts with distinguishable merozoites are seen in many nonfalciparum infections. Both older trophozoites and schizonts may have detectable pigment granules as the metabolic result of hemoglobin degradation. In addition, red blood cells infected with *P. vivax* and *P. ovale* are generally larger than uninfected red blood cells. In well-stained blood films, cells infected with either of these two species may show scattered pinkish granules in their cytoplasm (Schuffner's dots). Finally, cells parasitized with *P. ovale* may have a characteristic oval shape, with fingerlike projections (fimbria) extending from the margin of the erythrocyte. When fimbria are not present, *P. ovale* and *P. vivax*-infected cells are difficult to distinguish from each other and an educated diagnosis may have to be made based on the likely geographic origin of the malaria infection.

It is important to remember that mixed infections may occur and visualization of nonfalciparum mature forms on a smear does not preclude the diagnosis of an associated infection with *P. falciparum*.

The microscope used for malaria diagnosis should preferably be a binocular instrument with a mechanical stage and substage electrical illumination with a blue daylight filter. Both thin and thick films are best read directly under oil immersion at a magnification of 400 to 600×. Slide examinations should be performed in a consistent fashion, preferably by routine scanning of 200 oil immersion fields. A hand-operated counter is invaluable.

Definitive diagnosis of malaria should rest on identification of parasites in the blood. Because parasitemia may fluctuate in an individual patient, parasites may be undetectable during the early prodrome of acute malaria or in asymptomatic semi-immune persons. The diagnosis of malaria, therefore, cannot be excluded on the basis of a single negative blood smear. If clinical signs and symptoms suggest the diagnosis, repeat blood films should be examined. Rarely, in instances in which malaria is strongly suspected despite negative blood slides, a therapeutic trial of antimalarials may be indicated. Although indirect immunofluorescence antibody techniques and enzyme-linked immunosorbent assay (ELISA) tests have been developed for epidemiologic studies of malaria, they have no place in the diagnosis of acute infection.

TREATMENT

Each antimalarial drug has its own well-described pharmacologic activity against each stage of the *Plasmodium* sp. life cycle. Drugs active against circulating asexual parasites are those used in the treatment of acute infections (Table 25-2).

The choice of a particular antimalarial should be based on (1) the species of parasite, (2) the geographic origin of the parasite and the likelihood of drug resistance, (3) the level of parasitemia and the presence or likelihood of complications, and (4) the level of immunity of the host. Unfortunately, the global spread of multidrug-resistant *P. falciparum* over the past 25 years has severely impeded the treatment and control of this disease.

Chloroquine is the most widely available antimalarial. It is administered orally, is highly effective against sensitive parasites, and is in-

Table 25-2. Use of Antimalarial Drugs

	Drug[a]	Adult Dose	Pediatric Dose
TREATMENT *Plasmodium falciparum* (chloroquine resistant)			
	Quinine		
	PO	650 mg q8h × 3–14 days	10 mg/kg q8h × 3–10 days
	IV	600 mg in 300 ml normal saline over at least 1 hour; repeat in 6–8h if PO therapy still cannot be tolerated (max. dose = 1800 mg/day)	25 mg/kg/day; give half the dose in a one hour infusion with normal saline, give the other half 6–8 h later if PO therapy still cannot be tolerated (max. dose = 1800 mg/day)
	AND EITHER		
	Pyrimethamine-sulfadoxine (Fansidar)	75 mg pyrimethamine + 1500 mg sulfa. (3 tabs) as single dose	1.5 mg/kg pyrimethamine + 30 mg/kg sulfa. as a single dose
	or		
	Pyrimethamine-sulfalene (Metakelfin)		
	or		
	Tetracycline	500 mg q6h × 7–10 days	250 mg q6h × 7–10 days (for children over 8 years of age)
	or		
	Doxycline	100 mg q12h × 7–10 days	2 mg/kg q12h × 7–10 days (for children over 8 years of age). Max. dose = 100 mg q12h.
	ALTERNATIVELY, the following combination product can be used alone:		
	Mefloquine + pyrimethamine + sulfadoxine (Fansimef)	3 tablets PO × 1 (= total of 750 mg mefloquine + 75 mg pyrimethamine + 1500 mg sulfadoxine)	
Plasmodium vivax, P. ovale, P. malariae, and chloroquine sensitive P. falciparum	Chloroquine	600 mg base initially, followed by 300 mg in 6 h, then 300 mg once daily × 2 days	10 mg base/kg, followed by 5 mg/kg in 6 h, and 5 mg/kg once daily × 2 days
	or		
	Amodiaquine (Camoquine, Flavoquine)	600 mg base initially, followed by 200 mg in 6 h, then 400 mg once daily × 2 days	14 mg base/kg, followed by 7 mg/kg once daily × 2 days (> 50 kg use adult dose)

Table 25-2. Use of Antimalarial Drugs (*Continued*)

	Drug[a]	Adult Dose	Pediatric Dose
RELAPSE PREVENTION (of P. vivax and P. ovale only)			
	Primaquine (do not use during pregnancy; screen for G6PD deficiency if test is available)	15 mg base once daily × 14 days *or* 45 mg base once weekly × 8 weeks	0.3 mg base/kg once daily × 14 days *or* 0.9 mg base/kg once weekly × 8 weeks
PROPHLAXIS (see text for explanation of use)			
	Chloroquine	300 mg base/week	5 mg base/kg/week (> 50 kg use adult dose)
	Pyrimethamine-sulfadoxine *or* Pyrimethamine-sulfalene	25 mg pyrimethamine + 500 mg sulfa	0.5 mg/kg/week pyrimethamine + 10 mg/kg/week sulfa (> 50 kg use adult dose)
	Pyrimethamine	25 mg/week	0.5 mg/kg/week (> 50 kg use adult dose)
	Pyrimethamine-dapsone (Maloprim)	12.5 mg pyrimethamine + 100 mg dapsone (1 tab)/ week	0.25 mg/kg pyrimethamine + 2.0 mg/kg dapsone/ week (> 50 kg use adult dose)
	Doxycycline	100 mg/day	> 8 years old; 2 mg/ kg/day
	Mefloquine	250 mg base/week	5 mg base/kg/week (> 50 kg use adult dose)
	Amodiaquine	400 mg base/week	7 mg base/kg/week (> 50 kg use adult dose)
	Chlorquanide (Proquanil; Paludrine)	100–200 mg/day	1.5–3.0 mg/kg/day

[a]All drugs should be administered orally unless otherwise stated. All doses are expressed in milligrams (mg) of drug **base;** doses of equivalent **salts** will vary, for example, chloroquine phosphate or chloroquine sulfate.

[b]All antimalarials are given during malaria exposure and for six weeks after leaving the malarious area. Quinine, tetracycline, and primaquine are not recommended or adequately tested for use in prophylaxis.

expensive. It is of low toxicity in therapeutic doses and is generally well tolerated, even in babies. Chloroquine is not teratogenic and can be administered without harm to pregnant women. An annoying, though not life-threatening, adverse reaction found primarily among black Africans is severe pruritus, especially of the hands and feet. This itching reaction responds poorly to antihistamines but is self-limited. Chloroquine-associated retinopathy has been reported in individuals who have taken chloroquine in high doses for extended periods of time, primarily when used in the treatment of collagen vascular disease. It is very unlikely to occur in relief workers who take the drug as weekly chemoprophylaxis, even if taken continuously for several years.

All strains of *P. vivax, P. ovale,* and *P. malariae* worldwide are sensitive to chloroquine; it is the drug of choice for infections with these parasites (see Table 25-2 for dosage). Amodiaquine is a useful alternative. Many isolates of *P. vivax* from various parts of the world have been found to be highly resistant to pyrimethamine and other antifolates. Consequently, the sulfa/antifolate combinations should not be used to treat nonfalciparum malaria.

P. vivax and *P. ovale* infections acquired by mosquito bite may have persistent exoerythrocytic forms (hypnozoites), which can cause relapses months to years after the initial infection. Primaquine is a drug that *may* prevent these relapses (there are documented resistant strains in Southeast Asia); however, its use is not always necessary or desirable. In individuals with G6PD deficiency, primaquine causes a hemolytic anemia that may be severe depending on the genotype of the enzymatic deficiency. Asians in particular may experience marked life-threatening hemolysis following treatment with primaquine, while such severe reactions are uncommon in affected individuals from Latin America. In general, because the facilities for determining G6PD status are not available in relief settings, and because there is usually a continuous exposure to relapsing species of malaria, health providers in many refugee camps do not use primaquine as a radical curative agent. However, when the eradication of malaria from a particular relief setting is a goal, primaquine should be used. Primaquine should not be given to pregnant women or young children.

Chloroquine-Sensitive *Plasmodium Falciparum*

The number of countries in which chloroquine-resistant malaria is transmitted has expanded dramatically in the past five years (Table 25-3). There is every expectation that the list will continue to grow at the expense of the world's disadvantaged and homeless persons.

Chloroquine-Resistant *Plasmodium Falciparum*

Although there are recognized gradations of drug resistance, as a general guideline, individuals who acquire *P. falciparum* malaria in areas of known drug resistance should presumptively be treated with an alternative drug regimen. Quinine remains the mainstay of chloroquine-resistant *P. falciparum* therapy and should be given orally, if possible, 650 mg or 10 mg/kg every eight hours. Quinine acts rapidly on parasites in the peripheral circulation, but is a poor single-agent drug to cure malaria because of its frequent side effects of nausea, vomiting, vertigo, and tinnitus. Patients may require as little as 3 days or, as in infections from Southeast Asia, as much as 10 to 14 days of quinine. In all instances, quinine should be supplemented with a curative regimen of a tetracycline or a sulfonamide/antifolate combination—for example, pyrimethamine plus sulfadoxine (Fansidar) or Metakelfin. Quinidine, an isomer of quinine, is also an effective antimalarial.

The sulfa/antifolate combinations have been used for many years. Their major advantage is that a complete therapeutic dose may be given at one time, thus obviating concerns of patient noncompliance. Sulfa/antifolates have a number of disadvantages, however, including relatively high cost and possible severe side effects (see Prevention). These drugs should not be used in persons allergic to sulfonamides or in children under two months of age. Although some authorities remain concerned about teratogenic potential, at present, these combination drugs appear safe for use during pregnancy.

Fansidar-resistant *P. falciparum* was first recognized in Thailand during the early 1980s.

Table 25-3. Areas with Reported Chloroquine-Resistant Plasmodium Falciparum (as of June, 1985)

Africa	Asia	South America	Oceania
Angola	Bangladesh	Bolivia	Papua, New Guinea
Burundi	Burma	Brazil	Solomon Islands
Central African Republic	China (Hainan Island & southern provinces)	Colombia	Vanuatu
Comoros	India	Ecuador	
Gabon	Indonesia	French Guiana	
Kenya	Kampuchea	Guyana	
Madagascar	Laos	Panama (east of Canal Zone)	
Malawi	Malaysia	Peru	
Mozambique	Pakistan (Rawalpindi)	Surinam	
Namibia	Philippines	Venezuela	
Rwanda	Thailand		
Sudan (north)	Vietnam		
Tanzania			
Uganda			
Zaire			
Zambia (northeast)			

Since then, it has been reported in Southeast Asia, the Amazon basin of South America, and East African countries such as Kenya and Tanzania. The true prevalence and extent of Fansidar-resistance remains unknown, but health care workers should be aware that the drug combination may not always cure individuals with chloroquine-resistant malaria.

Tetracyclines (including doxycycline and minocycline), if given for at least seven consecutive days, cure infections with all strains of *P. falciparum*. Tetracyclines are slow acting and should always be administered along with a rapidly acting drug such a quinine. Clindamycin is another antibiotic with antimalarial activity.

Mefloquine (Lariam) is a new synthetic antimalarial that is chemically related to quinine. It has been field tested in Thailand, Brazil, and Zambia. To delay the emergence of widespread mefloquine resistance (drug-resistant isolates have already been identified), it will be marketed as a combination product with Fansidar called Fansimef. A single tablet of Fansimef will contain 250 mg of mefloquine + 500 mg of sulfadoxine + 25 mg of pyrimethamine. Three tablets will be administered in a single dose for treatment of multidrug-resistant *P. falciparum*, or one tablet per week will be used for suppression.

Pregnancy

In endemic areas, malaria occurs more frequently and with greater severity in pregnant women than among similarly aged women who are not pregnant. It is clear that maternal malaria is a major cause of placental dysfunction and resultant fetal malnutrition, low birth weight, and premature birth. It is generally agreed that pregnant women with malaria should always receive antimalarial therapy, as it is safer than the infection. However, the following antimalarials are relatively contraindicated for pregnant women: quinine (an abortefacient in high doses), tetracyclines (tooth and bone dysgenesis), and primaquine (a potentially lethal hemolytic agent for the developing fetus). Pregnant women with relapsing malaria should be carried to term on weekly suppression with chloroquine or amodiaquine. Treatment with Fansidar may be necessary, although it is sensible to give folinic acid supplementation along with any regimen during the first trimester of pregnancy; this does not affect the sulfa/antifolate antimalarial efficacy. Mefloquine and the Fansimef combination have not yet been assessed for use in pregnancy.

Complicated *Plasmodium falciparum*

Any patient with complicated *P. falciparum* infection, such as cerebral malaria, should be hospitalized. Prompt treatment should be initiated with a loading dose of parenteral quinine dihydrochloride (20 mg/kg body weight in normal saline infused over four hours, followed by 10 mg/kg every eight hours until the patient is able to take oral medication). Initial quinine therapy should be followed by an oral regimen of an appropriately curative drug such as tetracycline (see Table 25-2). Parenteral chloroquine, although widely available outside the United States, should be avoided because of its potential cardiotoxicity and incidence of sudden death, especially in children.

Most severely ill patients are dehydrated on arrival to a health facility and require frequent assessment of fluid and electrolyte balances, urine output, respiratory status, and transfusion requirements. Both intravenous quinine and high levels of parasitemia have been associated with hypoglycemia, especially in pregnant women, necessitating support of blood glucose in some severely ill patients. Corticosteroids and anticoagulant therapy are contraindicated in the treatment of acute, complicated *P. falciparum* malaria. Moribund patients, or those with greater than 20 percent parasitization of their red blood cells, may benefit from complete exchange transfusion with whole blood.

PREVENTION

Prevention and control of malaria should address each of the three components of malaria transmission: the mosquito vector, the parasite, and the human host. Medical entomologists and sanitarians have taught clinicians much about the complex epidemiology of malaria, however, control of anopheline mosquitoes has proved difficult to achieve.

Although the risk of exposure to malaria varies with the individual and the geographic region, malaria prevention should always be based on protection of the individual from the mosquito vector. Application of insect repellent, wearing protective clothing, including long-sleeved shirts and trousers, the use of mosquito netting and "knock-down" insecticides inside dwellings, and window screens are effective measures.

The judicious use of antimalarials to suppress clinical illness is a useful strategy for nonimmune travelers and for long-term workers in endemic areas. Prophylactic antimalarials may also be useful for selected groups of semi-immune persons who may be at high risk for complications such as pregnant women and young children. Because of the rapid spread of drug-resistant parasites, and occasional side effects of certain antimalarials, no drug currently exists that can guarantee malaria suppression in all situations. Therefore, a diagnosis of malaria should still be considered for any individual who becomes febrile while taking prophylactic drugs.

The choice of suppressive drug(s) will depend on the prevalence of drug-resistant *P. falciparum* in the area of exposure. It is important to assess the impact of potential disease on different populations, specifically between semi-immune residents of malarious areas, such as refugees from endemic areas, and nonimmune residents, such as relief workers. Because of acquired humoral immunity following multiple infections, so called semi-immune individuals may tolerate parasitemia without obvious acute ill effects. Furthermore, when symptomatic, they may be able to suppress the signs and symptoms of infection after the administration of a smaller dose of drug than is given to individuals who have never been infected. The practice of giving such semi-immune individuals lower doses of antimalarials, either for prophylaxis or treatment, should be discouraged because this may lead to increased prevalence of drug-resistant parasites in the area.

Well-documented cases of severe cutaneous side effects, including fatal Stevens–Johnson syndrome, have occurred during or following the use of Fansidar for chemoprophylaxis. Although the incidence of these reactions is low, health professionals should be watchful for such complications.

Side effects similar to those associated with Fansidar may be anticipated from other sulfonamide combinations such as Metakelfin. Maloprim is a combination tablet of dapsone plus pyrimethamine. It is probably not as effective as Fansidar for malaria suppression and there are well-documented reports of agranulocytosis associated with its use. Dosage for adults should not exceed one tablet per week.

Pyrimethamine alone and biguanide antifolates such as proguanil (Paludrine) and chlorproguanil (Lapudrine) have been used for many years for the suppression of malaria. Although these compounds appear to be safe, drug resistance to *P. vivax* and *P. falciparum* has been recognized in most areas of the world, and thus limits their usefulness.

Recent reports of fatal agranulocytosis and toxic hepatitis (Centers for Disease Control 1986) following the administration of amodiaquine suggest that its use as a suppressive drug be limited.

Tetracyclines are probably effective as chemoprophylactic agents; however, they have not been adequately field-tested for long-term use. Further, their potential side effects, such as photosensitivity and gastrointestinal upset, suggest that they should be reserved for treatment of acute malaria.

CONTROL

Although mosquito vector control may seem like the most sensible method for malaria prevention, achieving this end may prove an overwhelming task in the relief setting. Nevertheless, under the supervision of a trained sanitarian, it is useful to reduce the number of mosquito breeding sites by regulating all water sources and draining unnecessary water collection, in addition to the use of appropriate larvicides. Economic considerations, types of human habitation, regional climate, and professional assessment of biting behavior and pesticide susceptibility of the predominant anophelines should determine whether or not insecticides may be useful. Displaced persons and refugees should be encouraged to participate in all malaria prevention and control efforts. It is advantageous for such operations to be integrated with local government programs.

The control of malaria will eventually be achieved through the development and widescale administration of effective and safe vaccines. Human immunity to malaria generally appears to be both species- and parasite stage-specific. Initial research has identified the antigenic determinant on the surface of the sporozoite of *P. falciparum* with the expectation that circulating antibodies to this protein should prevent human infection. With recombinant DNA technology, potential immunogens are being prepared and standardized for field-testing of vaccines.

REFERENCES AND SELECTED READING

Bruce-Chwatt LJ: Essential Malariology. London, William Heinemann Medical Books Ltd, 1980.

Bruce-Chwatt LJ (ed): Chemotherapy of Malaria, 2nd ed. Monograph Series No 27, Geneva, World Health Organization, 1981.

Bruce-Chwatt LJ: Malaria and Pregnancy. Br Med J 1983;286:1457–458.

Centers for Disease Control: Agranulocytosis associated with the use of amodiaquine for malaria prophylaxis. MMWR 1986;35:165–66.

Centers for Disease Control: Revised recommendations for preventing malaria in travelers to areas with chloroquine-resistant *Plasmodium falciparum*. MMWR 1985;34:185–95.

Centers for Disease Control: Adverse reactions to Fansidar and updated recommendations for its use in the prevention of malaria. MMWR 1985;33:713–14.

Clyde DF, Miller RM, Dupont HL et al: Antimalarial effects of tetracyclines in man. J Trop Med Hyg 1971;74:238–42.

Clyde DF: Clinical problems associated with the use of primaquine as a tissue schizonticidal and gametocytocidal drug. Bull WHO 1981;59:391–95.

Editorial: Chloroquine-resistant malaria in Africa. Lancet 1985;1:1487–488.

Kramer SL, Campbell CC, Moncrieff RE: Fulminant *Plasmodium falciparum* infection treated with exchange blood transfusion. JAMA 1983;249:244–45.

Krogstad DJ, Pfaller MA: Prophylaxis and treatment of malaria. In Remington JS, Swartz MN (eds): Current Clinical Topics in Infectious Diseases, vol 3, pp 56–73. New York, McGraw-Hill, 1982.

Miller LH, Mason SJ, Clyde DF et al: The resistance factor to *Plasmodium* vivax in blacks: The Duffy blood group genotype FyFy. N Engl J Med 1976;302–04.

Miller LH: Malaria. In Warren KS, Mahmoud AAF (eds): Tropical and Geographical Medicine, pp 223–29. New York, McGraw-Hill, 1984.

Schwartz IK, Chin W, Newman J et al: Glucose-6-phosphate dehydrogenase deficiency in Southeast Asian refugees entering the United States. Am J Trop Med Hyg 1984;33:182–84.

Warrell DA, Looareesuwan S, Warrell MJ et al: Dexamethasone proves deleterious in cerebral malaria. N Engl J Med 1982;306:313–19.

Watkins WM, Sixsmith DG, Spencer HC et al: Effectiveness of amodiaquine as treatment for chloroquine-resistant *Plasmodium falciparum* infections in Kenya. Lancet 1984;1:357–59.

White NJ, Looareesuwan S, Warrell DA et al: Quinine pharmacokinetics and toxicity in cerebral and uncomplicated falciparum malaria. Am J Med 1982;73:564–75.

White NJ, Looareesuwan S, Warrell DA et al: Quinine loading dose in cerebral malaria. Am J Trop Med Hyg 1983;32:1–5.

White NJ, Warrell DA, Chanthavanich P et al: Severe hypoglycemia and hyperinsulinemia in falciparum malaria. N Engl J Med 1983;309–16.

WHO Working Group: Advances in Chemotherapy. Technical Report Series No 711. Geneva, World Health Organization, 1984.

26
Dengue Fever and Rickettsial Diseases

CYNTHIA S. WEIKEL

Dengue fever and the rickettsial diseases are caused by two distinct classes of microbes; the flaviviruses and small pleomorphic gram-negative bacilli, respectively. The geographic distributions of these diseases are not identical, thus it is imperative that health care workers in the field identify which diseases occur in their location.

Although the etiologic agents, geographic distribution, and pathogenesis of these conditions are diverse, extensive overlap in clinical manifestations (high fever, headache, myalgias and arthralgias, and gastrointestinal upset) may occur. At certain stages of the disease process, rashes are characteristic of both dengue fever and the rickettsial diseases. The pattern and clinical features of the rash may help to distinguish these illnesses, particularly if eschar formation (seen only with the rickettsial diseases) is present. The most important complications of dengue fever are bleeding and shock. These complications occur most frequently in children, and in those experiencing a second dengue infection within five years of a previous infection. Encephalitis, pulmonary edema, and infarction in multiple organ systems may be life-threatening in the rickettsioses, and major bleeding complications occur in severe, untreated rickettsial infections.

Antibiotic therapy with tetracyclines (including doxycycline) or chloramphenicol is potentially life-saving in the rickettsial diseases; no specific therapy is available for dengue fever. The key to the successful outcome of either infection is meticulous fluid and electrolyte management. At present, no consistently effective preventive therapy for either dengue fever or the rickettsioses is available. However, use of topical insect repellents containing high concentrations (30 to 50%) of the compound diethyltoluamide (deet) is recommended to decrease contact with the insect vectors (mosquitoes, ticks, fleas, lice, and mites) of dengue fever and the rickettsioses.

The remainder of this chapter addresses the clinical recognition, pathogenesis, diagnosis, management, and therapy of dengue fever and the rickettsial diseases. For more detailed discussions, the references by Halstead (1984a, b), Saah and Hornick (1985), and the WHO Working Group on Rickettsial Diseases (1982) should be consulted.

DENGUE FEVER

Dengue viruses are single-stranded, enveloped RNA Group B togaviruses or flaviviruses (the prototype flavivirus is yellow fever). The four distinct dengue viruses—types 1, 2, 3, and 4—all produce a similar disease in humans and are transmitted by certain species of day-biting *Aedes mosquitoes.* The usual vector, *Aedes aegypti,* is present in most tropical and subtropical areas between the latitude 45° north and 35° south (Halstead 1984a). Both humans and, occasionally, monkeys may perpetuate cycles of infection with these viruses. *Aedes aegypti* can acquire the virus from infected humans 6 to 18 hours before clinical illness occurs and then for the duration of the fever (Halstead 1984b). Following an infective blood meal and an incubation period of approximately two weeks, the mosquito may transmit the infection for the duration of its life. *Aedes* mosquitoes breed primarily indoors in water containers such as planters or ant traps (Halstead 1984a).

Illness due to dengue viruses ranges from mild to severe. Milder disease is referred to as dengue fever syndrome while severe hemorrhagic disease is called dengue shock syndrome. In young children, dengue fever is often an undifferentiated febrile illness accompanied by pharyngeal erythema, rhinitis, mild cough, and gastrointestinal symptoms. In older children and adults, classic dengue fever begins with an abrupt rise in temperature (to as high as 39° to 41°C) accompanied by frontal or retroorbital headache, backache, and pain in the muscles and joints. "Dengue facies" refers to the facial flushing, eyelid edema and conjunctival injection, and suffusion that may occur (Halstead 1984b). During the first two days of fever, a transient, blanching macular rash may be seen. On days 2 to 6 of illness, nausea, vomiting, lymphadenopathy, relative bradycardia, cutaneous hyperesthesia, marked anorexia, and constipation occur. Coincident with, or one to two days after the fever resolves, a generalized morbilliform, maculopapular rash begins centrally and spreads peripherally (sparing the palms and soles). This rash may be associated with a second rise in temperature (classic biphasic temperature curve). During the febrile period, laboratory studies reveal profound leukopenia with decreased polymorphonuclear leukocytes and relative lymphocytosis (Halstead 1970a). Occasionally, mild thrombocytopenia is present. Although rare with uncomplicated dengue fever, bleeding complications such as epistaxis, petechiae, purpura, or gastrointestinal bleeding may occur at any stage of the disease. Although the dengue fever syndrome is usually benign, prolonged asthenia, mental depression, and bradycardia may follow acute illness.

The onset of dengue hemorrhagic fever is similar to the dengue fever syndrome. However, after two to five days of illness (median four days) and sometimes at defervescence, a leaky capillary syndrome and abnormalities in hemostasis (thrombocytopenia, a prolonged bleeding time—more than five minutes—and an elevated prothrombin time) may develop. Deterioration may be rapid. In dengue hemorrhagic fever, hemoconcentration occurs (defined as hematocrit increased by 20%) and the platelet count is less than or equal to 100,000 platelets per cubic millimeter (Halstead 1970b, 1984b). If shock or a narrowed pulse pressure (systolic minus diastolic blood pressure of $\leq$ 20 mm Hg) is present, this subgroup is called the dengue shock syndrome. Physical examination reveals scattered petechiae, spontaneous ecchymoses, and bleeding at venipuncture sites. Patients may be irritable and complain of midepigastric pain. Gastrointestinal bleeding and vaginal bleeding occur in about 10 percent of cases, particularly in adults (Halstead 1984b). In a recent series of virologically confirmed cases from Indonesia, 70 percent of patients with a fatal outcome had signs of encephalitis (e.g., convulsions, somnolence), and 80 percent had gastrointestinal bleeding (Sumarmo et al 1983). In dengue shock syndrome, an enlarged liver may develop. If hypovolemia is corrected, convalescence may occur after a crisis period of 24 to 48 hours.

Dengue shock syndrome occurs in two major immunologic groups: initial dengue infections in infants less than one year of age, and dengue infections in children usually over one year of age. The pathogenesis of these severe dengue infections is explained by the presence in both groups of infection-enhancing antibody (Halstead 1970a, 1970b, and 1984a). The presence of serum antibody (IgG), which does not neutralize the dengue virus, allows the virus to parasitize and replicate in human mononuclear phagocytes efficiently, resulting in larger amounts of circulating virus. Infected mononuclear phagocytes become activated, thus leading to a release of proteolytic enzymes and activation of the complement and blood-clotting systems that result in the capillary defect and hemostatic abnormalities seen in this disease. In the case of infants under one year of age, infection-enhancing antibody is passively acquired from the mother during gestation. Infant dengue hemorrhagic syndrome/dengue shock syndrome occurs as early as 3 months of age, peaks at 7 to 8 months of age, and wanes by 12 months of age (Halstead 1984a). In children over one year of age, the vast majority of the cases of dengue shock syndrome are associated with secondary dengue infections occurring between three months and five years after the initial infection (Halstead 1970b, 1984a). The sequence of virus types encountered by the individual appears to be important with secondary infections due to dengue type 2 resulting in a higher incidence of shock (Halstead 1970b; Sangkawibha et al 1984). Females over the age of four and children with a good nutritional status (i.e., capable of making adequate serum antibody) are at greater risk for the dengue shock syndrome. Sequential infections with two different dengue virus types protect the individual against clinical disease with the third or fourth dengue virus types (Halstead 1970b).

Diagnosis of dengue virus infections depends on the measurement of specific antibodies or isolation of the virus by inoculation of serum or buffy-coat specimens into cell culture or certain mosquito species. The N test, or the measurement of virus neutralizing antibody, may provide the earliest and most specific answer (Halstead 1984b). However, these procedures are not likely to be available in the refugee setting.

No specific therapy is available to treat dengue viral infections (Halstead 1984b). Management is directed at maintaining adequate blood volume and blood pressure until the capillary defect heals, usually within 24 to 48 hours. Oral rehydration solutions may be used in patients without shock (see Chapter 15). If vomiting or hemoconcentration develop, parenteral fluid therapy with 5 percent glucose and one half lactated Ringer's solution should be initiated. Shock is a medical emergency. The patient's feet should be elevated and the head lowered. Fluids (e.g., lactated Ringer's, normal saline, plasma, albumin) should be administered rapidly until vital signs improve, urine output is at least 0.5 ml/kg/hour, and the hematocrit begins to decline. Vital signs should be monitored at 15-minute intervals, and urine output and hematocrit every one to two hours until stable. Oral rehydration should be substituted for intravenous therapy as soon as is clinically possible. Fluid therapy should be reduced when there is evidence that the capillary defect is repairing, to avoid precipitation of congestive heart failure due to resorption of tissue fluid "leaked" during the acute illness (Halstead 1984b). Sympathomimetic amines and salicylates should not be used.

Long-term control of dengue viral infections depends on health education and community projects aimed at reducing the breeding sites of *Aedes* mosquitoes (Halstead 1984a). Personal protection should focus on avoiding the bites of daytime mosquitoes by wearing appropriate clothing and using insect repellents. The most effective topical insect repellent currently available is diethyltoluamide (deet) (Medical Letter 1985). Other effective repellents are ethyl hexanediol and dimethyl phthalate. Topical repellents are easily removed from the skin by bathing or sweating and must be reapplied often to be effective. Table 26–1 lists available insect repellents and the concentrations of the most active ingredients in these repellents. The most effective concentrations of deet suggested for use are 30 to 50 percent. Diethyltoluamide is absorbed and 10 to 15 percent of each dose can be recovered in the urine. Toxic and allergic reactions (including anaphylaxis) to deet may occur, particularly in children in whom toxic encephalopathy and grand mal seizures have been reported. Fifty percent deet has been associated with local skin reactions including burning, erythema, and blisters. With 75 per-

Table 26-1. Insect Repellents

Product	Form	Major Ingredients
6-12 Plus (d-Con, subsidiary Sterling Drug)	Aerosol	25% ethyl hexanediol, 5% deet and isomers
	Stick	56% ethyl hexanediol, 9.1% deet and isomers
OFF (SC Johnson)	Aerosol	15% deet and isomers
Cutter insect repellent (Cutter)	Spray	17.9% deet and isomers, 12% dimethyl phthalate
Deep Woods Off (SC Johnson)	Aerosol, pump spray	20% deet and isomers
	Lotion	30% deet and isomers
OFF (SC Johnson)	Towelettes	32.3% deet and isomers
Cutter insect repellent (Cutter)	Stick	33% deet and isomers
	Cream	51.75% deet and isomers, 13% dimethyl phthalate
Repel (Wisconsin)	Spray	40% deet and isomers
Deep Woods OFF maximum strength (SC Johnson)	Liquid	100% deet and isomers
Jungle Formula ("Ole Time" Woodsman)	Liquid	75% deet and isomers
Jungle Plus ("Ole Time" Woodsman)	Liquid	100% deet
Muskol (Plough, Inc.)	Spray	25% deet and isomers
	Liquid, lotion	100% deet and isomers

(Adapted with permission from the Medical Letter, 1985;27:63.)

cent deet, up to 50 percent of individuals may experience local skin toxicity (Medical Letter 1985).

RICKETTSIAL DISEASES

The Rickettsiaceae are a family of hardy, small, pleomorphic gram-negative bacilli that are distinct from other bacteria in that they are obligate intracellular parasites. These organisms are maintained in nature through a cycle involving mammal reservoirs and insect vectors. Humans are incidental hosts except in the case of louse-borne epidemic typhus for which humans are the principal host and the human body louse *(Pediculus humanus corporis)* is the vector. In epidemic typhus, explosive epidemics may occur.

The rickettsial diseases are a large group of illnesses that are best organized into three disease categories: the spotted fever, the typhus group, and Q fever. The pathogenesis, epidemiology, clinical manifestations, and diagnosis of the spotted fever and typhus illnesses are similar. Although Q fever does overlap with the other rickettsioses in clinical manifestations and therapy, it is distinct in its pathogenesis, epidemiology, and diagnosis and will be discussed separately. Table 26–2 summarizes certain epidemiologic features and clinical manifestations of the rickettsial diseases.

Spotted Fever and Typhus Illnesses

These diseases are acquired when the appropriate infected vector (tick, louse, mite, or flea) deposits rickettsial-laden feces while feeding on the human host (Saah & Hornick 1985; Woodward & Osterman 1984). Minute abrasions at the site of arthropod attachment become contaminated with the fecal debris and infection is initiated. Less often, the organisms may enter by mucous membrane contamination. Once the skin is inoculated, local multiplication of organisms occurs, in some cases with formation of a local lesion or eschar in one to three weeks. These lesions begin as firm, erythematous papules (2 to 10 mm) that later ulcerate and form a black crust, which is the eschar. The rickettsia enter the blood from the local lesion where they penetrate endothelial cells of small capillaries and venules and multiply, leading to cell injury or death. This results in increased permeability of the blood vessels and leads to tissue edema and hemorrhage, and a vasculitis that is associated with fibrin thrombi leading to infarction of skin and, potentially, other organ systems including kidney, heart, brain, and adrenals. It is these key physiologic and pathologic features, increased capillary permeability, and vasculitis that help account for the major clinical manifestations of these diseases.

The clinical symptoms and signs of these rickettsioses are similar and will be discussed together (Saah & Hornick 1985; Woodward & Osterman 1984; WHO Working Group on Rickettsial Diseases 1982), with significant exceptions noted. A prodrome of malaise, headache, and mild fever may be described, but often onset of clinical illness is abrupt. One exception is endemic (murine) typhus in which the onset is gradual. Generally, the shorter the incubation period, the more severe the disease. In the rickettsial diseases associated with eschar formation, systemic illness usually follows the appearance of the eschar by three to seven days. In rickettsial diseases not associated with eschar formation, systemic symptoms and signs are the first manifestations of illness. The patient appears ill with major complaints of fever, chills, headache, which is quite severe and often frontal in location, myalgias and muscle stiffness often prominent in the neck and leg muscle groups, and arthralgias. Nausea, vomiting, and nonproductive cough may occur. Fevers may be sustained to above 39°C. By the fourth day of illness, most patients will have developed a rash that varies with the etiologic agent. Conjunctivitis and nonpitting edema are seen. In severe disease, encephalitis and pulmonary infiltrates secondary to increased capillary permeability and vasculitis may develop. Hepatomegaly with elevated liver function tests may occur. The course of illness may be complicated by superimposed bacterial infections (e.g., parotitis, pneumonia), skin ulcerations and gangrene, and disseminated intravascular coagulation with decreased platelets and elevated coagulation parameters. Untreated infection gradually resolves in about two weeks, but without antibiotic therapy, mortality is high.

The rashes associated with the rickettsial diseases are very important to early recognition and treatment of these infections. The rash of Rocky Mountain spotted fever appears peripherally on the hands, wrists, feet, and ankles (often involving the palms and soles) as macular, rose-colored, blanching lesions that rapidly spread centrally. If treatment is delayed and vasculitis develops, the rash becomes petechial and can progress to coalescent

Table 20-2. Summary of Certain Epidemiologic and Clinical Features of the Rickettsial Diseases

Disease	Organism	Geographic Area	Natural Cycle: Insect Vector	Natural Cycle: Animal Reservoir	Rash Distribution	Eschar
Spotted fever group						
RMSF[a]	*R. rickettsii*	Western hemisphere	Tick	Wild rodents, dogs	Extremities to trunk	Occasional
Boutonneuse	*R. conorii*	Africa, India, Mediterranean	Tick	Wild rodents, dogs	Trunk, extremities, face	Yes
Queensland tick typhus	*R. australis*	Australia	Tick	Wild rodents, marsupials	Trunk, extremities, face	Yes
North Asian tick typhus	*R. siberica*	Siberia, Mongolia	Tick	Wild rodents	Trunk, extremities, face	Yes
Rickettsialpox	*R. akari*	U.S., USSR, Korea, Africa	Mite	House mouse, other rodents	Vesicular; trunk, extremities, face; heals by crusting	Yes
Typhus group						
Epidemic typhus[a]	*R. prowazekii*	Highland areas of South America, Africa, Asia, eastern U.S.	Body louse	Man, flying squirrel[b]	Trunk to extremities	No
Brill–Zinsser	*R. prowazekii*	Worldwide based on immigration	None	Man (recurrence years after primary attack)	Trunk to extremities (may be absent)	No
Endemic (murine) typhus	*R. typhi*	Worldwide in pockets (urban, seaports, granaries)	Flea	Small rodents, especially rat	Trunk to extremities (present in 60 to 80%)	No
Scrub typhus	*R. tsutsugamushi*	South Pacific, Asia, Australia, Pakistan, USSR, Afghanistan	Mite	Wild rodents	Trunk to extremities (may be absent)	Yes
Others						
Q fever	*C. burnetii*	Worldwide	——	Cattle, sheep, goats, small mammals (inhalation of organism)	None	No

[a]Life-threatening rickettsioses.
[b]In the eastern United States, typhus exists as a zoonosis in flying squirrels.
(Adapted with permission from Mandell GL, Douglas RG, Jr, Bennett JE (eds): Principles and Practices of Infectious Diseases. New York, John Wiley, 1985.)

purpura with associated skin infarction most commonly seen on the extremities, scrotum and pressure points (Woodward & Osterman 1984). The rash of rickettsialpox, another spotted fever, appears as papules with central vesicles that heal wth crusting and may be confused with chickenpox. Among the typhus group, the rash of epidemic (louse-borne) and scrub typhus resembles that of Rocky Mountain spotted fever but begins centrally on the axillary folds and trunk and spreads peripherally. However, in Brill-Zinsser disease, a recrudescence of previous infection with *R. prowazekii* (epidemic typhus), rash may be absent. In scrub typhus, rash may also be absent in up to two thirds of patients (Saah & Hornick 1985). The rash of endemic (murine) typhus occurs in 60 to 80 percent of patients, may be present only briefly, and is distinct in that it occurs only on the thorax and abdomen.

The differential diagnosis of the rickettsioses is quite broad and includes atypical measles, meningococcal infection, typhoid fever and other enteric fevers, leptospirosis, infectious mononucleosis, dengue, and brucellosis.

Laboratory studies early in the infection are nondiagnostic and include mild anemia and leukocytosis. In severe disease, electrolyte disturbances (including decreased sodium and chloride), hypoalbuminemia, and azotemia occur.

Diagnosis and institution of therapy are dependent on a high index of suspicion and the ability to recognize an illness consistent with the rickettsial diseases in the appropriate epidemiologic and geographic setting. Definitive diagnosis relies on serologic studies, which are not likely to be available in the refugee setting. The Weil–Felix test is a nonspecific agglutination assay based on an early observation that serum from patients with typhus agglutinated certain strains of the bacterium *Proteus vulgaris* (OX–19, OX–2, and OX–K). In samples collected at the onset of illness, then two to six weeks later (convalescent) and assayed simultaneously, a fourfold rise in antibodies may be diagnostic. If only a convalescent serum specimen is available, a titer greater than 1:640 is suggestive of recent disease. Agglutination reactions with *Proteus* OX–19 and OX–2 are positive in patients with the spotted fevers except rickettsialpox and may be positive in the typhus group except for Brill-Zinsser disease. Although potentially helpful in diagnosis, the Weil–Felix is a nonspecific test and must be interpreted with caution because positive agglutination is seen in other nonrickettsial conditions such as relapsing fever. The most reliable test currently available to confirm a diagnosis is the indirect fluorescent antibody test using specific rickettsial antigens.

Effective therapy in the rickettsial diseases involves a two-pronged approach: antibiotic therapy and judicious supportive care. Early empiric antibiotic therapy is mandatory to reduce the morbidity and mortality incurred by these diseases. Both chloramphenicol (50 mg/kg/day divided over six to eight-hour intervals) and tetracycline (25 mg/kg/day given at six-hour intervals) or doxycycline (100 mg orally twice daily in adults) are effective (Saah & Hornick 1985; Woodward & Osterman 1984). Single-dose doxycycline therapy (100 mg) has been successful in treating epidemic (louse-borne) typhus (Perine et al 1974), but has been associated with relapse of infection in scrub typhus (Olson et al 1981). Single-dose therapy should not be used in Rocky Mountain spotted fever. If treatment is given very early in the course of the rickettsial infection, symptomatic relapse may occur rarely. Relapses repond to retreatment with tetracycline, doxycycline, or chloramphenicol (Saah & Hornick 1985). Antibiotics should be given intravenously in seriously ill patients or those with nausea and vomiting. Oral therapy should be substituted as soon as possible. Despite being only rickettsiostatic, these antibiotics lead to rapid clinical improvement and decreased temperature within two to three days. Antibiotics should be continued for two to three days after clinical improvement and defervescence occurs, which is generally a five- to seven-day course. (See Chapters 12 and 23 for usage precautions and further information on the dosages of chloramphenicol and the tetracyclines.)

Supportive therapy includes careful attention to blood pressure, volume and electrolyte status, nutritional support, and skin care. In severely ill patients, hypotension due to extravasation of fluid and protein from leaky capillaries may occur. Careful restoration of the blood volume with intravenous serum albumin and fluids is critical. In the presence of leaky capillaries, overzealous rehydration may precipitate pulmonary or cerebral edema, particularly if evidence of renal insufficiency (azotemia, oliguria) has occurred. Frequent turning of the patient is important to prevent decubiti and skin gangrene at pressure points. Critically ill patients may be helped by large doses of steroids given for several days at the start of therapy (Woodward & Osterman 1984). It is not recommended or necessary to use steroids in mild to moderate illness. Heparin has not been effective in correcting disseminated intravascular coagulation in these diseases.

At present, no reliable vaccines or consistently effective prophylaxis are available for preventive therapy. Limited data suggest that either chloramphenicol (3 g orally once a week) or doxycycline (200 mg orally once a week) may be partially effective in preventing scrub typhus among individuals exposed in hyperendemic areas. It is important to note that clinically apparent infection may develop after prophylaxis is discontinued (Olson et al 1980; 1981). In general, the use of prophylactic antibiotics is not suggested. Personal protection depends on the use of insect repellents, as described for dengue fever in Table 26–1. Attached ticks must be removed carefully with the head part intact. Ticks may be induced to release their grip by the application of petroleum jelly and then removed with forceps. Ticks should never be squeezed with the fingers as infected feces can contaminate the skin (Saah & Hornick 1985).

Q Fever

Q fever is caused by *Coxiella burnetii,* which differs from the other rickettsiae in several ways. This organism exhibits phase variation (i.e., it displays different antigens depending on the method of cultivation), and specific diagnosis is dependent on demonstrating serum antibodies to phase antigens. The Weil–Felix is negative in Q fever. *Coxiella burnetii* is not transmitted to humans by an arthropod vector and it rarely causes a rash.

Epidemiologically, *Coxiella burnetii* is established worldwide and maintained in nature by wild animals and domestic livestock. Infection is spread from animal to animal by ticks. Human infection is acquired by inhalating organisms from contaminated environments and, possibly, by ingesting unpasteurized milk. Placental and birth fluids of infected livestock are particularly infectious because the organism is concentrated in the placenta, birth fluids, and milk (Saah & Hornick 1985).

Q fever causes both acute and chronic clinical disease. Acute Q fever frequently presents with symptoms and signs indistinguishable from other rickettsial diseases, including severe headache, chills, myalgias, and high spiking fevers. Nausea, vomiting, diarrhea, and arthralgias may occur. Clinical features that distinguish Q fever from the other rickettsioses are the development of pneumonia or hepatitis, which may be the presenting features of the disease. Pneumonia is characterized as atypical (interstitial, not lobar) and similar to *Mycoplasma pneumoniae, Legionella pneumophila,* or psittacosis. The differential diagnosis of acute Q fever includes influenza, brucellosis, leptospirosis, typhoid and other enteric fevers, viral hepatitis, infectious mononucleosis, and cytomegalovirus infection.

Chronic Q fever or Q fever endocarditis is an insidious systemic disease manifested by symptoms and signs consistent with endocarditis (e.g., new or changing murmurs, fatigue, fever, embolic phenomena), but with negative blood cultures. Hepatomegaly and thrombocytopenia are not uncommon.

Fever in untreated acute Q fever lasts approximately 2 to 14 days, but convalescence may be prolonged. Diagnosis of Q fever requires a high index of suspicion and is presumptive in the appropriate clinical and epidemiologic setting. Serial serologic studies (usually a complement fixation test) are necessary for definitive diagnosis. In acute Q fever, antibody to phase 2 antigen increases; in chronic Q fever, antibody to phase 1 antigen exceeds antiphase 2 antibody.

The role of antibiotic therapy in altering the course of acute Q fever or preventing chronic Q fever is unclear. However, if acute Q fever is suspected, patients should be treated for two weeks with tetracycline (25 mg/kg/day orally in four divided doses) or doxycycline (100 mg orally twice daily in adults). Chloramphenicol (50 mg/kg/day orally in four divided doses) may also be used (Saah & Hornick 1985). Chronic Q fever requires prolonged therapy for two to five years and, perhaps, for life. The regimen most likely to succeed and optimal duration of treatment are not known (Tobin et al 1982). However, combinations of tetracycline and lincomycin, tetracycline and trimethoprim-sulfamethoxazole, or doxycycline and rifampin have been effective (Saah & Hornick 1985; Tobin et al 1982). At present, no preventive therapy is available for acute or chronic Q fever.

REFERENCES

Halstead SB: Observations related to pathogenesis of dengue hemorrhagic fever: Hypotheses and discussion. Yale J Biol Med 1970a;42:350–62.

Halstead SB, Nimmannitya S, Cohen SN: Observations related to pathogenesis of dengue hemorrhagic fever: Relation of disease severity to antibody response and virus recovered. Yale J Biol Med 1970b;42:311–28.
Halstead SB: Selective primary health care: Stategies for control of disease in the developing world: Dengue. Rev of Infect Dis 1984a;6:251–64.
Halstead SB: Dengue. In Warren KS, Mahmoud AAF (eds): Tropical and Geographic Medicine, pp 652–59. New York, McGraw-Hill, 1984b.
The Medical Letter: Insect repellents. 1985;27:62–64.
Olson JG, Bourgeois AL, Fang RCY et al: Prevention of scrub typhus: Prophylactic administration of doxycycline in a randomized double-blind trial. Am J Trop Med Hyg 1980;29:989–97.
Olson JG, Bourgeois AL, Fang RCY et al: Risk of relapse associated with doxycycline therapy for scrub typhus. In Burgdorfer W, Anacker RL (eds): Rickettsiae and Rickettsial Diseases, pp 201–10. New York, Academic Press, 1981.
Perine PL, Brooke S, Krause KW et al: Single-dose doxycycline treatment of louse-borne relapsing fever and epidemic typhus. Lancet 1974;2:742–44.
Saah AJ, Hornick RB: Rickettsiosis. In Mandell GL, Douglas RG Jr, Bennett JE (eds): Principles and Practices of Infectious Diseases, pp 1081–95. New York, John Wiley, 1985.
Sangkawibha N, Rojanasaphot S, Ahandrik S et al: Risk factors in dengue shock syndrome: A prospective epidemiologic study in Rayong, Thailand. Am J Epidemiol 1984;120:653–59.
Sumarmo H, Wulur H, Jahja E et al: Clinical observations on virologically confirmed fatal dengue infections in Jakarta, Indonesia. Bull WHO 1983; 61:693–701.
Tobin MJ, Cahill N, Gearty G et al: Q fever endocarditis. Am J Med 1982;72:396–400.
WHO Working Group on Rickettsial Diseases: Rickettsioses: A continuing disease problem. Bull WHO 1982;60:157–64.
Woodward TE, Osterman JV: Rickettsial diseases. In Warren KS, Mahmoud AAF (eds): Tropical and Geographical Medicine, pp 873–85. New York, McGraw-Hill, 1984.

27
Measles

PAUL J. EDELSON

EPIDEMIOLOGY

Measles is a widespread disease among infants and young children in underdeveloped countries. It carries considerable morbidity and a high case fatality rate. In some countries, measles accounts for one third of all deaths in children under five (Black 1984). As the African proverb says, "Count your children after measles has past. A child that gets out of measles is a child reborn."

To understand the pattern of measles in less developed areas, one needs to know something about the basic epidemiology of measles. Measles is sensitive to both population size and density (Black 1984). Because measles is highly contagious and there is no immune carrier state or extrahuman reservoir, measles spreads rapidly but abates quickly in a small population. It is generally considered that a minimum population of several hundred thousand is necessary to allow new cases to occur on a regular basis. Below this level, populations will often accumulate large number of susceptibles during long interepidemic periods punctuated by relatively brief, but extensive, outbreaks of disease. The substantial population shifts that characterize refugee movements can trigger rapidly developing and extensive epidemics of measles among such susceptibles.

Measles activity has three characteristic patterns. In "virgin soil" outbreaks, measles is introduced into small, isolated populations where the disease may not have been seen for generations. A universal point-source epidemic rapidly develops and nearly everyone in the community, regardless of age, is ill at the same time (Gear 1962). Case fatality rates are extremely high in this situation with up to 20 to 40 percent of the population succumbing. The very young and the old are most vulnerable. These high fatality rates reflect, in part, the cessation of normal community life; with so many sick individuals, there is no one to get food, water, or fuel, or to minister to the sick.

In most developed countries before the introduction of measles immunization, measles had a cyclical epidemic pattern. Peaks of activity occurred every three to four years as sufficient numbers of susceptible individuals accumulated to support a flare-up of disease. In these countries, school-aged children are the main targets, though measles is rarely fatal among this group.

In predominantly rural countries with low population densities, measles activity is present year-round with seasonal increases in activity associated with large gatherings or communal celebrations. For example, there is a yearly surge in measles activity during the African dry season when people visit one another and attend large regional festivals. During these times, considerable numbers of people gather from small villages and towns where a large pool of susceptibles may have accumulated over several years. In this setting, a few cases of measles can set off an explosion of disease activity. A similar risk exists when large numbers of displaced persons from relatively small communities are assembled in refugee camps or resettlement compounds. Physicians caring for displaced persons must therefore be prepared with strategies to prevent measles epidemics, which have high morbidity and mortality.

CLINICAL PICTURE

Measles in the developed world begins about 14 days after exposure with the classic "3 Cs" of cough, coryza, and conjunctivitis. It is during this prodromal period that patients are most likely to spread the disease to others, though they remain infectious for at least as long as their rash persists (about five days) and, in some severely ill children, probably for a longer period (Scheifele & Forbes 1972). About three days after the prodromal symptoms appear, the characteristic erythematous, macular rash develops on the face and upper chest, and rapidly progresses down the trunk and along the extremities in a centrifugal pattern. Fever develops a day or two before the rash, and both begin to resolve after about five days. The rash is so characteristic that it is generally considered diagnostic. Before the rash develops, the characteristic buccal exanthem of from a few to hundreds of tiny white lesions on reddish bases, or Koplik spots, develops, and is considered pathognomonic. In developed countries, measles is unpleasant but self-limited. The major complication of measles in these countries is encephalitis, occurring in one case in 1000. The case fatality rate in developed nations is about 1:10,000.

There is a more serious clinical variety of measles referred to as "black measles." The Muslim physician, Rhazes, taught that "measles which are of a deep red and violet color are of a bad and fatal kind." It is this form of measles that is particularly prevalent in underdeveloped nations today (Br Med J 1976). In the typical clinical case, an infant in the first or second year of life develops inflamed eyes, fever, a weak laryngitic cry, and a mottled rash. Over several days, the rash progresses from red to purple to nearly black and is accompanied by extensive peeling. Stomatitis with ulceration interferes with sucking, and the child may drink or eat little or nothing. By the second week, bloody diarrhea and dyspnea develop and, in the severest cases, the already weakened child becomes listless and unresponsive. For most of these children, this progression can be halted with routine nursing techniques.

Complications of measles are the result of extensive mucous membrane involvement, which is characteristic of measles, superimposed on malnutrition and sometimes worsened by folk approaches to the disease. Few of the complications of measles are caused by secondary viral or bacterial infection.

Severe measles typically involves five areas: the skin, the eyes, oral mucous membranes, and the respiratory and gastrointestinal tracts. The measles rash may vary from mild involvement of the neck and groin creases and a few scattered patches on the trunk, to severe confluent desquamation over most of the body. The severity of the rash is generally a good index of the severity of the disease as a whole. However, the full extent of the skin involvement may not be evident at first, but may develop over the course of two or three days. With extensive peeling, children may have difficulty regulating their temperature and controlling insensible water losses, much the same as burn patients. Secondary bacterial infection with staphylococci or streptococci can develop in the denuded areas.

Stomatitis is common and often involves both the lips and buccal mucosa. Swelling and soreness can make sucking impossible, and tissue sensitivity may make children refuse solid foods, particularly if they are highly spiced. Keratoconjunctivitis can be a serious complication, occasionally leading to corneal ulcerations and loss of sight. This complication has usually been associated with xerophthalmia caused by severe vitamin A deficiency, although some have suggested that it is due to secondary bacterial infection or to superimposed herpes simplex keratitis (Sanford-Smith & Whittle 1979).

The epithelium of the entire respiratory tract, from the sinus mucosa to the alveolar spaces, is involved in measles, and the pathophysiology is analogous to skin changes. Sinusitis and otitis media, although common, are generally not clinically significant. Laryngotracheobronchitis is also common, manifesting itself primarily as hoarseness in the older child and as a weak, throaty cry in the infant. Some children develop respiratory distress because of tracheal swelling and the accumulation of viscid secretions.

Pneumonia has been emphasized as an important and worrisome complication of measles, even in the developed world. The emphasis has usually been placed on superinfecting bacterial pneumonias. In fact, in developing countries, even among fatal cases, most pneumonia is not due to bacterial superinfection but results from the extensive inflammatory response and desquamation caused by the measles infection itself (DeBuse et al 1970).

Measles diarrhea generally develops during the period of desquamation and the weeks that follow. Although usually mild, it can be associated with a picture of dysentery and may represent an important route for protein loss with as much as 1.0 to 1.5 g of protein being lost daily in severe cases. This protein-losing enteropathy may also be associated with sugar malabsorption and lactose intolerance (Dossetor & Whittle 1976). In some patients, cryptosporidiosis has been identified in association with measles enteropathy (De Mol et al 1984), but in most cases, no enteric pathogen other than the measles virus can be recognized. Encephalitis is a complication of measles in underdeveloped countries and refugee settings just as it is in the developed countries.

The differential diagnosis of measles is not usually difficult, as there are few other agents that cause the typical mucosal prodrome and characteristic rash with fever. Mild or atypical cases may be due to drug reactions, particularly to sulfa drugs, whch may precipitate a Stevens–Johnson syndrome. Patients with rubella or typhus may develop a similar, but less extensive, rash with fever, but they are rarely as seriously ill as the measles patient. Dengue fever is not accompanied by mucosal involvement. In very hot, humid climates, an extensive heat rash, miliaria rubra, may precisely mimic the measles rash but without any of the accompanying symptoms. In some cases, pox virus infections, particularly monkeypox, may be confused with measles, but this infection is seen only in individuals living in remote jungle villages in west or central Africa and has little potential for presenting as epidemic human disease.

MANAGEMENT

Nutrition is the key to treatment of the child who is severely ill with measles. Approximately one in four children will lose 10 percent of his or her body weight, which may take months to regain once the illness resolves (Morley et al 1967). In addition to adequate nutrition, an effective overall therapeutic plan must include careful attention to fever control, meticulous nursing care of the skin and respiratory tract, and a clear understanding of the social attitude toward measles that prevails in the patient's community.

Although the importance of malnutrition in the development of severe measles is debated, there is no doubt that measles represents a major nutritional stress to the young child. The consequences of a prolonged interruption in feeding, along with the increased protein and calorie loss that measles causes, undoubtedly play an important role in measles deaths, and this condition may persist for months after the acute illness subsides (Koster et al 1981).

The main cause of poor food intake in measles is severe stomatitis. This may be compounded by folk beliefs that children with measles should be on restricted diets or should not be fed at all. The clinician's main contribution is to ensure that the child with measles is given adequate food and fluid. The child's inability to suck adequately can contribute to the development of maternal breast abscesses, which then further complicates nursing. Mothers should be taught how to express breast milk and feed it to their children with a cup or spoon. Children may be very weak, particularly if they have been sick for several days, and feeding may proceed very slowly, with one feeding taking an hour or more.

All children with measles should receive supplementary food. A mixture of edible oils and powdered milk or fish protein is an excellent protein supplement. Where honey or other naural sweeteners are available, they may be added to the protein mixture. Even very young infants are able to eat small amounts of this moistened mixture from the end of a spoon. Diarrhea should not be considered a reason to stop oral intake (see Intestinal Illness, Chapter 34). Children who cannot tolerate milk or solid foods should be managed temporarily with the World Health Organization's oral rehydration fluid until they are able to feed again (see Fluid and Electrolyte Therapy, Chapter 15). All children with measles should also receive a single immediate dose of vitamin A (see Chapter 18 for dosage recommendations) to prevent the complications of xerophthalmia. Because many of these children fail to achieve "catch-up" growth once the measles has resolved (Koster et al 1981), they should not be weaned for at least two months following measles.

Bathing to reduce high fever will help conserve precious calories and keep the skin free of bacterial pathogens. Meticulous respiratory care is essential to reduce the effort of breathing. Both the nose and pharynx should be kept clear, by suctioning if necessary. Tracheostomy has been used in very sick children but rarely produces a substantial clinical improvement, because there is no localized site of obstruction in the upper respiratory tract as there might be with epiglottitis or croup. An endotracheal or, better, a nasotracheal tube may be useful in maintaining good respiratory toilet. Most mothers, with guidance, can learn how to suction their infants. Humidified oxygen, if available, is often of benefit. Two excellent, practical guides to caring for children with measles are the text by King, King, and Martodipoero (1978), and that of Werner (1981).

Antibiotics are usually not needed for treatment of severe measles. Prophylactic antibiotics should not be used because they only predispose to bacterial superinfection (Weinstein 1955). Secondary bacterial skin infections should be treated with local care, and oral penicillin, 50 mg/kg/day in four divided doses. Children with minimal pneumonia do not require antibiotics. In children with more severe pneumonia, penicillin has been shown to reduce mortality more effectively than chloramphenicol (O'Donovan & Barua 1973) and should be given parenterally, 100 mg/kg/day in four divided doses. Tuberculosis, which may have a prevalence of up to 2.5 cases per 100 children in this age group (Kent 1973), may be reactivated by a measles infection. Pneumonia that does not resolve with penicillin should be treated presumptively as tuberculosis pending further diagnostic studies.

There is no evidence of benefit gained by the use of immune serum globulin in the treatment of measles. Steroids should not be used either. Digitalis has been used to manage cardiac failure in measles, however, most children in apparent failure are hypoalbuminemic and benefit more from cautious intravenous infusion of albumin or blood, particularly if they are anemic. Myocarditis has been reported to occur in measles, in which case the use of digitalis might be contraindicated as well. Although there is some preliminary evidence that the broad-spectrum antiviral agent ribavirin may be clinically effective, it does not seem likely that this will be a practical or cost-effective therapy in the near future (Fernandez 1980).

A practical approach to the management of endemic measles has been outlined by Scheifele and Forbes (1972). They emphasize well-organized out-patient management of most cases, using a specially designated "measles room" in which to see children without exposing other out-patients. Hospitalization and progressive nursing care are reserved for only the sickest infants (Table 27-1). They make the point that, in assessing the need for hospitalization, one should pay attention to the stage of the child's illness. For example, fever, dyspnea, and vomiting are all to be expected during the acute exanthematous phase, but would indicate serious complications if present several days after resolution of the rash.

Laboratory support to ensure adequate care of the measles patient in the field hospital setting need not be elaborate. For the care of measles patients, white blood cell counts and differentials and hematocrits should be done. Gram's stain and acidfast (AFB) stain of sputum should be available to allow monitoring of secondary bacterial infection. A microscope is also useful for identifying epithelial giant cells in nasopharyngeal mucus (Tompkins & Macaulay 1955). Scheifele and Forbes (1972) have shown how it can be helpful, prognostically, to monitor giant cell shedding, since their disappearance heralds resolution of symptoms over the subsequent three days.

Table 27-1. Admission Criteria for Hospitalization of Children with Measles

1. Moderate or severe bronchopneumonia. Mild pneumonia can be treated on an out-patient basis. Those with moderate to severe bronchopneumonia should be hospitalized. Extensive crepitations suggest bacterial superinfection.

2. Severe dehydration. Lesser degrees of dehydration can be corrected in the measles room with oral therapy.

3. Moderate to severe malnutrition. These patients should be admitted at any stage of measles. They are more likely to develop both viral complications and bacterial superinfections.

4. Laryngotracheobronchitis. Those with severe forms with upper respiratory obstruction at rest or who refuse to lie supine should be admitted. Milder forms may be observed in the measles room where mothers can be shown how to clear secretions and what signs of worsening to watch for.

5. Any other severe complication, such as anemia or convulsions.

6. None of the above, but the child looks inappropriately ill.

From Forbes CE, Scheifele DW The Management of Measles in Nairobi. East African Med J 1973;50:162 (Used with permission.)

CONTROL OF MEASLES OUTBREAKS

Measles is a highly transmissible disease with an attack rate of greater than 90 percent in exposed susceptibles (Panum 1846). It is spread by respiratory droplets, which allows rapid transmission through a susceptible population. Infected individuals are most contagious in the catarrhal phase, before the rash appears, thus making it impossible to control spread by isolating recognized cases. When outbreaks have developed among enclosed populations, such as in schools or hospitals, closing the institution to new admissions has been effective. There is no value in hospitalizing children for "quarantine" because admission of measles cases only increases the risk of infecting other hospitalized patients.

Measles vaccine is effective in halting outbreaks. A study from Finland (Ruuskanen et al 1978) has shown that even postexposure prophylaxis will reduce the rate of clinical measles. Among 74 exposed and presumed susceptible children who received postexposure prophylaxis, only five developed clinical disease. Although the Centers for Disease Control recommends the use of vaccine only during the first 72 hours following exposure (CDC 1982), the Finnish group's results suggest that there may be benefit in immunizing children up to 14 days after exposure, providing that prodromal symptoms have not yet begun.

Immunization during an epidemic may not be readily accepted by the community (Kaartinen 1984). Immune serum globulin (ISG), providing it includes measles antibodies, is also effective in limiting outbreaks, but the prevalence and level of measles antibodies vary widely among donor groups. In addition, ISG is expensive and requires special handling and refrigeration. If it is used, ISG should be given within six days of exposure as a single dose of 0.25 ml/kg IM. The subcutaneous injection of small amounts of whole blood is not recommended. Identification of susceptibles by history is generally reliable because the disease is well recognized by most adults in endemic areas.

PREVENTION

In some parts of the underdeveloped world, severe disease may occur in 80 percent of measles cases. Death rates from measles, as a percentage of all births, range from 1 to 3.7 percent (Black 1984), while case fatality rates in hospitalized patients are reported to be 15 to 20 times higher (Hull et al 1983). Overall, measles fatality rates are 400- to 4,600-fold higher in underdeveloped countries than those prevailing in Europe or the United States (Nolan et al 1982). There is no evidence that these rates reflect a unique genetic susceptibility of Asian or African people to the disease; similar rates were prevalent in Glasgow at the turn of the century (Chalmers 1930).

The major determinants in the prevalence of severe measles with high case fatality rates are malnutrition and overcrowding. Both of these factors are evident among displaced populations. In addition, the aggregation of large numbers of people from rural areas ensures a substantial pool of susceptibles at risk, should a case be admitted to the settlement. The conjunction of these three factors makes measles prevention a first-order priority in a refugee health program.

Measles control is accomplished by systematic immunization of susceptibles with live, attenuated vaccine. The impact of measles on a community can also be substantially modified by appropriate attention to adequate nutrition and to housing programs that diminish overcrowding.

Morley (1963) and Scrimshaw and colleagues (1966) were among the first to emphasize the importance of malnutrition as a determinant of severe measles in a population. In fact, it has been said that a community is malnourished as long as its children still die of measles. However, data implicating malnutrition in high case fatality rates have been easier to collect on a population basis than on an individual basis. It has been shown that populations with significant childhood malnutrition have high case fatality rates and that, on a population basis, supplemental nutrition programs can reduce those rates (Scrimshaw et al 1966). However, on a case-by-case basis, it has been difficult to show that the more severely malnourished child will have the most severe disease or is the likeliest to succumb (O'Donovan 1971).

Both age and crowding can also have substantial effects on measles morbidity and mortality rates. The best demonstration of the age dependence of measles mortality rates is from data collected in virgin communities in the Arctic, where all ages were susceptible and malnutrition was not a problem (Black 1984). Age-specific mortality rates were highest at the two age extremes, reaching a rate of 46.8 per 1000 in the infants (Table 27-2), approximately six times higher than the rate for the one- to two-year-old group, and 20 times higher than the rate for children ages 2 to 14 years.

Recent work in west Africa has emphasized

Table 27-2. Age-Specific Measles Mortality in the Virgin Communities of the Arctic, 1951–1982

Age (years)	Number of Cases	Number of Deaths	Rate per 1000
0–1	834	39	46.8
1–2	726	5	6.9
2–14	5929	10	1.7
15–34	5539	26	4.7
35–55	2869	42	14.6
55+	1231	56	45.5

(From Black FL: Measles. In Warren KS, Mahmoud AA (eds): Tropical and Geographic Medicine, pp 594–602. New York, McGraw-Hill, used with permission.)

the importance of crowding and family structure on the severity of measles (Aaby et al 1984). Although this work identified in aggregate a considerable age effect, and some evidence for an effect of malnutrition, the case fatality rate was most affected by the total number of cases occurring in the index case's living compound. The case fatality rate for isolated cases at all ages was 9.3 percent, but when other cases occurred in the same compound the case fatality rate was 23.5 percent, or about 2.5 times higher. Other studies by this group indicate that fatality rates are higher for twins (Aaby et al 1983) and in polygamous households (Aaby et al 1983b). These health workers conclude that intensity of exposure, as determined by contact rates, may be an important factor in the appearance of severe disease.

These studies imply that supplementary feeding programs and adequate housing are likely to decrease the impact of measles on a community. However, the single most effective way to control measles morbidity and mortality is by preventing it through immunization.

The key to designing an effective vaccination program is to identify those groups at highest risk for severe morbidity and morality from measles, and to assign vaccination priorities accordingly. In general, children beyond three years of age can be considered immune, unless they are from a virgin population, in which case every individual, regardless of age, should be considered susceptible. Although maternal antibody appears to wane more rapidly in underdeveloped countries, most infants will continue to have adequate antibody through the fourth to sixth months of life (WHO 1977). About 90 percent of children immunized at nine months of age will seroconvert (Ministries of Health 1983), but children immunized earlier may have a suboptimal response to the vaccine (Hull et al 1983) and, subsequently, must be reimmunized after the age of one year (Wilkins & Wehrle 1979). In resettlement situations where the risk of measles is high, all children between the ages of six months (when a child can sit up on his own) and three years should be immunized. Screening children for a history of measles should not be done routinely except when the supplies of vaccine are limited. Serologic studies have no place in a field immunization program. For further discussion of the importance of and methods of using measles vaccine, see Chapter 6.

REFERENCES

Aaby P, Bukh J, Smits AJ et al: High case fatality rate in twins with measles. Lancet 1983a;2:690.

Aaby P, Bukh J, Lisse IM et al: Measles mortality, state of nutrition, and family structure: A community study from Guinea-Bissau. J Infect Dis 1983b;147:693–701.

Aaby P, Bukh J, Lisse IM et al: Determinants of measles mortality in a rural area of Guinea-Bissau: Crowding, age, and malnutrition. J Trop Pediatr 1984;30:164–68.

Black FL: Measles. In Warren KS, Mahmoud AA (eds): Tropical and Geographic Medicine, pp 594–602. New York, McGraw-Hill, 1984.

British Medical Journal: Measles in the Tropics (editorial). Br Med J 1976;2:1339.

Centers for Disease Control: Measles prevention. MMWR 1982;31:217–24, 229–31.

Chalmers AK: The Health of Glasgow, 1818–1925. Glasgow, Bell & Bain, 1930, p 340. As cited in Morley D, Martin WJ, Allen I: Measles in east and central Africa. East Afr Med J 1967;44:497–508.

DeBuse PJ, Lewis MG, Mugerwa JW: Pulmonary complications of measles in Uganda. J Trop Pediatr 1970;16:197–203.

DeMol P, Mukashema S, Bogaerts J et al: Cryptosporidium related to measles diarrhea in Rwanda. Lancet 1984;2:42–43.

Dossetor JFB, Whittle HC: Protein-losing enteropathy and malabsorption in acute measles enteritis. Br Med J 1976;2:592–93.

Fernandez H: Ribavirin: A summary of clinical trials; *Herpes genitalis* and measles. In Smith RA, Kirkpatrick W (eds): Ribavirin: A Broad Spectrum Antiviral Agent, pp 215–30. New York, Academic Press, 1980.

Gear JHS: Measles in South Africa. Am J Dis Child 1962;103:261–64.

Hull HF, Williams PJ, Oldfield F: Measles mortality and vaccine efficacy in rural West Africa. Lancet 1983;1:972–75.

Kaartinen L: Ethiopia: Measles epidemic. Lancet 1984;1:39.

Kent PW: Tuberculosis in East Africa, East African Tuberculosis Investigation Centre, July 16, 1969. As cited in Forbes CE, Scheifele DW: The management of measles in Nairobi. East Afr Med J 1973;50:159–68.

King M, King F, Martodipoero S: Primary Child Care: A Manual for Health Workers. London, Oxford University Press, 1978.

Koster FT, Curlin GC, Aziz KMA et al: Synergistic impact of measles and diarrhoea on nutrition and mortality in Bangladesh. Bull WHO 1981;59:901–08.
Ministries of Health of Brazil, Chile, Costa Rica, and Ecuador, and the Pan American Health Organization (PAHO): Seroconversion rates and measles antibody titers induced by measles vaccination in Latin American children 6 to 12 months of age. Rev Infect Dis 1983;5:596–605.
Morley D: A medical service for children under 5 years of age in West Africa. Trans Roy Soc Trop Med Hyg 1963;57:79–88.
Morley D, Martin WJ, Allen I: Measles in East and Central Africa. East Afr Med J 1967;44:497–508.
Nolan TF, Goodman RA, Patriarca PA et al: Hospitalizations for measles 1970–1978. Am J Public Health 1982;72:1037–39.
O'Donovan C: Measles in Kenyan children. East Afr Med J 1971;48:526–32.
O'Donovan C, Barua KN: Measles pneumonia. Am J Trop Med Hyg 1973;22:73–7.
Panum PL: Observations Made during the Epidemic of Measles on the Faroe Islands in the Year 1846. Cleveland, Delta Omega Society (translation), 1940.
Ruuskanen O, Salmi TT, Halonen P: Measles vaccination after exposure to natural measles. J Pediatr 1978;93:43–46.
Sanford-Smith JH, Whittle HC: Corneal ulceration following measles in Nigerian children. Br J Ophthalmol 1979;63:720–24.
Scheifele DW, Forbes CE: Prolonged giant cell excretion in severe African measles. Pediatrics 1972;50:867–73.
Scrimshaw NS, Salomon JB, Bruch HA et al: Studies on diarrheal disease in Central America. VIII. Measles, diarrhea, and nutritional deficiency in rural Guatemala. Am J Trop Med Hyg 1966;15:625–31.
Tompkins V, Macaulay JC: A characteristic cell in nasal secretions during prodromal measles. JAMA 1955;157:711.
Walsh JA: Selective primary health care: strategies for control of disease in the developing world. IV. Measles. Rev Infect Dis 1983;5:330–40.
Weinstein L: Failure of chemotherapy to prevent the bacterial complications of measles. New Engl J Med 1955;252:679–83.
Werner D: Where There Is No Doctor: A Village Health Care Handbook. Palo Alto, CA, Hesperian Foundation, 1981.
Wilkins J, Wehrle PF: Additional evidence against measles vaccine administration to infants less than 12 months of age: Altered immune response following active/passive immunization. J Pediatr 1979;94:865–69.
World Health Organization: Measles immunity in the first year after birth and the optimum age for vaccination in Kenyan children. Bull WHO 1977;55:21–31.

28
Skin and Soft Tissue Infections

FRED GORDIN

Infections of the skin and underlying structures constitute a major health care problem in underdeveloped countries. Individuals in warm climates wear little protective clothing and are frequently barefoot. Thus, the natural barrier of the skin is frequently broken by minor trauma, abrasions, and insect bites. Because of these conditions, microorganisms easily gain access to the skin, resulting in higher rates of infection. Surveys of individuals in Africa, Central America, and Southeast Asia have shown infections of the skin to be the most common problem encountered in dermatology clinics, with rates as high as 30 percent reported (Pettit 1976). The situation among refugees is worsened by the frequent occurrence of malnutrition, lack of adequate housing, and poor sanitation, all of which increase the incidence and severity of infection. In one survey of more than 1000 children evacuated from Vietnam and Cambodia, skin infections were the single largest cause of disease, affecting 13 percent of the refugees (Swender & Sandler 1977). Two smaller surveys demonstrated skin infections in over 20 percent of the refugees.

Skin and soft tissue infections can range from a mild annoyance, such as tinea versicolor, to a life-threatening infection such as gas gangrene. A disease such as scabies is rarely a major problem to an individual in good health. In the refugee setting, however, scabies is frequently the primary factor in the development of pyoderma and other invasive diseases. The microorganisms involved in these infections vary widely by geography and climate.

SKIN INFECTIONS

Pyoderma

The most common causes of skin infections in tropical regions are bacteria. A direct correlation has been shown between increased heat and humidity and increased frequency of streptococcal pyoderma (Taplin et al 1973). A combination of less clothing being worn and a greater number of abrasions and insect bites is one explanation. The most common manifestations of pyoderma are described in the following subsections.

Impetigo

Impetigo is a superficial infection of the skin that usually presents as groupings of yellow crusted lesions. The initial appearance is one of vesicles, but these rapidly form pustules that drain spontaneously. The lesions are most commonly found on the face but can occur on any part of the body. Although children are affected most often, the disease is highly contagious and can affect adults as well. Impetigo can occur as a primary infection or in an area of prior skin abnormality, such as from scabies.

The diagnosis of impetigo is usually made on clinical grounds. Most individuals are free of systemic illness. After removal of the crust, a Gram's stain will frequently show gram-positive cocci. Group A streptococci have been shown to account for the majority of cases of impetigo (Dajani et al 1972). Although *Staphylococcus aureus* is often found, it is usually a secondary colonizer. Bullous impetigo is found in a small percentage of cases in which large, thin blisters rupture and leave a yellow crust. *S. aureus* is the pathogen in most of these cases.

Impetigo can be easily treated with a variety of antibiotics. Penicillin given orally, or as a single injection of benzathine penicillin, is the drug of choice. If *S. aureus* is suspected, the patient should receive an antistaphylococcal penicillin such as dicloxacillin or a cephalosporin. Erythromycin is an effective alternative. The lesions should be kept clean and covered to promote healing and prevent spread to others. If pruritus is a major problem, antipruritics may be of value.

Cellulitis

Cellulitis usually presents as a localized area of warmth, erythema, and tenderness. The skin is indurated and tense, with spreading margins. Usually there is a single area of involvement, but multiple regions can be involved. The extremities are most commonly affected, probably as a result of trauma to the skin. Tender regional adenopathy can occur, and fever and chills are common. The white blood cell count can range from normal to over 20,000.

An attempt should be made to determine the pathogen. If an abscess is present, a sterile needle should be used to drain it and the material sent for Gram's stain and culture, if available. If no collection of pus is present, sterile, nonbacteriostatic saline can be injected into the margin of the cellulitis with a 25-gauge needle and aspirated (Uman & Kunin 1975). Streptococci and staphylococci, either individually or in combination, account for the majority of infections. In children, *Hemophilus influenzae* can cause severe cellulitis with a reddish blue discoloration, usually on the face. These children may be bacteremic and sometimes have other serious hemophilus infections.

Therapy for cellulitis should be directed toward the likely pathogens mentioned above. In adults, penicillin is adequate unless staphylococcus is suggested by the presence of pustules or clumped gram-positive cocci on Gram's stain. Therapy can be given orally, but parenteral therapy is advised in systemically ill patients and those with facial cellulitis. If staphylococcus is suspected, a beta-lactamase–resistant penicillin or cephalosporin should be used. In children, consideration should be given to using ampicillin, chloramphenicol, or an appropriate second- or third-generation cephalosporin to cover *H. influenzae.* (Cephalosporins are expensive and may not be available in refugee camps.)

Several other important forms of cellulitis exist. Erysipelas is a distinctive form of streptococcal cellulitis that usually affects the face. The skin is very indurated and red with distinct borders. Fever and adenopathy are common. Penicillin is highly effective. Erysipeloid, caused by *Erysipelothrix rhusiopathiae,* is a painful, discolored cellulitis that frequently affects the fingers. This gram-positive bacillus causes disease in persons with environmental contact with animals and water. Penicillin, erythromycin, and tetracycline are effective therapy. *Vibrio species* have been associated with severe forms of necrotizing cellulitis in individuals exposed to warm seawater. Marked local destruction, and even sepsis and death, have been reported. If *Vibrio* cellulitis is suspected, therapy should include tetracycline or chloramphenicol. Gram-negative aerobes such as *Proteus, E. coli,* and *Klebsiella* can cause cellulitis, usually in immunocompromised persons. Aminoglycosides or third-generation cephalosporins should be used in these situations.

Furunculosis

Staphylococcus aureus is a frequent cause of localized skin abscess. Furuncles (boils) and carbuncles start as tender red nodules and develop into painful pustular lesions. Because infection may start in a hair follicle, areas of the body that are covered with hair are common sites for these infections. The patient may develop a surrounding cellulitis and systemic symptoms if the lesion is deep. Topical heat and drainage of fluctuant lesions will be adequate in most cases. Facial lesions should be treated with antistaphylococcal antibiotics to prevent intracranial complications. Individuals with cellulitis or constitutional symptoms will need systemic therapy and adequate surgical drainage.

Superficial Skin Infections

Cutaneous Mycoses

Ringworm or superficial fungal infections commonly occur in tropical and temperate regions. Common areas of infection are the head, groin, and feet. Infections most often appear as erythematous plaques with well-defined margins and central clearing. Scaling may be prominent. Alopecia may occur with tinea capitis due to infection of the hair follicle. A scraping can be made of the edge of the lesion and the specimen placed on a slide with 10 percent potassium hydroxide (KOH) solution. Hyphae may be seen. A variety of dermatophytes are responsible, and differentiation is not important. If treatment is desired, a variety of topical antifungals are available including miconazole and clotrimazole. Gentian violet and magenta paint are also effective. Recurrences are common.

Tinea versicolor (pityriasis) is a common infection with the yeast *Malassezia furfur.* The patient usually develops widespread changes of hypopigmentation and hyperpigmentation with fine scaling. Selenium sulfide (1% cream or shampoo) applied twice daily for a week is usually effective.

Cutaneous candidiasis is also common with lesions most common in moist areas such as the groin, skin folds, and under the breasts. Topical nystatin or any of the previously mentioned compounds should be effective.

Erythrasma

Erythrasma is an infection caused by the gram-positive bacillus *Corynebacterium minutissimum* and is common in the tropics. It presents as large, dry plaques with irregular borders, usually in the intertriginous areas. Lesions may be chronic, and scaling is prominent in older lesions. Gram's stains of scrapings are usually helpful in establishing the diagnosis (look for Gram positive rods). Oral erythromycin for five to seven days is effective therapy.

Ulcerative Skin Infections

Anthrax

Anthrax is usually acquired by contact with infected livestock or their products. The spores of the *Bacillus anthracis* are inoculated under the skin where they germinate. The initial clinical manifestation is a painless papule containing hemorrhagic fluid, which enlarges over several days. Edema, which can involve a wide area of surrounding tissue, creates a craterlike lesion frequently containing a black eschar. Pruritus may be intense, but there is little pain. Systemic symptoms are few except when potentially fatal bacteremia occurs. Diagnosis can be made by Gram's stain of the lesion, which will demonstrate large gram-positive rods. Penicillin is the drug of choice, but tetracycline, erythromycin, and chloramphenicol are also effective.

Diphtheria

Diphtheria can occur in either normal skin or areas with preexisting disease. The disease is acquired from contact with skin or respiratory tract secretions of infected persons. Cutaneous diphtheria presents as a shallow, ulcerative lesion with an adherent grayish crust or membrane. Mixed bacterial superinfections are common. Diagnosis may be on clinical grounds alone if culture facilities are unavailable. Although most patients with cutaneous diphtheria do well, treatment is important to present complications and spread of the disease (Koopman & Campbell 1975). If diphtheria is suspected, patients should receive antitoxin. Treatment with erythromycin or parenteral penicillin for ten days is recommended. Both patients and their contacts should be immunized.

Tularemia

Tularemia infection should be suspected in persons with a shallow ulcer accompanied by painful regional adenopathy. Contact with animals or ticks is reported in most cases. The infecting organism is a gram-negative bacillus. The initial lesion is a small, painful papule that rapidly ulcerates, and fever and constitutional symptoms are common. Diagnosis is made on clinical findings, although blood cultures may be positive. Streptomycin, tetracycline, or chloramphenicol should be given for one week.

Mycobacterial Infections

Mycobacterial infections of the skin frequently present as chronic ulcers. *Mycobacterium tuberculosis* is an uncommon cause of skin infection. However, tuberculosis of the skin can occur through primary inoculation or as a manifestation of disseminated disease. Therapy should include at least two active drugs, as outlined in Chapter 33. *M. ulcerans* can cause a slowly progressive ulcer that results in significant destruction of underlying structures (Clancey et al 1961). Lesions begin as nodules, which ulcerate with necrotic bases and undermined edges. There are no systemic symptoms. Acid-fast stains of material from the base should reveal numerous organisms. Chemotherapy is difficult and wide surgical debridement with skin grafting should be attempted. *M. marinum* usually causes small, indolent nodules that may ulcerate and frequently resolve without therapy. The organism is acquired from contact with salt water and is resistant to standard chemotherapy. The nodularity of the disease may be confused with sporotrichosis. *M. fortuitum* and *M. chelonei* are distinguished from the other mycobacteria by their rapid growth (seven days) in culture. Both of these organisms can cause skin lesions ranging from draining pustules to chronic ulcers. Amikacin, cefoxitin, and doxycycline have all been effective therapy. *M. leprae* is discussed in Chapter 29.

Cutaneous Leishmaniasis

Cutaneous leishmaniasis occurs in the Middle East, Africa, and parts of Central and South America. The disease is caused by various species of the protozoan *Leishmania,* which are transmitted to humans by the bite of a sandfly. The lesions can be single or multiple, and they progress from papules to shallow ulcers that slowly granulate. The ulcers have well-indurated margins and frequently fluid or crusting. Healed lesions often leave a permanent scar. In South America, mucosal involvement of the mouth and nose is not uncommon. Diagnosis depends on demonstration of the organism on either touch prep of the lesion or biopsy. A leishmania antigen skin test can be used to support a diagnosis. Treatment of leishmaniasis is usually with one of the pentavalent antimonials such as sodium stibogluconate or meglumine antimoniate. Pentamidine and amphotericin B have also been used in difficult cases.

Nodular and Subcutaneous Infections of the Skin

Mycetomas

Mycetomas are chronic granulomatous infections of the skin and subcutaneous tissues that can be caused by a variety of fungi and bacteria. Infections of the foot (Madura foot) are commonly caused by trauma to the skin. Characteristically, the patient presents with a large, painless, fungating lesion with multiple draining sinuses. Lesions may penetrate deep into the underlying tissue, including bone. Infections have frequently been present for many years with little effect on the overall health of the individual. Diagnosis can be confirmed by visualizing the grains of organisms from the draining sinuses. Medical therapy may be effective for the actinomycotic mycetomas caused by *Nocardia* and *Actinomyces* species (Mahgoub 1976). Combinations of streptomycin with either trimethoprim-sulfamethoxazole or dapsone have been effective in treating these organisms. The mycotic mycetomas are caused by a variety of fungi and are resistant to medical therapy. Amputation is not unusual in these cases.

Sporotrichosis

Sporotrichosis is caused by the fungus *Sporotrichum schenckii.* This soil organism is inoculated into the skin during minor trauma. Infection usually appears as a series of painless nodules, which spread proximally on an extremity. The nodules may eventually break down and form ulcers. Pus or biopsy material can be stained and cultured to identify the organism. Systemic symptoms are absent. Topical treatment with a saturated solution of potassium iodide (SSKI) will cure most cases. Therapy should be continued for at least three to four weeks after clinical cure.

Systemic Fungal Infections

Systemic fungal infections frequently involve the skin. Lesions caused by the fungus *Blastomyces dermatitidis* (blastomycosis) may be ulcerative or verrucous. Pulmonary disease is frequently present in these patients. Both *Coccidioides immitis* (coccidioidomycosis) and *Paracoccidioides brasiliensis* (South American blastomycosis) can cause similar skin lesions. Treatment with amphotericin B is needed for all three of these fungi.

Yaws and Pinta

Yaws and pinta are nonvenereal treponemal diseases that primarily affect the skin. Pinta is confined to Central and South America, whereas yaws is present in Africa and Southeast Asia. Both occur in warm, humid areas and are the result of person-to-person transmission of the organism. Yaws begins as a painless papule that enlarges, and is frequently accompanied by regional adenopathy. Lesions appear moist, and a dark-field examination is diagnostic. Secondary lesions appear over a period of months. Lesions may become nodular or ulcerate into underlying tissue. Pinta more commonly presents as a plaquelike lesion that may be scaly, with abnormal pigmentation. Serum tests for syphilis are positive in both of these diseases. Therapy for both yaws and pinta is a single injection of benazthine penicillin. Tetracycline and erythromycin are alternatives.

Other Organisms

A number of other organisms can cause subcutaneous infections. *Pseudomonas pseudomallei* is the cause of melioidosis, which can cause purulent and ulcerative nodular lesions. Patients may become septic, and pulmonary involvement is common. The disease is endemic in Southeast Asia. A number of worms have prominent skin involvement, the most important being the nematodes (or roundworms). Hookworms and strongyloides may both produce a transient rash and discomfort at the initial penetration site (usually the legs). Creeping eruption, or cutaneous larva migrans, represents an animal hookworm infection of humans. Patients have a migratory subcutaneous serpentine eruption. Of the various filarial species, *Loa loa* and *Onchocerca volvulus* are most likely to have skin manifestations. *Loa loa* causes migratory areas of inflammation and pruritus known as Calabar swellings. Swellings in onchocerciasis tend to be stationary and located over bony prominences. The guinea worm, *Dracunculus medinensis,* resides in the subcutaneous tissues and presents as a small blister from which the worm is extracted. Dermatitis can be a prominent feature of early schistosomal infection.

SOFT TISSUE INFECTIONS

Infections involving the subcutaneous tissues are usually severe and often life-threatening. These infections can be caused by a variety of both aerobic and anaerobic organisms with deep trauma frequently a predisposing condition. Surgical debridement is usually mandatory for accurate diagnosis and cure. The clinical features of some of the more important infections are outlined in Table 28–1 and briefly described below.

Infections of the Subcutaneous Tissues

Anaerobic Cellulitis

Anaerobic cellulitis is an infection of the subcutaneous tissues that can be caused by a variety of anaerobes. Organisms obtain access following trauma or contaminated surgery. Symptoms appear gradually over two or three days, and patients may show moderate systemic toxicity. Gas is frequently present, which may cause confusion with clostridial myonecrosis. Muscles should be visualized at the time of surgical debridement to determine whether there is any involvement. Causative organisms include *Clostridia, Bacterioides,* streptococci, and gram-negative species. Antibiotics should include penicillin, possibly with clindamycin and gram-negative coverage added for toxic patients.

Table 28-1. Clinical Features of Soft Tissue Infections

Criterion	Anaerobic Cellulitis	Synergistic Necrotizing Cellulitis	Necrotizing Fasciitis	Clostridial Myonecrosis	Anaerobic Streptococcal Myonecrosis	Tropical Pyomyositis
Onset	Gradual	Acute	Acute	Acute	Subacute	Gradual
Pain	Absent	Severe	Moderate to severe	Severe	Moderate	Minimal
Toxemia	Minimal	Severe	Severe	Very severe	Moderate	Moderate
Swelling	Minimal	Moderate	Marked	Marked	Moderate	Moderate
Skin	Little change	Scattered areas of necrosis	Pale red; areas of necrosis	Tense; necrotic	Tense; erythema	Little change
Exudate	Slight	Profuse; "dishwater pus"	Serosanguinous	Serosanguinous	Profuse; seropurulent	None
Gas	Marked	Minimal	Minimal	Marked	Slight	None
Smell	Foul	Foul	Foul	Variable; may be sweet	Slight, sour	None
Muscle involvement	None	Moderate	None	Marked	Moderate	Local abscess

(Modified with permission from Finegold SM: Anaerobic Bacteria in Human Diseases, p 401. New York, Academic Press, 1977.)

Synergistic Necrotizing Cellulitis

Synergistic necrotizing cellulitis is an infection that begins in the subcutaneous tissues and skin but may spread to involve muscles. Patients frequently have underlying medical problems including diabetes mellitus and renal disease. Involved areas of the skin are extremely painful, and patients may appear toxic (Stone & Martin 1972). Surgery is needed to determine the area of involvement and for radical debridement. Antibiotic coverage should be directed toward anaerobic streptococci, *Bacterioides,* and *Staphylococcus aureus.*

Necrotizing Fasciitis

Necrotizing fasciitis is a severe, life-threatening infection that can spread rapidly and involve large areas. Mortality rates are over 25 percent even with appropriate therapy. Patients have sudden onset of pain and discoloration of the skin. Skin necrosis with local areas of anesthesia may follow. Patients may appear toxic, and rapid surgical intervention is mandatory. Detailed bacteriologic studies have shown Group A streptococci and staphylococci to be the main pathogens in some cases, while multiple aerobes and anaerobes have been isolated in other patients (Giuliano et al 1977). Because of the severity of this disease, broad antibiotic coverage should be given until Gram's stain or culture results are available.

Infections of the Muscles

Clostridial Myonecrosis (Gas Gangrene)

Gas gangrene is a major illness among war casualties and other trauma victims. The disease is the result of muscle liquifaction due to a variety of clostridial toxins (Caplan & Kluge 1976). *Clostridia perfringens* is most commonly isolated, but other *Clostridia* species can account for this illness. Pain over the involved muscle is extreme. The patient appears very toxic and may have a number of cardiovascular and neurologic abnormalities. Laboratory data may be of little value in making the diagnosis. Although gas is usually present in the tissues, it may not be profound. Emergency surgical procedures are necessary in all cases in which gas gangrene is suspected. If muscle necrosis is present, widespread debridement is essential with amputation in selected cases. High-dose penicillin is the drug of choice. Chloramphenicol can be used as an alternative.

Anaerobic Streptococcal Myonecrosis

This infection resembles gas gangrene in its destruction of muscle. The disease begins more slowly, however, with pain being a late manifestation. Over time, the disease spreads more rapidly and can result in severe destruction of tissue. Surgical debridement is essential. Both anaerobic streptococci and staphylococci are important pathogens in this illness. Antibiotics should include penicillin and an antistaphylococcal antibiotic.

Tropical Pyomyositis

Pyomyositis is a localized muscle infection almost always caused by *Staphylococcus aureus.* It is endemic in tropical regions where it is most commonly seen in young males. It is presumed that trauma to the skin allows entry of organisms, which spread through the bloodstream to involve muscles. Most persons have a subacute presentation with fever, myalgias, and leukocytosis (Brown & Wheeler 1985). Pain and swelling of the involved muscle aid in the diagnosis. Frank erythema and warmth are unusual. Diagnosis can be confirmed by needle aspiration of the involved muscle. Blood cultures may be positive. Surgical drainage, combined with an antistaphylococcal antibiotic should result in complete cure.

INFESTATIONS

Scabies

Scabies is the single most common skin problem in many regions of the world (Gulati et al 1977). The adult mite, *Sarcoptes scabiei,* enters the skin and may go unnoticed for several weeks until a sensitization reaction begins. Although any region can be involved, the typical lesion is a papular eruption in the finger webs, flexor surfaces of the wrists, abdomen, axillary folds, and genital areas. Lesions can also appear as vesicles or nodules. Burrows are seen in two thirds of cases. Pruritus is common, especially at night, and lesions may become superinfected with bacteria from excoriations. A drop of mineral oil on the skin may help to visualize a burrow. If a microscope is available, a scraping of the lesion should be made and the mite or its eggs or feces, if present, can be seen. Lindane (Kwell), applied from the neck down and left on overnight, is the most effective therapy. This therapy is not advised for small children or pregnant women because of potential neurologic toxicity. Alternative treatments include 10 percent crotamiton or 5 to 10 percent sulfur ointment. Both of these should be applied two or three times daily to be effective. All family members should be treated at the same time to prevent spread and reinfection. Fomites are not important in transmission. If possible, however, bedding and clothing should be washed in hot water or stored in plastic bags for ten days.

Pediculosis

Pediculosis, or lice infestation, is less common than scabies. The body louse is involved in the transmission of typhus, but head and pubic lice are not involved in disease transmission. Most patients with lice complain of daytime pruritus, which can result in excoriation and superinfection. Diagnosis is usually made by visualization of the nit (or egg) attached to hair shafts. Nits appear as white, oval-shaped material firmly attached to the hair. A magnifying glass may allow the visualization of adult lice, which are 1 to 3 mm in size. Therapy with lindane shampoo for head and pubic lice, and lotion for body lice, is very effective. A second course of therapy may be needed after one week. Other effective treatments include benzyl benzoate (20 to 35% concentration), and pyrethrins (RID). Clothing should be treated as for scabies.

Myiasis

Myiasis, or infestation with fly larvae, can occur in preexisting wounds or as a primary event. Open wounds attract a variety of flies and can become breeding grounds for maggots. Many maggots attach only to decaying tissue, but nondiseased areas can also be affected. Careful surgical removal of the maggots is therapeutic. Some flies deposit their larvae into previously normal skin, which then appear as a furuncle. Removal is accomplished by suffocating the maggot with animal fat or petroleum jelly and waiting for the larvae to exit.

BITES

Human Bites

Human bites are frequently associated with infection. All bite wounds should be thoroughly cleansed and debrided. Most authorities give prophylactic antibiotics for all bites and advise against primary closure of the wound. Penicillin or a cephalosporin is reasonable for prophylaxis. Established infections may be due to streptococci, staphylococci, anaerobes, or the gram-negative bacillus *Eikenella corrodens.* Patients should be treated with parenteral penicillin or ampicillin combined with an antistaphylococcal antibiotic. Severe infections may need immobilization and surgical debridement. Tetanus immunization should be current.

Animal Bites

Animal bites may range from a small scratch to extensive crush injuries. Cleansing and debridement are essential to avoid infection, and wounds should be left unsutured. One study has demonstrated a benefit from antibiotic use in high-risk wounds, such as those on hands (Callahan 1980), but the role of prophylactic antibiotics is unclear. Infections seen less than 12 hours after the bite are frequently due to *Pasturella multocida* and can be treated with penicillin or tetracycline. Late appearing infections are usually due to streptococci or staphylococci and should be treated appropriately. Tetanus immunization should be up-to-date and consideration should be given to the use of rabies antitoxin and immunization.

Snake Bites

Poisonous snakes inhabit all regions of the world. Although most snakes are harmless, it is important to learn the characteristic markings of dangerous snakes in a given region. Most snake bites occur on the extremities, and pain at the bite site is usually the first sign of envenomation. Local changes may include diffuse swelling or the formation of large blebs, which sometimes contain serosanguinous fluid. Systemic toxicity includes hypotension, arrhythmias, neurologic abnormalities, and coagulopathies. All persons with snake bites should be observed for 24 hours. Antitoxin is the only effective therapy and should be given as soon as possible for individuals with systemic or severe local reactions. Because of the possibility of adverse reactions to the antitoxin, it should not be given prophylactically (Warrell 1984). Persons with snake bites should be kept calm and the affected extremity immobilized. Incision and drainage at the site of envenomation is of questionable value. The value of tourniquets is also in doubt but, if one is applied, it should be a tight arterial tourniquet that is loosened every 30 minutes and used for no more than two hours. Patients with systemic toxicity may need general support measures.

Arthropod Bites

Spider bites are usually harmless. There are, however, a number of spiders that can cause human illness. Antivenoms are available for the bite of spiders that can produce systemic illness and death, such as black widow and banana spiders. Other spiders, such as the recluse spiders, usually produce local skin destruction.

Scorpion stings can be life-threatening to children. Administering antivenom is useful. Ant and centipede stings often produce painful local lesions and, occasionally, systemic abnormalities. Bee stings can usually be treated with antihistamines and ice packs unless the patient has a hypersensitivity reaction, in which case epinephrine may be life-saving.

REFERENCES AND SUGGESTED READING

Brown JD, Wheeler B: Pyomyositis. Arch Intern Med 1985;144:1749–51.

Callahan M: Prophylactic antibiotics in common dog bite wounds: A controlled study. Ann Emerg Med 1980;9:410–14.

Canizares O: Clinical Tropical Dermatology. Oxford, Blackwell Scientific, 1975.

Caplan ES, Kluge RM: Gas gangrene. Arch Intern Med 1976;136:788–91

Clancey JK et al: Mycobacterial skin ulcers in Uganda. Lancet 1961;2:951–54.

Dajani AS et al: Natural history of impetigo. II. Etiologic agents and bacterial interations. J Clin Invest 1972;51:2863–71.

Finegold SM: Anaerobic Bacteria in Human Disease. New York, Academic Press, 1977.

Giuliano et al: Bacteriology of necrotizing fasciitis. Am J Surg 1977;134:51–57.

Gulati PV et al: Scabies in a semi-urban area of India: An epidemiologic study. Int J Dermatol 1977;16:594–98.

Koopman JS, Campbell J: The role of cutaneous diphtheria infections in a diphtheria epidemic. J Infect Dis 1975;131:239–44.

Mahgoub ES: Medical management of mycetoma. WHO Bull 1976;54:303–09.

Pettit J: Perspectives in dermatology: Malaysia. Int J Dermatol 1976;15:505–12.

Stone HH, Martin JD: Synergistic necrotizing cellulitis. Ann Surg 1972;175:702–11.

Swender PT, Sandler AP: Vietnamese and Cambodian orphans 1975: The first look. Clin Pediatr 1977;16:264–69.

Taplin D et al: Prevalence of streptococcal pyoderma in relation to climate and hygiene. Lancet 1973;1:501–03.

Uman SJ, Kunin C: Needle aspiration in the diagnosis of soft tissue infections. Arch Intern Med 1975;135:959–61.

Warrell DA: Venomous and poisonous animals. In Warren KS, Mahmoud A (eds): Tropical and Geographic Medicine, pp 517–34. New York, McGraw-Hill, 1984.

29 Leprosy

ROBERT H. GELBER

Leprosy, also referred to as Hansen's disease, is endemic in most underdeveloped countries in Africa, Asia, Latin America, and the Pacific. Almost all cases in the United States, Western Europe, Canada, and Japan are imported. Its frequency in a refugee setting varies a great deal depending on the refugee population and clinician awareness. Leprosy in the refugee setting is often dealt with by Western medical professionals who have had no professional exposure to the disease and who do not appreciate the specific cultural concerns regarding the disease in the refugee population being served. Clinicians are often confronted by a myriad of anachronistic social and immigration policies that place special barriers to recognized cases, preventing the patients' integration into a new society.

In many cultures, particularly Oriental cultures, people with leprosy are ostracized. Thus, it is not uncommon for patients to be banished from the family or isolated within the home without being allowed to share meals communally, enjoy conjugal relations, or share toilet facilities. In some cultures, leprosy is felt to be punishment for wrongdoing. Among Orientals, because of strongly held cultural beliefs concerning genetic transmission, family members of affected individuals are also stigmatized. Frequently, patients and family members deny the diagnosis, often becoming angry at professionals who insist on it and preferring to await the potential ravages of the disease rather than face its social consequences.

Leprosy presents with different faces in different locales. In India and Africa, 90 percent of patients are affected with the tuberculoid form while only 10 percent have the lepromatous form. In China and Southeast Asia, 50 percent of patients are tuberculoid and 50 percent are lepromatous; and in Mexico, 90 percent of patients are lepromatous and only 10 percent tuberculoid. Even in endemic countries there are unexplained clusterings of patients. For example, in Mexico the disease is virtually absent in the east coast states and the Yucatan but hyperendemic in certain west coast states. In endemic locales a particular village may have a high prevalence of disease, but one only a few miles away, without obvious differences in nutrition, hygiene, or other factors, has little or no disease. Hence, a knowledge of the patterns of disease in the refugee population being treated and the particular geographic patterns of its distribution may be very important in making individual and logistic decisions concerning this disease.

ETIOLOGY

The causative agent of leprosy, *Mycobacterium leprae,* is an obligate intracellular parasite. It has been demonstrated rarely to affect other primates, and although in Louisiana and Texas it frequently affects armadillos, it is a pathogen that remains essentially confined to humans. *M. leprae* cannot be grown on artificial media but multiplies in the feet of rodents (Shepard 1960) and may disseminate systemically in immunosuppressed mice, rats, and armadillos. When stained by Ziehl–Neelsen or FITE stains, it appears as an acid-fast rod (0.3 to 0.4 mm $\times$ 4 to 7 mm). A specific serologic test is also available, based on a phenolic glycolipid (PGI) in *M. Leprae* (Cho et al 1983). Among bacteria, *M. leprae*'s propensity to invade peripheral nerves in humans and armadillos is unique.

EPIDEMIOLOGY AND TRANSMISSION

The World Health Organization (WHO) estimates that worldwide there are 12 million cases of leprosy. The age of onset may be as early as two years, but it can affect individuals of any age. The male/female ratio of lepromatous leprosy is 2:1, while the sexes are equally disposed to tuberculoid leprosy. The incubation period for leprosy is uniquely long, averaging about 5 years, no fewer than 2 years, and occasionally 15 or more years.

The mode of transmission of leprosy remains uncertain. The most commonly held view of transmission is that infection is spread by nasal droplets (Rees et al 1974). After a few months of dapsone treatment or even a few days of rifampin treatment, nasal droplets no longer contain viable *M. leprae,* and patients are no longer infectious. Mosquitos and bed bugs living in the vicinity of leprosaria harbor *M. leprae* (Kirchheimer 1976), and mosquitos have been shown capable of transmitting experimental leprosy (Narayanan et al 1977). Skin-to-skin contact as a means of leprosy transmission has become a less likely explanation for disease spread. This is especially true because *M. leprae* is not found in the epidermis or superficial dermis but only in the deeper dermal tissue. On the other hand, the epithelium of patients may at times become denuded as a result of trauma and ulcerative reactions, allowing a potential route of egress for *M. leprae.* Direct dermal inoculation of leprosy has been documented, but it is unusual.

Leprosy transmission generally requires close, prolonged, intimate, and usually household contact with an untreated and, hence, infectious lepromatous case. It has been established in endemic locales that if there is a lepromatous case within the house, the chances that any other household member will become affected is about 10 percent (Worth & Wong 1971). In nonendemic locales, household spread appears considerably less likely. Thus, a family history of disease should stimulate a careful investigation of those placed at risk. Though tuberculoid leprosy is generally believed to be noncontagious, even if untreated, its presence in a household member should also stimulate careful examination for other affected household members. Casual contacts and medical personnel treating patients are not at risk. In hospital settings, no isolation procedures are required even for untreated lepromatous patients.

IMMUNOLOGY

Patients with lepromatous leprosy have a cellular immune defect that appears to be specific for *M. leprae.* They have appropriate dermal delayed hypersensitivity to tuberculin (Rea et al 1976). In lepromatous patients, lepromin skin tests (heat-killed *M. leprae*) do not develop induration at two to three days (Fernandez) or three to four weeks (Mitsuda) (Rees 1974). Thus, the anergy of lepromatous leprosy, unlike sarcoidosis, carcinomatosis, or Hodgkin's disease, is highly specific and not generalized. On the other hand, tuberculoid leprosy patients' peripheral blood lymphocytes recognize *M. leprae,* and these patients have positive lepromin skin tests.

Lepromatous leprosy patients commonly have a polyclonal hyperglobulinemia. This results in a wide variety of frequently confusing false-positive serologic tests, including VDRL, antinuclear antibodies, cryoglobulins, rheumatoid factor, autoantibodies to thyroglobulin, testicular germinal cells, and others.

PATHOLOGY

The specific clinicopathologic classification of leprosy patients provides a basis for initiating appropriate therapy and predicting prognosis and reactional states (Ridley & Jopling 1966; Ridley 1974). In lepromatous leprosy, the epithelium and most superficial layer of the dermis are spared. In the deeper dermis, the most striking feature on hematoxylin and eosin-stained sections are heavily vacuolated macrophages termed *foam cells;* on acid fast staining, numerous bacilli, often in large clumps or "globi," are readily apparent. In tuberculoid leprosy, acid-fast organisms are rare or entirely absent, and the cellular infiltrates are composed of epithelial cells, lymphocytes, and giant cells usually arranged in granuloma, frequently associated with microscopic dermal nerves and, at times, almost entirely replacing them. On occasion the pathology in tuberculoid leprosy will show no more than chronic nonspecific inflammation without evident granuloma formation.

CLINICAL SIGNS AND SYMPTOMS

Leprosy is a chronic infectious disease that most often is associated with minimal symptoms. Manifestations are confined to the skin, peripheral nerves, and upper respiratory tract. The skin rash is quite variable, almost never pruritic, and its appearance depends entirely on the patient's specific classification within the clinicopathologic spectrum.

Tuberculoid patients have one or a few hypopigmented hypoesthetic lesions with well-defined, sometimes slightly raised, and erythematous borders (see Figure 29–1A). These macules may be a few to over 30 cm in diameter and may present anywhere on the body.

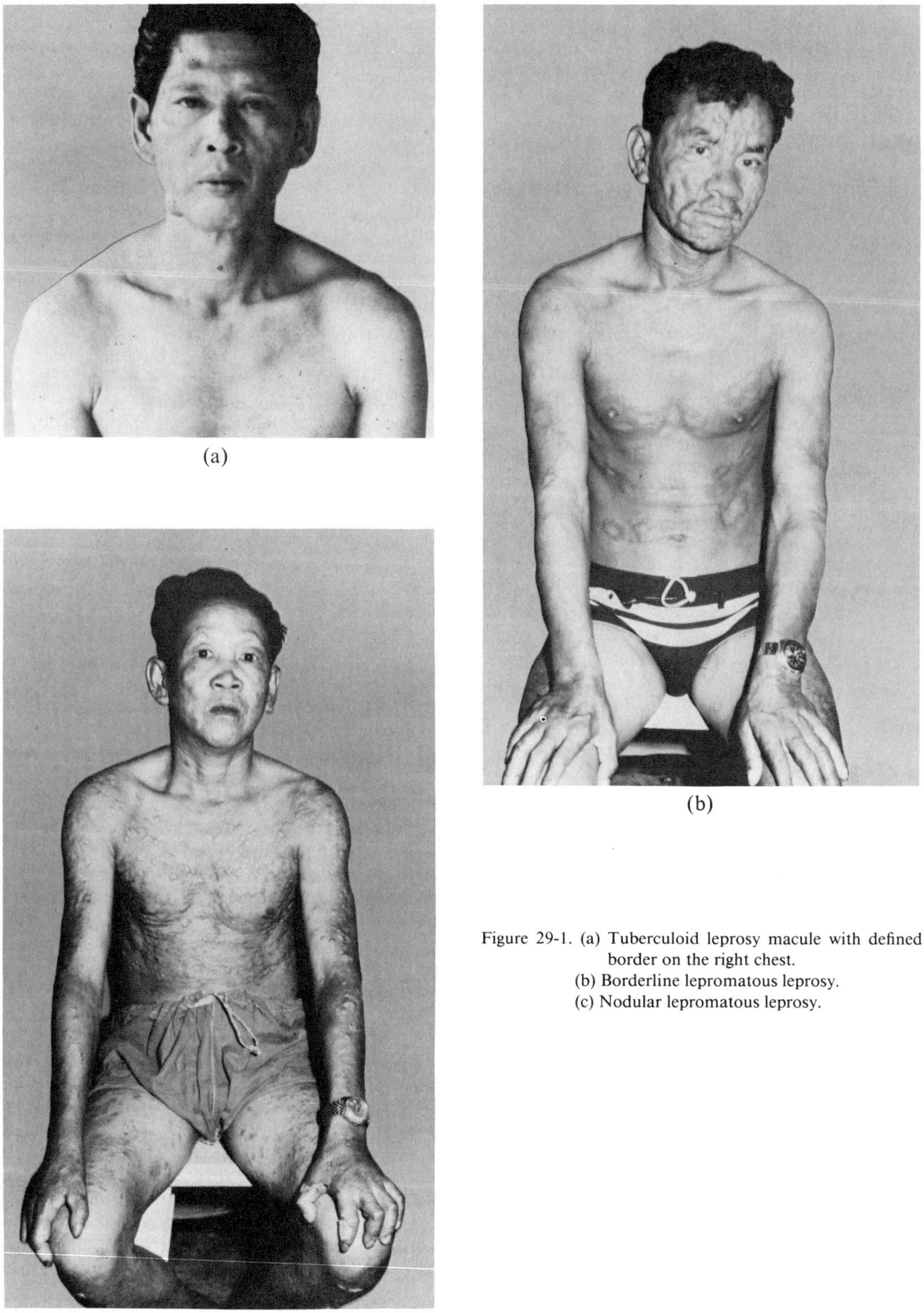

(a) (b) (c)

Figure 29-1. (a) Tuberculoid leprosy macule with defined border on the right chest.
(b) Borderline lepromatous leprosy.
(c) Nodular lepromatous leprosy.

Lepromatous leprosy patients present with nodular and infiltrated skin lesions (see Figure 29–1B). In this form of leprosy, eyebrows (initially the lateral margins) and eyelashes may be lost. In Asia, nodular disease predominates, and this diagnosis is generally easily made from the appearance of the skin. In Mexico and Central America, however, loss of body hair (except on the scalp) and diffuse dermal infiltration may result in a subtle shiny appearance to the skin with no obviously visible lesions; only by assessing dermal thickness by pinching the skin does the diagnosis become evident.

Patients in the middle of the leprosy spectrum are said to have borderline leprosy (see Figure 29–1C). Skin lesions of borderline leprosy have features of both polar forms of the disease, and patients may have both infiltrated plaques and hypopigmented macules wherein sensation is frequently better preserved than in tuberculoid lesions. The macular lesions of borderline leprosy are frequently described as "saucers on end," that is, erythematous, somewhat raised central lesions with hypopigmented edges.

Leprosy is the only bacterial disease with pathology of the peripheral nervous system. Dermal nerves are preferentially affected in tuberculoid lesions, and in both forms of leprosy the larger nerve trunks may be diseased. Leprous neuropathy may result in muscle weakness (myopathy) and sensory loss, particularly fine touch, pain, and temperature sensation. The ulnar nerve at the elbow is the most commonly involved peripheral nerve which, when severely affected, leads to the typical claw hand deformity of leprosy (fourth and fifth fingers) and the loss of dorsal interosseus musculature in the affected hand. If the peroneal nerve is affected, partial or complete foot drop may result. Except for a rare hereditary neuropathy (Charcot–Marie–Tooth disease), leprosy is the only human illness resulting in palpable, enlarged peripheral nerves. Hence, finding a definitely enlarged nerve makes the diagnosis of leprosy extremely likely.

Familiarization with the location of commonly affected nerves and their expected sizes is important for health care professionals working in refugee settings, because assessing peripheral nerve size may not have been part of their routine physical examination in the past. Literally any peripheral nerve may be enlarged in leprosy, but the most frequently detected are the posterior auricular, ulnar, superficial radial, peroneal, sural, and posterior tibial. The posterior auricular nerve is normally neither visible nor palpable, but the others can normally be detected by palpation. Certain consequences of the neuropathy of leprosy ought to suggest the diagnosis. These include acute or recurrent plantar ulcerations, lagophthalmos (incomplete eye closure), corneal scarring, loss of digits, and recurrent burns of the extremities.

Chronic nasal congestion secondary to bacterial invasion and consequent pathology of the nasal mucosa is a common symptom of untreated lepromatous patients. Nasal septal perforation or even nasal collapse leading to a saddle nose deformity, both secondary to nasal cartilage involvement, may be seen in lepromatous leprosy patients whose disease has been neglected.

FIELD EVALUATION

A careful history and physical examination should be taken and carefully recorded. Skin lesions should be described and attention to their loss of sensation should be assessed and documented. A stamp of the anterior and posterior body surface with a drawing of lesions and enlarged nerves affixed is very helpful to others who will subsequently see the patient. Clinical photographs are desirable. A family history of disease may be very productive.

Patient and family education in the refugee setting cannot be overemphasized if a long-term salutary outcome is to be obtained. Patients should hear that the diagnosis will not affect their longevity and be reassured about the risks of contagion. They need to be told that they will not be put away and that special precautions such as separate housing, dishes, toilets, and so on are not required. These lessons may be greeted by considerable cultural resistance and may require frequent repetition. Their acceptance will often depend on the feelings the refugee population has for the professional offering these judgments and the rapport established with the affected patient and his or her family.

Histologic and bacteriologic confirmation of the clinical diagnosis should be sought, if at all possible, where conditions allow. Biopsies should be done in clinically lepromatous patients, ideally from nodules or infiltrated plaques, and from the rim of lesions in patients appearing borderline or tuberculoid. A full-thickness, 3-mm punch biopsy of the skin with an inexpensive disposable punch does not require suturing. Formalin fixation is ideal for field conditions. The formalin bottles should have a tight (preferably screw-cap) top that will not allow evaporation or leakage. These will keep for many months, permitting sectioning and hematoxylin-eosin as well as acid-fast bacteria staining at some later date.

Skin smears are ideally done from four to six different sites. Ears, lesions, posterior elbows, and anterior knees are preferred sites. Smears may be done with a scalpel or razor blade. Sufficient pinching and blanching of the skin and subcutaneous tissue is required that an incision 2 to 3 mm in depth can be done without bleeding. A smear is done of the subcutaneous fluid. The site may be covered with a bandage or benzoine cotton. Smears should be heat fixed immediately and stained within hours. A moderately good microscope is required for evaluation. Both the density of bacteria (bacteriologic index, BI) and solid staining characteristic of bacteria (morphologic index, MI) are useful in initial patient assessment and in following the efficacy of therapy. With therapy, the organisms become beaded in weeks to months, whereas the actual number of bacilli decreases very slowly. In lepromatous leprosy it may require five to ten years for skin smears to become devoid of bacilli.

Detailed sensory mapping (preferably utilizing graded silastic monofilaments) and objective assessment of muscular strength are helpful. These provide a baseline and allow for objective assessment of any deterioration.

DIFFERENTIAL DIAGNOSIS

Skin lesions of tuberculoid leprosy are most commonly confused (especially by inexperienced observers) with tinea versicolor, vitiligo, and ringworm—all of which have intact sensation. Diseases that may clinically mimic lepromatous leprosy are lupus erythematosus, sarcoid, yaws, leishmaniasis, lupus vulgaris, systemic mycosis, and mycosis fungoides.

COMPLICATIONS

Complications of leprosy generally result directly or indirectly from peripheral neuropathy. These include plantar ulcerations, drop foot deformity, autoamputation of fingers and toes, claw hand deformity, interosseus wasting, burns of the extremities, inability to oppose the thumb, lagophthalmos, corneal scarring, and others. Counseling patients to avoid activities that result in injury is important. Amyloidosis and renal failure is a rare complication of lepromatous leprosy. Leprosy patients, on the whole, can be expected to realize normal longevity.

THERAPY

Compliance with therapy in leprosy, as in many other chronic diseases without debilitating symptoms, is a common problem. Poor compliance is found especially often in underdeveloped countries. Here, medical care and drugs are frequently available only haphazardly, and patients often are not well informed of their diagnosis and the need for long-term therapy. The disruption of life leading to the refugee state frequently results in an interruption in therapy for months or even years. Hence, in refugee settings health care providers may often encounter patients with the established diagnosis of leprosy whose therapy has been disrupted irregularly and often over long periods. Such patients are especially susceptible to drug-resistant relapse.

Drug therapy for leprosy must be directed against the causative bacillus and certain "reactional states" that frequently complicate the course of the disease. Availability of drugs for these purposes in refugee settings is often far from optimal and compromises must sometimes be made.

The lepromatous or multibacillary form of leprosy poses the greater problem for antimicrobial therapy because the number of organisms is far in excess of any other human bacterial disease (as much as 10^9 bacilli/gram of skin). Also, these patients lack specific protective cellular immunity for *M. leprae*. Therefore, patients with lepromatous or multibacillary leprosy require multidrug therapy for a very prolonged time.

Dapsone (4,4′-diaminodiphenylsulfone, DDS) is the mainstay of therapy for leprosy. It is highly active against *M. leprae* and the minimal inhibitory concentration, 3 μg/ml, is uniquely low. Dapsone is also relatively nontoxic, and most important for refugee settings, quite inexpensive. Unfortunately, dapsone has been used as monotherapy for leprosy worldwide since its introduction in 1943, and dapsone resistance is becoming an increasing problem (Pearson 1981). Resistance to all the other antimicrobials used to treat leprosy, though less common, has also been confirmed.

Fortunately, almost all of the primary dapsone resistance encountered so far is to low-dose dapsone, far less than that usually used (Gelber 1984).

Patients with all forms of leprosy should be given dapsone in adult doses of 100 mg once daily. Previously, leprologists built up to this dose slowly and discontinued dapsone when reactions occurred, but this no longer appears warranted. Dapsone is the only antimicrobial used in the therapy of leprosy that has been found safe in pregnancy. Dapsone decreases red cell survival and may cause actual anemia or exacerbate established anemia. This is particularly true for pregnant women, malnourished individuals, and for those with G6PD deficiency. Dapsone may be allergenic, and may cross-react with sulfonamides. With large doses, methemoglobinemia and sulfhemoglobinemia may occur. Within the first few weeks or months of therapy, a rare but serious condition termed the "sulfone syndrome" may necessitate discontinuation of dapsone and initiation of steroid therapy. This syndrome includes high fever, exfoliative dermatitis, lymphadenopathy, icterus, hemolytic anemia, and lymphocytosis with many atypical lymphocytes.

Unlike dapsone, which is bacteriostatic for leprosy, rifampin is bactericidal (Rees 1975). Rifampin has the significant drawback of being quite expensive. Rifampin causes urine to turn red, and patients should be advised to expect this. It may cause hepatitis and should be avoided in alcoholics and patients with established liver dysfunction. It may cause flulike symptoms and, rarely, severe thrombocytopenia and renal failure when given irregularly. Because of its potency for *M. leprae* and because erythema nodosum leprosum (ENL) is associated with the killing of bacteria, it was feared that rifampin would result in early and severe ENL; fortunately, this has not been the case.

Clofazimine has significant antimicrobial activity against *M. leprae* (roughly equivalent to that of dapsone) and mild efficacy in treating ENL. Recommended antimicrobial doses range from 100 mg three times weekly to 100 mg daily. Unfortunately, clofazimine results in a dose-dependent red-black discoloration of the skin, particularly within leprosy lesions and in sun-exposed areas, which may not completely resolve for a year or more following discontinuation. Gastrointestinal side effects from clofazimine are not uncommon but are usually mild.

Ethionamide or prothionamide are also effective against *M. leprae,* and are utilized in adults in daily doses of 250 to 500 mg. Many patients treated with these agents (especially ethionamide), experience unacceptable gastrointestinal intolerance, particularly with the higher dosage. These thioamides may also result in hepatic toxicity, especially if rifampin is administered concomitantly. Indeed, such a combination should be avoided in settings where liver function tests cannot be monitored.

REGIMENS

In the United States it is generally recommended that multibacillary (i.e., many bacteria in the skin are noted on smear) leprosy be treated with daily dapsone (100 mg) and daily rifampin (600 mg) for the first two to three years, and dapsone alone thereafter for life. Dosage adjustments are made for children by comparing the child's weight to a 60-kg adult. The WHO advocates triple-drug therapy for multibacillary leprosy. Their reasons include difficulty of routinely monitoring for drug resistance in endemic countries, concerns over the clinical significance of primary dapsone resistance in individual patients, and the potential for promoting dapsone resistance. The WHO (WHO Study Group 1982) recommends that for multibacillary disease, 100 mg of dapsone and 100 mg of clofazimine be taken daily. In addition, rifampin, 600 mg, and clofazimine, 300 mg, should be given once a month under supervision.

For those who will not accept clofazimine for cosmetic reasons, ethionamide or prothionamide, 375 mg daily, may be substituted. The monthly rifampin interval suggested by the WHO is primarily because of the high cost of daily therapy. For multibacillary leprosy, the WHO recommends that therapy be maintained for a minimum of two years or until skin smear bacteriologic negativity occurs (generally five to ten years). Viable drug-sensitive *M. leprae* may be found in tissues of lepromatous leprosy patients after many years of therapy (Waters et al 1977; 1978). The clinical significance of these "persisters" remains unclear, and some leprologists are not convinced of the prudence of ever discontinuing therapy for multibacillary disease.

In the United States, paucibacillary leprosy (few organisms seen) is treated with dapsone, 100 mg daily for five years. Some authorities advocate the addition of rifampin, 600 mg daily for the first six months. For paucibacillary leprosy, the WHO advocates dapsone 100 mg daily and rifampin 600 mg monthly, for a total duration of six months.

REACTIONS AND THEIR THERAPY

Reactional states may occur before therapy. However, they more commonly occur after the initiation of antimicrobial therapy, result in more disturbing symptoms than the uncomplicated untreated disease itself, and are blamed by the patient on the therapy being offered. This frequently will lead to the patient discontinuing therapy, losing faith in the prescribing professionals, and being convinced that their signs and symptoms represent clinical deterioration. To avert this situation, patients should be carefully advised at the time of diagnosis about symptoms of reactions and the possible need for additional therapy if these symptoms occur.

About half of the patients with lepromatous leprosy will develop some signs of ENL. Over 90 percent of ENL occurs after the initiation of chemotherapy, generally within the first year or two after therapy has commenced, and resolves spontaneously, generally after about five years of treatment. ENL thus appears to be associated with the killing of *M. leprae.* Histologically it is a vasculitis consisting of infiltrates of predominately polymorphonuclear leukocytes, thought to result from immune complexes (Gelber et al 1974). The most frequent manifestation of ENL is painful erythematous papules of the skin, which occur most commonly on the extensor surfaces of extremities but may occur anywhere on the body. In severe ENL, these skin lesions may pustulate and ulcerate. Individual ENL lesions last only a few days but may recur in repeated crops at various intervals. ENL, being a syndrome associated with a systemic vasculitis, may have protean clinical manifestations that also include fever, neuritis, lymphadenitis, uveitis, orchitis, anemia, arthritis, and glomerulonephritis.

Borderline leprosy patients may develop other lepra reactions. If these occur prior to therapy they are termed *downgrading reactions,* and if they develop while antimicrobial therapy is being given they are referred to as *reversal reactions.* Pathophysiologically, the former is believed to be due to loss of cellular immunity for *M. leprae,* and the latter to an increase in cellular responses. Manifestations include signs of inflammation in the skin (generally within previous skin lesions, though new lesional areas may also appear), inflamed nerves, and low-grade fever. The neuritis, if untreated for even 24 hours, can result in complete and irreversible nerve damage.

ENL is best treated initially with a short course of prednisone (40 to 60 mg/day). After a few weeks, the steroids are tapered off. If ENL recurs with tapering, the dose is increased. If ENL appears to be a chronic or recurrent problem necessitating consideration of long-term corticosteroids with their known complications, thalidomide, 100 to 300 mg nightly (if available), is advocated. It obviously should not be given to women in the childbearing years because of its propensity to cause serious birth defects and, in refugee populations, males given these tablets should be carefully counseled not to share them. This is particularly important since thalidomide's tranquilizing properties are often very attractive. If chronic steroids are necessary, the lowest dose necessary to minimize or eliminate symptoms of ENL should be sought. Clofazimine, 300 mg daily, has been found useful in enabling lower doses of corticosteroids to prevent ENL. Chloroquine has been found minimally effective against ENL and should be considered only when the other agents are not available.

Unlike ENL, in which short intermittent courses of corticosteroids are often effective and other agents are useful, other reactions (reversal and downgrading) can be treated effectively only by corticosteroids; discontinuation before two to three months is frequently associated with relapse. Thus, minor inflammation in skin lesions should be tolerated, especially if the patient is not particularly troubled by it, and therapy should be reserved for neuritis and inflammation threatening ulceration, especially on the face. If corticosteroids are required, 40 to 60 mg prednisone daily is initially recommended. Prednisone can usually be tapered off to 15 to 20 mg daily over a few weeks and maintained for two to three months before it is terminated.

OTHER THERAPEUTIC CONSIDERATIONS

Acute soft tissue and ulcerative infections should be treated vigorously with careful debridement and appropriate antibiotics, lest they result in destructive osteomyelitis. Avoiding weightbearing is essential for the healing of plantar ulcers. This may be accomplished by total bed rest, use of crutches, or optimally, a total-contact walking cast.

Patients with a history of plantar ulcers should be provided with shoes. Extra depth shoes or specially molded shoes may be required to prevent recurrence. Once ulcers are healed, patients should be encouraged to progressively ambulate very slowly since ulcer breakdown frequently occurs within the first or second week of weightbearing. Sites of old ulcerations frequently develop hard, thick calluses which provide a nidus for recurrent ulcerations. Patients should be instructed to keep these calluses trimmed carefully and soak the feet daily, preferably applying a moisturizing cream before drying them; this is useful in keeping the skin of the feet soft and supple so as to prevent recurrent ulceration.

Iridocyclitis of ENL may result in blindness. Treatment consists of atropine and steroid drops, in addition to systemic steroids. Patients with lagophthalmos and corneal insensitivity benefit from tear substitutes.

Reconstructive surgery for lagophthalmos and deformities of the hands and feet can be effective. Tendon transfers should be delayed for at least six months after the initiation of antimicrobial therapy and after signs of reaction have abated. Such surgery should be performed by those with training and experience in the specific problems of these patients, at facilities where intensive preoperative and postoperative physical therapy is available.

CONTROL AND PROPHYLAXIS

Sulfone prophylaxis of household contacts does not prevent the development of lepromatous leprosy and only partially reduces the subsequent prevalence of tuberculoid leprosy (Shepard et al 1979). Thus, sulfone prophylaxis is not generally recommended. Three BCG trials for the prevention of leprosy have been completed and have produced variable results. Thus, for now, BCG is not recommended. The WHO is embarking on vaccine trials of heat-killed armadillo-derived *M. leprae* (alone and in combination with BCG), which have shown some signs of promise in mice. *M. leprae*-specific products obtained by chemical purification, organic synthesis, or bioengineering offer perhaps even greater hope that a vaccine for leprosy might be available in the future.

It is recommended that household contacts of leprosy patients undergo annual physical examinations by experienced medical personnel. Because of the long and variable incubation period, these examinations should be done for at least five years after diagnosis of the index case.

Early serodiagnosis of leprosy, especially utilizing ELISA to PGI, is being vigorously pursued and may prove to be a valuable tool in leprosy control.

REFERENCES

Bloom BR, Godal T: Selective primary health care: strategies for control of disease in the developing world. V. Leprosy. Rev Infect Dis 1983;5:765–80.

Cho SN, Yanagihara DL, Hunter SW et al: Serological specificity of phenolic glycolipid I from *Mycobacterium leprae* and use in serodiagnosis of leprosy. Infect Immunol 1983;41:1077–83.

Gelber RH, Drutz PJ, Epstein WV et al: Clinical correlates of Clq precipitating substances in the sera of patients with leprosy. Am J Trop Med Hyg 1974;23:471–75.

Gelber RH: Primary dapsone-resistant leprosy in San Franciso. Int J Lepr 1984;52:471–74.

Kirchheimer WF: The role of arthropods in the transmission of leprosy. Int J Lepr 1976;44:104–07.

Narayanan E, Sreevatsa, Kirchheimer WF et al: Transfer of leprosy bacilli from patients to mouse footpads by *Aedes aegypti*. Leprosy in India 1977;49:181–86.

Pearson JMH: The problem of dapsone-resistant leprosy. Int J Lepr 1981;49:417–20.

Rea TH, Quismorio FP, Harding B et al: Immunologic responses in patients with lepromatous leprosy. Arch Dermatol 1976;112:304–10.

Rees RJW: The significance of the lepromin reaction in man. Prog Allergy 1964;8:224–58.

Rees RJW, McDougall AC, Weddell AGM: The nose in mice with experimental human leprosy. Lepr Rev 1974;45:112–20.

Rees RJW: Rifampicin: The investigation of a bactericidal antileprosy drug. Lepr Rev 1975;46:121–24.

Ridley PS, Jopling WH: Classification of leprosy according to immunity. A five group system. Int J Lepr 1966;34:255–73.

Ridley PS: Histological classification and the immunological spectrum of leprosy. Bull WHO 1974;51:451–65.

Shepard CC: The experimental disease that follows the infection of human leprosy bacilli into footpads of mice. J Exp Med 1960;112:445–54.

Shepard CC, Fasal P, Worth RM et al: Acedadapsone in the prevention of leprosy: Field trial in three high prevalence villages in Micronesia. Am J Trop Med Hyg 1979;28:559–63.

Waters MFR, Rees RJW, McDougall L et al: Ten years of dapsone in lepromatous leprosy. Clinical, bacteriological and histological assessment and the finding of viable leprosy bacilli. Lepr Rev 1977;45:288–98.

Waters MFR, Rees RJW, Pearson JMH et al: Rifampicin for lepromatous leprosy: Nine years' experience. Br Med J 1978;1:133–35.

World Health Organization Study Group: Chemotherapy of leprosy for control programmes. Tech Report Series 1982;675:7–33.

Worth RM, Wong TO: Further notes on the prevalence of leprosy in Hong Kong Chinese living with a lepromatous patient. Int J Lepr 1971;39:744–48.

30
Meningitis and Poliomyelitis

STANLEY E. READ

The identification and management of infections involving the central nervous system (CNS) in a refugee setting depend on the clinical diagnostic acumen of the clinician, a knowledge of the kinds of infections that are prevalent, and the use of the best therapeutic intervention techniques available. Two of the most important acute infectious diseases are meningitis and poliomyelitis. These two infections occur in all parts of the world but are particularly important as causes of infection of epidemic proportion in underdeveloped countries (Hassan-King et al 1979; Onile et al 1982; Robinson 1982; Miner & Edman 1978) and areas disrupted by wars or natural disasters.

The first, bacterial meningitis, is treatable and usually has a good outcome if appropriate therapy is instituted early, though undiagnosed and untreated bacterial meningitis is devastating. Bacterial meningitis in the refugee setting is most frequently caused by *Neisseria meningitidis,* an organism that can cause epidemics. Epidemic disease can be averted by mass immunizations (Tauny et al 1974).

The second, poliomyelitis, is caused by a virus and is not amenable to treatment at the present time. However, it is important to recognize this disease because of the potential for epidemic spread in the crowded conditions of a refugee camp. Poliomyelitis is preventable by early vaccination.

A third important CNS infection, cerebral malaria, occurs in parts of the world where *Plasmodium falciparum* malaria exists, and it is treatable (see Chapter 25).

BACTERIAL MENINGITIS

Presentation

The presentation of an individual with altered consciousness, fever, headache, and vomiting strongly suggests an infection involving the CNS. These symptoms, together with signs of meningeal irritation, should make the clinical diagnosis evident. In addition, irritation caused by the infection may trigger seizures.

The general health status of the patient must always be taken into consideration. For example, in individuals with malnutrition and gastroenteritis, clinical findings of fever and altered consciousness might be a result of those two processes alone or a result of meningitis. Severe malnutrition can result in less clearly defined clinical criteria for CNS infections. In addition, malnutrition makes the individual more susceptible to infections in general because of its effect on all aspects of the host defense system. In the case of children who have been adequately fed for several months but have a history of malnutrition, residual immunodeficiency may not be evident from clinical evaluation, yet these children will remain more susceptible to infections in general and to severe complications of these infections in particular.

Clinical Features

Clinical features include fever, altered consciousness, signs and symptoms of increased intracranial pressure, meningismus, other neurologic signs, and rash.

Fever may be of recent onset or it may have been present for several days. There may be a history of a preceding focus of infection, such as otitis media, or of an influenza-like illness before the onset of symptoms of meningitis.

Altered consciousness may vary from minimal signs such as drowsiness and irritability, to more profound changes eventually leading to coma. Convulsions may occur as the result of irritation caused by the inflammatory process. Seizures are usually generalized.

Signs and symptoms of increased intracranial pressure can include headache, vomiting, and loss of venous pulsations on fundoscopic examination. In infants, the fontanel should be checked for fullness or bulging. Edema of the optic disk is an unusual sign in acute meningitis.

Meningeal irritation can occur under many circumstances including bacterial, viral, or parasitic infections. The sign may be elicited by pain and limitation of movement of the neck, particularly flexion, or pain on straight leg raising. In its most extreme form, muscle spasm resulting in arching of the whole body (opisthotonus) may occur.

Other neurologic signs, such as focal signs, usually indicate a complication of the meningitis such as subdural, epidural, or parenchymal abscess.

Rashes are usually petechial or ecchymotic and suggest disseminated intravascular coagulation triggered by release of lipopolysaccharide by the bacteria. Rash is most commonly associated with sepsis caused by *N. meningitidis* but also occurs with *Streptococcus pneumoniae, Haemophilus influenzae,* and other bacterial and viral infections. Rash is uncommonly reported to be associated with meningococcal disease in Africa.

The classic signs of meningitis are frequently absent in the first month of life. Subtle changes such as poor feeding, bradycardia, respiratory difficulties such as apnea, and temperature instability are suggestive of meningitis.

Etiologic Agents

Etiologic agents will be discussed under two categories; organisms causing infection in the apparently healthy host and those infecting the malnourished or otherwise immunocompromised host.

Healthy Hosts

Neisseria meningitidis is the most common cause of bacterial meningitis in adults throughout the world, and perhaps the most common agent among all age groups in underdeveloped countries. There are several serogroups of meningococci. Of these groups, A and C are most often associated with epidemics, although they can also cause sporadic infections.

Streptococcus pneumoniae is probably the second most common cause of meningitis but is significantly less common than the meningococcus in crowded impoverished areas.

Haemophilus influenzae is the most common cause of meningitis in young children in the Western Hemisphere, Europe, and Japan. It occurs in young children in underdeveloped countries but is relatively uncommon. It rarely occurs in children over five years of age.

Immunocompromised or Immunoimmature Hosts (Neonates)

Individuals who are obviously malnourished can be expected to be immunocompromised in the refugee setting. In addition, others who appear to be well nourished may have residual defects in their defense system caused by previous malnutrition. These individuals are susceptible to systemic and CNS infections with the organisms indicated above and, in addition, may be infected by less common organisms.

Neonates (up to one month of age) represent a group in which the defense system is immature. They may also have additional profound defects in the development of their defense system if their mothers were serverely malnourished during pregnancy. Common organisms causing sepsis or meningitis in this group are shown in Table 30-1.

Diagnosis

The diagnosis of bacterial meningitis is based on the recognition of the clinical features and the diagnostic workup. The workup will depend on the health care facility and the availability of various tests.

The most basic situation is one in which a clinical diagnosis of bacterial meningitis is made but facilities or equipment for a lumbar puncture are unavailable. In such a case, a clinical decision is made and the most appropriate antibiotic available is chosen.

Table 30-1. Organisms Causing Meningitis

Normal host
N. meningitidis
S. pneumoniae
H. influenzae
Neonate
Group B streptococcus
E. coli
Listeria
Immunocompromised host
All of the above
S. aureus
Group A streptococcus
Klebsiella
Pseudomonas
M. tuberculosis
Cryptococcus
Toxoplasma

Table 30-2. Identification of Organisms

Organism	Gram Stain	Shape	Pattern
N. meningitidis	Negative	Cocci	Pairs
S. pneumoniae	Positive	Cocci	Short chains
H. influenzae	Negative	Mainly rods (variable)	Single
S. aureus	Positive	Cocci	Clusters
Groups A and B streptococcus	Positive	Cocci	Chains
E. coli	Negative	Rods	Single
Pseudomonas	Negative	Rods	Single
Klebsiella	Negative	Rods	Single

When basic laboratory facilities are available, but there are not bacteriologic cultures, following the clinical diagnosis of meningitis, a lumbar puncture is performed. The cerebrospinal fluid (CSF) is examined for the presence of white blood cells and the relative proportion of polymorphonuclear leukocytes (PMN) to mononuclear cells. A Gram's stain preparation is made for identification of bacteria (see Chapter 22 for technique; Table 30-2 for organism identification). One or more PMNs in the CSF is abnormal in any patient over one month of age. An increased number of PMNs compared to mononuclear cells is only suggestive of bacterial versus viral infection and is not particularly useful in making a therapeutic decision. A predominance of mononuclear cells suggests the possibility of tuberculous meningitis. An increase in the total number of peripheral blood leukocytes, particularly with an increase in PMNs and bands, suggests a bacterial infection.

The latex agglutination test (Bortolussi et al 1982) for detecting bacterial antigens is very sensitive and there are relatively few problems with cross-reactivity. In addition, it has the advantage of being simple to perform and can be done in the field. Kits are commercially available for the detection of antigens of *N. meningitidis* A and C, *S. pneumoniae, H. influenzae,* and groups A and B streptococci. The major disadvantage is that commercial kits are expensive. Tests are best done on the CSF, but antigens can also be detected in serum and in urine. There are problems with cross-reactions when testing.

A workup, when complete laboratory facilities are available, includes the following:

- All of the previously described procedures.
- CSF for isolation of bacteria and sensitivity testing.
- CSF glucose and protein levels. In bacterial infections, the CSF glucose is often less than half the level of the peripheral blood glucose; the protein content may be elevated, but this is less helpful in differentiating bacterial from other CNS infections.
- Culture of peripheral blood for isolation of bacteria.
- Countercurrent immunoelectrophoresis. This has no advantage over latex agglutination and it may be less sensitive for some antigens. Special equipment is necessary for the test system; but if the equipment is in place, it is less costly to do than latex agglutination.
- Blood and urine electrolytes. Inflammatory processes within the CNS may result in the syndrome of inappropriate secretion of antidiuretic hormone (SIADH); this can be monitored by following the electrolyte and fluid balance. Because the urine output is decreased in patients with SIADH, administration of routine maintenance fluid can result in fluid overload.

Differential Diagnosis

Viral Meningitis or Meningoencephalitis

In a refugee setting—and, in fact, in most situations—viral infection of the CNS is a diagnosis made by exclusion. If the patient has signs and symptoms of meningitis with inflammatory cells in the CSF, but no evidence of bacteria by Gram's stain, culture, or antigen testing, then it is assumed that a viral infection is present. One exception is if the patient has a history of antibiotic therapy that may obscure the isolation of bacteria. Because it is very difficult to prove that there were no bacteria present, however, such cases should probably be treated as bacterial meningitis.

Cerebral Malaria

Cerebral malaria is an acute medical emergency and the differential diagnosis of this, versus bacterial meningitis, cannot be made on the basis of clinical findings alone. If there is a reasonable chance of either infection, but no further diagnostic tests are available, then both should be treated (see Chapter 25). Cells can be found in the CSF in cerebral malaria but are usually fewer in number than in bacterial meningitis. The diagnosis is made by finding *P. falciparum* in the peripheral blood and no evidence of bacteria in the CNS. If there is any question of the etiology of the clinical signs and symptoms, even after laboratory testing, treat for both bacterial meningitis and malaria.

Tuberculous Meningitis

The onset of tuberculous meningitis is usually more insidious than that of other bacterial causes. Rarely, it presents with acute onset of fever, stiff neck, and altered consciousness, but these symptoms usually develop over days to weeks rather than rapidly over a few hours, which is more commonly seen with bacterial meningitis.

Tetanus

The neonate with tetanus may present with findings compatible with neonatal sepsis. Because the signs are often subtle, fever is frequently absent and altered consciousness is difficult to assess. The signs of irritability due to tetanus may be similar to those of sepsis. Even the tetanic spasm may be mistaken for opisthotonus, although it should be noted that this is very rarely a result of bacterial sepsis with meningitis in the neonate. If both diagnoses are possible, it is safest to treat both if appropriate medications are available (see Chapter 31).

Management

Antibiotics should be chosen to provide the best overall coverage for the most likely infecting organisms. The availability of antibiotics depends, to a great extent, on their cost.

In neonates, a combination of ampicillin and gentamicin is considered optimal for organisms most likely to cause sepsis and/or meningitis (see Table 30-3 for dosage schedule). If the organism is known to be the group B streptococcus, then either ampicillin or penicillin can be used alone. If other antibiotics are not available, chloramphenicol can be used in the dosages recommended in Table 30-3 but there are potentially severe side effects in the neonate.

Antibiotics for children and adults include the following:

- Chloramphenicol. The single antibiotic that most effectively treats the common infect-

Table 30-3. Neonatal Parenteral Antibiotic Dosages for Meningitis and Sepsis

Antibiotic	Birth to 7 days of age BW < 2.0 kg	BW > 2.0 kg	Over 7 days of age BW < 2.0 kg	BW > 2.0 kg
Ampicillin	50 mg/kg/dose q12h	50 mg/kg/dose q8h	50 mg/kg/dose q8h	50 mg/kg/dose q6h
Gentamicin	2.5 mg/kg/dose q12h	2.5 mg/kg/dose q12h	2.5 mg/kg/dose q8h	2.5 mg/kg/dose q8h
Penicillin G	50,000 IU/kg/ dose q12h	50,000 IU/kg/ dose q8h	50,000 IU/kg/ dose q8h	50,000 IU/kg/ dose q6h
Cloxicillin, oxicillin, methicillin, or nafcillin	50 mg/kg/dose q12h	50 mg/kg/dose q8h	50 mg/kg/dose q8h	50 mg/kg/dose q6h
Chloramphenicol[a]	25 mg/kg/day q24h	25 mg/kg/dose q24h	25mg/kg/dose q24	25 mg/kg/dose q12h

[From Peter G, Giebink GS, Hall CB, Plotkin SA (eds): Report of the Committee on Infectious Diseases. 12th ed. Elk Grove Village, IL, American Academy of Pediatrics, 1986, pp. 432–33.]

BW = Birth Weight

[a]Not recommended except under unusual circumstances. Can be used orally for meningitis after initial parenteral dose.

ing organisms from infancy through adulthood is chloramphenicol. It is probably the least expensive antibiotic in its class. Although penicillin is comparable in price, it does not cover as wide a range of bacteria as chloramphenicol.

Chloramphenicol can be given intravenously, intramuscularly, or orally (when the patient is capable of taking it by mouth); each route achieves comparable bood levels (Shann et al 1985). It is very well absorbed by the gastrointestinal tract. Several studies carried out in Africa indicate that chloramphenicol is effective in treating meningococcal meningitis. Most have used a five-day regimen starting with intramuscular antibiotic and then changing to oral (Whittle et al 1973). Studies on single-dose intramuscular chloramphenicol have shown that it can be effective in treating meningococcal meningitis, but this use is not recommended except in extreme circumstances (Wali et al 1979).

As many as 60% of *H. influenzae* organisms in certain parts of the world may be resistant to ampicillin. These strains are usually sensitive to chloramphenicol. If sensitivity testing is available, both drugs can be started initially, discontinuing one after sensitivities are known. In certain areas of the world where *H. influenzae* is known to be occasionally sensitive to ampicillin but resistant to chloramphenicol, the use of both concomitantly may be considered.

Campos and coworkers (1986) have reported multiply resistant *H. influenzae* type b organisms causing meningitis in Spain. Sixty percent of their 35 cases were resistant to ampicillin, 66% to chloramphenicol, an 57% to both antibiotics. All *H. influenzae* organisms were sensitive to cefotaxime. Acceptable alternatives include other appropriate second- or third- (not first-) generation cephalosporins such as cefuroxime, cefotaxime, or moxalactam. The combination of gentamicin and carbenicillin has also been shown to be effective against multiply resistant *H. influenzae* organisms (Mathies et al 1986; Uchiyama et al 1980).

A major disadvantage of chloramphenicol is that it cannot be used safely in neonates unless the facilities to do serum chloramphenicol levels are available. This is because of the unpredictability of the neonatal liver in handling this antibiotic. High levels of chloramphenicol and its products may accumulate, resulting in shock and the gray baby syndrome. Under exceptional circumstances, however, it can be used by modifying the dose, as shown in Table 30-3. There is an extremely small risk of an idiosyncratic reaction in any patient, with resultant aplastic anemia. Long-term use at high doses will result in reversible marrow depression.

- Penicillin is effective in the treatment of infections due to *N. meningitidis* and most *S. pneumoniae.* It is also effective in the treatment of infections due to groups A and B streptococci. However, *H. influenzae* is not sensitive to penicillin, so children under five years of age should be treated with ampicillin or chloramphenicol.
- Cloxacillin is a semisynthetic penicillin to which most *S. aureus* are sensitive. It is also effective against most streptococci.
- Ampicillin is effective in treating infections by *N. meningitidis* and most *H. influenzae* and *S. pneumoniae,* although ampicillin-resistant *H. influenzae* are increasing in many parts of the world. It is also effective against groups A and B streptococci and some *E. coli.*
- Gentamicin is an aminoglycoside that is effective against many gram-negative organisms including most *E. coli, Klebsiella,* and many *Pseudomonas.* It must be given intramuscularly or intravenously.
- Cefuroxime is a second-generation cephalosporin effective against *H. influenze, S. pneumoniae,* and *N. meningitidis.* It must be given intramuscularly or intravenously. It results in effective CSF levels, unlike many other cephalosporins. It is expensive.
- Sulfonamides are inappropriate therapy because of the emergence of resistant organisms. They can be used when the organism is known to be susceptible.

The dosage regimen for antibiotics is provided in Table 30-4. Duration of treatment in neonates with *E. coli* or other coliforms is three weeks—two weeks when other organisms are the cause of infection. Children and adults with *N. meningitidis* should be treated for five to seven days, and for seven to ten days for other organisms.

General management of patients includes the following:

- Fluid restriction to 60 to 70 percent calculated total fluid maintenance, to avoid the effects of possible inappropriate antidiuretic hormone (ADH) secretion. In the absence of the laboratory facilities to measure serum electrolytes and osmolarity, fluid restriction should be maintained until the patient has shown a distinct clinical improvement.

Table 30-4. Antibiotic Dosage Regimen

		Dosage (per day)				
		Adults		Children		
Antibiotic	Organism	Oral	Parenteral	Oral	Parenteral	Interval
Chloramphenicol	*N. meningitidis* *S. pneumoniae* *H. influenzae*[a]	50–100 mg/kg	50–100 mg/kg	50–100 mg/kg	50–100 mg/kg	q6h
Penicillin	*N. meningitidis* *S. pneumoniae*[b] Groups A and B streptoccocus	1–2 g	1.2–24 million U	25–50 mg/kg	100,000–500,000 U/kg	q6h
Cloxacillin	*S. aureus* Groups A and B streptococcus	2–4 g	2–9 g	50–100 mg/kg	100–200 mg/kg	q6h
Ampicillin	*H. influenzae*[a] *S. pneumoniae* *N. meningitidis* Groups A and B streptococcus *E. coli*[b]	2–4 g	2–12 g	50–100 mg/kg	100–400 mg/kg	q6–8h
Gentamicin	*E. coli* *Klebsiella* *Pseudomonas*[b]	Not available	3–5 mg/kg	Not available	3–7.5 mg/kg	q8h
Cefuroxime	*N. meningitidis* *S. pneumoniae* *H. influenzae*	Not available	2.25–9 g	Not available	50–240 mg/kg	q8h

[a]See important comments in the "Management" section of this chapter under Chloramphenicol and Ampicillin, about *H. influenzae* organisms resistant to multiple antibiotics.
[b]Not all strains.

- Appropriate seizure control.
- Antipyretics. Although there is controversy over the value of antipyretics, they probably help in febrile seizure control and make the patient more comfortable.

Complications

Septic shock can occur with any of the major bacterial infections, although it is most commonly seen with infections due to *N. meningitidis*. There is no known effective management for this complication, although in major centers, intensive care management and support are attempted. The use of antibodies to lipopolysaccharide (endotoxin) may be a useful adjunct in the management of this problem in the future.

Other complications include the following:

- CNS abscess—subdural, epidural, parenchymal
- Osteomyelitis
- Pericarditis
- Septic arthritis
- Hydrocephalus
- Deafness

Prevention

Prophylaxis

Family members and other close contacts are at increased risk of developing meningococcal meningitis. To eliminate the *N. meningitidis* organism and prevent the chances of invasive disease, it is recommended that prophylactic antibiotics be given. The drug of choice is rifampin (10 mg/kg, up to 600 mg, twice daily for two days), given as soon as the index case is documented. If the organism is known to be sulfonamide sensitive, then this may be used. Minocycline may also be used, although there is a high incidence of nausea, ataxia, and tinnitus. The index case should be treated before discharge from the hospital to eliminate the carrier state. Antibiotics used in the treatment of meningitis, such as penicillin and chloramphenicol, are not effective in eradicating nasopharyngeal carriage.

Contacts under five years of age have an increased risk of developing *H. influenzae* meningitis. The recommended prophylaxis is rifampin (20 mg/kg, up to 600 mg, daily for four days). The index case should also be treated with rifampin.

Vaccines

Meningococcal Polysaccharide Vaccines

Vaccines are available against groups A and C meningococci and are under investigation for groups Y, W135, and 29E (Greenwood et al 1980a; Greenwood et al 1980b; Gold et al 1975) (see Chapter 6). The group A and C vaccines provide at least 90% protection in children and adults against meningococcal disease due to these specific strains and the protection lasts for at least two years. The group A vaccine is effective in infants as young as three months, but group C vaccine does not protect infants under 18 to 24 months of age.

The vaccine is recommended for epidemic control, for travelers to areas where epidemics are occurring, and for household contacts of affected persons.

Pneumococcal Polysaccharide Vaccine

This vaccine (Clemens & Shapiro 1984) contains polysaccharides from 23 of the most common serotypes of *S. pneumoniae* representing 85 to 90 percent of cases of pneumococcal sepsis and meningitis. It is usually not available in the refugee setting.

H. influenzae Type b Polysaccharide Vaccine

A new type b polysaccharide vaccine (Peltola et al 1977) appears to be effective for children two years of age and older. The vaccine is expensive, however, and is unlikely to be available in the refugee setting in the near future.

POLIOMYELITIS

Poliomyelitis is still a common infection wherever vaccination programs are absent or incomplete. It occurs primarily during the summer and fall in temperate climates, and year-round in warm climates. The introduction of vaccines has changed the incidence of polio dramatically in developed countries. For example, in 1955 the United States had an annual incidence of paralytic polio of 10 to 14 per 100,000. Following the introduction of inactivated polio vaccine and, later, attenuated live vaccines, the incidence fell to 0.5 per 100,000 within five years, and by 1980 it was 0.003 per 100,000 (Robinson 1982).

As the result of lameness surveys conducted during the late 1970s, it became apparent that control of paralytic polio was not being achieved in many countries with poor health care structures. The incidence of paralytic disease in these countries is two to three times greater than it was in developed countries during epidemic periods (Ofosu-Amaah et al 1977). The problem, in part, appears to be the age of the vaccine target population. In some underdeveloped countries, 90 percent or more are infected by all three serotypes of the virus by the end of the second year of life and most paralytic disease occurs before this time.

Presentation

Most infections with poliomyelitis virus are asymptomatic, with no sequelae, and are recognized only by the demonstration of antibodies to the viruses on serologic surveys. The mode of acquisition is the fecal–oral route, usually as the result of fecal contamination of water supplies.

Clinical Features

Minor Illness (Abortive Poliomyelitis)

The diagnosis of minor illness is presumptive on clinical grounds and is based on the occurrence of a brief clinical illness with symptoms such as malaise, anorexia, nausea, vomiting, headache, sore throat, constipation, and abdominal pain occurring during a known poliomyelitis outbreak.

Aseptic Meningitis (Nonparalytic Poliomyelitis)

Individuals with nonparalytic polio display the same symptoms as those with abortive poliomyelitis, along with more severe CNS signs and symptoms suggestive of meningitis or meningoencephalitis including meningeal signs with nuchal rigidity. There may be changes in the deep tendon reflexes and transient loss of bladder control.

Paralytic Poliomyelitis

In addition to the signs and symptoms of abortive and nonparalytic poliomyelitis, paralytic poliomyelitis presents with weakness of one or more muscle groups; either skeletal or cranial. This may be followed by a symptom-free interlude of several days followed by a recurrence of symptoms with paralysis.

Diagnosis

The diagnosis of the index case usually depends on the recognition of muscle weakness or paralysis accompanying a febrile illness with evidence of CNS infection and meningismus. Other illness in the community consistent with the spectrum of disease described above tends to substantiate the likelihood of poliomyelitis.

If facilities to differentiate between bacterial and viral infection of the CNS are not available, it should be initially assumed that a bacterial illness is present, and appropriate therapeutic steps should be taken.

If laboratory facilities are available for ruling out bacterial infection, then antibiotics need not be given and supportive care, as well as appropriate public health intervention techniques, are indicated. Laboratory tests in acute poliomyelitis are as follows:

- Gram's stain of CSF, CSF bacterial culture, and CSF tests for bacterial antigens.
- CSF leukocyte count is usually fewer than 500 cells per cubic millimeter. Initially these are predominantly PMNs, later changing to mononuclear cells. CSF glucose is normal to elevated. Protein content is normal in the early stages but later becomes elevated.
- Viral serology shows a rise in antibody titer to the specific type of polio virus over a two-week period.
- Viral cultures from the CSF and stool can be positive, particularly in the early stages of the disease.

Differential Diagnosis

Diseases to be considered in the differential diagnosis of nonparalytic poliomyelitis include bacterial meningitis, aseptic meningitis due to other viruses, and tuberculous meningitis. Those to be considered in paralytic poliomyelitis include Guillain-Barre syndrome, peripheral neuritis, bacterial meningitis with muscle weakness, demyelinating types of encephalomyelitis, and other conditions such as pseudoparalysis, trauma, congenital syphilis, and scurvy.

Management

No specific treatment is available. General management includes supportive care including strict attention to fluid and nutritional intake, analgesics and hot soaks for pain and muscle spasms, prevention of early deformity by careful positioning and passive range of movement, management of bladder and bowel management, and psychosocial support. If there is bulbar involvement, respiration may become a major problem. Depending on the available facilities, mechanical respirator support may or may not be possible. (See Chapter 21 for a discussion of physical rehabilitation.)

Prevention

Primary prevention of polio in a refugee setting, and the prevention of spread once polio has been identified, follow the same principles (Robinson 1982). It can probably be assumed that most individuals over two years of age have been infected by the wild types of virus and are immune. Therefore, the best strategy for rapid control is to vaccinate infants between three months and two years of age, as they are the most likely to be susceptible. Older children and adults may be vaccinated after the primary group. Improved community and family sanitation and hygiene will limit the circulation of wild polioviruses. Infants whose mothers have antibodies to all three polio serotypes will be protected by passive antibodies for about the first three months of life. There is no benefit from gamma globulin given as a preventive measure to exposed persons.

Two kinds of polio vaccine are available: inactivated (Salk) and live, attenuated (Sabin). Both contain all three types of polio viruses. Most experience throughout the world has been with the live, attenuated vaccine, which has proved to be effective with a three-dose regimen. However, this vaccine is susceptible to the deleterious effects of heat and must be kept frozen. Inactivated, more heat-stable vaccines that have greater antigen content and may invoke an adequate antibody response with one or two doses are being studied. Further studies are necessary to determine which preparation (or combination) will be most effective in the refugee setting (see Chapter 6).

REFERENCES AND SELECTED READING

Bortolussi R, Wort AJ, Casey S: The latex agglutination test versus counterimmunoelectrophoresis for rapid diagnosis of bacterial meningitis. CMAJ 1982;12:489–93.

Campos J, Garcia-Tornel S, Gairi JM et al: Multiply resistant *H. influenzae* type b causing meningitis: Comparative clinical and laboratory study. J Pediatr 1986;108:897–902.

Clemens JD, Shapiro ED: Resolving the pneumococcal vaccine controversy: Are there alternatives to randomized clinical trials? Rev Infect Dis 1984;6:589–600.

Gold R, Lepow ML, Goldschneider I et al: Clinical evaluation of group A and group C meningococcal polysaccharide vaccines in infants. J Clin Invest 1975;56:1536–47.

Greenwood BM: Selective primary health care: strategies for control of disease in the developing world. XIII. Acute bacterial meningitis. Rev Infect Dis 1984;6:374–89.

Greenwood BM, Bradley AK, Blakebrough IS et al: The immune response to a meningococcal polysaccharide vaccine in an African village. Trans Roy Soc Trop Med Hyg 1980;74:340–46.

Greenwood BM, Whittle HC, Bradley AK et al: The duration of the antibody response to meningococcal vaccination in an African village. Trans Roy Soc Trop Med Hyg 1980;74:756–60.

Hassan-King M, Greenwood BM, Whittle HC et al: An epidemic of meningococcal infection at Zaria, northern Nigeria. 3. Meningococcal carriage. Trans Roy Soc Trop Med Hyg 1979;73:567–73.

Miner WF, Edman DC: Acute bacterial meningitis in Cairo, Arab Republic of Egypt, 1 January 1971 through 31 December 1975. Am J Trop Med Hyg 1978;27:986–94.

Ofosu-Amaah A, Kratzer JH, Nicholas DD: Is poliomyelitis a serious problem in developing countries? Lameness in Ghanaian schools. Br Med J 1977;1:1012–14.

Onile BA, Montefiore DG, Alausa OK et al: Bacterial meningitis: The first documentation of an epidemic in southern Nigeria. Trans Roy Soc Trop Med Hyg 1982;76:41–44.

Peltola H, Kayhty H, Sivonen A et al: *Haemophilus influenzae* type b capsular polysaccharide vaccine in children: A double-blind field study of 100,000 vaccinees 3 months to 5 years of age in Finland. Pediatrics 1977;60:730–37.

Robbins FC, Nightingale EO: Selective primary health care: strategies for control of disease in the developing world. IX. Poliomyelitis. Rev Infect Dis 1983;5:957–68.

Robinson DA: Polio vaccination—A review of strategies. Trans Roy Soc Trop Med Hyg 1982;76:575–81.

Shann F, Linneman V, Mackenzie A et al: Absorption of chloramphenicol sodium succinate after intramuscular administration. New Engl J Med 1985;313:410–14.

Tauny A de E, Galvao PA, de Morais JS et al: Disease prevention by meningococcal serogroup C polysaccharide vaccine in preschool children: Results after 11 months in Sao Paulo, Brazil. Pediatr Res 1974;8:429.

Uchiyama N, Greene GR, Kitts DB et al: Meningitis due to *H. influenzae* type b resistant to ampicillin and chloramphenicol. J Pediatr 1980;97:421–24.

Wali SS, MacFarlane JT, Weir WRC et al: Single injection treatment of meningococcal meningitis. 2. Long-acting chloramphenicol. Trans Roy Soc Trop Med Hyg 1979;73:698–702.

Whittle HC, Davidson N McD, Greenwood BM et al: Trial of chloramphenicol for meningitis in northern Savanna of Africa. Br Med J 1973;3:379–81.

31
Tetanus

MARGARET EDWARDS

Tetanus, a preventable disease, is still a major cause of death in underdeveloped countries. Although precise numbers are not available, worldwide death due to tetanus has been estimated at 500,000 annually with 50 percent occurring in neonates (Stoll 1979; Beatty 1983; Lulkus et al 1984). Recent community surveys of neonatal tetanus lend credence to the view that tetanus is underreported in many countries and its actual incidence worldwide is much higher, with neonatal mortality due to tetanus approaching 1 million annually (Stanfield and Galazka 1984).

Tetanus in developed countries is a rare occurrence. The incidence in the United States for the past decade has been fairly steady at fewer than 100 cases per year. The majority of cases occur in adults over 50 years of age (MMWR 1981). Recently cases have been reported in neonates born at home to unimmunized women (Adams 1979) and children of immigrants from a refugee setting (Lyons 1981). In Great Britain, a similar trend is seen. Death due to tetanus, even in technically sophisticated settings, is high. In the United States in 1977, 32 of 77 reported cases had a fatal outcome (Stoll 1979). In Great Britain, the case fatality rate in the decade 1970–1979 was 10 percent (Edmondson and Flowers 1979).

The pattern of tetanus occurrence in underdeveloped countries is strikingly different. In Bangladesh in 1977, 78 percent of all cases of tetanus occurred in children less than one year of age, and 27 percent of all infant deaths were due to tetanus (Stoll 1979). Neonatal mortality from tetanus in some parts of Bangladesh is 24/1000 live births (Rahman, S. 1980). Tetanus is 10 to 500 times more common in underdeveloped countries in all age groups than in developed countries (Senecal 1978).

The setting that fosters tetanus is composed of a wide range of factors, including climate, custom, economics, and education. In industrialized nations, even before the availability of vaccine, tetanus rates declined as peoples' livelihood shifted from a rural to an urban setting and principles of hygiene were followed (Stanfield and Galazha 1984; Collacott 1981). In tropical settings, shoes and protective layers of clothing are often not worn. Local custom may mandate procedures such as circumcision or ear piercing, which are performed under unhygienic conditions (Senecal 1978). The practice of delivery under the care of midwives without medical training in sterilization techniques puts both mother and infant at risk for tetanus. Women contract tetanus from septic abortions and from puerperal infection. Neonates are exposed when unclean implements are used to sever the cord; contaminated roots or fibers are used to tie the cord; and substances such as soil, dung, or ashes are used to dress the umbilicus.

PATHOGENESIS

Clostridium tetani is a ubiquitous organism found in the intestines of animals and humans and commonly in soil, particularly cultivated soil. It produces a potent exotoxin, tetanospasmin, which is responsible for the clinical entity known as tetanus. *C. tetani* is an obligate anaerobe. It is a gram-positive rod that may have a drumsticklike contour due to a terminal spore. The spores are hardy and, if protected from sunlight, can survive in soil for years. Heating at 120°C for 15 to 20 minutes kills the spores, which are resistant to antiseptics and boiling. In an anaerobic milieu such as injured, infected, or necrotic tissue, the spores give rise to the vegetative form of *C. tetani,* which elaborates the toxin.

The toxin is a 150,00 dalton protein in its dimer form. It is lethal to humans in minute amounts. It binds to nerve cell membranes and is taken up by sensory, motor, and autonomic nerve fibers, where it is transported centrally within the nerve cell along the axon at a rate of about 250 mm a day. The toxin is clinically silent until it crosses the synaptic cleft. There, it prevents the release of the neurotransmitters gamma-aminobutyric acid and glycine from presynaptic inhibitory neurons (Kerr 1979;

Griffin 1981). The uncontrolled firing of motor neurons produces the muscle rigidity and spasms associated with the clinical disease. Strychnine, which blocks the action of inhibitory transmitters postsynaptically, produces a similar clinical syndrome.

Generalized tetanus follows a wide distribution of the toxin in the lymphatics and blood, thereby exposing nerves distant to the wound site. Muscles innervated by shorter nerves, such as the paraspinous and bulbar muscles, are the first to be affected.

Although its major manifestation is that of disinhibition, it has been shown that, in high concentrations, tetanospasmin causes a flaccid paralysis through inhibition of acetylcholine release at the neuromuscular junction. In severe generalized tetanus, cardiovascular instability, profuse sweating, peripheral vasoconstriction are presumed to reflect the interference of toxin with sympathetic control.

The diagnosis of tetanus is based on the history, symptoms, and signs. Culture results are not helpful because, even when culture facilities are available, only 30 percent of wounds are culture positive (Bartlett 1984).

The history may include injury ranging from sever trauma to minor abrasions or lacerations. Tetanus has resulted from puncture wounds, fractures, abrasions, burns, frostbite, intramuscular infections, skin testing, elective surgery, bite wounds, gastrointestinal infections, abortion, childbirth, omphalitis, and chronic otorrhea. Necrotic tissue infection and the presence of a foreign body encourage the proliferation of *C. tetani.* However, in some studies as many as 40 percent of cases had no wound identified (Edmondson 1980). The afflicted individual has a history of inadequate immunization (partial, lapsed, or never immunized). The interval between initial infection and first symptoms varies from 2 to 56 days, but is usually a few weeks. The time from the first symptoms to the first generalized spasm is usually 24 to 72 hours. The shorter the incubation period and more rapid the onset of symptoms, the more serious the disease and the graver the prognosis.

CLINICAL FEATURES OF THE DISEASE

Tetanus can present in four ways. The most common is generalized tetanus. Trismus ("lockjaw") and dysphagia, the most common presenting complaints, are followed by stiffness of back and abdominal muscles, progressing to persistent rigidity. Superimposed are painful tetanic muscle spasms with marked extension of the back (opisthotonus), flexion of the arms, clenching of the fists, plantar flexion of the toes, and the well-known facial grimace termed *rhisus sardonicus.* Spasms can be precipitated by almost any stimulus such as a light touch, a current of air, a noise, or a bright light. These excruciating spasms may be strong enough to produce fractures of the vertebral bodies and, in children, long bone fractures and avulsion fractures of the sternum (Cockshott 1974). Consciousness is not impaired; the patient remains alert and anxious during the spasms. Laryngeal and respiratory muscle spasms may compromise respiration and can cause sudden airway obstruction. Other findings include diaphoresis, tachycardia, and low-grade fever.

Tetanus can also present as a milder, more localized infection. Symptoms include stiffness and pain in the muscle groups immediately adjacent to the wound. This may progress to generalized tetanus, or it can be a mild, slowly developing disease with a mortality of about 1 percent.

Cepahlic tetanus presents as a weakness of muscle groups supplied by one or more of the cranial nerves, often the seventh, subsequent to injury of the face or head. Cephalic tetanus is rare and has a poor prognosis.

Tetanus neonatorum, the severe generalized tetanus of the newborn, presents within seven to ten days of birth. Initially, there are complaints of irritability and poor sucking, progressing to facial grimacing, generalized rigidity, and spasms. The usual portal of entry is the umbilicus. Generally, the spasms become more frequent and severe in the three days following the first spasm. The clinical picture stabilizes for about one week and symptoms begin to abate on days 10 to 14. Complete recovery of those who survive usually occurs within four weeks with, perhaps, some residual stiffness. However, mortality is 60% (Beatty 1983).

The clinical pattern of tetanus is usually distinct enough to preclude other diagnoses. Strychnine poisoning mimics tetanus, as mentioned above. Dystonic reactions to phenothiazines can be confused with tetanus, but the facial grimacing is not actually like the *rhisus sardonicus* and, if the drug is discontinued or an antidote is administered (i.e., an antihistamine), the reaction clears. Other causes of jaw stiffness and dysphagia such as dental abscess, peritonsillar abscess, and retropharyngeal abscess should be ruled out. The possibility of meningitis or encephalitis should be considered. The spinal fluid in tetanus is normal.

TREATMENT

There are four basic principles in the treatment of tetanus: to neutralize toxin not yet bound to nerve cells and remove *C. tetani* producing the toxin; to prevent spasms; to minimize spasms that do occur; and to prevent and treat complications.

Human tetanus immunoglobulin (TIG) is the safest means of neutralizing toxin. It is given in a single intramuscular dose (3000 to 10,000 U). As little as 500 U may be effective, and this dose has been used in neonates (Adams 1979). It is imperative to administer the immunoglobulin as soon as possible because, once the toxin has entered the nerve cell, it cannot be inactivated. The half-life of TIG is 25 to 30 days, and protective levels after one injection are maintained for about four weeks (Edmondson 1980). Equine antiserum is used when TIG is not available. The recommended dose (10,000 U) is administered intramuscularly. Anaphylaxis or serum sickness occurs in about 5 percent of patients given equine antiserum.

Penicillin effectively kills *C. tetani*. Procaine penicillin (1.2 million U once a day) or penicillin G (1 million U every six hours) for ten days is recommended in adults. For neonates, procaine penicillin or penicillin G (100,000 U/kg IV in four divided doses) is recommended. Tetracycline is an acceptable alternative in adults and children over the age of eight years.

Once antitoxin has been administered, the wound site should be meticulously cleaned, necrotic tissue excised, abscesses drained, and any foreign body removed. Omphalectomy in cases of omphalitis and hysterectomy in cases of septic abortion have been performed.

A possible source of human tetanus immunoglobulin is a compatible blood donor who has had a booster toxoid within one month. One unit of whole blood (450 cc) is estimated to have 2500 to 10,000 U of antitoxin (Lall 1979).

Because antitoxin and antiserum do not cross the blood–brain barrier, intrathecal use of antiserum in an attempt to bind any extracellular toxin in the CNS has been tried with conflicting results (Neequaye & Nkrumah 1983; Singh et al 1980; Sedaghatian 1979; Bhandari 1980; Hughes-Davies 1979). Great care must be exercised using this mode of therapy because the preservative (phenol, in particular) used in antiserum designed for intramuscular or intravenous use can be neurotoxic. Improved survival has been reported with an intrathecal dose (200 U) of equine antiserum (Sanders 1979). In neonates 100 U intrathecally was used (Singh et al 1980). It is useful in treating spasms to classify the severity of the symptoms. In mild tetanus the patient has mild trismus, infrequent, short spasms, and little dysphagia. In moderate tetanus both the frequency and severity of spasms are greater. Trismus and dysphagia are marked, but respiration is adequate during spasms. In severe tetanus frequent and prolonged spasms occur that interfere with adequate respiration. Patients presenting in one stage may progress to more severe stages. Therefore, careful observation is essential, with readiness to intervene in case of respiratory compromise.

A secure airway is crucial. In mild cases, intubation or tracheostomy is not necessary. Careful sunctioning, use of an oropharyngeal airway, and oxygen administration may be adequate. In more severe cases, staff and conditions permitting, tracheostomy or intubation may be the only way to secure the airway. In neonates, endotracheal intubation is preferred.

Spasms are provoked by even mild external stimuli so, to the extent possible and without interfering with good nursing care, a quiet environment with subdued lighting is recommended for the tetanus patient. Control of spasms through muscle relaxation and sedation can be accomplished through use of various sedatives and tranquilizers. A combination is often required. Phenobarbital (50 to 100 mg every three to six hours for adults; 2 to 3 mg/kg dose every eight hours for children) can be used, keeping in mind that respiratory suppression is a side effect of the barbiturates. In children, a paradoxical effect of irritability and hyperactivity may result. Phenothiazines are muscle relaxants and may be used (200 to 300 mg/day in adults; 2 mg/kg/day divided into three or four doses in children). With prolonged use of phenothiazines, increased dosages may be needed to maintain an effect. Muscle rigidity is an undesirable side effect. Diazepam in adult dosages (40 to 120 mg/day) is a very effective muscle relaxant. The dosage can be adjusted for children (0.04 to 0.2 mg/kg every two to four hours to a maximum of 0.6 mg/kg in an eight-hour period). Higher dosages are often required to control spasms. Hypotension and respiratory depression are the major side effects of diazepam. Other medications used to ameliorate spasms include paraldehyde and chloral hydrate. When respirators and trained personnel are available, tetanus spasms are controlled through curare paralysis and mechanical ventilation. This has lowered mortality considerably (Trujillo 1980; Edmondson 1980).

In neonates, pyridoxine (100 mg IM or IV daily) has been used when mechanical ventilation is not possible, with improved survival rates (Hajailay et al 1983; Godel 1982; Daud et al 1981). The theoretical basis for pyridoxine use is that, as a cofactor in the production of gama-butyric acid, it increases the amount of the inhibitory transmitter, thereby reducing uncontrolled neuronal activity.

Nutritional and fluid support are of vital importance. Patients with muscle spasms have increased energy needs. In addition, insensible fluid losses through sweating and salivation are great (as much as 3.8 liters per day for adults). The patient should not take liquid or food by mouth until respiratory status and spasms are stabilized. Nasogastric tube feedings may be instituted. At least 60 kcal/kg/day for adults and 140 kcal/kg/day for neonates should be provided.

MANAGEMENT OF COMPLICATIONS

Even in technically sophisticated settings, the basis of treatment is attentive, round-the-clock nursing care. Positioning and sunctioning the patient to prevent aspiration, turning to prevent decubiti, documenting the time and duration of spasms, bowel care for constipation, and bladder care to alleviate urinary retention are essential to prevent complications.

Sympathetic overactivity, a poor prognostic sign, is common in severe tetanus. It is characterized by unpredictable runs of tachycardia and hypertension with peripheral vasoconstriction. Beta-blockers such as propanolol have been used to treat these episodes. Caution must be exercised because these sympathetic bursts are paroxysmal, and sudden hypotension and bradycardia are also known to occur in the tetanus patient.

The most common complications (and causes of death) are respiratory, secondary to aspiration and pneumonia. Other complications include sepsis, pulmonary embolism (in the paralyzed patient), gastric dilatation, ileus, bone fractures, hypotension from fluid depletion, pulmonary edema from presumed myocarditis, and sudden cardiac arrest. High fever should provide a search for concomitant infection.

PREVENTION

What measures can be taken to prevent tetanus? Certainly, decreasing the risk of exposure to tetanus spores is helpful. Lower limb wounds are a common portal of entry, so wearing shoes may help. Unclean birth practices expose the neonate, so education of expectant mothers and midwives and distribution of sterile ligatures and blades are suggested (Woodruff et al 1984). In one study training of traditional birth attendants in Bangladesh reduced neonatal tetanus mortality in certain areas from a rate of 24 per 1000 to 5.6 per 1000 live births (Rahman, S. 1982). Prompt medical attention to wounds with debridement, copious irrigation, gentle instrumentation, and appropriate use of antibiotics is part of tetanus prevention.

In the final analysis, active immunization supplemented with passive immunization is the only sure way to prevent tetanus. Tetanus toxoid, a formaldehyde-treated toxin, is a safe means of inducing protective levels of antitoxin (0.01 μ/ml). The aluminum salt-adsorbed form is recommended. Side effects of the toxoid are usually local swelling, redness, and tenderness. Serious side effects are rare. Ten cases of serious side effects such as anaphylaxis, serum sickness, prolonged urticaria, and glomerulonephritis were reported after 2.5 million injections of toxoid in Denmark (Simonsen et al 1984). The only contraindication to toxoid is a history of neurologic or severe hypersensitivity reaction to a previous dose (MMWR 1981).

There is some evidence for the existence of protective levels of antitoxin acquired naturally, but these cannot be relied on to provide immunity. Therefore, any unimmunized person should be considered unprotected.

Worldwide, various regimens of toxoid administration have been used. The following sequence is currently recommended by the Centers for Disease Control (CDC) Immunization Practices Advisory Committee. For infants, tetanus toxoid incorporated into a diphtheria-pertussis-tetanus vaccine (DPT) is given by intramuscular injection at 2, 4, and 6 months. Booster doses are given at 18 months, between four and six years of age, and thereafter every ten years. Children under seven years of age not previously immunized should be given a series of three primary doses of toxoid at four- to eight-week intervals followed by a booster dose 6 to 12 months after the final dose. If the fourth dose is after the fourth birthday, the four- to six-year booster is omitted. For children over seven years of age, toxoid is given in the adult diphtheria-tetanus toxoid combination. The second dose is given four to eight weeks after the first dose and the third dose is given 6 to 12 months after the second. Boosters are recommended every ten years. Interruption of the sequence does not require starting over (MMWR 1981).

Prevention of neonatal tetanus can be accomplished effectively by immunizing the mother, since maternal antitoxin crosses the placenta. In Bangladesh, after an immunization program for pregnant women was instituted, there was a 1.3/1000 live birth neonatal mortality rate from tetanus in the study area compared with a control area rate of 24.1/1000 (Rahman, S. 1982). An unimmunized pregnant woman should have two tetanus toxoid immunizations, at least one month apart and at least two weeks prior to delivery, in order for the infant to benefit. The earlier in the pregnancy the toxoid is administered, the better (Rahman, M. et al 1982). This two-dose regimen provides protection for a while, but by the third year after immunization, 22 percent of those immunized are no longer protected. After these first two doses, single-dose boosters are sufficient during subsequent pregnancies (Kessel 1984). Administering two doses of toxoid to nonpregnant women in a rural area of Bangladesh afforded a 75 percent lower mortality among 4- to 14-day-old infants (the age when tetanus death are most likely to occur) (Black et al 1980). It has been pointed out that prevention of neonatal tetanus in this manner will decrease postabortion and postdelivery tetanus. The unprotected newborn may also be given prophylactic TIG (250 U) or equine antiserum (750 U), but high cost limits the widespread use of this method. Prophylactic use of antibiotics is much less effective.

In tetanus prophylaxis of wounds the immunization status, plus the nature of a wound (i.e., clean or dirty), determines whether tetanus toxoid alone, or tetanus immune globulin, is recommended. After a basic series of three immunizations, a booster dose will result in a rapid rise in circulating antibody in three to five days, regardless of the time interval between the booster and the primary series (Stoll 1979). Persons sustaining minor, clean wounds who seek medical attention within 24 hours of injury, and have had a primary series with a final injection of booster within the past ten years, need no additional tetanus prophylaxis. If the wound is minor and clean and the past immunization is that of two injections or less, or the immunization history is uncertain, or the last tetanus toxoid injection was given more than ten years earlier, tetanus toxoid (0.5 cc) is administered but TIG is withheld.

Tetanus-prone wounds are those that are severe, neglected, or more than 24 hours old. Tetanus toxoid should be given to individuals with these types of wounds if they have uncertain immunization history, fewer than three previous immunizations, or three or more immunizations, the last being administered more than five years before injury. Tetanus immune globulin is used in individuals with fewer than two immunizations, an uncertain immunization history, or two prior immunizations and a wound more than 24 hours old. The dose of TIG is 250 U IM. If only equine antitoxin is available, the dose is 3000 to 6000 U; 1000 to 3000 U may suffice in children. When toxoid and immune globulin are given at the same time, separate syringes and sites should be used. An attempt should be made to complete the primary series in those who have had fewer than two prior injections.

It is important to note that, even after having the most severe forms of tetanus, survivors do not usually develop an immune response to protect them against subsequent *C. tetani* infection. Do not neglect to immunize the patient with tetanus. The first dose of toxoid may be given during the acute illness.

REFERENCES AND SELECTED READING

Adams JM, Kenny JD and Rudolph AJ: Modern management of tetanus neonatorum. Pediatrics 1979;67(4):472–77.

Bartlett JG: Tetanus. In Strickland GT(ed): Hunters Tropical Medicine (6th Ed), pp 361–63, Philadelphia, Saunders, 1984.

Beatty HN: Tetanus. In Petersdorf RG et al (ed): Harrison's Principles of Internal Medicine, pp 1003–6, New York, McGraw Hill, 1983.

Bhandhari B: Intrathecal antitetanus serum in management of tetanus neonatorum. Indian J Med Res 1980;72:685–87.

Black RE, Huber DH and Curlin GT: Reduction of neonatal tetanus by mass immunization of nonpregnant women: duration of protection provided by one or two doses of aluminium-adsorbed tetanus toxoid. Bull World Health Organization 1980;58(6):927–30.

Cockshott P. Tetanus. In Cockshott P and Middlmiss H (eds): Clinical Radiology in the Tropics, pp 67–69, London, NY, Churchill Livingstone, 1974.

Collacott RA: Neonatal tetanus in St. Kilda. Scottish Med J 1981;26(3):224–27.

Crossley K, Irvine P, Warren JB et al: Tetanus and diptheria immunity in urban Minnesota adults. JAMA 1979;242(21):2298–300.

Dastur FD, D'sa JA, Badami PV et al: Immunizing against tetanus - a continuing problem. J Postgrad Med 1980;26(1):22–27.

Dastur FD, Awatramani VP, Dixit SK et al: Response to single dose of tetanus vaccine in subjects with naturally-acquired tetanus antitoxin. Lacet 1981;2:219–22.

Dand S, Mohammad T, Ahmed A: A prospective study at the Department of Child Health. Kyber Medical College, Peshawar, on the outcome of neonatal tetanus. J Pakistan Med Assoc 1981;31:419–23.

Edmondson RS: Tetanus. Br J Hosp Med 1980;23:596,599–602.

Edmondson RS, Flowers MW: Intensive care in tetanus: Management, complications, and mortality in 100 cases. Br Med J 1979;1:1401–404.

Furste W, Parsons JN and Cabrera H: Tetanus prevention. Comprehensive Therapy; 1981:7(9):49–57.

Galbraith NS, Forbes P and Tillet H: National surveillance of tetanus in England and Wales 1930–1979: J Infec, 1981;3(2):181–91.

Griffin JW: Local tetanus. John Hopkins Med J 1981;146(2):85–88.

Hajailay R, Sharon R, Agarwal VK et al: Pyrodoxine therapy in tetanus neonatorum. Indian Ped 1983;20:935–39.

Hughes-Davies TH: Letter. Med J Aus 1979;2(6):308.

Islam MS, Rahaman MM, Aziz KM et al: Birth care practice and neonatal tetanus in a rural area of Bangladesh. J Trop Pediatr 1982;28:299–302.

Kerr JH: Current topics in tetanus. Intens Care Med 1979;5:105–10.

Kerr JH: Insensible fluid losses in severe tetanus. Intens Care Med 1981;7:209–12.

Kessel E: Strategies for the control of neonatal tetanus. J Trop Pediatr 1984;30:145–49.

Lall JC, Gupta HL and Jaspal D: Treatment of tetanus neonatorum with special reference to hyperimmune blood transfusion. Indian Pediatr 1979;6(8):693–95.

Lutkus ER, Hirsch AF and Wood JP: Tetanus. Ann Emergency Med 1984;13:186–88.

Lyons DP, Rybak LP: Otogenic tetanus: case report and literature review. J Laryngol Otol 1981;95:627–29.

MMWR: Mortality and Morbidity Weekly Report. 1981;30(32):392–405.

Neequaye J and Nkrumah FK: Failure of intrahecal antitetanus serum to improve survival in neonatal tetanus. Arch Dis Child 1983;18:276–78.

Rahman M, Chen LC and Chakraborty J: Use of tetanus toxoid for the prevention of neonatal tetanus. Bull WHO 1982;11(2):261–76.

Rahman S: The effect of traditional birth attendants and tetanus toxoid in reduction of neonatal mortality. J Trop Pediatr 1982;28(4):163–65.

Sanders RKM: Letter, British Medical Journal 1979;1:49.

Schofield F: Selective primary health care: strategies for control of disease in the developing world. XXII. Tetanus: a preventable problem. Rev Infect Dis 1986;8:144 56.

Sedaghatian MR: Intrathecal serotherapy in neonatal tetanus: A controlled trail. Arch Dis Child 1979;54:623–25.

Senecal J: Tetanus. In Jelliffe DB, Stanfield JD (eds): Diseases of Children in the Subtropics and Tropics, pp 696–704, London, Edward Arnold, 1978.

Simonsen O, Kjeldsen K and Heron I: Immunity against tetanus and effect of revaccination 25 to 30 years after primary vaccination. Lancet 1984;1:240–242.

Singh AK, Bansal A, Goel SO et al: Intrathecal antitetanus serum (horse) with steroid in the treatment of neonatal tetanus. Arch Dis Child 1980:15:527–31.

Sixth International Conference on Tetanus (proceedings), Lyons, 1981. J Trauma 1982;22(12):1032–35.

Smucker CM, Swint JM and Simmons GB: Prevention of neonatal tetanus in India: A prospective cost-effectiveness analysis. J. Trop Pediatr 1984;30:227–36.

Stanfield JP, Galazka A: Neonatal tetanus in the world today. Bull WHO 1984;62(4):647–69.

Stoll BJ: Tetanus. Pediatr Clin NA 1979;26(2):415–31.

Trujillo MJ: Tetanus in the adult: Intensive care and management experience in 233 cases. Crit Care Med 1980;8(7):419–23.

Weinstein L: Tetanus. In Feigin R, Cherry J (eds): Textbook of Pediatric Infectious Diseases, pp 843–51, Philadelphia, Saunders, 1981.

Woodruff AW, Grant J, El Bashir EA et al: Neonatal tetanus. Mode of infection, prevalence, and prevention in southern Sudan. Lancet 1984;1:378–79.

32

Respiratory Tract and Ear Infections

GIFFORD S. LEOUNG

Acute respiratory infections (ARI) and diarrheal diseases are the most common causes of morbidity and mortality among children throughout the world. They account for 20 to 40 percent of all childhood out-patient services and 12 to 35 percent of pediatric hospital admissions. The average number of deaths from ARI among the 88 WHO member nations from 1970 to 1973 was 666,000 annually. If the crude mortality rate for these deaths were extrapolated to include nonreporting countries, the estimated number of deaths worldwide from ARI would approach 2.2 million per year. The annual incidence of lower respiratory tract infections in children under five years of age in the United States is about 35 per 1000—about half that in underdeveloped countries. The incidence can be up to 15 times greater in malnourished children. The case-fatality ratio of ARI is greater than 10 percent in some rural underdeveloped areas. It is estimated that ARI worldwide accounts for 6.3 percent of deaths from all causes, while it is about 12.2 percent in Africa, and 13.4 percent in underdeveloped Asian countries.

Acute respiratory infections constitute a complex and heterogeneous group of conditions with a variety of manifestations. If serologic types are considered, there are more than 300 different viral, bacterial, fungal, and parasitic etiologic agents responsible for respiratory illness. Decisions need to be made concerning hospitalization, antibiotic use, what supportive care to give, and what public health measures need to be taken. Evaluation of the patient will aid in these decisions and should include how much distress the patient is in; whether there is an upper or a lower respiratory infection; whether the infection is viral or bacterial; the patient's general state of health or disability; the state of immunocompetency; what support services are available in the home; and what dangerous or adverse sequelae can be expected in the course of treatment or nontreatment.

Specific therapy should be applied when the causative agent is identified. When identification of the organism is not possible, treatment should proceed against the presumptive pathogen(s). The range of possible organisms is large, but the list of probable organisms can be narrowed down. Fluid and nutrition management, along with measures for symptomatic relief, can sometimes influence the outcome of treatment as much as antibiotics. The decision to admit a patient for observation and treatment depends not only on the state of debility but also on the margin of safety present, if the patient does not respond quickly, and the out-of-hospital support available.

For efficiency of therapy and management, the microbial causes of respiratory disease have been divided into nine anatomic sites of infection (see Table 32-1). The following sections discuss diagnosis and treatment of respiratory disease affecting each of these sites.

PHARYNGITIS

Viral Pharyngitis

Sore throat or scratchy irritation of the throat is a common complaint in patients with a cold or influenza. The pharyngeal symptoms are usually mild and are associated with cough and nasal congestion. The pharynx may show a mild erythema, usually without exudates. Cervical lymph nodes are not markedly enlarged or painful. Sore throat symptoms usually resolve in four to five days.

Pharyngeal symptoms caused by adenovirus may mimic acute streptococcal disease in many respects. Fever, chills, headache, and malaise are common. Examination of the pharynx may reveal marked erythema and exudate. Conjunctivitis, occurring in 30 to 50 percent of cases, helps distinguish between adenovirus and streptococcal infections.

Primary infection by herpes simplex virus in severe cases can very closely mimic streptococcal pharyngitis. Severe sore throat, cough, fever, and tender anterior cervical adenopathy are often present. The pharynx examination may show erythema, exudate, and vesicles or shallow ulcers characteristic of herpetic infections.

Table 32-1. Viral and Bacterial Agents in Acute Respiratory Tract Infections

Clinical Entity and Etiologic Agents	Population at Risk	Distinctive Findings	Diagnostic Tests
Pharyngitis			
Viral agents Influenza Adenovirus Herpes simplex type I ECHO virus Coxsackie A21 Epstein-Barr virus Cytomegalovirus	All ages	Pharyngeal erythema and exudate; adenopathy inconstant Vesicles and ulcers may occur with HSV I or coxsackie	None
Bacterial agents			
Streptococcus pyogenes	All ages; Peak incidence in young school-age children	Pharyngeal erythema, enlarged tonsils with gray-white exudate; tender, enlarged lymph nodes	Culture of exudate on blood agar plate; latex agglutination of swab specimen
Corynebacterium diphtheria	Children	Mild cases: firmly adherent membrane on soft palate initially white, blue-gray Severe cases: rapidly progressing membrane; swelling of tonsils, uvula, cervical nodes; "bull-neck"	Culture on tellurite or Loeffler's medium, Gel diffusion of antibody-soaked filter paper in peptone maltose agar
Bordatella pertussis	Children <12 years of age	1st stage: low-grade fever, coryza, conjunctivitis 2nd stage: coughing fits with inspiratory whoop	Pernasal swab inserted into posterior pharynx and plated on Bordet-Gengou medium
Laryngotracheobronchitis (Croup)			
Parainfluenza virus 1,2,3 Influenza A Respiratory syncytial virus Enteroviruses	Children 3 months to 3 years	Dyspnea, inspiratory stridor, hoarseness, cough suggestive of a dog's or seal's bark, retractions on inspiration	Posterior-anterior x-ray film of neck showing narrowed tracheal shadow in subglottic area
Epiglottitis			
Hemophilus influenza	All ages but usual range 1 to 6 years with peak at 2 to 4 years	Anxiety, tachypnea, tachycardia, dysphagia, drooling, "cherry red" epiglottis	Lateral soft tissue x-ray of neck showing an enlarged epiglottis; "thumb" sign
Sinusitis			
Streptococcus pneumoniae *Hemophilus influenzae* Anaerobic bacteria *Staphylococcus aureus* [a] *Staphylococcus pyogenes* [a] *Branhamella catarrhalis* [a] Gram-negative bacteria [a]	All ages	Tenderness over affected sinus; sinus opacity on transillumination	Sinus x-ray films

Table 32-1. (*continued*)

Clinical Entity and Etiologic Agents	Population at Risk	Distinctive Findings	Diagnostic Tests
Otitis media *Streptococcus pneumoniae* *Hemophilus influenzae* Streptococci (groups A and B)[b] *Staphylococcus aureus*[b] *Bordatella catarrhalis*[b]	Children; peak age under 3 years	Red, bulging tympanic membrane, purulent discharge from canal	Dampening of motion by pneumonic otoscopy
Bronchiolitis Respiratory syncytial virus Parainfluenza virus Rhinovirus Adenovirus Influenza	Under 2 years of age	Restlessness, dyspnea, wheezing with ronchi and rales	Chest x-ray films showing depressed diaphragm
Bronchitis Adenovirus Rhinovirus Coronavirus Influenza virus Parainfluenza virus Respiratory syncytial virus Mycoplasma pneumoniae Bordatella pertussis *Streptococcus pneumonia* *Hemophilus influenzae*	All ages	Bronchial breath sounds, ronchi, rales, wheezes	Sputum smear and culture; Chest x-ray film to exclude infiltrates
Pneumonia			
Viral Influenza virus Parainfluenza virus Adenovirus Respiratory syncytial virus Rhinovirus	All ages; viral agents more common in children	Tachypnea, cyanosis, rales, ronchi	None
Bacterial			
S. pneumococci	All ages	Purulent sputum	Sputum smear and culture, CIE of sputum, latex agglutination of pleural fluid
M. pneumoniae	Younger adults		CIE on sputum; culture on enriched medium
S. aureus and gram-negatives	Nosocomial infection and immunocompromised hosts		Routine smear and culture; CIE on pleural fluid for staphylococcus
Anaerobic organisms	Aspiration pneumonia		Infiltrate in dependent area of lung
L. pneumophilia	All ages		Culture on charcoal yeast extract medium
H. influenzae			ELISA testing on sputum; CIE and latex agglutination

[a]These organisms combined are the etiologic agents for approximately 20% of cases of sinusitis.
[b]These organisms combined are the etiologic agents for approximately 15% of cases of otitis media.

Herpangina is caused by coxsackieviruses and presents with small vesicles on the soft palate, uvula, and anterior tonsillar pillars, which rupture and become small ulcers. It occurs primarily in small children and may present as a severe febrile illness with marked sore throat and dysphagia. Abdominal pain may also be seen.

Exudative tonsillitis or pharyngitis occurs in approximately 50 percent of the cases of infectious mononucleosis due to Epstein-Barr virus. Fatigue, malaise, headache, generalized lymphadenopathy, and splenomegaly are associated with the pharyngitis of infectious mononucleosis.

Streptococcal Pharyngitis

Infection with *Streptococcus pyogenes* is the bacterial agent of most concern when considering pharyngitis. In addition to being the most common bacterial infection in childhood, it can have serious postinfection sequelae. Colonization is common. Carriage rates vary; as high as 35 percent in school children but much lower in adults. Although all age groups are susceptible, the disease occurs mainly in children with peak incidence during the first few years of school, probably because of the effects of crowding.

Strep throat usually manifests by acute onset of sore throat, fever, and malaise, sometimes with headache. Young children may have additional symptoms of nausea, vomiting, and abdominal pain. Sinusitis and otitis are common complications in children under three years of age. Physical findings include fever to 38°C, erythema and edema of the pharynx; enlarged, hyperremic tonsils with a gray-white exudate; and enlarged, tender lymph nodes in the submandible and anterior cervical chains.

The best means of diagnosis is a culture of the pharynx and tonsils plated on sheep blood agar looking for beta hemolysis. Commercial kits that use immunologic methods for group A beta hemolytic strep identification are also available, but their reliability is unsubstantiated. It is estimated that only 15 percent of all patients with acute pharyngitis will require antibiotic therapy for symptomatic streptococcal infection.

In untreated patients with uncomplicated disease, the signs and symptoms of strep pharyngitis may resolve in approximately one week. The rationale for therapy is to prevent spread of the streptococcus to the sinuses or the middle ear, and to prevent the complications of acute rheumatic fever (ARF), which is estimated to cause 25 to 40 percent of all cardiovascular disease in the poor, crowded areas of the world. The incidence of ARF in untreated patients is 1 to 3 percent. The onset of ARF is approximately three weeks after the onset of pharyngitis (a range of one to five weeks). Carditis is the only manifestation of ARF that may potentially cause long-term disability or death; it can occur within the first three weeks of an attack of ARF. Carditis is seen in 40 to 50 percent of patients with their first episode of ARF. It has a higher incidence in young children.

Glomerulonephritis may occur after pharyngeal infection with certain serotypes of group A streptococci (serotypes 1, 3, 4, 12, 25). It is not possible to determine the serotype from the clinical presentation. Glomerulonephritis occurs most commonly in children between the ages of 3 and 7 years, but patients over 50 years constitute 5 to 10 percent of cases. Therapy for pharyngitis will not prevent the development of nephritis but it will prevent ARF and control spread of the nephritogenic strain.

The treatment of choice is a single injection of benzathine penicillin (1.2 million U IM; 600,000 U for children weighing less than 30 kg). If oral therapy is administered, pencillin V (125 mg or 250 mg four times daily) should be given for ten days. For the penicillin-allergic patient, erythromycin (20 to 40 mg/kg/day up to 1 g given four times daily) is acceptable. The tetracyclines and sulfonamides are much less effective than penicillin or erythromycin. Cephalosporins may be used. Patients with a history of ARF should be given prophylaxis with benzathine penicillin (1.2 million U IM, monthly). Sulfadiazine (1 g/day; 500 mg/day in patients weighing less than 30 kg) or penicillin V (125 or 250 mg daily) are acceptable, but less effective, prophylaxis. Erythromycin (250 mg/day) can be used in patients allergic to the preceding regimens.

Nonstreptococcal Bacterial Pharyngitis

Diphtheria

Though diphtheria is rare where successful immunization programs exist, the attack rate in susceptible populations is greater than 90 percent (by direct contact or droplet aerosol from infected individuals). There is usually a fever and mild sore throat, which may be insidious in onset. The throat may first appear only red, but gray or white spots soon appear. The spots coalesce and form a membrane that may cover the tonsils, soft palate, and uvula. The membrane is initially thin, white, and filmy. This becomes thick and gray or black due to capillary dilatation and seepage of blood into the membrane. The membrane's borders are sharply defined, and it is so strongly adherent to the mucosa that attempts at removal can cause bleeding.

In cases of moderate severity, the symptoms begin to spontaneously subside by the fifth or sixth day. The most severe cases tend to occur in young children in whom "malignant" or "bull-neck" diphtheria occurs. The onset is abrupt with the membrane rapidly covering the pharynx and extending to the nose. There is marked swelling of the tonsils, uvula, and cervical nodes. The swelling sometimes forms a distinct collar, the so-called bullneck. The temperature may rise to 41°C, with a rapid, weak pulse. Mental status changes may range from excitation to stupor.

Diphtheria toxin causes cardiac impairment in nearly 50 percent of patients. In patients with ECG changes, the mortality is 28 percent (100% in cases with untreated atrioventricular or left bundle branch block). Diphtheria paralysis (10 to 20% of patients) does not last more than ten days, and recovery is usually complete.

The appearance of the pharynx does not help distinguish diphtheria from other infections. Cultures on tellurite agar or Loeffler's medium offer the best yield; a gel diffusion test using filter paper soaked in antitoxin incubated for 24 hours will detect diphtheria toxin by producing a line of precipitate on the peptone maltose agar plate.

Treatment consists of the administration of antitoxin and antibiotics. Therapy should not be delayed because the antitoxin works only on toxin that is free in the circulation and has no effect on toxin attached to cells. Antitoxin should be given intravenously; the amount varies with the severity of disease (40,000 U in the average case of less than 48 hours duration; 80,000 U in severe cases or those of more than three days duration; 100,000 to 120,000 U in severe or bull-neck cases). Therapy with penicillin or erythromycin should be given for ten days. This decreases the number of carriers of *Corynebacterium diphtheriae.* Patients should also be immunized with diphtheria toxoid at one week, one month, and two months after onset of illness. Nonimmune contacts should be immunized and given benzathine penicillin (1.2 million U IM) or a seven-day course of erythromycin. Close contacts that cannot be kept under surveillance should receive benzathine penicillin intramuscularly and 10,000 U of antitoxin. Because of the number of asymptomatic carriers, the interruption of transmission is the main goal for control of this disease. Two doses of the toxoid usually provide a high level of immunity.

Pertussis

Pertussis has a worldwide distribution. It is highly contagious through aerosolized droplets, with an attack rate of greater than 90 percent in susceptible populations. The illness most commonly occurs in children under 12 years of age, although it does occur in a milder form in adults. Children under 1 year of age account for 50 to 60 percent of all deaths from pertussis. The illness has three stages: the catarrhal or prodromal stage, the paroxysmal or spasmodic stage, and the convalescent stage. The first stage has nonspecific symptoms including coryza, conjunctivitis, and low-grade fever. This stage is highly contagious and indistinguishable from other upper respiratory infections. The second stage lasts two to four weeks and is characterized by paroxysms of coughing that terminate in an inspiratory whoop. The inspiratory whoop is caused by air being drawn in through a narrowed glottis. Coughing fits may be sever enough that vomiting occurs. The convalescent stage usually lasts about one month, although occasional mild coughing may continue for months.

The diagnosis in the refugee setting is usually made based on this clinical pattern. If culture facilities are available, a pernasal swab is inserted into the posterior pharynx through the nostril and the patient is asked to cough. Organisms on the cilia will lodge on the swab during a cough. When plated onto Bordet-Gengou medium, *Bordatella pertussis* appears as small silver colonies with a small zone of hemolysis in four days.

The white blood cell count may be helpful in diagnosing pertussis since leukocytosis (20,000–50,000 cells/mm^3) is common. This is especially true at the end of the catarrhal and during the paroxysmal stage.

Treatment with erythromycin, tetracycline, or chloramphenicol is effective when given early in the disease; once the patient reaches the paroxysmal stage, there is no effect on clinical course. Erythromycin (35 to 50 mg/kg/day in four divided doses for 14 days) given early shortens the course of disease and renders patients noninfectious, thus reducing transmission. Immunization is the only means of controlling this disease. Efficacy of the killed, whole-cell vaccine ranges from 63 to 95 percent. Although multiple doses are needed for maximum protection, studies have shown that two doses, separated by two to six months, will elicit a serologic response equivalent to that seen with the routine protocol.

Miscellaneous

Spirochetes and anaerobic bacteria can cause pharyngitis with or without tonsillitis. There may be a purulent exudate and a foul odor. Peritonsillar abscess should be considered in patients with severe pain, dysphagia, swelling of the peritonsillar area, and displacement of the tonsil. Oral penicillin is effective therapy but will not replace surgical intervention if an abscess is present. Gonococcal pharyngitis is usually asymptomatic or mild but, if undiagnosed, it may serve as a source of continued transmission. Spectinomycin and ampicillin are not effective in pharyngeal disease; trimethoprim-sulfamethoxazole may be given for those cases that do not respond to penicillin or tetracycline.

LARYNGOTRACHEOBRONCHITIS (CROUP)

Croup is primarily a disease of children aged three months to three years, with a peak occurrence in the second year of life. It is caused by a variety of viruses and, occasionally, by *Mycoplasma pneumoniae.* Most cases begin with typical upper respiratory tract infection systems of cough, sore throat, rhinorrhea, and fever followed by dyspnea, inspiratory stridor, hoarseness, and deepening cough. The cough is variously described as a seal's or dog's bark, or the yelping of a fox. Retractions of the chest wall are common. Examination of the chest will show inspiratory stridor, poor air exchange, and diminished breath sounds; rales, ronchi, and wheezing may also be noted. Croup characteristically has a fluctuating course, often improving during the day and worsening at night. Most children improve in three to four days, although the upper tract signs may continue longer.

Laboratory examination in croup is not particularly distinctive; the white blood cell count may be elevated in a severely stressed child. In a refugee setting, the diagnosis is made on the clinical pattern. The key distinction to be made is between croup and epiglottitis, since the latter is much more dangerous.

Because of the naturally fluctuating course, therapy is difficult to evaluate. Antibiotics have no role unless there is evidence of concomitant bacterial infection. The usefulness of steroids remains controversial. The mainstay of treatment has been the administration of cool, moist air. Nebulized racemic epinephrine or phenylephrine temporarily provides clinical improvement by reducing stridor and retraction. Their use may be helpful in reducing fatigue and respiratory failure, thereby reducing the need for intubation. Since both drugs have a short duration of action, a child in respiratory distress who displays significant improvement while on these drugs will usually deteriorate in a few hours if repeat doses are not given.

EPIGLOTTITIS

Epiglottitis (acute bacterial supraglottitis) is best thought of as an acute cellulitis of the epiglottis with involvement of the surrounding structure (aryepiglottic folds and the arytenoids). The significance of this disease is the potential for sudden airway obstruction.

The typical patient is a preschool-age child with an illness consisting of fever and sore throat of 6 to 12 hours duration. Dysphagia and respiratory distress follow. The child is usually anxious, has a rapid heart rate without rapid respiration, often sits forward, and drools. Inspiratory stridor and hoarseness are often present. Examination shows an inflamed pharynx, an edematous "cherry red" epiglottis, and decreased breath sounds. Although direct visualization of the epiglottis may provide the diagnosis, care must be employed because manipulation of the posterior pharynx with a tongue blade may trigger airway obstruction. Laboratory examination shows a mild leukocytosis, and blood and pharyngeal cultures usually grow *Hemophilus influenzae.*

The main differential consideration for *H. influenzae* epiglottitis is croup. The important differentiating points are that croup has a more gradual onset, is usually preceded by an upper respiratory infection, has a more characteristic barklike cough, does not produce the dysphagia and drooling that accompany epiglottitis, and croup is more common in children less than two years of age.

Because airway obstruction is the major risk, precautions to maintain an open airway are the first order of business. Direct laryngoscopy of patients with suspected epiglottitis should be done in an operating room with intubation facilities available. There has been ongoing debate as to whether all patients with epiglottitis should be intubated immediately. Recently, there has been some agreement that, if facilities are available, intubation is a reasonable course since the mortality is 33 to 80 percent in patients in whom obstruction occurs. Most airways can be removed in two to three days after institution of appropriate antimicrobial therapy. Because ampicillin-resistant *H. influenzae* is now common, initial therapy should include ampicillin (200 mg/kg/day) and chloramphenicol (75 to 100 mg/kg/day) in four divided doses, pending culture and sensitivity results.[a] If cultures are not available, chloramphenicol alone should be used. Therapy should continue for seven to ten days. All family contacts under four years of age should be given prophylaxis with rifampin (20 mg/kg/day to a maximum of 600 mg/day, in a single dose for four days). The patient should also be given rifampin before discharge to prevent reintroduction of the organism into the household.

SINUSITIS

Acute sinusitis is an inflammatory process of the epithelial lining of the sinuses usually caused by bacteria. The most common bacterial agents include *S. pneumoniae* and *H. influenzae,* which cause over 50 percent of all cases. Anaerobic bacteria are also common. *S. aureus, S. pyogenes, B. catarrhalis,* and aerobic gram-negative bacteria represent approximately 20 percent of cases and various viruses cause the remaining cases.

Facial pain, purulent discharge, headache, nasal obstruction, inability to smell, and a nasal quality to the voice are common presenting complaints of acute sinusitis. Postnasal discharge, fever, and tenderness over the involved sinus are less constant features. Concomitant infection of adjacent sinuses is common. Maxillary sinusitis may be associated with dental infections, frontal sinusitis with frontal lobe abscesses, and frontal or ethmoid sinusitis with frontal bone osteomyelitis. Transillumination of the frontal or maxillary sinuses sometimes provides valuable information. Opacity of a sinus is good evidence of active inflammation. Transillumination is less helpful in a patient with chronic sinusitis. The most sensitive test for acute sinusitis is a sinus x-ray study. Culture of the nasal drainage will not accurately reflect sinusitis etiologic agents because of contamination by nasal flora.

Antibiotic regimens should cover the major etiologic agents. A ten-day course of therapy with ampicillin or trimethoprim-sulfamethoxazole is suggested.[a] Nasal decongestants, such as phenylephrine 0.25 to 0.50 percent can be helpful as supportive therapy. Needle aspiration for the purposes of drainage and microbiologic identification should be considered in patients who are severely ill or not responding to treatment. Dental care may be appropriate if periodontal disease is a contributing factor to the infection.

Chronic sinusitis results from inadequately treated acute sinusitis. The diagnosis is made in the same way as for acute illness. Chronic sinusitis is treated with the same drugs as acute sinusitis, but the duration of treatment is usually two weeks or more. Creation of an artificial ostium or submucosal resection may improve drainage from the affected sinus.

OTITIS MEDIA

Otitis media, or inflammation of the middle ear, is the most frequent diagnosis recorded in children under three years of age. By age three, two thirds of all children have had at least one episode, and one third have had three or more episodes of otitis media. The incidence declines with age except for a slight rise between ages five and six years.

S pneumoniae and *H. influenzae* are the most common bacterial agents, as documented by aspiration of middle ear effusions, and cause more than 50 percent of all cases. A small percentage of patients with *H. influenzae* otitis media are severely ill with concomitant bacteremia and meningitis. Streptococci (groups A and B), *S. aureus, B. catarrhalis,* and gram-negative organisms cause approximately 15 percent of cases. Fluid aspirated from about one third of patients with middle ear effusion will be sterile for a variety of reasons, including fastidious organisms; other microbes such as viruses, chlamydia, and mycoplasma; or prior antimicrobial therapy.

Acute otitis media is defined by the presence of fluid behind the tympanic membrane in association with symptoms of fever, ear pain, or drainage. In younger children, lethargy and irritation may accompany the more specific complaints. Redness of the tympanic membrane may be an early sign but is not enough for diagnosis (crying alone can cause an ear to

[a] See footnotes [a–c] on page 263 for important information on treatment of resistant strains of *H. influenzae.*

appear red). Presence of fluid is best determined by moving the eardrum with a column of air (pneumatic otoscopy). Initial therapy should cover *S. pneumoniae* and *H. influenzae* and, in newborns and immunocompromised hosts, gram-negative agents should be considered. A ten-day course of ampicillin is the regimen of choice.[a] Other effective regimens include trimethoprim-sulfamethoxazole or combinations of a sulfonamide and penicillin or erythromycin. If patients do not respond within two to three days, needle aspiration for organism identification and drainage of fluid should be considered if cultures are available. There is no evidence thus far that decongestants or antihistamines offer any additional advantage to the correct antimicrobial therapy.

In patients with recurrent otitis media, underlying causes such as sinusitis, immune system defects, allergies, or tumors should be considered. Suggested prophylactic regimens for patients with frequent bouts of otitis media include ampicillin (250 mg/day as a single dose) or sulfasoxazole (500 mg twice daily). The same regimens can be used for patients with chronic otitis media. If effusions remain for more than three months, myringotomy and placement of tympanostomy tubes can be considered if available.

BRONCHIOLITIS

Bronchiolitis is a clinical syndrome that occurs in children under two years of age. Air trapping is suggested by tachypnea, decreased breath sounds, low diaphragm, and little or no bronchospasm. Respiratory syncytial virus is the major cause of bronchiolitis, followed by parainfluenza virus. Rhinovirus, adenovirus, and influenza virus play smaller roles as etiologic agents. Bacterial causes of bronchiolitis are uncommon, but *Mycoplasma pneumoniae* has been isolated. Typically, bronchiolitis patients present with mild respiratory symptoms, and increasing tachypnea and difficulty in air exchange. Restlessness, retractions, wheezing, and ronchi or rales may be noted. Dyspnea usually lasts three to four days. Improvement is seen within seven days, although complete recovery may take several weeks. The white cell count is usually normal or mildly elevated. The diagnosis is made on clinical grounds and lack of evidence for a pneumonic process.

The mainstay of therapy is the administration of humidified air and supportive therapy. Bronchospasm is usually not responsive to bronchodilator therapy and steroids are not effective. Antimicrobial therapy is not warranted because the illness is almost always caused by viruses. Secondary bacterial infection is rare.

Mortality is less than 1 percent, even in patients who appear to be seriously ill. Death is usually associated with underlying disease such as cystic fibrosis or congenital heart disease. Complications include recurrent bronchospasms and abnormal pulmonary function tests. Rarely, bronchiolitis obliterans may develop; this is more common after adenovirus infections. Patients who develop this condition usually have bronchopneumonia along with bronchiolitis that persists for weeks. The chronic disease presents with atelectasis, bronchiectasis, recurrent pneumonias, and hyperinflation.

ACUTE BRONCHITIS

Acute bronchitis in an inflammation of the tracheobronchial tree. Etiologic agents include adenovirus, rhinovirus, coronavirus, influenza, parainfluenza, and respiratory syncytial viruses. A small number are caused by nonviral agents such as *M. pneumoniae* and *B. pertussis. S. pneumoniae* and *H. influenzae* have been cultured from patients with acute bronchitis, but their roles as etiologic agents remain unclear since they can be found as normal flora in some patients.

Cough is the predominant feature of acute bronchitis. Although bronchitis may begin with the nasal and pharyngeal components, these symptoms tend to decrease while the cough persists. The cough is initially dry but turns more purulent as the disease progresses. Ronchi and course rales may be heard. Bronchitis is a diagnosis of exclusion. Other diagnoses should always be considered because the clinical picture can be caused by many conditions. Chest x-ray studies are generally normal and smears and culture of the sputum are usually not helpful since bacterial agents cause a minority of cases.

Treatment of acute bronchitis is mostly symptomatic. Antibiotic therapy is recommended only when sputum examination or history suggest infection with *M. pneumoniae* or *B. pertussis.* Both agents can be treated with erythromycin, and tetracycline is useful only against *M. pneumoniae.*

[a] See footnotes [a–c] on page 263 for important information on treatment of resistant strains of *H. influenzae.*

ACUTE PNEUMONIA

The development of acute pneumonia suggests either a defect in host defenses, challenge by a particularly virulent organism, or an overwhelming inoculum. Infectious agents gain access to the lower respiratory tract through inhalation of aerosolized organisms, aspiration of upper airway flora, or by hematogenous spread. Factors that suggest the possible etiologic agent and, thereby, therapy include the clinical setting of the pneumonia, the status of host defense mechanisms, the exposure to specific pathogens, the age of the patient, the presence of underlying chronic illness, and any recent illness or dental manipulation.

Sputum examination and culture are the main sources for making an etiologic diagnosis. Mucopurulent sputum is most commonly found in cases of bacterial infections. Most atypical pneumonias present with scant or watery sputum. A Gram's stain of sputum should be done. Less than 10 epithelial cells per high-powered field and the presence of more than 25 polymorphonuclear cells indicate that the specimen is sputum rather than saliva. Although morphology and staining characteristics of all bacteria should be noted, an effort should be made to identify a predominant organism since that is the most likely culprit. Sputum cultures should be done if available.

Pleural effusions and positive blood cultures each occur in approximately 20 to 30 percent of all cases of bacterial pneumonia. When pleural fluid, examined by smear or culture, or blood cultures are positive, the specific etiologic agent can be treated. Counterimmunoelectrophoresis (CIE) can be used on sputum or pleural fluid specimens for identification of certain organisms. Chest tube drainage of persistent pleural effusions may be necessary. Other complications of bacterial pneumonia such as bacteremia, meningitis, abscess formation, or empyema require prolonged high-dose antibiotics and drainage procedures as indicated.

Bacterial Pneumonia

Most of the cases of bacterial pneumonia are caused by *S. pneumoniae*. *Legionella pneumophilia* is now being recognized more frequently when proper serologic and culture techniques are used. *H. influenzae* is the cause

Table 32-2. Therapy for Pneumonias[a]

Organism	Drug of Choice	Alternative Drug
Streptococcus pneumoniae[b]	Bicillin 1.2 million U bid IM followed by oral penicillin for 10 days	Erythromycin in penicillin-allergic patients; cephalosporin if allergy does not include bronchospasm, urticaria or hypotension
Legionella pneumophila	Erythromycin 500 mg to 1 g qid for 2 weeks	Tetracycline 500 mg to 1 g qid for 2 weeks
Hemophilus influenzae[c]	Ampicillin 100 mg/kg/day (4 divided doses); chloramphenicol in areas of beta-lactamase-positive isolates	Trimethoprim(TMP)-sulfamethoxazole (SMZ) 1 double-strength tablet (160 mg TMP/800 mg SMZ) bid for 10 days
Mycoplasma pneumoniae	Erythromycin 500 mg qid for 7 days	Tetracycline 500 mg qid for 10 days (do not use for children under 8 years of age)
Staphylococcus aureus	Nafcillin 1 g every 4 hours	Cephalosporin (see above caution) or vancomycin in penicillin-allergic patients
Gram-negative organisms	Aminoglycoside for 10 days	Trimethoprim-sulfamethoxazole or chloramphenicol
Anaerobic organisms	Penicillin 500 mg qid or clindamycin 600 mg qid for 2 weeks	Metronidazole 500 mg every 6 hours

[a]See Chapter 23 for more complete dosing information.
[b]See footnote [a] on page 260 for information on resistant strains of *S. pneumoniae*.
[c]See footnotes [a–c] on page 263 for treatment information on resistant strains of *H. influenzae*.

of a significant number of cases, especially in children under five years of age. The true incidence is uncertain, however, as it is often difficult to recognize this organism on Gram's stain. *S. aureus,* gram-negative organisms, and mixed aerobic–anaerobic infections account for the remainder of cases. Viruses play a more prominent role in children, particularly respiratory syncytial, parainfluenza, and adenoviruses. Therapy for bacterial pneumonia is listed in Table 32-2.

Atypical Pneumonia

The atypical pneumonia complex is typified by infection with *Mycoplasma pneumoniae.* The age group at greatest risk ranges from young children to young adults, particularly those congregating in enclosed spaces. White cell counts are greater than 10,000 in about 20 percent of patients. Infiltrates seen on chest x-ray films are more prominent than physical examination would suggest. Constitutional symptoms usually resolve within one to two weeks, although complete resolution may take several more weeks. Other agents include *Coxiella burnetii* (Q fever) and *Chlamydia psittaci* (psittacosis). *Chlamydia trachomatis* has been described as a pulmonary pathogen in neonates and infants. Viral causes include influenza A and B, adenovirus, and, to a lesser extent, rhinovirus, enterovirus, parainfluenza, and respiratory syncytial viruses.

Aspiration Pneumonia

Aspiration can occur in any patient with altered consciousness or abnormal gag or swallowing reflexes. Consequences of aspiration include chemical pneumonitis (particularly from the low pH of the gastric fluid), obstruction of the bronchus (from particulate matter that may result in distal pneumonitis or atelectasis), and bacterial pneumonitis from aspirated organisms. Bacterial infection may be insidious and appear after several days. Fever, productive cough, and weight loss are seen in these patients, commonly with necrotizing pneumonitis, abscess, and empyema. Because oropharyngeal flora are aspirated, the infections are usually anaerobic or mixed aerobic–anaerobic. The organisms most commonly responsible for pneumonia are streptococcal species and anaerobes. For hospitalized patients, or those on antibiotics, *S. aureus* and gram-negative organisms must be considered.

Pneumonia in Immunocompromised Hosts

In addition to bacterial pathogens, fungi, protozoa, parasites, and viral agents contribute to the list of potential etiologies. Up to 70 percent of pneumonias in immunocompromised hosts are caused, in whole or in part, by gram-negative organisms. Bronchoscopy and/or biopsy may be required to make the diagnosis in these patients. Search for abdominal or other occult abscesses should be considered if there is no response to empiric therapy.

TUBERCULOSIS

Tuberculosis is a major problem as a cause of pneumonia (see Chapter 33) in refugee camps. It may present as an acute illness or insidiously with few symptoms except transient fever and malaise. Tuberculosis should be considered in patients with suspected bacterial pneumonia who do not respond to routine bacterial therapy. Chest x-ray studies may show only hilar adenopathy in children, whereas findings in adults range from nonspecific infiltrates to cavitary lesions. Acid-fast staining of the first morning sputum is usually sufficient for diagnosis if adequate specimens are obtained.

PARASITIC PULMONARY DISEASE

A number of parasites that may not include the lungs as the primary focus of infection nonetheless pass through the lung as part of their life cycle and cause pulmonary symptoms. For example, *Ascaris lumbricoides* and hookworm pass through the lungs and enter the alveoli, causing symptoms of pneumonitis. *Strongyloides* infection, or autoinfection, also produces a clinical picture similar to that of hookworm. Infection with *Toxocara,* microfilaria, and schistosomiasis can cause pneumonitis presenting as asthma, bronchiolitis, or pneumonia. Paragonimiasis may cause a syndrome similar to tuberculosis.

RAPID DIAGNOSTIC TECHNIQUES

A number of immunologic techniques that require less time than a culture of the organisms have been employed to make specific bacterial

Table 32-3. Techniques Used for Rapid Diagnosis

Organism	Specimen
Streptococcus (group A)	Throat swab: LA[a]
Streptococcus pneumoniae	Sputum: CIE[b]
	Pleural fluid: CIE, LA
Hemophilus influenzae	Sputum: CIE, LA
	Pleural fluid: CIE, LA
Legionella pneumophilia	Sputum: ELISA[c]
	Tissue: direct FA[d]
Staphylococcus aureus	Pleural fluid: CIE

[a] LA = latex agglutination.
[b] CIE = counterimmunoelectrophoresis.
[c] ELISA = enzyme-linked immunosorbent assay.
[d] Direct FA = direct fluorescent testing.

identification in various diseases (Table 32-3). The methods include counterimmunoelectrophoresis, latex agglutination, and enzyme-linked immunosorbent assay (ELISA). Usually, these methods require only minutes to hours to perform. In a refugee setting, the best tests are simple to perform, are easy to interpret, do not require extensive technical training, and are inexpensive. The sensitivity varies according to the test involved and the antigen used. Clinical correlation of the immunologic tests is variable. The main advantages are speed of results, possible identification of organisms in patients who began antibiotic therapy before presentation to health services, and usefulness when cultures are not available.

REFERENCES AND SELECTED READING

Barrett-Connor E: Parasitic pulmonary disease. Am Rev Respir Dis 1982;126:558–63.
Berman S, McIntosh K: Selective primary health care: strategies for control of disease in the developing world. XXI. Acute respiratory infections. Rev Infect Dis 1985;7:674–91.
Brown HW: Basic Clinical Parasitology. New York, Appleton-Century-Crofts, 1975.
Centers for Disease Control: Diphtheria, tetanus, and pertussis: Guidelines for vaccine prophylaxis and other preventive measures. MMWR 1985;34(27):405–26.
Chretien J, Holland W, Macklem P et al: Acute respiratory infections in children. New Engl J Med 1984;310(15):982–84.
Feingold M, Klein JO, Haslam GE Jr et al: Acute otitis media in children. Am J Dis Child 1966;111:361–65.
Hewlett EL: Selective primary health care: strategies for control of disease in the developing world. XVII. Pertussis and diptheria. Rev Infect Dis 1985;7:426–33.
Hitze KL: The problem of acute respiratory infections (ARI) in the world. Bull Int Union Tuberc 1978;53(4):303–06.
Howard JE, Nelson JD, Clahsen J et al: Otitis media of infancy and early childhood. Am J Dis Child 1976;130:965–70.
Mandell G, Douglas RG, Bennett J (eds): Principles and Practices of Infectious Diseases. New York, John Wiley, 1985.
Medical Letter: Rapid office diagnostic tests for streptococcal pharyngitis. The Medical Letter 1985;27:50.
Moffet HL: Pediatric Infectious Diseases. Philadelphia, JB Lippincott, 1975.
Nissenson AR: Poststreptococcal acute glomerulonephritis: Fact and controversy. Ann Intern Med 1979;91:76–86.
Pan American Health Organization: Acute Respiratory Infections in Children. Washington DC, World Health Organization, 1983.
Pennington J: Respiratory Infections: Diagnosis and Management. New York, Raven Press, 1983.
Siegel D: Management of community-acquired pneumonia in outpatients. West J Med 1985;142:45–48.
WHO (memorandum): Clinical management of acute respiratory infections in children. Bull WHO 1981;59(5):707–16.
WHO (memorandum): A programme for controlling acute respiratory infections in children. Bull WHO 1984;62(1):47–58.

33

Tuberculosis: The Patient and the Program

GARY SLUTKIN

Tuberculosis is caused by *Mycobacterium tuberculosis.* It is transmitted from person to person via the respiratory tract and most commonly causes disease in the lungs. Symptoms include cough, fatigue, fever, chills, night sweats, and weight loss. The cough may be productive of sputum, which is occasionally bloody. Mortality of untreated pulmonary tuberculosis is high; approximately 25 percent of such cases die within one year and 50 to 65 percent within five years (Styblo 1978; Gryzbowski & Enarson 1978).

In 15 to 20 percent of patients, organs other than lungs are affected. Extrapulmonary sites of disease include the lymph nodes (most commonly of the neck, called scrofula); bones and joints (most often of the thoracic or lumbar spine, called Pott's disease); genitourinary tract; gastrointestinal tract, pericardium, peritoneum, and skin. Extrapulmonary involvement is commonly seen in children and may result in meningitis, diffuse disseminated disease, and death (Miller 1982).

The World Health Organization estimates that about 10 million persons develop tuberculosis annually and 3 million of these die (WHO 1982a). The incidence among Southeast Asian refugees entering the United States in 1979 was more than 700 per 100,000 (CDC 1981). Case rates for Somali refugees have been 400 to 900 per 100,000 in several camps. This compares with rates of 200 to 400 per 100,000 for some of the most seriously affected countries of Asia and Africa, and an overall rate of 11 per 100,000 in the United States (Hershfield 1979). Refugee populations not only originate from countries with high prevalence of tuberculosis, they frequently have increased incidence of the disease from intense crowding, undernutrition, and stress from other diseases. Historically famine has been associated with very high rates of mortality from tuberculosis.

In refugee camps, tuberculosis competes for attention with more acute causes of mortality, particularly during early relief efforts. However, programs should be established quickly to limit spread. By 1983, tuberculosis had emerged as the third leading cause of death in Somali refugee camps, responsible for 9.2% of all deaths and 25.0% of adult deaths.

ESTIMATING THE MAGNITUDE OF THE TUBERCULOSIS PROBLEM

The extent of the tuberculosis problem in a community can be estimated using three indices: mortality (deaths); morbidity (cases); and the rate of infection, as demonstrated by skin test reactivity (Styblo 1976). It is not necessary to systematically estimate the magnitude of the problem before beginning the camp tuberculosis program.

Mortality

Most data on deaths from tuberculosis are derived from treatment centers. Because treatment usually prevents death, mortality data may be underestimated where many cases and deaths occur without patients ever entering the medical care system. Underestimation may be less of a problem in refugee camps if population movement in and out of the camp is limited, and if the health care system is effectively attracting cases. A "rule of thumb" frequently used for underdeveloped countries is that the tuberculosis mortality is approximately 50 percent of the morbidity (Styblo & Rouillion 1981).

Mortality from tuberculosis in children is even more likely to be underestimated. Because pulmonary, meningeal, and miliary tuberculosis have such diverse manifestations in children, and bacteriologic confirmation is rarely obtained, tuberculosis is usually not recognized as the cause of death.

Camp ____________

Date ____________

PATIENT DEMOGRAPHICS AND SITE OF DISEASE

	SEX			SITE			
Age	Male	Female	TOTAL No. (%) Patients	Pulm. Smear ⊕	Pulm. Smear ⊖	Extra Pulm.	TOTAL No. (%) Sites
0-4							
5-9							
10-19							
20-29							
30-39							
40-49							
50+							
TOTALS No. (%)							

Figure 33-1. Patient demographics and site of disease form.

Morbidity

Tuberculosis morbidity can be estimated by collating data from area clinics and health posts, or from prevalence studies in the community. However several problems exist in the accurate determination of case rates based on morbidity reports from refugee camps.

First, an accurate figure for the population of a refugee camp may not be available. Second, the actual number of cases under treatment may change rapidly with population movements, thereby rates may reflect migration patterns rather than newly developing cases. Further, donor funded health programs may attract patients from neighboring villages where there may be less access to services.

To obviate these problems, the number of cases should be collected from clinics and health posts at least every six months (see sample form, Figure 33-1). Mean case numbers and rates from several camps or clinics can be used to compare individual reports. Overreporting (and therefore overtreating) can be suspected from units where fewer than three fourths of the pulmonary cases are confirmed by positive sputum smears.

Extrapulmonary tuberculosis is expected to account for 20 to 40 percent of total cases of tuberculosis in children, and from 10 to 30 percent in adults. Higher rates of extrapulmonary disease suggest possible underreporting of pulmonary disease.

The reliability of morbidity estimates based on clinical data is often limited by the vigor of case finding and the reliability of diagnosis. For example, reported rates of tuberculosis in similar Somali refugee camps during 1982 ranged from 285 to 2100 per 100,000 population, although it is unlikely the true disease rates varied this much. As diagnosis and case finding became more uniform and microscopy more reliable, the variability decreased.

Screening of the entire population or a randomly selected sample is the most direct and reliable method for estimating the actual prevalence of tuberculosis. Unfortunately, thousands of persons must be screened to obtain accurate data. Most prevalence studies fail because of incomplete collection of sputums.

How are prevalence surveys conducted? One method is to systematically request two or more sputum samples from each person over 15 years of age. Accuracy is reduced if only one specimen per person is requested, or if only persons admitting to symptoms are tested. Although radiologic surveys are another possible method of prevalence screening, they are cumbersome, expensive, and completely unreliable unless accompanied by sputum smears of all persons with abnormal chest x-ray studies. It has been suggested that prevalence of tuberculosis can be estimated by doubling the incidence, given that the mean duration of the disease is two years. However, this relationship may be less reliable because of the unusual population dynamics in refugee camps.

PREVALENCE AND INCIDENCE OF INFECTION

Data on rates of tuberculosis infection in children can be derived from tuberculin skin test surveys. These provide a relatively simple and inexpensive estimate of the magnitude of the tuberculosis problem while not relying on clinic case finding for reliability. Since previous BCG vaccination may cause positive tuberculin skin tests, such surveys are not valid for populations in which BCG has been widely used.

Tuberculin skin test surveys should record the child's age, presence or absence of BCG scar, and test results. The surveys should focus on young children, since infection rates for adults in many underdeveloped countries approach 100 percent. Although multiple puncture tests have the advantage of requiring neither refrigeration nor handling of syringes and needles, the intradermal method [using 5 tuberculin units strength purified protein derivative (PPD) antigen] is preferred.

The age-specific prevalence of infection can be derived from a single survey. For example, in one survey of Somali refugee camp children, 48.3 percent of 773 children ages 5–13 (mean 9.9) years had positive skin tests. This means that on the average 5% of each age group was newly infected each year. However, this serves as only the first approximation of the annual rate of infection (ARI), since some age groups may have been infected more commonly than others, or it may be that all age groups may have been infected more in certain years. For example, the infection rate might have increased significantly in the last few years.

Because of the year to year variation, it is necessary to perform a second skin test survey in the same population several years later in order to evaluate age cohorts. The annual rate of (new) infections (ARI) can then be derived to help estimate the present transmission of tuberculosis (Bleiker & Styblo 1978; Nybóe 1957).

Tuberculin surveys are highly recommended. A single survey gives a useful guide to the magnitude of the tuberculosis problem and also provides a baseline for future studies. A second study allows calculation of the ARI, which quantitates ongoing transmission. An effective program will decrease ARI long before an effect on morbidity is seen. The ARI has also been used to give rough estimates for the annual incidence of smear positive tuberculosis (55 × ARI/100,000 persons of all ages) and prevalence (110 × ARI/100,000), and the annual incidence of tuberculous meningitis (5 × ARI/100,000 children less than 4 years of age). However, these relationships have not been tested in refugee camps and might be unreliable as a result of variations over time in the magnitude of transmission.

TRANSMISSION OF *M. TUBERCULOSIS* AND PROGRESSION TO DISEASE

Infection with *Mycobacterium tuberculosis* is spread from a person with untreated pulmonary disease to a susceptible host. The mechanism of spread is airborne droplets produced by coughing, talking, or sneezing. A new infection begins with the inhalation of the tubercle bacillus suspended within a droplet. Extrapulmonary tuberculosis is not infectious because the tubercle bacillus is not aerosolized into the environment.

The infectivity of the source case is directly related to the presence (and number) of microorganisms, as demonstrated on microscopic examination of stained sputum. Individuals on chemotherapy become noninfectious rapidly (within 2 weeks for most persons), even though it may take weeks to months for the organisms to no longer appear on the sputum smear (Rouillon et al 1976). On the average, 25 to 50 percent of a patient's close contacts are infected, with higher percentages seen in crowded conditions. This can result in ten or more persons becoming infected from each untreated case of pulmonary tuberculosis.

Tuberculosis is initiated when an infective droplet is inhaled into the lung of a susceptible host. In most cases, the infection will be contained by the immune response and the presence of infection noted only if a tuberculin skin test is applied and found to be positive. However, the microbe has spread by lymphatics and blood to other parts of the lungs and other organs, even among asymptomatic infected individuals.

Five to 10 percent of newly infected individuals will develop the clinically apparent disease. Tuberculosis can result from direct progression within months of an initial infection or can be a reactivation of a latent focus seeded years earlier. The risk of reactivation is lifelong for all infected persons who have not had chemotherapy because the microorganism can persist in a latent stage for decades. Most of the factors controlling reactivation are not known, although other infections, such as measles, and undernutrition appear to contribute. Measles vaccine and other live virus vaccines may suppress a skin test (Starr & Berkovich 1974) but they do not reactivate tuberculosis.

PULMONARY TUBERCULOSIS

Symptoms

The most common symptoms of pulmonary tuberculosis is a persistent cough. This cough may be dry, productive of sputum, or bloody. Other pulmonary symptoms, such as chest pain and shortness of breath, may also be present. Common systemic symptoms include fever, chills, night sweats, fatigue, weakness, and weight loss.

The symptoms of tuberculosis may be acute or indolent. It is common for patients in less developed countries to ignore a chronic cough. Medical attention may be sought late, perhaps only after the onset of hemoptysis or after months of progressive wasting. Experts constantly stress the need to educate health workers and the community as to the importance of identifying and evaluating persons with a chronic cough.

Diagnosis

An accurate diagnosis of pulmonary tuberculosis is important for several reasons. The diagnosis of tuberculosis carries the commitment of completing a therapeutic regimen usually lasting 6 to 12 months. This commitment includes pursuing a patient who defaults on treatment. Lack of commitment to therapy because of uncertain diagnosis will lead to premature discontinuation of therapy for some patients, resulting in relapse to the infectious state. A false diagnosis of tuberculosis can lead to unnecessary adverse drug reactions, lifestyle disruptions, and wasteful diversion of resources. With confidence in the diagnosis, health care providers can concentrate their efforts on those patients who would otherwise deteriorate clinically and infect others.

The diagnosis of tuberculosis requires clinical recognition of the symptoms and signs of disease, and the correct use of diagnostic tests. Tuberculin skin testing is of limited value in less developed countries when used for the diagnosis of an individual patient.

Chest radiography is frequently unavailable because equipment is expensive, cumbersome, and difficult to maintain. Furthermore, diagnosis of pulmonary tuberculosis made on the basis of "suspicious" radiographic shadows, but unconfirmed by sputum bacteriology, can be misleading or lead to overdiagnosis. The latter results in the unnecessary treatment of persons who do not have tuberculosis. Although some of the more characteristic radiographic findings of pulmonary tuberculosis are described below, it is recommended that radiography be used primarily to aid in diagnosing cryptic pulmonary cases and in nonpulmonary problems (i.e., trauma or bone infection). If screening chest radiography is used, the suspected diagnosis must be confirmed by sputum bacteriology.

The most reliable and widely accepted method for diagnosis of pulmonary tuberculosis is the bacteriologic examination of sputum samples of patients with symptoms of pulmonary tuberculosis. Sputum microscopy is frequently the only diagnostic tool available but is sufficiently specific to provide a reliable diagnosis. Although less sensitive than culture, diagnosis by sputum microscopy identifies the most infectious cases.

The recommended approach to the diagnosis of tuberculosis in refugees is to examine sputum smears by direct microscopy of all patients with symptoms compatible with tuberculosis. A generally accepted method is to collect two or three sputum samples from all persons with a cough of three or more weeks' duration, hemoptysis, unexplained weight loss, and persistent fever and children who fail to gain weight as expected.

Whether to treat presumptive cases in which the diagnosis has not been confirmed is dependent on local resources and priorities. In general, if the laboratory is proficient at smear microscopy, repeated negative results usually means that an alternative diagnosis is more likely. Referral for chest radiography may be indicated in some of these cases. Alternative diagnoses include asthma, bronchitis, bacterial pneumonia, lung abscess, empyema, tropical eosinophilia, paragonomiasis, or meliodosis (in Southeast Asia). These alternative diagnoses should be sought and consideration given to empiric antibiotic therapy. If symptoms persist, sputum examinations can be repeated weeks later. For patients who continue to deteriorate, empiric antituberculous therapy may be indicated. If there is a lack of confidence in the laboratory, proficiency should be improved and quality control assured with the help of a reference laboratory.

Sputum Bacteriology

The only way to prove a diagnosis of tuberculosis conclusively is by demonstrating the tubercle bacillus from the involved site of disease. Therefore, persons who are suspected of having pulmonary tuberculosis should have a bacteriologic evaluation of their sputum or lower respiratory tract secretions. A complete diagnostic examination of sputum samples for *M. tuberculosis* includes microscopic examination of a strained smear, incubation in culture medium for growth, definitive identification of the organism, and drug susceptibility if growth is demonstrated.

Under ideal circumstances, sputum cultures, combined with identification procedures, are more specific than sputum smear results. In the refugee setting, however, a smear that demonstrates acid-fast bacilli (AFB) is sufficiently predictive of tuberculosis that culture confirmation is not required. Failure to obtain culture growth from the sputum of a coughing patient with a positive smear may be more likely the result of inadequate laboratory conditions for culture than a false positive smear.

Facilities for culturing *Mycobacteria* are difficult to set up and maintain. Major limitations are unreliable electricity, which makes temperature control for culture maintenance difficult, and the absence of skilled personnel. Direct smear microscopy is the most practical method for diagnosis of pulmonary tuberculosis because it is relatively inexpensive, does not require highly trained personnel, and does not have the operational disadvantages of cultures and chest radiography.

Approximately 50 to 70 percent of sputum specimens that are culture positive will also yield a positive smear examination. In one study, two sputum smears were nearly as good as one sputum culture (Bailey 1967). A first sputum smear will detect only about 70 to 85 percent of patients in whom a diagnosis could be made by examining several smear specimens. Most of the additional yield is generated by the next two specimens. The collection of two or three specimens is widely practiced (Toman 1979).

When should the sputum samples be collected? Because a cough is often most productive when one first awakes, a practical approach is to collect one specimen at the clinic and then send the patient home with two collection containers and instructions to collect first-morning sputums for the following two days.

Microscopy for AFB is only as good as the sample obtained, the equipment used, and the microscopist. Quality control of the laboratory is essential to avoid missing, or erroneously diagnosing, cases. Methods of checking the laboratory include rereading of slides, the use of test slides, and submission of part of a split specimen to a reference laboratory. If national laboratory facilities are accessible, but not part of the refugee program, it may be helpful to request reference slides or an agreement for periodic checking of specimens.

A widely used method of staining is described in Chapter 22. Culture facilities and susceptibility studies are usually not technologically appropriate in the refugee camp setting. A reference laboratory may be helpful in the performance of these tests for unusual clinical problems or for epidemiologic studies.

Chest Radiography

Almost any radiographic finding can be seen in pulmonary tuberculosis. The most common finding in adults is fibronodular infiltrates in the upper lobes and the superior segments of the lower lobes. Progressive scarring may lead to loss of upper lung volumes with retraction and elevation of one or both hila. Cavitation is characteristic of advanced disease. Other common findings include pleural effusions, single or multiple nodular densities, or mid-lung to lower-lung field infiltrates. In children, the most common radiographic findings are mid-lung or lower-lung infiltrates, hilar adenopathy, and pleural effusions.

These findings, although typical of pulmonary tuberculosis, are not specific for this disease. The differential diagnosis includes bacterial, viral, or parasitic pneumonias, and malignancy (Chapter 32 provides detailed tables on possible etiologies of pneumonia and lung abscesses). Chest x-ray findings usually do not completely resolve after either therapeutic or spontaneous "cure." The clinician must therefore be wary of incorrectly diagnosing active pulmonary tuberculosis even when the radiographic findings appear typical. Progression in size of abnormalities over time and the presence of cavitation suggest current disease.

Tuberculin Skin Testing

The most reliable tuberculin skin testing procedure is to inject 0.1 cc of 5 TU purified protein derivative (PPD) intradermally (Mantoux method). The test is read in 48 to 72 hours; a reading of 10 mm or more of induration indicates infection. Five millimeters is considered positive for infant and child household contacts who have not had BCG. Remember that at its best a positive skin test can only indicate infection, and not disease. Even large test readings do not indicate that the patient has active tuberculosis. Multiple puncture methods of application (e.g., Heath, Tine) cannot be standardized because the amount of antigen injected varies by tester (Comstock 1975). Prior BCG administration can result in sensitization and, although very large reactions are more likely to occur with true exposure to tuberculosis, there is no reliable method of differentiation. Besides the problem of BCG, false-positive reactions may be seen as a result of prior exposure to nontuberculous ("atypical") *Mycobacteria,* which commonly exist in the soil and water of tropical climates (Glassroth et al 1980).

A serious error is that of discounting a diagnosis of tuberculosis because of a negative tuberculin skin test. Reasons for a false-negative test include errors of antigen administration, improper reading of results, loss of antigen potency, patient undernutrition, current or recent viral illness or immunization, or advanced age. Up to 20 percent of persons with severe tuberculosis will have a negative tuberculin test. False-negative and false-positive test results are too common for the skin test to be of use for diagnosis.

EXTRAPULMONARY TUBERCULOSIS

Mycobacterium tuberculosis can cause disease in any organ of the body, usually as a result of reactivation of a dormant site that was seeded earlier. Favored sites of reactivation other than the lung and pleura include the lymph nodes, bones and joints, and the genitourinary tract. Less frequently, disease involves the gastrointestinal tract, peritoneum, pericardium, or skin. Meningeal and miliary disease, with resultant high morbidity and mortality, are particularly prevalent in very young children.

The symptoms, signs, and diagnostic approach differ by site of disease. For a number of reasons, an empiric approach to treatment for extrapulmonary tuberculosis is most often taken in underdeveloped countries. The tuberculin skin test has the same diagnostic problems as discussed for pulmonary disease. A negative skin test should not be used to exclude the diagnosis of tuberculosis at any site. Radiologic studies may be less helpful than for pulmonary disease, and bacteriologic sampling is more difficult and often yields false-negative information. Empiric therapy is often justified for lymphatic and spinal tuberculosis because clinical features are sufficiently characteristic.

An evaluation for pulmonary tuberculosis should accompany the diagnostic evaluation of known or suspected extrapulmonary disease since 10 to 40 percent of patients with extrapulmonary disease will have pulmonary disease as well.

Lymphatic Tuberculosis

Scrofula, or tuberculosis of the lymph nodes of the neck, is especially common in children. Anterior cervical lymph nodes are most often involved, but disease can be present in the posterior cervical, supraclavicular, and submandibular regions. Axillary or inguinal disease is less common. Involved lymph nodes are usually painless and enlarge slowly. They may appear slightly erythematous on inspection and feel minimally warm to the touch. Palpation usually reveals a nontender, fluctuant-to-firm mass. Thick, cheesy (caseous) or thin, milky drainage may occur spontaneously.

The most important differential diagnostic consideration is bacterial adenitis complicating an upper respiratory, dental, or scalp infection. Lymphoma is also an important consideration, especially for older patients. Less common considerations include fungal disease, secondary syphilis, or trypanosomiasis. The mouth, pharynx, teeth, gums, and scalp should be examined carefully. Most experts recommend giving a trial of antimicrobials (e.g., penicillin, ampicillin, erythromycin, or tetracycline) to cover the common skin and oropharyngeal pathogens before embarking on more aggressive diagnostic approaches or initiating antituberculous therapy.

Aspiration can be performed for relief of symptoms if the diseased node is fluctuant, tense, and painful. Acid-fact organisms are occasionally demonstrated on smears or cultures from aspirated material. Fifty percent of acid-fast stains of excised biopsy specimens will be positive, and almost all should be positive by culture (Huhti et al 1975).

Bone and Joint Tuberculosis

The most common site for tuberculosis of the skeletal system is the spine (Pott's disease), although any joint or bone can be affected. Spine involvement is usually in the low thoracic or upper lumbar region in adults, and the upper or lower thoracic region in children. Pott's disease characteristically presents with a progressive gibbous (or hunchback) deformity without significant pain or tenderness.

After the spine, the most common bony involvement is the weight-bearing joints of the hip and knee. Joint involvement presents as an acute or chronic arthritis with slowly progressive limitation of motion. Pain and tenderness may be present, not infrequently with a chronic or acute effusion. A chronic draining fistula tract may also be seen but is not diagnostic.

The radiographic appearance of spinal tuberculosis is sufficiently characteristic (in the high-prevalence setting) to be diagnostic. Findings include destructive changes of the disk space and adjacent vertebrae, especially anteriorly, with disk space narrowing. This results in "anterior wedging" with angulation and deformity. A bacteriologic diagnosis of spinal tuberculosis is usually unnecessary and impractical in developing countries.

The differential diagnosis of acute and chronic monoarticular arthritis is broader. Pyogenic bacterial infections caused by *Staphylococcus aureus* and streptococcal species are most common. If possible, aspirated fluid should be obtained and examined by Gram's stain and AFB techniques (see Chapter 22). From knee aspirations, acid-fast bacilli may be seen in 20 to 50 percent of smears and 50 to 70 percent of cultures from the tuberculous joints. If the aspiration is negative, empiric antimicrobial therapy directed against staphylococcal and streptococcal organisms is usually indicated before one embarks on antituberculous therapy.

Genitourinary Tract Tuberculosis

This form of tuberculosis can result from renal reactivation and spread down the collecting system. In men, the prostate, epididymis, or seminal vesicles can be involved. Disease may present as acute or chronic cystitis, prostatitis, epididymitis, or as a scrotal mass. Dysuria and frequency are reported by 30 to 60 percent of patients with 20 to 30 percent experiencing gross hematuria. In women, genital tract disease most commonly involves the fallopian tubes. Acute or chronic pelvic pain, menstrual irregularities, and infertility may be present.

A bacteriologic diagnosis of tuberculosis is not possible when the required cultures and histology are unavailable. There are many causes other than tuberculosis for the genitourinary clinical syndromes mentioned above. Staining of urine for AFB is too insensitive to be useful and non-pathogenic *Mycobacteria* may yield false-positive results. Cultures of first-morning urine specimens may be helpful but only if species identification can be done.

Gastrointestinal Tract Tuberculosis

The ileocecal and ascending colon are the most common sites of intestinal tuberculosis. Patients may experience chronic abdominal pain, distention, constipation (less commonly diarrhea), and intestinal obstruction (from fibrosis). Peritoneal tuberculosis may present with ascites, fever, and constitutional symptoms. Chronic peritoneal disease with scarring can evolve to cause a "doughy" texture to the abdomen on palpation. The same difficulties in bacteriologic diagnosis apply as mentioned for genitourinary tuberculosis.

Meningeal Tuberculosis

Tuberculous meningitis, often seen in conjunction with widely disseminated disease, is the most common cause of death from tuberculosis in children. Permanent neurologic sequelae are common for disease treated late, whereas untreated disease is almost always fatal. Meningitis develops when a tuberculous lesion in the cerebral cortex grows to invade, or rupture into, the subarachnoid space.

The onset of symptoms may be acute, resembling bacterial meningitis, but is most often insidious. Young children present with apathy, drowsiness, or irritability. Fever is almost always present, and vomiting is seen in over half of all cases. Older children complain of headache.

Since the disease commonly involves other sites simultaneously, the patient may have pulmonary or abdominal complaints as well. Signs of meningeal irritation such as nuchal rigidity (resistance to neck flexion) and positive Kernig's and Brudzinski's signs (see Chapter 12) may sometimes be seen after a few weeks of a nonspecific febrile or wasting illness.

Differentiation of early tuberculous meningitis from common childhood infections may be difficult. A spinal tap should be performed whenever meningitis is suspected. Characteristic findings of tuberculous meningitis include a white cell concentration of 100 to 500 (range of 10 to 1000) cells per cubic millimeter, a normal to low glucose concentration, and an elevated protein level. A predominance of lymphocytes is the most common clue that tuberculous meningitis is present, but this finding is also seen with viral meningitis or partially treated bacterial meningitis. A further difficulty is that polymorphonuclear leukocytes may be predominant early in 25 to 35 percent of cases of tuberculous meningitis.

A definitive diagnosis is made by bacteriologic examination of the spinal fluid. The thin film that develops on the surface of the specimen after standing should be smeared and stained by Gram's stain and for acid-fast organisms. If enough time is spent examining the slide(s), acid-fast organisms can be found in 25 to 50 percent of cases. Culture yield is 45 to 90 percent but, even if cultures are available, treatment should not be delayed when significant suspicion of tuberculous meningitis exists (Kennedy & Fallon 1979).

Evidence for pulmonary tuberculosis should be sought in the child and the family. Family members should be examined, since the presence of tuberculosis in a family member more strongly suggests tuberculosis as the cause of meningitis in the child.

Presumptive therapy should be considered for tuberculous meningitis when a child with meningitis of unknown etiology presents with a predominance of lymphocytes in the spinal fluid. If a child's condition fits the above description, and tuberculosis is known to be present in the household, then initiation of antituberculous therapy is indicated. If the child is suffering from an acute febrile illness, possible bacterial etiologies of meningitis should be presumptively treated as well. Tuberculous meningitis is the first consideration in chronic meningitis or any meningitis that does not respond to therapy for the usual pyogenic causes.

Disseminated (Miliary) Tuberculosis

Widespread generalized tuberculosis results from hematogenous spread to all organs. The diagnosis of miliary tuberculosis is complicated by the lack of specificity of the signs and symptoms. Untreated miliary disease is almost always fatal.

Disseminated tuberculosis is most common in young children but can occur at any age. The disease may present as a low-grade chronic infection or as acute overwhelming sepsis. Anorexia, fatigue, weight loss, and fever each occur in about 80 percent of patients, while lymphadenopathy, hepatomegaly, and splenomegaly are each seen in about 15 to 30 percent of cases. Less frequently, choroid tubercles in the fundi or cutaneous lesions may be seen. Headache, cough, or abdominal pain may represent central nervous system, pulmonary, or intestinal involvement.

Chest radiography most often shows a characteristic pattern resembling millet seeds, from which the disease derives its name. Cavitary pulmonary lesions, which may have been the source of the disseminated infection, may also be seen on chest x-ray studies. Bacteriologic diagnosis might be obtained from sputum, urine, or spinal fluid specimens. The highest yield is from lung, bone marrow, or liver biopsy.

The Child Under Five Years with an Undiagnosed Febrile Illness or Wasting

When diagnostic facilities are limited, a young child with a chronic febrile illness or wasting should be suspected of having pulmonary, miliary, or meningeal tuberculosis. If an alternative diagnosis cannot be found, and if therapeutic trials of antibacterial agents have been unsuccessful, empiric antituberculosis chemotherapy should be considered. This diagnosis is more likely if pulmonary tuberculosis is present in a family member, caretaker, or other close contact.

TREATMENT OF TUBERCULOSIS

Principles of Therapy

There are two basic requirements for successful therapy of tuberculosis: more than one antituberculous drug must be used to treat the disease and therapy must be prolonged for months to years. Although the task of killing all of the *M. tuberculosis* organisms is difficult, several regimens are available that offer 90 to 99 percent clinical and microbiological cure rates (Chaulet 1983).

The use of more than one antituberculous drug is required to prevent emergence of drug resistant organisms during therapy.

Prolonged therapy is required because of the ability of the *M. tuberculosis* organism to divide slowly and intermittently. This slow division demands that effective antimicrobial agents be present in adequate concentration over a long period of time. Discontinuing chemotherapy prematurely will result in relapse and return to the infectious state.

Drug resistance may also emerge when disease recurs after premature discontinuation of drugs. Unfortunately, alternative drugs needed for retreatment may not be available locally and, if these patients are started on a second course of the same therapy, disappointing results often follow. A patient who has been treated unsuccessfully may spread this less treatable form of the disease to others, further magnifying the problem for the community.

The basic requirement of taking daily medication for 6 to 12 months poses a significant problem for the patient. Most patients will view such prolonged therapy as unnecessary. Even if initially convinced, the patient's commitment frequently wanes after he or she begins to feel better. Keeping the patient on therapy for the full course is one of the most important and difficult jobs for the health worker.

Drugs for Tuberculosis

Table 33-1 lists several of the most commonly available antituberculous drugs along with recommended doses, common side effects, antimicrobial activity, and costs. Isoniazid (INH), rifampin, and streptomycin are the most active agents. Rifampin and pyrazinamide have the special ability to sterilize persistent populations of organisms usually responsible for relapse and, as a result, are useful in short-course therapy regimens. Thiacetazone, a relatively weak antituberculous drug, is commonly used in less developed countries because it is inexpensive.

Drug Regimens

Antituberculous drugs are combined to form chemotherapy regimens. Table 33-2 lists some of the best tested and most widely used daily treatment regimens according to duration of therapy, cost, and success rate. Most of these regimens may be modified to biweekly programs (Table 33-1) after an initial one to two months of daily treatment. This can be done without sacrifice of efficacy if compliance is ensured by direct observation of ingestion of all drugs.

Until recently, standard therapy in the United States consisted of 18 months of INH and ethambutol since it was inexpensive, safe, and 96 to 99 percent effective. However, the difficulty in keeping persons on therapy for such a long period of time has stimulated therapeutic trials in short-course chemotherapy. Good success has been achieved with a nine-month course of therapy when rifampin is added. When pyrazinamide is included in the initial phase, and rifampin continued for the duration, treatment can be shortened to six months (Stead & Dutt 1982). These short-course chemotherapy regimens are frequently unavailable in less developed countries because of the high cost of rifampin. Recent decreases in the cost of rifampin may resolve the problem.

The most widely used regimens in less developed countries have been the 12-month protocols using INH and thiacetazone (Table 33-2, regimens c, d, and e) because this is the least expensive combination. Ninety to 96 percent success rates have been achieved in East Africa with regimen e (Table 33-2) (East African British Medical Research Council 1970).

The availability of more expensive drugs in refugee camps in Southeast Asia allowed health workers to use regimen i (Table 33-2). Since 1983, the CDC has been supervising a modification of regimen n (Table 33-2), which includes ethambutol for the full six months of therapy with ingestion of each dose being directly observed. In Somalia, the Ministry of Health's Refugee Health Unit (RHU) has written guidelines for treatment with a modification of regimen e (Table 33-2) including 3 months of streptomycin injections (Refugee Health Unit 1982).

Adverse Reactions to Tuberculostatic Drugs

The most common adverse reactions to tuberculostatic drugs are listed in Table 33-1. To assist the clinician in properly responding to these adverse reactions, when taking the patient's history, it is helpful to attempt to char-

Table 33-1. Commonly Used Antituberculosis Drugs

		Dosage[a]			Antimicrobial Activity		Cost/Day ($US)	
Drug (Symbol)	How Supplied	Daily Dose	Twice Weekly Dose	Most Common Adverse Reactions	Cidal	Sterilizing	UNIPAC[b]	Average Country[c] 1978
Isoniazid/INH (H)	Tabs: 300 mg, 100 mg Suspension: 100 mg/5 ml	5–10 mg/kg up to 300 mg	15 mg/kg up to 900 mg	Mild CNS[d] symptoms peripheral neuritis, hepatitis	+++	++	0.004	0.003
Thiacetazone (T)	Combination tabs H300 + T150, H100 + T50	3–5 mg/kg up to 150 mg	NA	GI[e] intolerance, hepatitis	+	+	0.006	NA
Streptomycin (S)	For injection 5.0 or 1.0 g vial	15 mg/kg to 1 g IM	25 mg/kg to 1 g IM	8th nerve damage[f], kidney damage	+++	+	0.1	0.1
Ethambutol (E)	Tabs: 400 mg	15–25 mg/kg	50 mg/kg	Optic toxicity, skin rash	++	++	0.04	0.34
Rifampin (R)	Caps: 300 mg, 150 mg	10 mg/kg to 600 mg	10 mg/kg to 600 mg	GI intolerance, fever, skin rash, hepatitis	+++	+++	0.16	0.95
Pyrazinamide (Z)	Tabs: 500 mg	20–25 mg/kg to 2 g	50–70 mg/kg to 3 g	Hepatitis, arthralgias	+	+++	0.14	0.35

[a]All doses orally (po) unless otherwise indicated.
[b]UNIPAC, UNICEF Catalog 1986.
[c]Average cost to countries surveyed Chaulet P.: BIUAT 1978;53:247.
[d]Central nervous system.
[e]Gastrointestinal.
[f]Potentiated by thiacetazone.

Table 33-2. Selected Antituberculosis Drug Regimens

Duration of Therapy (months)	Cost (US$) UNIPAC[a] 1986	1978 Average[b]	Success Rate (%)[c]	Regimen[d]	Text Reference Letter[e]
18	18	(185)	96–99	18HE	(a)
	40	(56)	96–99	18 HS	(b)
12	2	(3)	80	12 HT	(c)
	4	(6)	84–92	1 SHT/11 HT	(d)
	6	(9)	90–96	2 SHT/10 HT	(e)
8–9	18	(85)	95–99	2 SZRH/6 HT	(f)
	18	(175)	95–99[f]	3 ERH/6 HE	(g)
	24	(175)	95–99[f]	3 ZRH/6 HE	(h)
	34	(275)	95–99	2 ERH/7 RH	(i)
	36	(275)	95–99	2 SRH/7 RH	(j)
6	10	(45)	80	1 SZRH/5 HT	(k)
	20	(85)	85–93	2 SZRH/4 HT	(l)
	20	(170)	80–95	6 RH	(m)
	30	(190–210)	95–99	2 EZRH/4 RH[g]	(n)
	32	(190–210)	95–99	2 SZRH/4 RH[g]	(o)
	28	(190–210)	95–99	2 ZRH/4RH	(p)
	24	(190–210)	95–99	6 SRH	(q)

[a]UNIPAC, UNICEF Catalog 1986.
[b]Average cost to countries surveyed, Chaulet P: BIUAT 1978;53:247.
[c]Several sources including Chaulet P: BIUAT 1983;58:26; Tubercle 1974;55:211; Fox W: Chest 1979;76:285.
[d]Daily regimens; see Table 33-1 for drug symbols; the number preceding the letters indicates the number of months used (for example, 2 SHT/10 HT indicates two months of daily streptomycin (S), isoniazid (H), and thiacetazone (T), followed by ten months of isoniazid plus thiacetazone).
[e]These regimens are referred to in text by the letter given.
[f]Limited data.
[g]Twice or three times weekly HR for last four months reduces cost to $20–25.

acterize the possible adverse reactions as either intolerance, toxicity, or hypersensitivity.

Intolerance may consist of complaints of mild dizziness or lightheadedness, as is often experienced with INH. Mild gastrointestinal (GI) complaints may occur with many of the oral agents, particularly thiacetazone. Problems of drug intolerance usually require little more than reassurance. Occasionally, it is helpful to alter the drug routine, such as taking INH at bedtime if dizziness is a problem. Similarly, thiacetazone can be taken with meals or in divided doses to help decrease GI side effects. The common, but usually unnecessary, practice of concomitant use of iron or vitamin supplements may contribute to intolerance, resulting in GI upset from the iron or complaints related to the ingestion of a large number of pills at one time. Simple drug intolerance does not lead to organ damage and is not life-threatening. However, if patient complaints are not properly attended to, treatment failure may result from patient noncompliance or default.

Toxicity refers to specific organ damage, which can be progressive if the offending medication is continued. Fortunately, toxicity occurs relatively infrequently with tuberculostatic chemotherapy. The organs most commonly damaged when toxicity does occur include the liver, eyes, and eighth cranial nerve.

Hepatitis from INH occurs in 2 to 3 percent of exposed persons over 50 years of age, 1 percent of patients from 21 to 50 years, and rarely in those under 20 years of age. Hepatitis due to rifampin is even less common but may be seen with doses of 15 mg/kg or more. Care should be taken to give children and small adults a dose of 10 mg/kg, rather than the full 600-mg adult dose. Weight charts posted in the clinics are useful for determining proper dosage.

The first clinical signs of hepatitis are persistent loss of appetite, nausea, and fatigue. Jaundice appears later. Gastrointestinal complaints that are temporally related to drug ingestion are more likely due to simple intolerance. It is reassuring if the problems are relieved by taking the drug with meals, or by changing the time of day the drug is administered. On the other hand, if complaints last several days and persist throughout the day hepatotoxicity should be suspected. Drug doses should be checked, one or more drugs discontinued, and the patient followed closely. The appearance of jaundice is an absolute indication to discontinue all medications.

Hearing loss or vestibular dysfunction may be a result of eighth nerve damage from streptomycin. This toxicity is also dose dependent. It is more common when streptomycin is being given concomitantly with thiacetazone or in elderly patients or patients with renal failure. Early symptoms of streptomycin toxicity that should alert the health worker to discontinue the drug include tinnitus or complaints relating to balance. It is prudent to question patients receiving streptomycin regularly about these symptoms, especially those over 50 years of age. Note should also be made of these patients' gait. An early sign of gait disturbance is difficulty in turning 180 degrees after walking in a straight line.

Optic neuritis from ethambutol is rare in persons receiving 15 mg/kg/day, but the incident increases to 1 to 2 percent for patients receiving 25 mg/kg/day. An early sign of this toxicity is the inability to distinguish red from green.

Peripheral neuritis due to INH presents as numbness or tingling of the distal extremities. It can be prevented by giving small doses (5 to 10 mg/day) of pyridoxine and is treated with larger doses (50 to 100 mg/day).

Hypersensitivity reactions, or drug allergies, usually present as unexplained fever or rash. Streptomycin and thiacetazone (and another antituberculous drug, not discussed here, called PAS) are the most frequent offenders, although any drug can be responsible. If symptoms persist with no other known cause, it may be necessary to discontinue therapy since life-threatening complications, though rare, can occur. Rechallenge to determine a regimen the patient can tolerate can be performed under controlled circumstances after symptoms resolve.

Monitoring for Treatment Failure by Monthly Sputum Examination

Failure of therapy for pulmonary tuberculosis is best defined bacteriologically by the failure of sputum smears (and/or cultures) to convert to, or remain, negative on therapy. To detect treatment failure, it is therefore necessary to have a program for periodic sputum reevaluation during therapy. The most useful protocol calls for a monthly sputum examination for all patients who had a positive sputum at the beginning of therapy. This is easy for the health worker to use and record, allows detection of individual treatment failures, and facilitates program evaluation. Some programs stop collecting sputums after 1 or 2 negative results. This risks overreliance on a single lab result (which may be from saliva) and late failures may also be missed.

Protocols should be developed for appropriate response to suspected or confirmed treatment failures. The most common cause of unsuccessful therapy is irregular drug ingestion or premature cessation of therapy. Direct observation of medication administration should, therefore, always precede attempts to change the drug regimen.

Occasionally, initial drug resistance is responsible for treatment failure. In most refugee situations, drug susceptibility testing is not available to guide drug changes, reserve drugs may be in limited supply, and expensive retreatment may be inappropriate. If the drug protocol requires change, two or more drugs should be added or substituted at the same time to avoid further drug resistance. Expert consultation is advisable to assist in the development of alternative protocols when drug resistance is identified or suspected.

GOAL AND METHODS OF TUBERCULOSIS CONTROL

The goal of a communicable disease control program is to decrease morbidity and mortality by decreasing transmission of the responsible pathogen. For tuberculosis, transmission of the tubercle bacillus is interrupted by finding those persons who are most infectious and rendering their sputum free of viable bacilli by treatment (Sutherland 1981).

An integrated case finding and treatment program is the only reliable method of tuberculosis control. Although individual patients may benefit, BCG vaccination and INH chemoprophylaxis have a negligible overall effect on interrupting transmission in the community (Gryzbowski 1979; Styblo & Meijer 1976).

The basic case finding and treatment program requires that patients who present with symptoms suggestive of tuberculosis have their sputum microscopically examined for acid-fast bacilli. Further, the program should ensure that those individuals with positive sputums are started on, and complete, an adequate course of antituberculous chemotherapy. The essential components of an effective tuberculosis control program are as follows:

- The ability to make a reliable microscopic diagnosis.
- A regular and reliable source of drugs.
- A health care system with personnel who are educated and motivated to perform the necessary tasks.
- An efficient and accurate record-keeping system.
- A program of ongoing tuberculosis education for health care workers, patients and their families, and the community.
- A system for ongoing evaluation of program effectiveness.

The ability to make a reliable diagnosis requires a microscope, staining materials, and a competent technician. A technical guide for sputum examination is listed in the reference section (International Union Against Tuberculosis 1978). The laboratory should be tested periodically to ensure quality control.

A regular supply of drugs must be ensured. Aside from the adverse impact on individual patient care, interruption of the drug supply has a profound and lasting negative effect on the motivation of patient and health worker.

Each of these program components should be in place before an existing tuberculosis control program is expanded. It may be helpful to start with a pilot project so that solutions for common problems such as noncompliance and default can be defined. The program can then be expanded after a "working model" has been developed and evaluated.

Although periodic attention to case finding is common, the effectiveness of most tuberculosis programs is limited by failure to keep patients on therapy. A well-run treatment program will develop a good local reputation and attract new cases; a poorly run program will have the opposite effect.

Passive Case Finding

Case finding activities in refugee camps should consist of microscopic examination of sputum from patients who present to the clinic with symptoms of tuberculosis. Health workers must be trained to recognize tuberculosis symptoms and should be urged to query patients specifically regarding these symptoms, even if the visit is for another reason. Continuing education and support for health workers are necessary to maintain their skills and interest.

Supervisory personnel will find it useful to check laboratory records of sputum requests periodically to compare the number and yield of positives from individual health workers and clinics, or for one clinic over time.

Two other methods for increasing case finding are a change of protocol to include sputum examination of patients with a two-week (instead of four-week) history of cough, and community education programs that provide information on the symptoms of tuberculosis, that completion of therapy leads to cure, and that tuberculosis is not a cause for shame.

Active Case Finding

Active case finding refers to more direct seeking out of cases in the community. A nonselective house-to-house search is usually the least efficient use of resources for case finding. Rather, initial efforts should focus on high-risk groups such as patient contacts or individuals in sections of the community known to have a high prevalence of tuberculosis. The assistance of elders or community leaders may be enlisted for referral of persons with symptoms suggestive of tuberculosis.

Increasing active case finding does not always represent optimal use of limited tuberculosis program resources. Before increasing case finding activities the camp medical officer should determine how well the treatment program is keeping people already registered on therapy, determine the yield of current case finding activities, and check that most patients on therapy have a proven diagnosis (e.g., were bacteriologically positive). There is no benefit to further overloading a treatment program that is not succeeding at its current patient load. It may be more worthwhile to have less patients (who are more certainly proven to have TB), in particular during early stages of program development.

Case Holding: Minimizing Noncompliance and Default

All too often, discussions about tuberculosis treatment focus on the choice of drug regimen without paying sufficient attention to the more essential and urgent problem of keeping patients on therapy (case holding). Aside from inefficient use of resources, lack of attention to these problems may increase drug-resistant tuberculosis in the community. The most common reasons for unsuccessful therapy are patient noncompliance and default, with 40 to 50 percent of patients in less developed countries discontinuing therapy prematurely (WHO 1982b).

When a patient is started on antituberculous drugs, he should be registered and close records kept on his clinic attendance. Time should be spent with the patient and his or her family to provide information about the disease to answer all questions, and to stress the need for adherence to the treatment plan.

It is helpful to remember that patient adherence to a drug regimen represents "abnormal" behavior; taking daily medication for 6 to 12 months is something most people have not done before. Furthermore, patients with tuberculosis frequently note the benefits of chemotherapy slowly and, when they do feel better, doubt the need for continued use of medication.

There is no simple way to maximize case holding but a number of steps can be taken to encourage adherence to the drug regimen including:

- Education of health workers, patients and their families, and the community should be ongoing. Health workers should be taught to stress that tuberculosis is infectious and, although it is cured by complete chemotherapy, but both disease and infectivity recur if treatment is abandoned.
- Medications should be free of charge to the patient.
- The treatment regimen should be as simple as possible with all medications given at once instead of in divided doses.
- Whenever possible, administration of drugs should be directly observed by the health workers. Unfortunately, medication picked up promptly on the day of appointment does not mean that it will actually be taken by the patient. Medications are often sold or taken home to be shared with a sick family member. Direct observation of the ingestion of medication is the only way to ensure that medications are actually taken. When daily streptomycin injections are given, the ingestion of oral medications should be observed during the visit.
- The routine use of iron and vitamin pills should be discouraged particularly if they add to confusion and cost or are suspected as a cause of adverse reactions.
- The clinic should be accessible; outlying drug distribution posts can be considered if proper supervision can be ensured.
- Patient waiting time at the clinic should be minimal.
- The clinic should be a pleasant place to visit; shelter from the sun or rain is helpful and sufficient space and chairs should be provided so that patients need not be hurried out of the clinic.
- Health workers should respond rapidly when patients miss appointments. A daily attendance register (see Record Keeping) is critical for promptly identifying these patients. The importance of staying on therapy is made clear to the patients and their families when a health worker visits within 24 to 48 hours of a missed appointment. Program supervisors should regularly question health workers about defaulters and about the problems encountered and steps taken to bring the patient back into the treatment program. Weekly or monthly conferences on problem patients can be helpful.

It can be helpful to involve the community with patients who refuse therapy. Educating (or reeducating) patients and their families and community leaders is an important responsibility for health workers. The importance of regular and uninterrupted drug ingestion must be emphasized.

Record Keeping

Registration Book

There are a myriad of possible record keeping systems. One system that worked well in some Somali refugee camps called for two separate books in each clinic; one for registration and another for attendance.

Initially, pertinent patient information is recorded in the registration book. Each patient is given one page on which is recorded the patient's name, number, age, sex, address, site of disease, presence or absence of prior therapy, initial weight, initial sputum smear date and result, and the signature of the health care worker initiating therapy. Some clinics include the patient's signature as if a treatment contract were being signed. The patient's presenting symptoms can also be recorded here. Clinics might find it helpful to provide space on each page for a medical officer or program supervisor's signature. Supervisors can review all patients registered or, perhaps, those who are started on therapy without a positive sputum

TUBERCULOSIS ATTENDANCE BOOK (Sample Page)

• = Shot given
√ = Pill given

				Treatment Completed at First of Month		January												
Patient No.	Name	Site / Smear	Meds	# Shots Finished	Weeks After Shots Finished	1	2	3	4	5	6	7	8	9	30	31	Sputum Date / Result	Weight
1	Patient's name	Pulm ⊕	SM TB-1*	60	8	√	√	√	√	√		√					1/2 ⊖	65
2	"	Pulm ⊕	SM TB-1	60	8	√	√										1/4 ⊕	62
3	"	Pulm ⊕	SM TB-1	60	7	√	√	√	√	√							1/4 ⊖	70
4	"	Pulm ⊕	SM TB-1	60	6	√	√	√	√	√							1/4 ⊖	65
5	"	Pulm ⊖	SM TB-1	60	4	√	√	√	√	√							1/4 ⊖	55
6	"	Pulm ⊕	SM TB-1	60	4		√										1/4 ⊕	44
7	"	Lymph	SM TB-1	60	2	√	√	√	√	√		√					ND	30
8	"	Pulm ⊕	SM TB-1	60	1	√	√	√	√	√		√					1/5 ⊖	25
9	"	Lymph	SM TB-1	58	0	•√	•√	√	√	√							ND	28
10	"	Spine	SM TB-1	52	0	•√	•√	•√	•√	•√		•√					ND	32
11	"	Pulm ⊖	SM TB-1	45	0	•√	•√	•√	•√	•√		•√					1/7 ⊖	30
12	"	Pulm ⊕	SM TB-1	44	0	•√		•√				•√					1/7 ⊕	45
13	"	Pulm ⊕	SM TB-1	30	0	•√			•√								1/7 ⊕	51
14	"	Lymph	SM TB-1	30	0	•√	•√	•√	•√	•√		•√					ND	45
15	"	Spine	SM TB-1	28	0	•√	•√	•√	•√	•√		•√					ND	42

* TB-1 = isoniazid + thiacetazone

Figure 33-2. Tuberculosis attendance book sample form.

result. Such review helps to minimize overzealous empiric therapy.

The registration book is not referred to on a regular basis. Rather, it is used for collecting demographic data, for specifying occurrence of different types of tuberculosis, and for such program assessment functions as monitoring the percentage of pulmonary tuberculosis patients treated with and without positive sputum smears (See Figure 33-1).

Attendance Book

Attendance information is best recorded in one book rather than on separate cards. Figure 33-2 shows a sample page from an attendance book. On this form the most important registration information is also included at the top. The attendance and bacteriologic status of the patient is clearly displayed and nurses or health workers will be guided to their most important tasks: to keep patients on therapy and to collect monthly sputum results (for pulmonary patients). Supervisors should use this record to monitor individual patients, health workers, and overall program progress. Problem patients and program failures are identified by sputum results such as those that fail to convert or stay negative.

Laboratory Log

The laboratory should keep a log of sputums received and microscopy results. Entries should include the patient's name, birthdate or age, address, date received, health post or clinic name, container number, and result. There should be a regular dispatch of results to the clinic, preferably by written list. Supervisory personnel should regularly check the laboratory record against the clinic records to ensure reliable communication. Supervisors can also use the laboratory log to calculate the "yield" from sputum samples as follows:

Sputum yield (%)

$$= \frac{\text{No. of positive sputums}}{\text{No. of sputums examined}} \times 100$$

The yield can be used to evaluate overall case finding activities and differences between health workers or clinics.

Records for Supervisors

Local or regional supervisors should regularly collect information on who is being treated and how well the treatment program is working. Figure 33-1 is a sample form for collecting data on age, sex, and site of disease, which can be collated from clinic registration books. This information should be used to determine differences between camps and trends over time. Camps or clinics found to be treating mostly smear-negative patients should better focus case finding activities and reevaluate laboratory diagnosis. Figure 33-3 is a sample form that can be used to collect information from an attendance book to evaluate a treatment program.

EVALUATING THE TREATMENT PROGRAM

Evaluation of the treatment program is the pivotal point in effective tuberculosis control. Such evaluation should precede all decisions on expansion of case finding activities or changes in the choice of therapeutic regimen (Chaulet 1982).

The only reliable method for evaluating the treatment program is by tabulating the results of therapy for a cohort of patients. For example at the beginning of 1986, it may be worthwhile to collect the results for all patients begun on therapy between 1 Jan 1984 to 31 Dec 1984, since all of these patients are expected to have completed therapy by Jan 1986. Preliminary analysis may be made earlier. (For example in mid 1985 analysis could be done to 12 months for half the patients and to 6 months for the other half.)

Following a form, such as Fig 33-3, each patient is categorized as to status at month 3, 6, and 12. For patients who are still on therapy it is critical to record last sputum smear (or culture) because this is the only way to reliably determine outcome. An abbreviated evaluation

Camp ______________

Date ______________

OUTCOME OF THERAPY FOR SMEAR POSITIVE PATIENTS

Begun on Therapy ______________ to ______________

	Number of Patients with Noted Status at:		
	Month 3	Month 6	Month 12
ON THERAPY			
Smear positive			
Smear negative			
Smear not done			
NOT ON THERAPY			
Lost			
Moved			
Died			

Figure 33-3. Outcome of therapy for smear-positive patients form.

would record only final outcome for each patient, but it is frequently useful for the program to determine the rate of loss by quarter. For example an analysis of outcome for 5 camps in Somalia showed that 2.2%, 13.8%, 30.3%, and 43.2% of patients were lost by months 3, 6, 9, and 12 respectively. This rate of loss for the first 6 months was surprisingly low. An evaluation of sputum conversion by quarter is useful if there is lack of confidence in the regimen used (which is common among expatriates for the thiacetazone containing regimen).

Program efficacy is a function of the success of the drug regimen, for those who completed therapy, and overall case holding. Data on compliance may also be derived from the attendance book.

If sputum conversion occurs less frequently than expected, it is likely that the tuberculosis program's drug delivery system is deficient. More emphasis on direct observation of drug ingestion is likely to be necessary, and program alterations designed to increase case holding should be considered. *Mycobacterium tuberculosis* drug resistance is a less common cause of poor program results than non-compliance and default.

OTHER PREVENTIVE MEASURES

The most effective strategy for preventing tuberculosis in communities is to find pulmonary tuberculosis patients and treat them with a complete course of chemotherapy. In this way, the sputum of infectious cases is rendered noninfectious, transmission is interrupted, and new infections are prevented. Immunization with BCG vaccine and chemoprophylaxis with INH have reduced the likelihood of tuberculosis for susceptible individuals. However, neither of these methods effectively interrupts transmission, and both offer less overall community benefit than case finding and treatment (Gryzbowski 1979).

BCG

Bacillus Calmette Guerin (BCG) vaccine is derived from attenuated strains of *Mycobacterium bovis.* Presently used in many countries, BCG is given early in life with the rationale that a nonvirulent mycobacterial infection will produce immunity and thereby prevent progression of a native tuberculosis infection to disease. Some suggest that it is useful in preventing more serious forms of the disease, such as tuberculosis meningitis in children.

The benefit of BCG vaccination is in question because clinical trials report a range of protection from 0 to 80 percent (Luelmo 1982). Explanations for this variability of results include differences in vaccine strains, virulence of local *M. tuberculosis* organisms, environmental exposure to other nonpathogenic mycobacteria, and study methods used.

The present WHO policy for countries with a high tuberculosis prevalence is to vaccinate all newborns when feasible; otherwise, all children under one year of age should be vaccinated. BCG has been included in the WHO Extended Programme on Immunization (EPI) and is therefore usually administered outside of the tuberculosis program.

The decision on whether or not to use BCG will most often be made by national or international authorities. Health workers are advised not to argue against the use of BCG because it is safe, inexpensive, and possibly of value for young children. However, it is important to urge that BCG immunization not be relied on as the sole means of tuberculosis control.

INH Preventive Therapy (IPT) for Child Contact

Isoniazid taken daily for 12 months gives 70 to 90 percent protection against future tuberculosis among previously infected persons, while 6 months of IPT provides 50 to 60 percent protection (Coleman & Slutkin 1984). However, because dozens to hundreds of persons (depending on the risk group) must receive IPT for each case of tuberculosis prevented, widespread use of IPT is unjustified in countries with limited resources. Resources are better spent on finding and treating current cases of tuberculosis.

Household contacts of persons with pulmonary tuberculosis have a high risk of contracting the disease and should be evaluated. This is particularly true of children under five years of age who are good candidates for IPT. Under these circumstances, IPT is used to prevent disease in the most susceptible individuals. Young children can be given INH simultaneously with the adult index case. Contacts of persons with extrapulmonary disease need not receive IPT.

LESSONS LEARNED IN SOMALI REFUGEE CAMPS

The experience with an INH-thiacetazone-streptomycin regimen in Somali refugee camps is instructive. Initially, individual camp programs were run by many different voluntary and government agencies. Although treatment protocols were originally mandated by the Somali government, health workers had little confidence in the prescribed regimens. This resulted in premature and unnecessary manipulation of the drug regimen and frequent use of expensive reserve drugs (rifampin). The following factors are the reasons for this lack of confidence:

- Health workers lacked prior experience with the locally recommended regimen.
- Information was not readily available on the expected or achieved efficacy of the mandated regimen.
- Health workers had unrealistic expectations for rapid clinical response of tuberculosis.
- Bacteriologic evidence of response was often not being systematically collected.
- Supervision of the ingestion of medication was inadequate.

Early in 1983 a program was started in the Hiran region of Somalia to address these problems. The program included the following steps:

- Explanation to health workers and others that the regimen was expected to be 90 percent effective based on data obtained in Kenya.
- Emphasis on the importance of proper record keeping.
- Emphasis on the importance of direct observation of ingestion of medication.
- Commitment to maintaining patients on therapy for adequate periods of time.
- Regional agreement on a uniform approach to therapy using an algorithm as a basic guide. The use of reserve drugs came under more strict control of regional authorities.
- Commitment to adequate documentation of the progress of patients on therapy by monthly sputum AFB smears for appropriate patients.
- Centralized supervision of data collection.
- Closer overall program supervision by the government's regional refugee health coordinator.

The results of the program were that 90 percent of patients who complied with the prescribed regimen converted to negative sputum AFB smears after six months of therapy; most treatment failures were found to be due to patient noncompliance. These results stimulated additional confidence in the drug regimen. The focus shifted from manipulating drugs to observing medication ingestion and case holding.

An often difficult issue for health workers is the withholding of potentially more effective drugs from patients when area protocols do not call for their use. This issue commonly emerges in refugee camp tuberculosis programs because treatment regimens most often are mandated by national or international authorities. Occasionally, health workers have temporary access to more expensive, and possibly more efficacious, drugs not included in the protocols. Health workers are urged to establish guidelines to closely limit the use of reserve drugs for the following reasons:

- Certain drugs, especially rifampin, can develop a local reputation as a "magic cure," leading to the development of a black market trade for the drug and disappointment when access to the expensive drug is cut off.
- The community learns when different tuberculosis programs or clinics use different drug regimens; this may result in a lack of faith in programs that adhere to national recommendations.
- It is the organization of services and the ability of a program to keep patients on therapy that are most critical to successful therapy. Poorly organized services will yield poor results regardless of the drug regimen.

Tuberculosis programs in refugee camps frequently suffer from lack of consistent attention. This may be unavoidable because many acute problems take precedence. However, disruptions should be minimized because tuberculosis accounts for a substantial proportion of disease and death in most refugee camps. Patients lost from the program will be responsible for further spread and possible drug resistance.

The best way to insure a continuously functional program is to be sure that the essential elements are in place (ie. the drug supply, microscopy, the clinic dispensing system), establish an attendance register early that can be easily used and supervised, institute regular supervision by camp and regional medical officers. Outside consultation may be helpful to assist in program organization and evaluation, and when changes in the drug regimen are considered.

REFERENCES

Bailey GVJ, Savic D, Gothe GE, et al: Potential yield of pulmonary tuberculosis cases by direct microscopy of sputum in a district of South India. Bull WHO 1967;37:875–92.

Bleiker MA, Styblo K: The annual tuberculosis infection rate and its trend in developing countries. Bull Int Union Tuberc 1978;53:295–98.

Centers for Disease Control: Tuberculosis among indochinese refugees: an update.

Chaulet P: The chemotherapy of tuberculosis in 1983. Bull Int Un Tuberc 1983;30:603–06.

Chaulet P: Applicability of short course chemotherapy to national tuberculosis control programs of the developing countries. Geneva, WHO, 1982.

Coleman DL, Slutkin G: Chemoprophylaxis against tuberculosis. West J Med 1984;140:106–10.

Comstock G: False tuberculin test results. Chest 1975;68:465–69.

Daniel TM: Selective primary health care: strategies for control of disease in the developing world. II. Tuberculosis. Rev Infect Dis 1982;4:1254–65.

Des Prez RM, Goodwin RA: Mycobacterial diseases. In Mandell G, Douglas RG, Bennett W (eds): Principles and Practice of Infectious Diseases, 2nd ed, pp 1383–1406. New York, Wiley, 1985.

East African British Medical Research Council: Isoniazid with thiacetazone in the treatment of pulmonary tuberculosis in East Africa. Tubercle 1970;51:353–58.

Eilersten E: Epidemics of primary tuberculosis and their significance. Acta Tuberc Scand 1959;37:203–10.

Glassroth J, Robins AG, Snider DE, Jr.: Tuberculosis in the 1980s. New Engl J Med 1980;302:1441–50.

Gryzbowski S: Strategy for worldwide control of tuberculosis. Chest 1979;76:812–15.

Gryzbowski S, Enarson DA: The fate of cases of pulmonary tuberculosis under various treatment programmes. Bull Int Un Tuberc 1978;53:70–75.

Hershfield E: Tuberculosis in the world. Chest 1979;76 (suppl):805–15.

Huhti E et al: Tuberculosis of the cervical lymph nodes: A clinical, pathological and bacteriological study. Tubercle 1975;56:27–36.

Kennedy DH, Fallon RJ: Tuberculous meningitis. JAMA 1979;241:264.

Luelmo F: BCG vaccination. Am Rev Respir Dis 1982;125:70–72.

Miller FJW: Tuberculosis in children. London, Churchill Livingston, 1982.

Nyboe J: Interpretation of tuberculosis infection age curves. Bull WHO 1957;17:319–39.

Refugee Health Unit, Somali Ministry of Health: Guidelines for health care in refugee camps. Unit. Kingdom, Oxfam Press; 1982.

Rouillon A, Perdrizet S, Parrot R: Transmission of tubercle bacilli: The effects of cheomotherapy. Tubercle 1976;57:275–99.

Starr S, Berkovich S: Effect of measles, gammaglobulin-modified measles, and measles vaccine on the tuberculin test. N Engl J Med 1974;284:1255–57.

Stead WW, Dutt AK: Chemotherapy for tuberculosis today. Am Rev Respir Dis 1982;125(Suppl):94–101.

Styblo K: Surveillance of tuberculosis. Int J Epidemiol 1976;5:63–68.

Styblo K: Epidemiology of tuberculosis. Bull Int Un Tuberc 1978;53:141–48.

Styblo K, Meijer J: Impact of BCG vaccination programmes in children and young adults on the tuberculosis problem. Tubercle 1976;57:17–43.

Styblo K, Rouillion A: Estimated global incidence of smear positive pulmonary tuberculosis. Unreliability of officially reported figures on tuberculosis. Bull Int Un Tuberc 1981;56:118–26.

Sutherland I: The epidemiology of tuberculosis: Is prevention better than cure? Bull Int Union Tuberc 1981;56:127–34.

Toman K: Tuberculosis, case finding and chemotherapy. Geneva, WHO 1979.

World Health Organization: Magnitude of the tuberculosis problem in the world. Geneva, WHO 1982a.

World Health Organization: Report of a joint IUAT/WHO study group. WHO Tech Report Series No. 671, Geneva, WHO 1982b.

34
Intestinal Illness

JEAN W. PAPE
RAVI BALASUBRAMANYAN
JON E. ROHDE

Intestinal illness is one of the leading afflictions of refugee populations and the poor in underdeveloped countries. The environmental conditions faced by these populations include overcrowding, lack of an adequate water supply, lack of proper waste disposal, and poor personal hygiene—all factors that contribute to the incidence of intestinal illness.

Effective treatment of intestinal diseases requires a complete understanding of the setting in which they occur, the target population they strike, and the specific agents that produce illness.

MAGNITUDE OF THE PROBLEM

Intestinal diseases can produce a variety of clinical symptoms, including diarrhea, abdominal cramps, bloating, vomiting, and occasionally, fever. However, of these, the primary and most significant manifestation of intestinal illness is diarrhea.

Although diarrhea can affect every age group, adults usually suffer fewer than one episode of diarrhea per year. Even when adults harbor organisms, serious disease seldom results. The highest incidence of diarrhea is in childhood, particularly in countries with impoverished populations. Among refugees, children are highly exposed to environmental pathogens, lack adequate immunity, and suffer most from malnutrition. In 1980, the World Health Organization (WHO) estimated that children under five years of age (a population of some 338 million) together experienced about 1 billion episodes of diarrhea, about 2.2 per child per year. The highest incidence of diarrhea is in children under two years of age. In those under one year of age, 12 or more episodes per year have been recorded.

The percentage of hospital bed occupancy by patients with diarrhea is as high as 65 percent of the pediatric service in some hospitals. High incidence of disease and high case fatality rates combine to make diarrhea the largest single cause worldwide of death in children under age five. In 1980, every minute ten children died of diarrheal diseases, an estimated 5 million deaths in total. High case fatality rates reflect the greater propensity of dehydration in the very young. In addition, malnourished and bottle-fed children have a much higher rate of both diarrheal diseases and death than age-matched peers who are better nourished and exclusively breastfed.

Diarrheal diseases are caused by a large number of pathogens, viruses, bacteria, and parasites. Whatever the etiology of the infecting agent that produces diarrhea, acute fluid and electrolyte losses pose the most serious threat to life. Our experience in the past five years in treating over 20,000 diarrhea patients in a rehydration unit serving the underprivileged population of Port-au-Prince, Haiti, has provided numerous useful insights for the care of large numbers of patients with minimal staff and facilities in refugee camps.

DETERMINANTS OF THE DISEASE

Definition of Diarrhea

The term *diarrhea* comes from the Greek roots *dia* and *rhein,* which mean "through" and "flow," respectively. A precise definition of diarrhea is difficult because consistency and bulk of stools may vary between cultures and depend very much on diet. For practical purposes, diarrhea may be defined as the passage of two or more liquid stools daily, that is, stools that conform to the shape of the container in which they are collected. Diarrhea is arbitrarily divided into acute and chronic, a helpful distinction since some infectious agents are associated primarily with one form or the other. Most acute diarrhea resolves within four to ten days; chronic diarrhea usually lasts more than three weeks.

General Causes of Diarrhea

Diarrhea is the manifestation of a myriad of disorders. In addition to a host of infectious causes, noninfectious causes include inflammatory bowel disease, adverse reactions to drugs, lactose intolerance, tropical and nontropical sprue, carcinomas, and various endocrine states (Zollinger–Ellison syndrome, hyperthyroidism, adrenal insufficiency, and others). Infections anywhere in the body may be associated with diarrhea. For example, gastroenteritis may be the presenting symptom in as many as 30 percent of patients with malaria.

Determinants of Acute Infectious Diarrhea

Determinants of acute infectious diarrhea include the infectious agent and host factors (see Table 34-1).

The Infectious Agent

Inoculum Size

In general, a large inoculum ($>10^5$ organisms) is required to cause disease by most infectious agents transmitted in solid or liquid food. However, only a small inoculum is needed to cause gastroenteritis by *Shigella, Entamoeba histolytica,* and *Giardia lamblia.* Therefore, these agents can be transmitted from person to person without an intermediary vehicle of transmission such as food or water.

Pathophysiologic Mechanisms of Diarrhea

To produce disease, infectious agents must establish contact with the intestinal mucosa and usually bind or adhere to the cells or mucus layer. Once adherence has occurred, pathogenic organisms may interact directly with the target cells *(Shigella, Salmonella)* or indirectly through newly formed toxins (*Vibrio cholera,* toxigenic *Escherichia coli*) or preformed toxins *(Staphylococcus aureus)* (see Table 34-2). Tissue invasion or destruction and toxin production are two main mechanisms by which infectious agents cause gastroenteritis. These two properties are not mutually exclusive. Hence, infectious diarrhea is the result of either secretion of fluid into the intestinal lumen (noninflammatory diarrhea) or invasion and/or destruction of the ileal or colonic mucosa (inflammatory diarrhea).

Table 34-1. Determinants of Acute Infectious Diarrhea

A. Infectious agent
   1. Inoculum size
   2. Pathogenicity
      a. Noninflammatory diarrhea
      b. Inflammatory diarrhea
B. Host Factors
   1. Gastric acidity
   2. Small bowel motility
   3. Resident bacterial flora
   4. Immune mechanisms

Table 34-2. Pathophysiologic Mechanisms of Diarrhea

A. Noninflammatory
   1. Toxin-producing
      Vibrio cholera, ST and LT *Escherichia coli, Staphylococcus aureus, Bacillus cereus,* etc.
   2. Non-toxin-producing
      a. Invasion of enterocytes (rotaviruses, Norwalk agent)
      b. Other *(Giardia lamblia, Strongyloides stercoralis, Cryptosporidium)*
B. Inflammatory
   1. Invasion and destruction of intestinal mucosa *(Shigella* sp, nontyphoid *Salmonella, Campylobacter jejuni,* enteroinvasive *E. coli, Vibrio parahemolyticus)*
   2. Invasion of intestinal mucosa with penetration beyond the lamina propria *(Salmonella typhi, Yersinia enterocolitica, Entamoeba histolytica)*

Noninflammatory Diarrhea. Noninflammatory diarrhea is caused by either toxin-producing or non-toxin-producing agents.

Toxin-producing diarrhea (TPD) (with *V. cholera* as the prototype) is caused by an enterotoxin released by the infecting organism. *V. cholera* and some *E. coli* are capable of producing toxins that activate specific intestinal enzymes (adenyl cyclase or guanylate cyclase. These, in turn, increase the level of specific cyclic nucleotides (cAMP and cGMP, respectively). This process results in a decreased absorption of sodium and an active secretion of chloride and bicarbonate ions in the lumen of the small bowel. To maintain isotonicity within the small intestine, there is an outpouring of electrolyte-rich fluid. The colon, with its limited absorption capacity (~300 ml/day), is unable to absorb the magnitude of fluid coming from the small bowel, resulting in a high-output, watery diarrhea, characteristic of TPD.

Other bacteria associated with food poisoning *(S. aureus, Clostridium perfringens)* produce toxins that include diarrhea by a mechanism that is still unclear.

Noninflammatory diarrhea can be produced by non-toxin-producing agents such as viruses and parasites.

Viruses (rotaviruses, Norwalk agent) invade the enterocytes, changing the architecture of the intestinal mucosa. The highly specialized columnar epithelium of cillus tips is destroyed, and cuboidal secretory cells from the crypts migrate rapidly upward to take their place. This causes a reduction of absorption and an increased secretion of fluids and electrolytes, resulting in watery diarrhea.

The pathophysiologic mechanisms of diarrhea caused by *G. lamblia, Strongyloides stercoralis,* and *Cryptosporidium* are not well understood. However, the architecture of the intestinal mucosa is not destroyed by these agents.

Inflammatory Diarrhea. Inflammatory destruction of the intestinal mucosa is the other process by which microbes produce diarrhea. This mechanism (with *Samonella* and *Shigella* as prototypes) alters absorption of intestinal fluids and produces leakage of protein and inflammatory cells. The diarrheal stool is usually of small volume, bloody, mucoid, and may be associated with tenesmus. In some cases, bacteria *(Salmonella typhi)* go beyond the lamina propria and are able to get into the peripheral circulation, causing major systemic symptoms.

Inflammatory diarrhea can be distinguished from noninflammatory diarrhea by microscopic examination of fresh stools for polymorphonuclear leukocytes (PMNs). The presence of PMNs suggests an inflammatory process secondary to invasion or destruction of intestinal mucosa. The absence of PMNs is characteristic of noninflammatory mechanisms.

Host Factors

Numerous factors contribute to host defense against the infectious agents that cause gastroenteritis. These factors include gastric acid, small bowel motility, resident flora, and secretory immune defense mechanisms.

Gastric Acidity

Intestinal bacteria are generally sensitive to an acid pH; elimination of gastric pH in postgastrectomy patients or neutralization of gastric pH by sodium bicarbonate will predispose patients to develop infections with *Salmonella* organisms. Cholera is found five to ten times more frequently in patients with previous gastrectomy or achlorhydria.

Small Bowel Motility

It has been suggested that diarrhea itself is a normal physiologic means for ridding the intestine of infectious organisms. For example, the use of antiperistaltic drugs such as diphenoxylate hydrochloride with atropine (Lomotil) has been shown to increase the severity of shigellosis in adults, increase colonic damage in *Clostridium difficile* diarrhea, and prolong most other diarrhea.

The Normal Bacterial Flora

By nutritional competition and production of substances that inhibit bacterial growth, the normal bacterial flora are essential for resisting enteric pathogens. Alteration of the natural bacterial flora by antibiotics predisposes to enteric infections in experimental animals and humans.

Immune Mechanisms

The role of the immune system in the control of gastrointestinal infections has not been well defined. Intestinal antibodies (coproantibodies) have been shown to decrease the adherence of *V. cholera* to intestinal mucosa. Patients with selective IgA deficiency have an increased frequency of giardiasis. Systemic antibodies against numerous infectious agents (rotaviruses, Norwalk agent, *V. cholera, E. histolytica*) can be found. Patients with acquired immune deficiency syndrome (AIDS), who exhibit a profound defect in cellular immunity, are particularly prone to colitis with cytomegalovirus and protozoa such as *Cryptosporidium* and *Isospora belli.* The general immune system plays an important role in preventing enteric pathogens from gaining access to the blood and lymphatics. The lamina propria—with its arsenal of plasma cells, lymphocytes, and polymorphonuclear leukocytes—constitutes the last line of defense. This is why bacteremia is a rare event even in the setting of inflammatory diarrhea.

CLINICAL EVALUATION OF PATIENTS WITH DIARRHEA

Diarrhea is the major symptom of intestinal infection. It can be acute or chronic and of varying degrees of intensity. Chronic diarrhea tends to be mild (fewer than five stools per day) or moderate (five to ten stools per day). In the majority of chronic cases, no etiologic agents can be found. Parasites such as *G. lamblia, E. histolytica,* and *S. stercoralis* are the agents most commonly identified with chronic diarrhea. Coccidia (*Cryptosporidium* and *I. belli*) are frequent causes of chronic diarrhea in immunosuppressed patients. Acute diarrhea is more likely to be severe (more than ten stools per day) with rapid progression to dehydration. Most bacteria and viruses cause acute diarrhea. A useful clinical classification is to separate infectious diarrhea into inflammatory and noninflammatory categories.

Clinical Manifestations of Noninflammatory Diarrhea

Noninflammatory diarrhea accounts for more than 80 percent of all cases of infectious gastroenteritis. Toxigenic *E. coli* and rotavirus alone each account for about 15 to 20 percent of all cases among children less than two years of age. Where it has been carefully looked for in underdeveloped countries, *Cryptosporidium* has sometimes been found in a similar percentage of cases. Agents in this group primarily affect the small bowel. Inflammatory cells (PMNs and monocytes) and red blood cells are not present in the stools of patients with this type of diarrhea. Clinical manifestations of agents causing noninflammatory diarrhea are outlined in Table 34-3. No single item is pathognomonic but, taken as a group, a pattern emerges. Diarrhea is usually more prominent as a symptom in patients with noninflammatory diarrhea and tends to be watery without blood or mucus.

Dehydration is the hallmark of noninflammatory diarrhea and is particularly severe in infections caused by *V. cholera* and some enterotoxigenic *E. coli.* High fever (>38°C) is uncommon in this group, in contrast with patients with inflammatory diarrhea. Mild crampy abdominal pain is common with all the agents, but severe abdominal pain is rare. Vomiting is also rare with these agents, except for *S. aureus* food poisoning and rotavirus, in which case it usually precedes the diarrhea. The incubation period varies from 16 to 72 hours for most of these agents, except for those associated with food poisoning, which cause disease after a short incubation period.

Clinical Manifestations of Inflammatory Diarrhea

In contrast to noninflammatory diarrhea, inflammatory diarrhea is characterized by various degrees of invasion or destruction of the intestinal lining of the ileum and colon. Hence the terms *colitis* and *enterocolitis* are often used to point out the specific target sites. The presence of inflammatory cells (PMNs and/or monocytes) is the hallmark of inflammatory diarrhea. Variable amounts of red blood cells and mucus may be present as well. Clinical manifestations of agents causing inflammatory diarrhea are outlined in Table 34-4. In mild cases, and during the small bowel phase of shigellosis, for example, the stools may be watery and the disease may be mistaken for a noninflammatory type of diarrhea. However, the presence of inflammatory cells in the stools is the clue to the diagnosis. In the classic dysenteric syndrome, the stools may be grossly bloody and tenesmus may be present.

Fever (>38°C) is a common feature of enteroinvasive agents. With shigellosis, fever is seen early in the course. The onset of shigellosis is usually abrupt. Associated findings in children include convulsions and respiratory symptoms. Abdominal cramps are common in gastroenteritis due to enteroinvasive agents. Ninety-five percent of patients with *Campylobacter* and up to 65 percent of patients with *Yersinia enterocolitica* may complain of abdominal pain, which in some cases may simulate an acute abdomen. Abdominal pain, headache, and vomiting are also common complaints of patients affected with *Vibrio parahaemolyticus* gastrointestinal infection.

Bacteremia is uncommon with most enteroinvasive agents. However, bacteremia and systemic symptoms can occur when organisms invade beyond the lamina propria. For example, when diarrhea is present with *S. typhi* and *Y. enterocolitica,* a mixture of monocytes and PMNs may be found in the stools. This contrasts with the marked predominance of PMNs in the stools of patients with other forms of in-

Table 34-3. Clinical Manifestations of Noninflammatory Diarrhea

	Onset	Incubation Period (hours)	Fever[a] (>38°C)	Abdominal[a] Pain	Vomiting	Other Associated Symptoms/Signs	Duration of Symptoms (days)	Stools		WBCs in Stools
								Volume	Morphology	
Toxin-producing agents										
V. cholera	Abrupt	24–72	Uncommon	Uncommon	Rare	———	Variable	Severe	Watery, no blood, no mucus	Absent
E. coli (heat labile, heat stable)	Abrupt	24–96	Uncommon	Uncommon	Rare	———	3	Moderate to severe	Watery, no blood, no mucus	Absent
S. aureus	Abrupt	1	Uncommon	Uncommon	Very common	———	1	Moderate	Watery	Absent
Non-toxin-producing agents										
Rotaviruses (type I,II)	Insidious	16–36	Uncommon	Uncommon	Very common	Pharyngeal erythema	2–3	Moderate	Watery	Absent
Norwalk agent	Insidious	24–48	Uncommon	Uncommon	Common	———	2–3	Moderate	Watery	
G. lamblia	Variable	1–4 weeks	Uncommon	Common (cramps) may mimic duodenal ulcers	Uncommon	Bloating, flatulence malabsorption	Variable	Moderate	Watery	Absent
Cryptosporidium	Variable	?	Uncommon	Rare	Rare	———	Variable	Moderate to severe	Watery	Absent

[a]Rare, 10 percent; uncommon 30 percent; common, 50 percent; very common, 90 percent.

Table 34-4. Clinical Manifestations of Inflammatory Diarrhea

	Onset	Incubation Period (hours)	Fever (>38°C)	Abdominal Pain	Vomiting	Other Associated Symptoms/ Signs	Stools		Duration of Symptoms (days)	WCBs in Stools
							Volume	Morphology		
Shigella	Abrupt	24–72	Common	Common (cramps)	Uncommon	Convulsions + respiratory symptoms in children	Moderate	Watery, odorless, w/blood + mucus	3–20	Polys
Enteroinvasive *E. coli*	Abrupt	48–72	Common	Common (cramps)	Uncommon	———	Moderate	Watery, odorless, w/ blood + mucus	3–7	Polys
Salmonella enteriditis	Variable	12–72	Common	Common (cramps)	Common	———	Moderate	Loose, foul-smelling green +/- blood + mucus	5–7	Polys
Vibrio parahemoliticus	Abrupt	16–72	Common	Common (cramps)	Common	Headache	Moderate	Watery +/- blood + mucus	2–3	Polys
Campylobacter jejuni	Abrupt	48–96	Common	Common (severe) may develop acute abdomen	Uncommon	———	Moderate	Watery, blood and mucus common	2–4	Polys
Yersinia enterolitica	Abrupt	16–48	Common	Common (severe) may develop acute abdomen	Uncommon	Migratory polyarthritis, Reiter's syndrome, *E. nodulum*	Moderate	Watery blood and mucus common	7–21	Polys, mono
Salmonella typhi	Insidious	Days	100%	Uncommon unless complications develop	Uncommon	Bacteremia, headache, cough, epitaxis	Mild diarrhea 1st 2 weeks	Watery, blood + mucus only if complications develop	7–21	Mono, polys
Entamoeba histolytica	Variable	Days	Uncommon	Uncommon	Uncommon	———	Moderate	Watery w/blood + mucus	4–21	Polys

flammatory diarrhea. Fecal leukocytes and variable amounts of blood and mucus are commonly associated with *E. histolytica* colitis, which mimics *Shigella* dysentery. However, the insidious presentation, the more chronic nature of *E. histolytica* colitis, and the absence of high fever are helpful distinguishing characteristics.

Specific Evaluation of Patients with Diarrhea

The main goal of the history and physical examination is to quickly assess the patient's hydration status, nutrition level, and the presence of associated diseases. As the history and the physical examination are being obtained and recorded, oral rehydration therapy (ORT) should be initiated (see Chapter 15). If the patient cannot drink, ORT can be delivered by nasogastric tube. For patients with persistent vomiting, ileus, or shock, intravenous therapy with Ringer's lactate or normal saline with 5 percent dextrose should be begun at once.

History

A set of six questions is helpful in assessing the severity, character (watery versus inflammatory), and type (acute versus chronic) of diarrhea:

1. Does the patient actually have diarrhea, that is, frequent liquid stools? If the frequency is more than every hour, this indicates an acute condition that will quickly lead to dehydration. The character of the stools is also helpful. Are the stools bloody, mucoid, or watery?
2. How long has the diarrhea lasted? Has it lasted for three or more weeks?
3. Is vomiting present? If so, how frequently? Is vomiting present at every meal? If so, ask the parents to show how the child is positioned when eating. Since the supine horizontal position favors vomiting, the child should preferably be sitting on his mother's lap. If the child is bottlefed, ask to see the size of the feeding bottle hole. Children fed from a bottle with a large hole may be prone to vomit. If feeding position and bottle hole size are correct, the presence of vomiting may suggest some specific infectious process, for example, rotavirus. Vomiting by itself is rarely an indication for intravenous fluids and cessation of oral intake. In our experience, only 1 percent of vomiting is serious enough to interfere with oral rehydration.
4. When was the last time the child passed urine? Was the urine light or concentrated? The passage of urine is one of the best estimates of dehydration status. Urine passed more than eight hours before evaluation suggests severe dehydration.
5. Is fever present? If so, is it associated with convulsions? In our experience, 90 percent of dehydrated children present with fever (>38°C). It is not necessary to do an elaborate laboratory workup for every patient with fever since it usually returns to normal within 12 hours of rehydration. Convulsions may be present in young infants with *Shigella* infections or just with high temperature (>40°C) rectally). Rectal temperature is preferable to axillary temperature as the skin may be cold due to poor circulation.
6. Has any oral rehydration solution been given? Is the child receiving any drug (particularly antibiotics)? The use of antibiotics (ampicillin and lincomycin in particular) may be associated with diarrhea, and occasionally with antibiotic-associated colitis.

Physical Examination

The patient's vital signs are taken immediately. These include rectal temperature, pulse, respiratory rate, and, when possible, blood pressure.

Weight, height, weight for height, and weight for age percentile will help determine nutritional status (see Chapter 14). Weight of patients is also helpful in initiating therapy.

If and when urine is available, obtain a specific gravity because this correlates well with dehydration status. A value of less than 1.010 indicates good hydration, while values over 1.020 are a source for concern. Register all the data on a flowsheet such as that supplied in Figure 34-1. If facilities and staffing permit, vital signs are taken every hour for the first six hours. To follow the progress of rehydration, weight is obtained every six hours. A rough evaluation of fluid losses in infants is estimated as follows: 30 cc per stool, 15 cc per urination or vomiting. For a child above one year of age, double these estimates. Total input is recorded.

Determination of the State of Dehydration

The characteristics of mild and severe dehydration are easily recognized, and moderate

Name ______________ Age ____ Sex ____ Degree of Dehydration ____ % Date ______

Other Medical Problems: ______________

30 cc per stool
15 cc per urination
15 cc per emesis

Hour of Evaluation	Weight	Temperature	BP	Pulse	Resp. Rate	Urine Specific Gravity	Output			Estimated Total Output	Intake			Estimated Total Intake	Comments
							Urine	Stool	Emesis		PO	IV	Other		

Figure 34-1. Twelve hour rehydration form.

dehydration is best defined as those cases that fall in between. When the patient's original weight is known, it is helpful to evaluate the state of dehydration: a 4 to 5 percent body weight loss corresponds to mild dehydration, 6 to 7 percent to moderate dehydration, and 10 percent or more to severe dehydration. This is usually not useful, however, because the original weight of patients living in low socioeconomic settings is rarely known. In addition, the age group most susceptible to diarrheal diseases is likely to have rapid weight gain or loss over short periods of time, making this information, when available, almost useless for evaluating the degree of dehydration.

There are specific guidelines that correlate with three clinically evaluable degrees of dehydration (Table 34-5). Of all the signs, mental status and urine flow are the best guidelines to evaluate degrees of dehydration (i.e., mild, moderate, or severe). If two or more signs of severe dehydration are present, the patient

Table 34-5. Determination of the State of Dehydration

Signs and Symptoms	State of Dehydration		
	Mild	Moderate	Severe
Mental status	Alert, thirsty	Irritable, thirsty	Depressed (lethargic, stuporous, rarely comatose)
Urine flow	Normal	Reduced and concentrated	None in the last 8–12 hours
Pulse	Normal	Rapid	Rapid, weak
Respiration	Normal	Deep	Deep and rapid
Tears	Present	Absent	Absent
Mucous membranes	Moist	Dry	Very dry
Eyes	Normal	Sunken	Deeply sunken
Anterior fontanels[a]	Normal	Sunken	Very sunken
Skin elasticity	Pinch reacts immediately (1 second)	Pinch reacts slowly (2 seconds)	Pinch reacts very slowly (>2 seconds)

[a]Useful in infants until fontanels close at 9 to 18 months of age.

should be considered to have severe dehydration. Similarly, two or more signs of moderate dehydration are evidence of the presence of such dehydration. Of all the signs, skin elasticity is the most unreliable indicator of dehydration status in malnourished populations. Indeed, marasmus is usually associated with decreased skin elasticity, whereas obese infants may not show a decreased skin elasticity even in the presence of moderate dehydration.

Mild Dehydration

There is usually no difficulty in determining that a patient has mild dehydration; by all criteria, the patient is normal. Such patients only present with a history of diarrhea and may be thirsty.

Severe Dehydration

In our experience, markedly depressed mental status (lethargy, stupor, or coma) and no urination in the last 8 to 12 hours before evaluation are indicators of severe dehydration. Very sunken anterior fontanels in patients less than 18 months old as well as absent lacrimation in all children are additional helpful signs. Deep and rapid respiration in the absence of pneumonia (greater than 50 breaths per minute) is a manifestation of metabolic acidosis, which often accompanies severe dehydration.

Moderate Dehydration

It is a matter of clinical judgment to determine moderate dehydration, since such patients present, to some degree, with all the signs and symptoms of patients with severe dehydration. Lethargy and reduced urine flow are not as marked as for patients with severe dehydration. However, when in doubt as to whether a patient is moderately or severely dehydrated, it is best to consider him or her severely dehydrated.

MANAGEMENT OF PATIENTS WITH DIARRHEA AND DEHYDRATION

The management of patients with diarrhea and dehydration is outlined in Table 34-6. The main acute threat of diarrhea is dehydration, but in the long run, its contribution to undernutrition may be even more important. Infants and young children are particularly susceptible to dehydration due to diarrhea. In children under two, about 10 percent of diarrheal episodes are serious enough to cause dehydration, and 1 percent are life-threatening. Undernutrition, a frequent complication of gastroenteritis, predisposes to serious infections and further diarrhea. Factors that contribute to the reduction of mortality in patients with severe dehydration are prompt initiation of rehydration therapy, proper utilization of oral therapy (ORT), early and continual feeding, recognition and treatment of associated disease, and integration of the mother as part of the therapeutic team.

Table 34-6. Six Steps for the Management of Patients with Diarrhea and Dehydration

1. Start giving ORT before any evaluation (If patient cannot take ORT, start IV Ringer's lactate. See Chapter 15.)
2. Assess degree of dehydration
   a. For mild to moderate dehydration, give ORT (see Chapter 15).
   b. For severe dehydration or if patient is unable to drink, start or continue Ringer's lactate.
3. Assess for associated diseases
   a. Clinical evaluation to rule out otitis media, pharyngitis, pneumonia, measles, meningitis.
      (1) If cause for fever found, treat accordingly.
      (2) If cause for fever not found, do laboratory evaluation.
   b. Laboratory evaluation—Should include malaria smears, methylene blue stain, stools for ova and parasites (to rule out *E. histolytica, G. lamblia*), and fecal leukocytes (see Chapter 22) for evidence of *Salmonella or Shigella* infection.
4. Rehydration phase (first 4 to 6 hours)
   a. Evaluate and record vital signs and frequency of stools, urine, vomiting, input, and estimated output every hour if feasible. Do not stop breastfeeding.
5. Maintenance phase (after the first 4 to 6 hours)
   a. If child was receiving IV Ringer's lactate and able to drink, change to ORT if passing urine.
   b. If child was receiving ORT, continue ORT, adjusted to severity of diarrhea.
6. Feeding
   a. Continue breastfeeding. For nonbreastfed children, start diluted artificial milk. For all children, start high-calorie food. Continue extra food for at least several days after diarrhea stops.

Prompt Initiation of Rehydration Therapy

Fluid replacement is the first and only effective treatment for dehydration from any cause. While assessing a patient for dehydration status and associated diseases, one should provide ORT to test the ability of the patient to drink; if he or she is able to drink, ORT should be continued by the mother or attending parent while clinical assessment is in progress. (Chapter 15 provides further details on oral rehydration, and fluid and electrolyte therapy.) If the child cannot drink for any reason (severe dehydration, frequent vomiting, depressed sensorium, etc.), an intravenous line with Ringer's lactate should be set up immediately. Remember that a few minutes' delay can be fatal for a patient with severe dehydration.

Early and Continued Feeding

General Considerations

Of all common illnesses, diarrhea has the most adverse effect on nutrition. Anorexia induced by fluid and electrolyte losses, fever, and withholding of food due to cultural beliefs all reduce nutritional intake. In addition, during the diarrheal process, there is a decreased absorption of nutrients by 20 percent for carbohydrates and up to 50 percent for fat. Moreover, protein loss in the gut has been documented in both inflammatory *(Shigella)* and noninflammatory (enterotoxigenic *E. coli*) diarrhea. There is a disadvantage in "resting" the bowel during and following diarrheal episodes. Indeed, fasting can further reduce the absorptive capacity of the intestine. When all these detrimental nutritional mechanisms come into play, a child with diarrhea may lose up to 5 g/kg of body mass per day. Young children in impoverished regions may have diarrhea for as many as 60 days during the course of a year; this can account for an annual deficit of up to 75 percent of their expected growth. Hence, good nutrition during the diarrheal process is essential.

Feeding

During the Rehydration Phase

- For breastfed children, breastfeeding should not be stopped during the four- to six-hour rehydration period.
- For nonbreastfed children, artificial milk should be avoided during this short period.

During the Maintenance Phase

- For breastfed children, breastfeeding should be continued on demand.
- For nonbreastfed children, the artificial milk normally used should be resumed but should be diluted with an equal volume of plain water.
- High-energy food, including fat, should be encouraged for all children.

During the Convalescent Period

All previously consumed food should be resumed, including artificial milk at full strength for nonbreastfed children. This period is usually associated with a rise in appetite, which should be exploited. The goal is to regain or exceed pre–illness weight. Nutritional intervention during this period may be the most effective means of avoiding nutritional deficit. There is evidence that adequate feeding during this period may reduce the susceptibility to further episodes of diarrhea by 50 percent.

Recognition and Treatment of Associated Diseases

Another factor contributing to death in patients with diarrhea is the presence of associated infections, which may be present in up to 12 percent of patients with acute diarrhea. The most frequent infections are otitis media, pneumonia, pharyngitis, malaria, measles, meningitis, and *Salmonella* (usually *S. typhi*) bacteremia (see Table 34-7). The presence of pneumonia, malaria, meningitis, and typhoid fever worsen the prognosis by 20-fold or more. Very high fever (>40°C), or prolonged fever—that is, an elevated temperature (>38.5°C) that persists beyond 12 hours after the patient has been rehydrated—is an indication that an associated infection may be present.

Clinical Clues

Otitis Media and Pharyngitis

Otitis media and pharyngitis can be readily ruled out by clinical examination.

Table 34-7. Associated Infections in Patients Presenting with Acute Diarrhea[a]

Infection	Percentage of Patients with Each Type of Infection
Otitis media	31.0
Pneumonia	26.0
Pharyngitis	20.0
Malaria	11.0
Measles with pneumonia	5.0
Meningitis	5.0
Typhoid fever	2.0

[a]Twelve percent of 8459 patients with acute diarrhea seen at the Rehydration Unit of the State University Hospital, Port-au-Prince, Haiti, had associated infections in 1980–82.

Pneumonia

While rapid breathing (greater than 50 breaths per minute) can be seen in both lower respiratory infections and acidosis, the depth of respiration is a useful clue to the presence of acidosis. The respiratory rate should then decrease gradually as the patient is being rehydrated. Persistence of rapid breathing in a patient in the absence of other signs of severe dehydration is an indication of pneumonia or septicemia. Very early, when the patient is dehydrated, there may be no abnormal auscultatory sounds; the presence of rales usually becomes evident once the patient is fully rehydrated. Patients with measles should be watched for the presence of associated pneumonia.

Malaria

Wherever malaria is endemic, it should be considered in patients who have prolonged fever.

Meningitis/Septicemia

Clinical suspicion of meningitis or septicemia should arise in the presence of either prolonged fever or abnormally low temperature ($<36°C$), rapid breathing and normal auscultatory sounds, vomiting, altered mental status, and normal urine flow. In a young patient (18 months or younger), bulging of the anterior fontanels is an important sign of meningitis. In this setting, a rapid feeble pulse may indicate hypovolemic shock and septicemia. Once diagnosed, these conditions should be treated immediately.

Advanced Malnutrition

Malnutrition is frequently associated with diarrheal diseases in underdeveloped countries, particularly in the zero- to five-year age group. In Bangladesh refugee camps, advanced malnutrition affected 11 percent of all children and 20 percent of the zero- to five-year age group. Although incidence of infection does not vary significantly by nutritional status, the severity of disease as measured by stool output, duration, or electrolyte abnormalities is far greater in the malnourished. The malnutritional status of patients with diarrhea correlates with mortality rates. In the rehydration unit of the State University Hospital of Haiti, 15 percent of patients had second- or third-degree malnutrition, and this group accounted for 84 percent of all deaths.

Chronic Diarrhea

For patients with chronic or persistent diarrhea, stools for ova and parasites and a modified Ziehl-Neelsen stain on the stools are performed. Direct examination of the stool for ova and parasites is done to look for *E. histolytica* (more likely if the methylene blue stain for leukocytes is positive), *G. lamblia,* and *S. stercoralis.* The modified Ziehl–Neelsen stain is done to look for *Cryptosporidium* (more likely if the methylene blue stain for leukocytes is negative).

Integration of the Mother as Part of the Therapeutic Team

There are numerous advantages in involving mothers directly in the care of their children. The mother's full-time presence will reduce the need for costly medical personnel, and she is the person most interested in the well-being of her child. Mothers learn by doing and, once trained, continue therapy at home and become effective community educators and role models in their neighborhoods. Mothers who are successful in providing ORT to their children are the most effective promoters of ORT in their communities. During the period that the mother provides active care to her child under supervision, she learns how to make ORT solution and perform basic hygienic practices such as washing hands and breasts with soap and water before nursing. Because she is not physically separated from her child at any time, breastfeeding practices can continue, which eliminates the danger of the mother's milk drying up. As noted earlier, many children in the underdeveloped world have diarrhea for 60 days or more each year during the first three years of life. Hence, it is quite likely that the practical knowledge gained by the mother will be put to use for the same child or a sibling. A mother who has previously rehydrated her child under guidance is likely to initiate ORT early at home in subsequent episodes. Since the great threat of diarrheal diseases is dehydration, rehydration early in the course of the disease is the most effective intervention. In recent years, more than two thirds of mothers have started rehydration before bringing their children to our hospital. Severe dehydration on admission has dropped from 27 percent to under 5 percent as a result. Mothers are the key to the success of ORT.

Table 34-8. Indications for Antimicrobial Therapy

Cause	Treatment of Choice	Children	Adults	Alternative Therapy	Children	Adults
Cholera	Tetracycline	50 mg/kg/day	250 mg every 6 hours for 5 days	Erythromycin	30 mg/kg/day in 3 doses for 5 days	250 mg every 6 hours for 5 days
Shigella dysentery	Trimethoprim (TMP), sulfamethoxasole (SMX)	TMP 10mg/kg/day + SMX 50 mg/kg/day in 2 doses for 5 days	TMP 160 mg + SMX 800 mg every 12 hours for 5 days	Tetracycline	50 mg/kg/day in 4 doses for 5 days for children and adults	
Acute amebic dysentery	Metronidazole	30 mg/kg/day for 5 to 10 days	750 mg every 8 hours for 5 to 10 days	Dehydroemetine, Hydrochloride	1–1.5 mg/kg up to a maximum of 90 mg for 3 to 5 days for children and adults	
Acute giardiasis	Metronidazole	15 mg/kg/day for 5 days	250 mg every 8 hours for 5 days	Quinacrine	7 mg/kg/day in 3 doses for 5 days	100 mg every 8 hours for 5 days

ADDITIONAL THERAPY

Additional therapy in the form of antibiotics, absorbents (kaolin), a combination of both (kaomycin), and antimotility drugs are unnecessary, potentially harmful, and add to the cost of therapy. Their major disadvantage is in distracting from the most simple, effective treatment: rehydration.

Antibiotics

The natural history of about 90 percent of all acute gastroenteritis is that the diarrhea stops by itself. Antibiotics are usually not indicated and may actually be harmful by causing diarrhea or antibiotic-associated colitis. Antibiotics will, however, decrease the severity and duration of cholera, severe *Shigella* dysentery, and severe infections due to *Campylobacter* or *Yersinia* (see Table 34-8). Each of these agents requires a specific antibiotic. In most refugee camps, bacterial cultures are not available. Even when cultures can be obtained, results are not available for two days, and by that time diarrhea will have stopped in most cases without any specific intervention. In addition, stool cultures are expensive and may cost 40 to 50 times more than rehydration treatment. When resources permit, stool cultures should be used only for inflammatory diarrhea, that is, after a positive methylene blue stain, or when epidemics of cholera are suspected and confirmation by culture is needed. Additional indications for antimicrobials are acute giardiasis and amebic dysentery.

Other Drugs

Antimotility drugs (opiates, Lomotil, loperamide) decrease gut motility; they may prolong the course of diarrhea and worsen systemic symptoms.

Absorbent drugs (kaolin-pectin) have no effect on the duration or severity of diarrhea.

CONCLUSION

Control of diarrheal diseases in refugee camps requires major improvements in sanitation, water supplies, and overcrowding. Early rehydration and feeding also produce marked reduction in diarrheal mortality and morbidity. Malnutrition can be reduced if caloric intake, particularly through breastfeeding, is continued during diarrheal attacks and increased during the convalescent period. Severe dehydration—the major cause of diarrheal death—can be avoided by training mothers with the concept that the treatment of diarrheal diseases does not begin in the clinic but in the home.

REFERENCES AND SELECTED READING

Black RE et al: Longitudinal studies of infectious diseases and physical growth in rural Bangladesh. Pattern of morbidity. J Epidemiol 1982;115(3):305–14.

Carpenter CJ: The pathophysiology of secretory diarrhea. Med Clin North Am 1982;597–610.

Dupont HL, Hornick RB: Adverse effect of Lomotil therapy in shigellosis. JAMA 1973;226:1525–28.

Gardner P et al: Health priorities among Bangladesh refugees. Lancet 1972;834–36.

Hirschhorn N: The treatment of acute diarrhea in children; an historical and physiological perspective. Am J Clin Nutr 1980; 33:637–63.

Hornick RB et al: Fecal leukocytes in diarrheal illness. Ann Intern Med 1976;76:697–703.

Pape JW et al: Management of diarrhea in Haiti: Mortality reduction in 8,443 hospitalized children. Proceedings of the Int Conference on Oral Rehydration Therapy. Washington DC, Agency for International Development 1983;87–89.

Pape JW et al: *Cryptosporidium* in Haitian children. Presentation at the American Federation of Clinical Research, Washington DC, 1985.

Parker RL et al: Oral rehydration therapy (ORT) for childhood diarrhea. Popul Reports [L] 1980;8:41–75.

Rohde JE: Therapeutic interventions in diarrhea. Food Nutr Bull 1981;3(4):34–38.

Rohde JE: Selective primary health care: Strategies for control of disease in the developing world. XV. Acute diarrhea. Rev Infect Dis 1984;6(6):840–53.

Rosenberg IH et al: Malabsorption associated with diarrhea and intestinal infections. Am J Clin Nutr 1977;30:1248.

Sack BR et al: The current status of oral therapy in the treatment of acute diarrheal illness. Am J Clin Nutr 1978;31:2251–57.

Scientific Working Group: Diarrheal diseases control programme: A manual for the treatment of acute diarrhoea. Publication No WHO/CDC/SER/80. 2 Rev 1. Geneva, World Health Organization, 1984.

Snyder JD, Merson MH: The magnitude of the global problem of acute diarrheal disease: A review of active surveillance data. Bull WHO 1982;60(4):605–13.

35
Common Intestinal Parasites

THOMAS C. JONES

The tropical environments in general, and refugee and other poverty-plagued populations in particular, are characterized by numerous intestinal protozoa and helminths (commonly called parasites). Helminths differ remarkably from protozoa; the former are complex small animals with digestive, nervous, muscular, and reproductive systems, and the latter are single-celled microbes. They are considered together because they are commonly diagnosed by microscopic inspection of stool specimens. In the case of helminths, one looks for the eggs resulting from the reproductive process of the worms; in the case of protozoa, one looks for the tissue-invasive form of the single-cell (trophozoite) or the protected form (cyst).

There are two important protozoal causes of illness among refugees: *Entamoeba histolytica,* the cause of amebiasis, and *Giardia lamblia,* the cause of giardiasis. *Cryptosporidium,* a recently identified protozoa, may also contribute to illness among refugees, but this has not yet been documented. Nine helminths are of importance among refugees—the roundworms, *Ascaris lumbricoides,* hookworm, *Strongyloides stercoralis, Trichuris trichuria,* and pinworm; the flat worms, *Taenia sp.* and *Hymenolepis nana;* and the flukes, *Schistosoma sp.* and *Clonorchis sinensis.* Their presence depends on exposure to the infection prior to entering the refugee setting, living conditions in the camp or settlement, and personal habits of the refugees, including food and water preparation. For example, clonorchis is seen only in the Orient among those who eat raw freshwater fish; schistosomiasis occurs among those who swim in contaminated water; pinworm and *Hymenolepis* are present in areas where crowding of young children occurs. The dominant intestinal parasites may change as the environment or conditions of a refugee setting change. In Thailand, among the first Cambodian refugees to arrive in large numbers at border camps, the important intestinal parasites were *E. histolytica,* hookworm, *Ascaris,* and *Strongyloides.* When the camps were better established, contaminated water and crowded conditions persisted and the most common parasites were *Giardia lamblia* and *Hymenolepis nana.* To demonstrate the magnitude of the problem, in one Cambodian refugee camp 40 percent of submitted stool specimens were positive for some parasite; *E. histolytica, Giardia, Ascaris,* hookworm, *Hymenolepis, Strongyloides,* and *Trichuris* being the most common. Many refugees had two or three different parasites at the same time; the record was six in one patient.

Many of these organisms have infected the refugee for many years and there is little need for rapid treatment. Parasite eradication is an important component of a public health program in the refugee setting, but there are few indications for vigorous therapeutic programs when resources are limited. Control of measles, meningitis, and malaria, and improvement of nutritional status are far more important. When facilities allow, careful case identification and treatment will improve overall patient well-being and allow beneficial results of effective nutrition programs. The most important infections to treat are heavy parasitemia by *Ascaris,* hookworm, or *Strongyloides,* and symptomatic disease due to ameba, *Giardia,* or *Hymenolepis.* Following are descriptions of the diseases caused by these parasites and their management.

PROTOZOA

Amebiasis *(Entamoeba histolytica)*

Amebiasis is transmitted by food and water contaminated with fecal matter. *Entamoeba histolytica,* the organism that causes amebiasis, is ingested by a human host and goes to the large intestine where damage is caused (Ravdin & Jones 1985).

Symptoms vary. Chronic cyst carriers may be asymptomatic whereas other patients have vague complaints of occasional, diffuse, crampy abdominal pain often alternating with diarrhea and constipation. The ameba can invade the submucosa and create symptoms of colitis (diarrhea with pus and blood). In severe cases, perforation of the bowel with peritonitis, or amebic liver abscess may occur. Therefore, all patients suspected of amebiasis should be checked for liver tenderness and hepatomegaly.

Definitive diagnosis can be difficult to make. Fresh stool samples, smears obtained by proctoscopy, aspirates of abscesses, or tissue sections can all be used. Observation of the *E. histolytica* cysts or the straight-line movement of the trophozoites in fresh specimens without fixative is helpful in making the diagnosis. On microscopic examination, the organism can easily be confused with nonpathogenic ameba (see Chapter 22). Differential diagnosis of amebic dysentery includes shigellosis, appendicitis, diverticulitis, and ulcerative colitis.

The two most common complications of amebiasis are peritonitis and liver abscess. Surgical drainage of even large amebic liver abscesses is usually not required because they respond well to medication. Metronidazole is the drug of choice for serious disease. In severely ill patients, emetine and chloroquine may also be indicated. Diiodohydroxyquin is recommended, when available, to eradicate the cyst stage in the intestine, thus preventing recurrent invasive infection.

Giardiasis *(Giardia lamblia)*

Giardia lamblia is a pear-shaped, multiflagellar protozoal parasite (Wolf 1978). It spreads through fecal–oral contamination from human to human, and by infected animals such as beavers. Drinking water contaminated with infected stool is a common cause of outbreaks of giardiasis. Once ingested, the parasite populates the duodenum and jejunum. No extraintestinal stage is known. Although young children have the highest prevalence rates, all age groups are affected. *Giardia lamblia* is one of the most common intestinal parasites and is found in all parts of the world. In the United States, giardiasis is prevalent within the homosexual community, in rural mountainous areas, and in day care centers.

In endemic areas, more than two thirds of those harboring the parasite may be asymptomatic. However, patients affected from point source outbreaks usually display symptoms. In these cases, watery diarrhea may have a rapid onset. Stools are foul smelling and fatty but without pus or blood. Crampy epigastric abdominal pain, anorexia, nausea, vomiting, and a low-grade fever may be present. Typically, the acute symptoms persist for a few weeks but they may last for months. Recurrent episodes of epigastric pain, flatulence, and soft stools may occur separated by symptom-free periods.

Diagnosis is made by identifying the cyst or the trophozoite in the stool. Unless a preservative such as formalin is used, stools should be examined within one hour. Many stool specimens may be needed to identify the parasite in those chronically infected. Metronidazole and quinacrine are the drugs of choice (Medical Letter 1982).

Cryptosporidiosis

Cryptosporidiosis is a newly recognized intestinal protozoal infection that is very common in tropical and subtropical areas and is increasingly recognized as a cause of diarrhea in visitors to these areas (Soave 1985). The organism is a small coccidian parasite (3 to 4 μ in diameter) that infects mucosal cells of the intestinal tract. It induces watery diarrhea without dysentery, similar to that seen in giardiasis. In otherwise healthy individuals, the disease is self-limiting and lasts one to two weeks. In immunosuppressed patients, perhaps including those nutritionally deficient refugees, however, the illness can be prolonged and is associated with marked morbidity. The presence of the organism can be documented by doing a Ziehl–Neelsen acid-fast stain on the stool (Ma & Soave 1983). Symptomatic patients usually have large numbers of organisms in their stool. There is no effective therapy at present.

HELMINTHS

Nematodes (roundworms)

Ascaris lumbricoides

This large (15 to 20 cm) roundworm is the most common intestinal parasite in the world, with an estimated worldwide prevalence of 1 billion infections (Marsden 1982). If a roundworm this large is seen in the stool, it is pathognomonic of *Ascaris*. The parasite is transmitted through the fecal–oral route, contaminated soil being a key intermediate vehicle since several days for egg maturation are required in this environment. Ingested eggs hatch in the small intestine. Larvae migrate through the bowel wall and, through hematogenous and lymphatic channels, spread to the lungs. There they transverse the alveoli, migrate up the trachea, are swallowed, and travel down the esophagus to the small intestine. Here the adults mature and, depending on their number, may produce obstruction of the abdominal viscera.

The symptoms of ascaris infection vary. Most infections are asymptomatic or cause only vague abdominal discomfort. Inflammatory reaction in the lungs sometimes occurs, leading to a set of clinical findings termed the Loeffler syndrome. This is manifested by dyspnea, transient fever, cough, eosinophilia in sputum and peripheral blood, and diffuse opacities on chest x-ray studies. These signs and symptoms are usually transient and resolve spontaneously. In children, large tangles of worms may cause bowel obstruction. The worms occasionally may be seen in vomitus. Biliary tract obstruction is sometimes seen when worms gain access to the common bile duct. Patients with this disorder usually complain of acute, colicky epigastric pain, nausea, and vomiting. Jaundice is a late manifestation.

Diagnosis of ascariasis is made by identifying large worms in the stool or by viewing *Ascaris* eggs by microscopic examination of fresh stool (see Chapter 22). Mebendazole, pyrantel pamoate, and piperzine are effective in therapy. Therapy should be cautious when a large number of worms are present because a bolus of worms may cause intestinal obstruction even after drug treatment. One should first ensure proper hydration and effective intestinal motility to avoid this complication.

Hookworm (*Ancylostoma duodenale* and *Necator americanus*)

Hookworms are small (1 cm) parasites distributed widely in temperate and tropical areas (Marsden 1982). Their eggs hatch in warm, moist soil. Larvae become infective after five days and penetrate the skin of unprotected feet. Lymph channels bring the parasite to the lungs where they travel through the alveoli and up the trachea. There, they are swallowed and lodge in the proximal portion of the small intestine. A single hookworm consumes about 0.2 ml of blood per day, which leads to the most common sign of hookworm infection—iron-deficiency anemia. The anemia and hypoalbuminemia, also often present, represent an imbalance between blood loss and dietary intake. Severe infections can lead to a 2-g per 100-ml hemoglobin concentration and resultant high-output congestive heart failure. Usually, however, the infection is associated with few symptoms such as nonspecific abdominal pain. It may present as "ground itch," an intensely pruritic, erythematous papular vesicular rash on the plantar surfaces and other cutaneous sites of larvae penetration. Pulmonary involvement may resemble Loeffler's syndrome, as described in the section on *Ascaris*. Diagnosis is made by observing the hookworm eggs in the stool (see Chapter 22). Mebendazole and pyrantel pamoate provide effective therapy.

Strongyloides stercoralis

Strongyloides stercoralis is a small (1 to 2 mm) worm with a complex life cycle (Masur & Jones 1982). The infection begins with penetration of the skin by free-living larvae found in contaminated soil. Continuous reinfection is possible because the eggs can hatch before leaving the host's bowel. This enables larvae to penetrate intestinal walls or perirectal regions, enter the lymphatic channels, and travel to the lungs where they continue the same cycle as the hookworm parasite. Thus, *Strongyloides* is unique in that infection by only a few larvae can lead to an overwhelming increase in the worm population from secondary autoinfection.

About one third of patients with *Strongyloides* infection are asymptomatic. Symptoms include "ground itch," which occurs when the larvae enter the skin; eosinophilic pneumonia during migration, which resembles Loeffler's syndrome; and burning, colicky midepigastric pain, which may simulate peptic ulcer disease. Diarrhea with mucus is often present. Nausea, vomiting, weight loss, and eosinophilia are seen. Protein-losing enteropathy may lead to hypoproteinemia severe enough to cause edema suggestive of nephrotic syndrome. Five to 20 percent of patients with *Strongyloides* infection will develop a generalized pruritic urticarial rash, which often begins in the perineal region and extends to the trunk and thighs. Autoinfection can lead to massive larval invasion of the lungs and other tissues, particularly in immunocompromised hosts such as those who have been given corticosteroids or are malnourished.

Diagnosis is made by identifying the larvae on microscopic examination of freshly passed stool or aspirated duodenal material. Concentrating the stool specimen can be helpful. Several examinations may be necessary to rule out disease. Thiabendazole or mebendazole can be used for treatment.

Whipworm *(Trichuris trichuria)*

About 500 million people are infected with whipworm worldwide (Marsden 1982). The small worm (40 mm) is spread directly by fecal–oral contamination. The eggs are ingested on contaminated food and attach to the mucosa of the cecum and colon.

The infection is often asymptomatic. Heavy worm loads can lead to diarrhea, an irritable colon syndrome, and rectal prolapse. Diagnosis is made by viewing whipworm eggs in the stool. Mebendazole is effective therapy.

Pinworm *(Enterobius vermicularis)*

Pinworm is spread by fecal–oral contact among individuals in crowded areas and, particularly, among children. Infection causes uncomfortable rectal itching (pruritis ani). Diagnosis is made by identifying eggs or adult female worms on the perirectal region. This is best done by use of cellophane tape touched to the perirectal region and then attached to a glass slide for microscopic examination. Therapy is a single dose of mebendazole or pyrantel pamoate.

Flatworms

Tapeworm *(Hymenolepis nana)*

Hymenolepis nana (2 to 4 cm) is a common parasite in large pediatric populations living in areas where poor sanitation exists (Jones 1985). Transmission is by the fecal–oral route and patients are often asymptomatic. Severe infections produce diarrhea, abdominal pain, and anorexia. Some children are irritable and, rarely, have seizures (thought to be from a yet unidentified neurotoxin absorbed from the worms). Diagnosis is made by identifying the characteristic eggs in the stool (see Chapter 22). Praziquantel and niclosamide are effective. Reinfection in crowded areas is common.

Taenia sp and Diphyllobothrium latum

Tapeworm gastrointestinal infections will result from eating contaminated rare or raw beef *(Taenia saginata)*, pork *(T. solium)*, or fish *(Diphyllobothrium latum)* (Jones 1985). These diseases are not serious and cause few symptoms except colicky abdominal pain. *D. latum* may cause a megaloblastic anemia. They are diagnosed by identifying proglotids of the worm, or characteristic eggs, in the stool. Treatment is with niclosamide or praziquantel.

One serious problem occurs in the refugee setting. If some individuals in the area have *Taenia solium*, and poor sanitation allows spread through fecal–oral contamination of the intermediate stage of the infection to other humans, the disease cysticercosis develops. This is most commonly characterized by central nervous system signs and symptoms such as seizures due to the presence of small cysts throughout the tissue. Therapy is not very effective but, in some cases, praziquantel may be helpful. Treatment should be done in a hospital setting because seizures can be more severe and frequent in the first weeks after therapy is started.

Trematodes (Flukes)

Chinese liver fluke *(Clonorchis sinensis)*

The Chinese liver fluke *(Clonorchis sinensis)* is a 15-mm fluke that infects about 1 million people in the Far East. The eggs are passed in the stool and contaminate the water of communities without proper sanitary facilities. Eggs are then ingested by specific snails. Larvae hatch in the snails, are released into the water, and penetrate a specific fish. Human infection is acquired by consuming these raw or inadequately prepared infected fish. After ingestion, the larvae travel through the ampulla of Vater. The bile ducts are then the site of maturation for the adult worms.

Infection is usually asymptomatic. Moderate infections may cause fever, epigastric pain, leukocytosis, and eosinophilia. An enlarged and tender liver, low-grade fever, and episodic jaundice due to intermittent cholangitis may follow.

Diagnosis is made by identifying the eggs in feces. Stool concentration techniques may be required to increase the likelihood of detection. The drug of choice is praziquantel. Some authorities have suggested that chloroquine phosphate be used, but this only stops egg laying and, therefore, is of no value in treating the disease.

Schistosomiasis

Schistosomiasis, also called bilharziasis, affects over 200 million people worldwide (Mahmoud 1984). Three species cause various forms of the infection: *Schistosoma mansoni, S. haematobium*, and *S. japonicum*.

The life cycles of these parasites are complex. *S. haematobium* eggs leave the host's body in the urine, whereas *S. mansoni* and *S. japonicum* exit in the stool. After hatching, the larvae enter a specific freshwater snail, which serves as an intermediate host. After maturation, the free-swimming cercaria penetrates the skin of humans who swim or walk in contaminated water. Within one day of invasion of the host's skin, "swimmer's itch," a pruritic papular rash, may appear. After entering the bloodstream, schistosomule travel to the lung, the liver, and finally the abdominal mesenteric veins, where they mature and remain. *S. haematobium* migrates to vessels around the urinary bladder. The gravid female deposits her eggs in the host's venules from which the eggs migrate into the lumen of the bowel or bladder, or they move with the flow of blood to other organs.

The disease symptoms are related to the presence of the egg' in various body tissues as well as the host's inflammatory response. Patients with few worms may remain asymptomatic. For those with heavy infections, three clinical stages can be recognized. A few weeks after infection, a symptoms complex resembling serum sickness may develop. Symptoms include fever, chills, sweating, headache, and cough associated with eosinophilia in the peripheral blood. An acute enterocolitis may be seen at the time of egg migration through the bowel wall (beginning four to five weeks after infection). Months to years after the initial infection, chronic gastrointestinal or urinary tract symptoms can develop. Hepatic fibrosis can lead to symptoms of portal hypertension. *Schistosoma haematobium* infection may result in urinary tract problems including recurrent bleeding and infection, bladder stones, ureteral obstruction, and bladder malignancy.

Definitive diagnosis can be made only by identifying the eggs in stool, urine, or biopsy specimens. The most effective therapy is single-dose praziquantel or, for *S. mansoni,* oxamoquine. Complete cure is not necessary because symptoms are related to the magnitude of the worm burden and multiplication does not occur in the host. Early treatment of all those infected will prevent most major complications of the disease.

Prevention is a very important aspect of schistosomiasis control. This can be accomplished by destroying the snail intermediate host with molluscacides, preventing snail infection by constructing privies, and treating human infection.

REFERENCES

Arfaa F: Selective primary health care: strategies for control of disease in the developing world. XII. Ascariasis and trichuriasis. Rev Infect Dis 1984;6:364–73.

Gilles HM: Selective primary health care: strategies for control of disease in the developing world. XVII. Hookworm infection and anemia. Rev Infect Dis 1985;7:111–18.

Jones TC: Cestodes (tapeworms). In Mandell G, Douglas G, Bennett J (eds): Principles and Practice of Infectious Diseases, vol 2, pp 1579–83. New York, John Wiley, 1985.

Ma P, Soave R: Three-step stool examination for cryptosporidiosis in ten homosexual men with protracted diarrhea. J Infect Dis 1983;147:824.

Mahmoud AAF: Schistosomiasis. In Warren K, Mahmoud AAF (eds): Tropical and Geographical Medicine, p 443. New York, McGraw-Hill, 1984.

Marsden P: Helminthic diseases. In Wyngaarten JB, Smith LH (eds): Cecil and Loeb Textbook of Medicine. Philadelphia, WB Saunders, 1982.

Martinez-Palomo A, Martinez-Baez M: Selective primary health care: strategies for control of disease in the developing world. X. Amebiasis. Rev Infect Dis 1983;5:1093–102.

Masur H, Jones TC: Parasitic diseases. In Grieco M (ed): Infections of the Immunocompromised Patient, pp 406–37. New York, Yorke Medical Books, 1982.

Medical Letter. Drugs for parasitic infections. Med Lett Drug Ther 1982;24:2.

Ravdin J, Jones TC: Amebiasis. In Mandell G, Douglas RG, Bennett J (eds): Principles and Practice of Infectious Diseases, vol 2, pp 1506–12. New York, John Wiley, 1985.

Soave R, Ma P: Cryptosporidiosis: Traveler's diarrhea in two families. Arch Intern Med 1985;145:70–72.

Stevens DP: Selective primary health care: strategies for control of disease in the developing world. XIX. Giardiasis. Rev Infect Dis 1985;7:530–35.

Warren KS: Selective primary health care: strategies for control of disease in the developing world. I. Schistosomiasis. Rev Infect Dis 1982;4:715–26.

Wolf MS: Giardiasis. New Engl J Med 1978;298:319.

36
Urinary Tract Infections

WARREN D. JOHNSON, JR.

Urinary tract infections (UTI) are among the most common of medical problems. About 5 percent of adult women have a UTI annually, and 10 to 15 percent have an infection at some time during their lives (Kunin 1972; Kaye 1972; Sanford 1976; Andriole 1980). Infections of the urinary tract are much less common in males, except during infancy and in adults with prostatic disease. The high incidence of UTI and the relative ease with which they can be diagnosed and treated make them important in a refugee population. The approach to the diagnosis and treatment of UTI taken in this chapter assumes the availability of a light microscope and antibiotics.

Urinary tract infections are almost always caused by bacteria; viruses and fungi rarely infect the urinary tract. The term *pyelonephritis* refers to involvement of the kidney, while *cystitis* refers to bladder infections. The normal urinary tract is free of bacteria and the urine is sterile. Bacteria usually gain access to the urinary tract by the ascending route, through the urethra into the bladder and then to the ureters and the kidneys. The short length of the female urethra is the major reason that UTI is much more common in females than in males. Occasionally, bacteria may reach the urinary tract by a hematogenous route or by the lymphatics.

Enterobacteriaceae are by far the most common pathogens in the urinary tract (Stamm et al. 1982; Komaroff 1984). *Escherichia coli* accounts for over 80 percent of uncomplicated infections. *Staphylococcus saprophyticus,* which is often misidentified as *S. albus* or *S. epidermidis,* is the second most common cause of lower urinary tract infection in many series. There is an increased frequency of infections due to *Proteus, Enterobacter, Klebsiella, Pseudomonas,* and enterococci in patients with recurrent infections or those associated with either anatomic abnormalities or urethral instrumentation.

The prevalence of UTI is higher in females than males at all ages except during infancy. The latter finding is attributable to the higher prevalence of urinary tract anomalies in infant males. The prevalence of bacteriuria in girls of school age is 1.2 percent; it is 0.03 percent in boys of the same age (Kunin 1972; Kaye 1972; Gillenwater et al 1979). The prevalence of bacteriuria increases about 1 percent per decade in females. The prevalence in young, nonpregnant females is 1 to 3 percent and up to 10 percent in elderly females. Asymptomatic bacteriuria occurs in 4 to 7 percent of pregnant females and, of those, up to 20 percent will develop symptomatic pyelonephritis during their pregnancies. The prevalence of UTI is 5 to 10 percent in males of prostatic disease age.

CLINICAL MANIFESTATIONS AND DIAGNOSIS

The diagnosis and treatment of UTI in a refugee setting will necessarily be restricted to symptomatic patients, since routine urinalyses and cultures will not be performed. The epidemiology dictates that most symptomatic patients will be young females, and the most common symptoms will be dysuria and frequency. Although the prevalence of infection is highest in elderly persons, they usually constitute a small percentage of the refugee community.

The classic signs and symptoms of a urinary infection are easily recognized. Cystitis is associated with lower tract symptoms such as dysuria, frequency, urgency, and suprapubic discomfort. The urine occasionally contains blood as a result of damage to the bladder mucosa. Fever is usually absent or low grade. Acute pyelonephritis is typically associated with fever, flank pain, and symptoms of cystitis. Although useful when present, the correlation between the presence of symptoms and the finding of large numbers of bacteria in the urine ($>10^5$ bacteria per milliliter) may be poor. For example, in recent studies only 48 percent of college students with dysuria and frequency of less than three weeks duration had greater than 10^5 bacteria per milliliter of clean-catch, midstream voided urine (Stamm

Table 36-1. Etiology and Diagnoses in Female College Students with Acute Dysuria and Frequency, in the United States

Diagnosis	Percentage
Bladder bacteriuria	53
Renal bacteriuria	12
Chlamydia trachomatis infection	7
Pyelonephritis or stone	3
Vaginitis (candida, trichomonas)	7
Genital herpes virus infection	2
Other (diabetes, pregnancy)	3
No pathogen identified	13
Total	100

Table 36-3. Microscopic Quantitation of Bacteriuria

	Urine Unstained (per ml)	Urine Stained (per ml)
Unspun urine	$>10^{6a}$	$>10^{5a}$
Centrifuged urine	$>10^{5a}$	$<10^{4b}$

[a]The finding of more than one bacterium per high-power (430X) microscopic field indicates this bacterial concentration.
[b]The inability to find at least one bacterium per high-power microscopic field indicates fewer than 10^4 organisms per milliliter.

et al 1982). Of the patients with significant bacteriuria ($>10^5$ bacteria per milliliter urine), 25 percent had renal infection as determined by the presence of antibody-coated bacteria in the urine, and 75 percent had infection confined to the bladder. As shown in Table 36-1, of women with dysuria, 53 percent will be found to have bladder bacteriuria (cystitis), 12 percent renal bacteriuria (pyelonephritis), 7 percent *Chlamydia,* and 3 percent acute pyelonephritis or stone. The remaining 25 percent will have other nonbacterial causes of their infection. Thus, at least 75 percent of dysuric women have bacterial urinary tract infections that are easily treated, and over half of the infections are limited to the bladder.

The correlation between the specific signs and symptoms and the site of infection within the urinary tract may also be poor. Table 36-2 indicates that, although the classic upper tract signs and symptoms are most common in patients with bacteriuria of renal origin, they may also occur in patients with infection limited to the bladder (Sanford 1976). Conversely, about one third of patients with asymptomatic bacteriuria ($>10^5$ organisms per milliliter of urine) or with symptoms of cystitis have renal bacteriuria.

We have usually relied on urine cultures to diagnose infection of the urinary tract. However, the technology required and the expense of cultures make it unlikely that they will be available in a refugee setting. The microscopic examination of urine for the presence of bacteria detects 85 percent of all bacteriurias and is our most reliable diagnostic test after the culture (Platt 1980). The presence of at least one bacterium per high-power field in a clean-catch, midstream, Gram's-stained, uncentrifuged urine correlates with 10^5 or more bacteria per milliliter of urine (Table 36-3) (Kaye 1972; Platt 1980). Conversely, there are probably fewer than 10^4 bacteria per milliliter of urine if there is less than one bacterium per field in stained and centrifuged urine sediment.

Table 36-2. Correlation Between Symptoms and the Site of Urinary Tract Infection

Clinical Manifestations	Renal Bacteriuria (%)	Bladder Bacteriuria (%)
Symptoms and signs suggesting lower urinary tract infection:		
Frequency	98	70
Burning	68	70
Suprapubic pain	68	51
Symptoms and signs suggesting upper urinary tract infection:		
Loin pain	48	19
Fever	44	4
Rigors	32	15
Nausea and vomiting	24	8
Hematuria (macroscopic)	20	12

Urine can also be examined without staining or centrifugation if these techniques are not available. Leukocytes will be present in the urine of about two thirds of patients with UTI. Stamm et al examined uncentrifuged urine in a hemocytometer chamber and found the critical number to be eight or more white blood cells (WBC) per cubic millimeter in symptomatic patients (Stamm et al 1982). This figure corresponds to two to five WBCs per high-power field in centrifuged sediment. The absence of pyuria, particularly in asymptomatic patients, does not exclude infection.

MANAGEMENT OF SYMPTOMATIC URINARY TRACT INFECTION

The treatment goals in the management of UTI are to relieve the patient's symptoms and to prevent renal damage or the spread of infection to other sites. A number of effective and relatively nontoxic orally administered antimicrobials are available for treatment of uncomplicated UTI (Table 36-4). Sulfisoxazole, tetracycline, and ampicillin are the least expensive and most readily available agents. Most patients with symptomatic lower tract infection can be treated with a single-dose oral regimen (Wong et al 1985; Fihn & Stamm 1985). Table 36-5 presents a simplifed scheme for the management of acute dysuria and frequency in adult females. This group will constitute the majority of patients with UTI. Cure rates of greater than 90 percent are obtained in adult female patients who do not have fever, flank pain, or a history of prior UTI. The best studied single-dose regimens include sulfisoxazole (1 g), amoxicillin (3 g), and trimethoprim-sulfamethoxazole (160 mg + 800 mg in one tablet). There is no evidence to support the use of bactericidal over bacteriostatic drugs. Furthermore, it is the concentration of drug in the urine, not in the blood, that correlates best with a favorable outcome (Kunin 1972; Kaye 1972).

Table 36-4. Oral Antimicrobial Agents for Uncomplicated Urinary Tract Infections

Sulfisoxazole
Tetracycline
Ampicillin
Trimethoprim-sulfamethoxazole
Amoxicillin
Nitrofurantoin
Cephalexin

Table 36-5. Management of Dysuria and Frequency in Adult Females[a]

Single-dose antimicrobial therapy with either:
Sulfisoxazole (1 g)
Ampicillin (3 g)
Tetracycline (2.5 g)
Microscopic urine examination (bacteria, pyuria) within 1 week, or earlier if symptoms persist
Relapses or persistent infection are treated orally for 2 weeks with same antimicrobial
Reinfection (more than 2 to 4 weeks after initial infection) treated with repeat single-dose therapy
Frequent symptomatic infections (relapse or reinfections) may be reduced by antimicrobial prophylaxis but only when the drug is being administered

[a]Excludes patients with flank pain, fever, or a history of recurrent infections.

Effective therapy decreases the urine bacterial count within one to two days. A symptomatic response can occur without eradicating the infection. Therefore, a microscopic examination of the urine should be done within one week of the single-dose treatment. A majority of women with renal bacteriuria will relapse within two weeks of their single-dose therapy (Komaroff 1984). If evidence of infection persists or relapse occurs, a two-week course of oral therapy is indicated. The same drug may be used (e.g., tetracycline 250 mg every six hours) because the development of resistance is unlikely after a single dose of medication. Reinfections and recurrent infections occurring more than two to three weeks after therapy can be treated with repeat single-dose therapy. If patients have frequent symptomatic infections, they may be placed on antimicrobial prophylaxis (Komaroff 1984). One tablet of trimethoprim-sulfamethoxazole daily is very effective, but infections may recur when the antimicrobial is discontinued. Trimethoprim-sulfamethoxazole and nitrofurantoin are particularly useful in recurrent infections because resistant strains emerge less frequently than with other agents.

Patients presenting with high fever, rigors, or hypotension may have bacteremia associated with their pyelonephritis. They should be hospitalized, if possible, and treated with parenteral antibiotics, which cover the common

Table 36-6. Prevalence of Infection and Surgically Correctable Lesions in the Urinary Tract

	Prevalence of UTI Based on Urine Culture (%)[a]	Percentage of Infected Patients Recommended for IVP and Cystoscopy (%)[b]	Percentage of IVP–Cystoscopy Patients with Surgically Correctable Lesions (%)	Percentage of Infected Patients with Detectable and Surgically Correctable Urinary Tract Lesions (%)
Females				
Preschool	<4	20	60[c]	12
School age	1–2	20	10–15[c]	2–3
Adult	1–3	<1	4–5	<0.05
Elderly	30–40	10–20	1–5	1
Males				
Preschool	<0.5	100	20–35[d]	20–35
School age	<0.05	100	50–75[d]	50–75
Adult	<0.1	100	50–75	50–75
Elderly	5–10	100	8[e]	80

[a]Clean-catch, midstream urine with greater than 10^5 bacteria per milliliter of urine.
[b]Cystoscopy and intravenous pyelogram are recommended for all infected males and for females who have either persistent or relapsing infection or more than three reinfections in one year.
[c]Vesicoureteral reflux is most common but is usually not corrected unless evidence of renal damage is present.
[d]Meatal stenosis is most common; passage of catheter into the urethral orifice will correct the lesion in many patients.
[e]Prostatism is the most common abnormality.

causes of pyelonephritis. In adults, gentamicin (3 mg/kg/day) and ampicillin (6 to 8 g/day) are effective agents. If the patient has a dramatic response to therapy (afebrile within 24 hours), the gentamicin can be discontinued after one week and therapy completed with oral ampicillin (2 g/day).

Although the facilities to perform intravenous pyelography and cystoscopy are usually unavailable in the refugee setting, it is relevant to consider what diagnoses can be missed. These procedures would be recommended for females who either relapse promptly after therapy, have persistent infections, or have three or more reinfections within a one-year period (Table 36-6). Some girls, and all boys, of preschool age should have an intravenous pyelogram and cystoscopy after their first infection. Surgically correctable lesions can be detected in 2 to 12 percent of preschool and school-age girls and in 20 to 80 percent of males with UTI ($>10^5$ bacteria per milliliter of urine). The lesion in girls is usually vesicoureteral reflux, which is rarely corrected unless evidence of renal damage is present. Adult women will usually have urethral diverticula or, less likely, reflux. Meatal stenosis is the most common abnormality in boys and may be detectable on examination, especially when observing the patient's urinary stream. Passage of a catheter into the orifice of the penis may correct the stenosis. Prostatism is the most common abnormality detected in adult males. A synthesis of these prevalences and probabilities indicates that, despite the limitations in the refugee setting, optimal medical care can be provided to well over 95 percent of patients with UTI if antimicrobials and a microscope are available.

SPECIAL SITUATIONS

Pregnancy

If conditions within the refugee setting permitted a limited screening program for asymptomatic bacteriuria, pregnant women would be the highest priority. The prevalence of asymptomatic bacteriuria is highest during the first trimester of pregnancy and ranges from 4 to 7 percent. Symptomatic pyelonephritis will develop in 20 percent of these women during pregnancy. Premature delivery, morbidity, and infant mortality may result. Treatment of asymptomatic bacteriuria will reduce the occurrence of acute pyelonephritis in the pregnant female by 75 percent.

Catheters

A single catheterization will result in bacteriuria in 1 to 2 percent of patients. Bacteria gain access to the bladder within three to four days in more than 90 percent of patients with open, indwelling catheter drainage systems. It is axiomatic that, in the presence of an indwelling urinary catheter, infection is inevitable even with closed systems. These infections cannot be prevented or cured with antimicrobials as long as the catheter remains in place. Therapy is indicated for these patients only when symptoms that suggest acute pyelonephritis with potential bacteremia are present. Similarly, it is not possible for antibiotics to cure a patient with congenital or acquired abnormalities that interfere with the normal flow or urine through the urinary tract (strictures, stones). Reflux of urine from the bladder back into one or both ureters may also prevent cure.

Children

It is important to note that infants and children with UTI frequently do not have dysuria and frequency. They may present with constitutional symptoms (anorexia, malaise, irritability), with abdominal discomfort and nausea, or with fever. A urinalysis is indicated in the child with recurrent abdominal symptoms, particularly if diarrhea or vomiting are not present.

REFERENCES

Andriole VT: Current concepts of urinary tract infections. In Weinstein L, Fields BN (eds): Seminars in Infectious Diseases, vol III, pp 89–130. New York, Thieme-Stratton, 1980.

Fihn SD, Stamm WE: Interpretation and comparison of treatment studies for uncomplicated urinary tract infections in women. Rev Infect Dis 1985; 7:468–78.

Gillenwater JY, Harrison RB, Kunin CM: Natural history of bacteriuria in school girls. A long-term case control study. N Engl J Med 1979;301:396–99.

Kaye D: Urinary Tract Infection and Its Management, pp 1–290. Chicago, CV Mosby, 1972.

Komaroff AL: Acute dysuria in women. N Engl J Med 1984;310:368–75.

Kunin C: Detection, Prevention and Management of Urinary Tract Infections, pp 1–230. Philadelphia, Lea & Febiger, 1972.

Platt R: Diagnosis and management of urinary tract infections. Infect Dis Practice 1980;3:1–6.

Sanford JP: Urinary tract symptoms and infections. Annu Rev Med 1976;26:485–98.

Stamm WE et al: Diagnosis of coliform infection in acutely dysuric women. N Engl J Med 1982;307:463–68.

Wong ES et al: Management of recurrent urinary tract infections with patient-administered single-dose therapy. Ann Intern Med 1985;102:302–07.

37

Sexually Transmitted Diseases in Refugee Medicine

JONATHAN W. M. GOLD

Sexually transmitted diseases (STDs) occur throughout the world and rank as major health problems in many impoverished areas, including the refugee setting. In such areas, complications of STDs are very common and often more severe than in developed regions. Furthermore, in the refugee setting, resources for diagnosing and treating these diseases may be minimal. A careful physical examination and medical history, and knowledge of infections common to the local area may be the best diagnostic tools available. Laboratory facilities for definitive diagnosis may be nonexistent or may be limited to staining material and a microscope. Access to bacteriologic cultures and serologic tests will be very limited. This chapter discusses the diagnosis and treatment of the major STDs and associated syndromes in the refugee setting, taking into account the limited availability of laboratory facilities and medical supplies.

GONORRHEA

Neisseria gonorrhoeae is a major health problem throughout the world but is especially so in underdeveloped countries. It can cause urethritis, epididymitis, pelvic inflammatory disease (PID), perihepatitis, purulent conjunctivitis, arthritis, tenosynovitis, meningitis, proctitis, and pharyngitis. Many individuals with gonorrhea have asymptomatic infections of the urethra (males) or cervix. Without cultures, such infections may not be recognized unless symptoms of gonorrhea occur in a sexual contact. Sexual contacts of individuals with gonorrhea should be identified and treated. Coinfection with *Chlamydia trachomatis* is very common in patients with genital gonorrhea.

In males, dysuria, and urinary urgency and frequency accompanied by a purulent urethral discharge (urethritis) suggest gonorrhea, *Chlamydia* infection, or urinary tract infection. In females, urethritis is not a prominent symptom because the endocervix is the primary site of infection. Epididymitis may occur, presenting with severe pain and swelling of the epididymis.[1] Purulent conjunctivitis due to *N. gonorrhoeae* occurs in neonates born to mothers with gonorrhea, and it may also occur in adults.[2] Arthritis and tenosynovitis can occur in sexually active females with gonococcal bacteremia. The extensor tendons of the hands and large joints are typical sites. There is redness of the skin over the involved tendon, which is painful on movement. Small pustules containing intracellular gram-negative diplococci may be seen. Organisms are difficult to detect by Gram's stain or even culture of infected joint fluid. Without cultures, gonococcal meningitis is difficult to distinguish from meningococcal meningitis. Asymptomatic gonococcal anorectal infection is common in women with endocervical infection; however, proctitis may occur. Symptomatic proctitis is particularly common in homosexual men. Gonococcal pharyngitis occurs in individuals who have oral sex with an infected partner. Cultures are required to prove these diagnoses. Perihepatitis (Fitz–Hugh-Curtis syndrome) usually occurs in women infected with *N. gonorrhoeae.* Right upper quadrant pain in a patient with gonorrhea is the main symptom. *Chlamydia* infection may also cause this syndrome. A few cases have occurred in men.

Definitive diagnosis of gonococcal infection requires a laboratory capable of isolating the organisms in culture. A Gram's stain of infected material, however, is of high diagnostic

[1] In addition to the STDs *N. gonorrhoeae* and *Chlamydia,* gram-negative enteric organisms (especially *E. coli*) and *M. tuberculosis* are potential infectious causes of epididymitis.

[2] Other causes of purulent conjunctivitis include *Chlamydia, Streptococcus pneumoniae, Hemophilus,* and viruses (enteroviruses and adenoviruses).

value in cases of urethritis, epididymitis, conjunctivitis, and PID. Numerous polymorphonuclear cells with many intracellular gram-negative diplococci are seen.[3]

Oral tetracycline, 500 mg four times a day for seven days, or doxycycline, 100 mg twice a day for seven days, are effective against genital gonorrhea (and also against *Chlamydia* and *Mycoplasma*). They are also effective in pharyngeal gonorrhea but not in rectal gonorrhea. Tetracyclines are contraindicated in pregnancy. Single-dose therapy consisting of 1.0 g of probenecid taken orally followed by either 4.8 million U of procaine penicillin (2.4 million U in each buttock), 3.0 g of amoxicillin, or 3.5 g of ampicillin is effective and has the advantage of avoiding compliance problems. Concurrent *Chlamydia* infections require tetracycline therapy.

A single dose of spectinomycin, 2.0 g IM, is effective against genital and rectal gonorrhea, but not against pharyngeal gonorrhea.

Disseminated infection (arthritis, tenosynovitis, and meningitis) is treated for seven to ten days with intravenous penicillin, 10 million to 20 million U a day, or ampicillin, 2.0 g IV every four to six hours. Intravenous treatment for three days followed by oral penicillin, 500 mg four times a day, or ampicillin, 500 mg four times a day, may be used if the patient is responding well. Penicillin, 10 million to 20 million U IV plus topical penicillin, and frequent saline eyewashes are used to treat gonococcal conjunctivitis. Silver nitrate prophylaxis of all newborns prevents gonococcal conjunctivitis.

Penicillin-resistant gonococci are increasingly prevalent, especially in Southeast Asia. Tetracycline, spectinomycin, cefoxitin, and ceftriaxone are usually effective against these organisms.

SYPHILIS

Syphilis occurs throughout the world. *Treponema pallidum,* the spirochete that causes syphilis, enters through mucous membranes or abraded skin during sexual contact, or it may pass transplacentally to infect the fetus, causing congenital syphilis. The incubation period of syphilis is that period between exposure and the development of the chancre. This is usually 10 to 90 days but it may be as short as 3 days. The chancre, characteristic of primary syphilis, appears at the site of inoculation (penis, anus, vulva, cervix, mouth, tongue, etc.) as a painless papule that rapidly breaks down to form a painless, indurated, shallow, gray-based ulcer with raised edges. Usually there is only one chancre. Painless localized lymphadenopathy is present. Microscopic examination of fresh material is the best method for diagnosis of primary syphilis. The coiled motile spirochetes are seen by use of indirect lighting techniques (dark-field or phase contrast), which are usually not available in a refugee setting. Construction of an indirect light source by movement of the mirror or light source of the microscope may provide the needed contrasts to visualize the motility of these organisms. Serologic tests for syphilis are positive in only 70 percent of cases at this stage. An untreated chancre heals in 1 to 12 weeks.

Secondary syphilis occurs six weeks to six months after infection, at the time of dissemination of organisms through the body. Symptoms vary, but typically there is fever, malaise, anorexia, rash (macular, maculopapular, or even pustular), and generalized lymphadenopathy. Pharyngitis, arthralgias, and central nervous system involvement including headache, signs of meningitis, tinnitus, and visual disturbances occur in a substantial minority of patients. Uncommon manifestations include hepatitis, glomerulonephritis, and nephrotic syndrome. Serologic tests are positive in nearly 100 percent of cases at this stage, and the patient is most infectious at this time.

After this secondary stage, syphilis becomes latent: there are no signs or symptoms of illness, but infection is still present. Relapses may occur during the first four years (especially during the first year); this is early latent syphilis. During late latent syphilis (after four years) transplacental infection may occur, although sexual transmission does not.

Tertiary syphilis is a slowly progressive disease. The best known are cardiovascular syphilis, neurosyphilis, and gummas, which are inflammatory masses that can occur anywhere in the body.

Congenital syphilis is the result of transplacental infection. Infected infants have mucusitis (rhinorrhea, called snuffles), desquamative maculopapular rash, which involves the palms and soles, and osteochondritis. The secretions teem with spirochetes and are potentially infectious. It is necessary to recognize and treat syphilis in the pregnant woman prior

[3]In contrast, in so-called nonspecific urethritis (caused by *Chlamydia* or *Mycoplasma*) the Gram's stain shows polymorphonuclear leukocytes, epithelial cells, and a variety of gram-negative and gram-positive organisms.

to the fourth month of pregnancy to prevent congenital syphilis.

There are two types of serologic tests for syphilis. Nontreponemal reaginic antibody tests (VDRL, RPR, ART) measure antibody against cardiolipin. This antigen is not a part of the treponeme, and the antibody is not specific for syphilis, but is very easy to measure and is a very sensitive indicator of treponemal infection. It is not completely specific because it may be detected in a number of other illnesses including mononucleosis, malaria, intravenous drug addiction, and collagen vascular disease. The rapid plasma reagin (RPR) test is a card test that may be available in refugee situations. Specific treponemal tests (FTA-abs, MHA-TP, TPI) are more difficult to perform but are specific since they measure antibody directed against treponemal antigens. Reaginic antibody tests are positive in 70 to 80 percent of cases of primary syphilis, and in nearly 100 percent of cases of secondary syphilis and early latent syphilis. They may become negative in late syphilis after many years, even if untreated. With treatment, nontreponemal antibody titers decline to negative or very low levels. In contrast, specific treponemal tests remain positive for life in most individuals. Both types of antibody are induced by other treponemal diseases that occur in the tropics, such as yaws, pinta, and bejel. (See Chapter 22 for further discussion of serologic tests for syphilis.)

Treatment of primary, secondary, and early latent syphilis (less than one year) is by injection of a single dose of benzathine penicillin, 2.4 million U IM, or by use of procaine penicillin, 600,000 U per day for eight days. Syphilis of more than one year's duration, late latent syphilis, and tertiary syphilis (except neurosyphilis) are treated with 2.4 million U of benzathine penicillin given intramuscularly each week for three weeks (total dose, 7.2 million U). This is the treatment given to individuals with positive serologic tests for syphilis who were not treated previously. Neurosyphilis, documented by a positive cerebrospinal fluid (CSF) serology, was formerly treated with the three-dose regimen of benzathine penicillin. This is probably quite effective; however, the currently recommended treatment is penicillin G, 2.0 million to 4.0 million U IV every four hours for ten days. Other possible regimens include procaine penicillin, 2.4 million U IM daily for ten days with 500 mg of probenecid daily (it is unlikely that the buttocks of many individuals will tolerate this). Individuals treated for syphilis may experience fever, chills, malaise, and other discomforts within 24 hours of treatment (Herxheimer reaction).

Pregnant women with syphilis are treated with penicillin as outlined above. Congenital syphilis is treated with 50,000 U/kg of penicillin G in two divided doses daily for ten days, or with procaine penicillin G, 50,000 U/kg IM daily for ten days.

Penicillin-allergic patients may be treated with tetracycline, 500 mg four times daily, or erythromycin, 500 mg four times daily. The duration of treatment is 15 days for primary, secondary, and early latent syphilis, and 30 days for late latent or tertiary syphilis. Tetracycline should not be given to pregnant women. Erythromycin is used to treat syphilis in penicillin-allergic pregnant women, but infants born to these women should be treated with penicillin after birth since penicillin is the only effective treatment of the infected neonate.

Regimens for gonorrhea are effective treatments of syphilis during the incubation period. This is important because coinfection with gonorrhea and syphilis is common.

HERPES

There are two strains of herpes simplex virus, types I and II, either of which can cause herpes labialis (fever blisters, cold sores) or herpes progenitalis (genital herpes). Genital herpes is usually caused by the type II virus. It is characterized by red-based vesicles that recur at intervals varying from weeks to many years. Itching and burning typically occur in the affected area before eruption of the vesicles. Usually there are several vesicles.

Primary herpes simplex infections may be associated with fever, rigors, lymphadenopathy, meningismus, and urinary retention. The characteristic history of recurrent lesions is highly suggestive of herpes, although other infections (including syphilis and chancroid) must be considered. In the refugee situation, viral cultures will certainly be unavailable. A Wright's or Giemsa stain of material from the base of the vesicle may show characteristic multinucleated giant cells.

The lesions require no treatment. Sexual relations must be avoided until the lesions heal to prevent transmission. If available, acyclovir ointment applied five or six times a day with a finger cot may decrease the duration of symptoms. In pregnant women, active genital herpes simplex infection at the time of delivery is an indication for cesarean section to prevent devastating neonatal infection.

CHANCROID

Chancroid is caused by *Hemophilus ducreyi,* a gram-negative coccobacillus. Chancroid is characteristically a small, sharply demarcated ulcer that, in contrast with the chancre of syphilis, is very painful, bleeds easily, and is not indurated. Most cases are recognized in men, but women with chancroid are often asymptomatic and may infect many individuals unless the infection is diagnosed and treated. The incubation period after exposure is usually short (typically 2 to 5 days, but it may range from 1 to 14 days). The lesion starts as a papule that becomes a pustule and breaks down to form the ulcer. There is usually one ulcer, but there may be more. Painful unilateral adenopathy is characteristic.

The diagnosis of chancroid is confirmed by a Gram's stain of the ulcer (which may be difficult to interpret) or of material aspirated from an involved lymph node (which is usually easier to interpret). The Gram's stain shows large numbers of gram-negative coccobacilli in a "school of fish" pattern.

Treatment is with trimethoprim-sulfamethoxazole (160 mg of trimethoprim, 800 mg of sulfamethoxazole twice daily for ten days); or with erythromycin, 500 mg four times daily for ten days. Fluctuant nodes should be aspirated. Sexual partners should also be treated.

CHLAMYDIAL INFECTIONS

Different immunotypes of *Chlamydia trachomatis* are responsible for nongonococcal urethritis, proctitis, and lymphogranuloma venereum, which are major STDs. Perinatal pneumonia and inclusion body conjunctivitis due to this organism are acquired during passage through the birth canal of an infected mother. Trachoma, a major cause of blindness, is also caused by *C. trachomatis.* Trachoma is not sexually transmitted but is spread in unsanitary conditions by flies and by eye rubbing with dirty hands.

In males, *C. trachomatis* causes urethritis and epididymitis. In homosexual men it also causes proctitis. In women it can cause urethritis, cervicitis (which may be asymptomatic), and PID. Coinfection with *N. gonorrhoeae* is common in patients with urethritis or epididymitis.

Definitive diagnosis of chlamydial infection is made by culture or by immunofluorescence to detect the organisms. A Gram's stain of urethral discharge can be characteristic. Polymorphonuclear leukocytes are seen with a variety of gram-positive and gram-negative cocci and bacilli.[4]

The treatment of nongonococcal urethritis and other genitourinary infections due to *Chlamydia* is oral tetracycline, 500 mg four times a day for seven days, or doxycycline, 100 mg twice a day for seven days. Erythromycin, 500 mg four times a day for seven days, or sulfisoxazole, 500 mg four times a day for ten days, are also effective. (See the section on treatment of PID.)

Lymphogranuloma venereum (LGV) is endemic in Asia, Africa, and South America. It is caused by certain specific serotypes of *C. trachomatis.* The disease consists of three phases. The first phase is characterized by the primary lesion (frequently not recognized), a painless papule, vesicle, or ulceration occurring in the genital, perineal, or rectal area within three weeks of exposure. This is followed by the characteristic regional adenopathy (two to six weeks after infection) consisting of painfully enlarged inguinal nodes that become matted. Overlying skin becomes fixed and then breaks down as the nodes suppurate. The "groove sign" is produced by the inguinal ligament surrounded on either side by swollen tissue. This second stage is sometimes accompanied by signs of systemic illness including fever, chills, anorexia, headache, and arthralgias. The third stage is characterized by the formation of scar tissue with strictures, ulcerations, and fistulas in the perineum, scrotum, urethra, and rectal area.

In the refugee setting, a presumptive diagnosis of LGV is frequently made from the clinical picture. Definitive diagnosis of LGV requires serologic testing or isolation of *Chlamydia* from the lesion.

Drugs used in the treatment of LGV are given for at least 14 days. Drugs that may be used include oral tetracycline, 500 mg four times a day; erythromycin, 500 mg four times a day; and sulfa drugs such as sulfamethoxa-

[4]In contrast, a Gram's stain of the urethral smear in gonorrhea shows numerous gram-negative intracellular diplococci.

zole alone, 1.0 g twice a day, or trimethoprim-sulfamethoxazole, 160 mg/800 mg twice a day. Fluctuant nodes are drained with a needle and syringe. The response to treatment is not dramatic. Symptoms improve, but the lesions heal slowly. Surgical correction of strictures and fistulas may be necessary.

GRANULOMA INGUINALE

Granuloma inguinale (donovanosis) is especially common in India, New Guinea, central Australia, and the Caribbean. It is caused by *Calymmatobacterium granulomatis,* a gram-negative rod that, on Wright's stain, has bipolar staining resembling a safety pin. Large mononuclear cells filled wtih these organisms are characteristic. The lesions start as nodules, which break down in the genital, inguinal, and perianal regions to form beefy, exuberant ulcers. Diagnosis is confirmed by finding the Donovan bodies in Wright's or Giemsa stains of a small piece of freshly excised infected tissue.

Treatments include oral tetracycline, 500 mg every six hours; erythromycin, 500 mg every six hours; or chloramphenicol, 500 mg every eight hours. Gentamicin, streptomycin, and trimethoprim-sulfamethoxazole are also effective. Treatment with any drug is continued until the ulcers heal (at least three weeks).

COMMON SEXUALLY TRANSMITTED DISEASE SYNDROMES

As noted earlier, when laboratory facilities are limited, the diagnosis of STDs is based on physical examination, medical history, and knowledge of infections that are prevalent in the region. Specific infections may be endemic in the refugee camp. The accuracy of diagnosis can be improved if there is access to a microscope with Gram's and Wright's stains. These methods also apply to the diagnosis of syndromes that occur in association with STDs. These syndromes include urethral discharge, genital ulcers with or without lymphadenopathy, and pelvic inflammatory disease. Conjunctivitis (caused by *N. gonorrhoeae* or *C. trachomatis*) and congenital and neonatal infections (such as syphilis and herpes simplex) are important consequences of some STDs; they were discussed earlier in this chapter and elsewhere in this book.

Urethral Discharge

Gonorrhea and infection with *Chlamydia* and *Mycoplasma* are associated with urethritis, which is most easily recognized in males. The discharge in gonorrhea is generally more purulent and associated with more severe dysuria than that of nonspecific urethritis. The Gram's stain of the urethral discharge in gonorrhea shows numerous polymorphonuclear cells with many intracellular gram-negative diplococci. In nonspecific urethritis (caused by *Chlamydia* or *Mycoplasma*), the Gram's stain shows polymorphonuclear leukocytes, epithelial cells, and a variety of gram-negative and sometimes gram-positive organisms. Urinalysis and Gram's stain will help distinguish urinary tract infections. Tetracycline, 500 mg four times a day for seven days, or doxycycline, 100 mg twice a day for at least seven days, are effective treatments for all three infections.

Genital Ulcers and Lymphadenopathy

Genital ulcers may be due to trauma or to a variety of STDs. In many cases, it is possible to be reasonably certain of the cause, but presentations are not always clear-cut. Patients with herpes simplex have the characteristic red-based, painful vesicles that recur and are frequently preceded by itching or burning. The chancre of syphilis is usually painless with a firm base, does not bleed, and is accompanied by painless inguinal lymphadenopathy. Chancroid is a small, very painful ulcer with a non-indurated base that bleeds easily and may be associated with painful lymph nodes, which become fluctuant. Lymphogranuloma venereum (LGV) is associated with painfully enlarged nodes that become matted and start to drain, producing sinuses. The ulcers of granuloma inguinale are beefy and indurated.

Microscopic examination may reveal viral inclusions of herpes simplex (on Wright's or Giemsa stain), pleomorphic gram-negative coccobacilli characteristic of chancroid (on Gram's stain), intracellular safety-pinlike inclusions (Donovan bodies) seen in snips of affected tissue in granuloma inguinale (on Wright's or Giemsa stain). Identification of the spirochete that causes syphilis requires dark-field examinations or special silver stains that are probably unavailable in the refugee setting.

The treatment of each infection is discussed above. Herpes simplex ulcers do not require treatment. If ulcers do not resolve within a week, consideration should be given to treatment for syphilis or chancroid. When ulcers are associated with suppurative nodes, the nodes should be aspirated through healthy skin and treatment with trimethoprim-sulfamethoxazole (one double-strength tablet twice a day) or tetracycline, 500 mg four times a day, should be given for one week. If they do not resolve, further evaluation is necessary. Consideration should be given to treatment for syphilis in all ulcerative lesions that do not respond. The patient's sexual contacts should also be treated.

Pelvic Inflammatory Disease

Pelvic inflammatory disease (PID) is responsible for severe discomfort and may lead to sterility. Severe, acute lower abdominal pain and excruciating pain on moving the cervix and on adnexal palpation (often impossible because of the pain) are characteristic. Ruptured ectopic pregnancy, appendicitis, peritonitis, and pelvic abscesses must be considered in the differential diagnosis. A Gram's stain of purulent cervical discharge showing intracellular gram-negative diplococci suggests that the patient has gonorrhea. However, the microbiology of PID may be complicated, and the syndrome can also be caused by *Chlamydia,* gram-negative enteric bacteria, and anaerobic bacteria.

Current recommendations for treatment of PID include procaine penicillin, ampicillin, or amoxicillin, as described for uncomplicated gonorrhea with the addition of 1.0 g of probenecid. If available, a single dose of cefoxitin, 2.0 g IM, can be used. This is followed by doxycycline, 100 mg orally twice a day for 10 to 14 days. More seriously ill patients require individualized, intravenous therapy.

OTHER SEXUALLY TRANSMITTED DISEASES

A number of other diseases are considered to be sexually transmitted under certain circumstances. Hepatitis, amebiasis, salmonellosis, shigellosis, giardiasis, and campylobacteriosis are sexually transmitted, especially among homosexual men. Scabies, pubic lice, and body lice can be transmitted during intimate contact. These illnesses are discussed elsewhere in this book.

Acquired immune deficiency syndrome (AIDS) is caused by a newly discovered retrovirus (human T-lymphotropic-III or lymphadenopathy-associated virus). In the United States and Europe, most cases have occurred in homosexual men and intravenous drug abusers. However, in underdeveloped countries, especially in Haiti and Central Africa where AIDS is also endemic, cases are spread heterosexually as well. AIDS is characterized by a profound loss of immune function, which renders patients very susceptible to tumors (Kaposi's sarcoma) and infections including pneumonia and to gastrointestinal, central nervous system, and systemic infections. The diagnosis of these complications requires sophisticated laboratory facilities; thus, diagnosis of AIDS in the refugee setting may be difficult.

REFERENCES

Holmes KK (ed): Sexually Transmitted Diseases. New York, McGraw-Hill, 1984.

King M (ed): Medical Care in Developing Countries. London, Oxford University Press, 1966.

Mandell GL, Douglas RG, Bennett J (eds): Principles and Practice of Infectious Diseases, 2nd ed. New York, John Wiley, 1985.

Meheuz AZ: Practical approaches in developing nations. In Holmes KK (ed): Sexually Transmitted Diseases, pp 998–1008. New York, McGraw-Hill, 1984.

Morbidity and Mortality Reports: Sexually transmitted diseases treatment guidelines 1982. MMWR; 31(Suppl):33–60.

St John RK, Brown ST, Tyler CW: Pelvic inflammatory disease. Am J Obstet Gynecol 1980;138:845–47.

World Health Organization: *Neisseria gonorrhoeae* and gonococcal infections. WHO Technical Report Series No 616. Geneva, World Health Organization, 1981.

World Health Organization: Social and health aspects of sexually transmitted diseases: Principles of control measures. WHO Public Health Paper No 65. Geneva, World Health Organization, 1977.

APPENDIX A
Periodicals and Other Resources

This appendix is meant to supplement the references and suggested reading sections provided at the end of each chapter. The reader is referred especially to the end of Chapter 1, which provides an extensive list of useful reading material on refugee and international health care.

Appropriate Technology. London, Intermediate Technology Publications Ltd.
Bulletin of the World Health Organization. Geneva, World Health Organization.
Diarrhea Dialogue. London, Appropriate Health Resources Technology Action Group (AHRTAG).
Disaster Preparedness in the Americas. Washington, DC, Pan American Health Organization.
Disasters: The International Journal of Disaster Studies and Practice. London, International Disaster Institute.
Glimpse. Dacca, International Centre for Diarrheal Disease Research.
International Health News. Washington, DC, National Council of International Health.
Medical File. London, International Planned Parenthood Federation.
Population Reports. Baltimore, The Johns Hopkins University.
Refugee Abstracts. Geneva, International Refugee Integration Resource Centre.
Refugee Reports. Washington, DC, American Council for Nationalities Service.
Refugees. Geneva, United Nations High Commission on Refugees.
Salubritas. Washington, DC, American Public Health Association and the World Federation of Public Health Associations.
Tropical Doctor. London, Royal Society of Medicine.
UNHCR Information. Geneva, United Nations High Commission on Refugees.
WHO Chronicle. Geneva, World Health Organization.
World Health Forum. Geneva, World Health Organization.

MISCELLANEOUS RESOURCES

Army Handbook of Practical Radiography. London, Her Majesty's Stationary Office, 1963.
The Refugee Child and the Child-to-Child Programme. London, Institute of Child Health, undated.
Seaman J (ed): List of suppliers. Disasters 1981;5:327–32. Lists names and addresses of suppliers of assorted useful equipment for disaster relief operations or refugee camps.
Walsh JA, Warren KS: Strategies for Primary Health Care. Technologies Appropriate for the Control of Disease in the Developing World. Chicago, University of Chicago Press, 1986.
Warren KS, Mahmoud AA (eds): Geographic Medicine for the Practitioner: Algorithms in the Diagnosis and Management of Exotic Diseases. Chicago, University of Chicago Press, 1978.
Wood E: Community Health Worker's Manual. Nairobi, African Medical and Research Foundation, 1982.

Transparency Teaching Sets. Below is a partial list of the slide teaching sets available from Teaching Aids at Low Cost (TALC), 30 Guilford St, London WC1N 1EH, UK:

- Childhood development in African children
- Charting growth in small children
- Common skin diseases of children in the tropics
- Communication in health (ways for a health worker to improve communication)
- Diarrhoea management
- Foods of West Africa
- Helminths
- Microscopic diagnosis of tropical diseases
- Malnutrition
- Management in child health
- Management of severe kwashiorkor
- Nutrition rehabilitation
- Primary child care (ten sets of slides to be used with M. King's book: *Primary Child Care*)
- Protein-calorie deficiency
- Xerophthalmia

APPENDIX B
Organizations

African Medical and Research Foundation, Nairobi, Kenya.
Agency for International Development (AID), Center for Development Information and Evaluation, Rm 209, SA 18, Washington, DC 20523.
American Council for Nationalities Service, 815 15th St NW No 610, Washington, DC 20005.
American Friends Service Committee, 1501 Cherry St, Philadelphia, PA 19102.
American Public Health Association, 1015 15th St NW, Washington, DC 20005.
American Refugee Committee, 310 4th Ave S, Rm 410, Minneapolis, MN 55415.
Appropriate Health Resources Technology Action Group (AHRTAG), 85 Marylebone High St, London W1M 3DE, UK.
Australian Counter Disaster College, Mount Macedon, Victoria 3441, Australia.
British Leprosy Relief Association, Slade Hospital, Headington, Oxford OX3 7JH, UK.
Bureau for Overseas Medical Service, London School of Hygiene and Tropical Medicine, Keppel St, London WC1 7HT, UK.
CAMA Services, PO Box C, Nyack, New York, NY 10960.
CARE, 660 First Ave, New York, NY 10016.
Caritas Internationalis, Palazzo San Calisto 16, 00120 Rome, Italy.
Catholic Relief Services (CRS), 1011 1st Ave, New York, NY 10022.
Center for Immigration Policy and Refugee Assistance, Georgetown University, Washington, DC.
Center for Population and Health, Columbia University Medical Center, 60 Haven Ave, New York, NY 10032.
Centers for Disease Control (CDC), US Department of Health and Human Services, Atlanta, GA 30333.
Centre for Disaster Studies, James Cook University of North Queensland, Townsville, Queensland 4811, Australia.
Centre for World Development Education, 128 Buckingham Palace Rd, London SW1 W9SH, UK.
Church World Service, 475 Riverside Dr, New York, NY 10115.
Concern, 1 Upper Camden St, Dublin 2, Republic of Ireland.
Cornell Medical Center, Division of International Medicine, 525 E 68th St, New York, NY 10021.
Disaster Management Center, University of Wisconsin-Extension, 432 N Lake St, Madison, WI 53706.
Emergency Relief Office, World Health Organization, 20 Ave Appia, 1211 Geneva 27, Switzerland.
Federal Emergency Management Agency (FEMA), Emergency Management Institute, National Emergency Training Center, 16825 S Seton Ave, Emmitsburg, MD 21717.
Food and Agriculture Organization of the United Nations (FAO), Via delle Terme di Caracalla, 1-000100 Rome, Italy.
Hellen Keller International, 15 W 16th St, New York, NY 10011.
Hesperian Foundation, PO Box 1692, Palo Alto, CA 94302.
Indochinese Language Resource Center, 1607 NE 41 Ave, Portland, OR 97323.
Institute for Child Health, 30 Guilford St, London WC1, UK.
Institute for Food and Development Policy, 2588 Mission St, San Francisco, CA 94110.
INTERACTION (American Council for Voluntary International Action), 200 Park Ave S, New York, NY 10003.
Intermediate Technology Publications, 9 King St, London WC2E 8HN, UK.
International Centre for Eye Health, 27–29 Cayton St, London EC1V9EJ, UK.
International Committee of the Red Cross (ICRC), Medical Division, 17 Avenue de la Paix, CH 1211 Geneva, Switzerland.
International Development Research Centre, PO Box 8500, Ottawa K1G 3H9, Canada.
International Development Services, Control Data Co, PO Box 0, Minneapolis, MN 55440.
International Disaster Institute, 85 Marylebone High St, London W1M 3DE, UK.
International Health Programs Project, American Public Health Association, 1015 15th St NW, Washington, DC 20005.
International Planned Parenthood Federation, 18–20 Lower Regent St, London SW1Y 4PW, UK.
International Refugee Integration Resource Center, 5–7 Ave de la Paix, 1211 Geneva 10, Switzerland.
International Rescue Committee (IRC), 386 Park Ave S, New York, NY 10016.
INTERTECT, PO Box 10502, Dallas, TX 75207.
Johns Hopkins University, School of Hygiene and Public Health, 615 N Wolfe St, Baltimore, MD 21205.
Liverpool School of Tropical Medicine, Pembroke Place, Liverpool L3 5QA, UK.

Medecins Sans Frontieres (MSF), 161 Boulevard Lefebvre, 75015 Paris, France.
MEDEX Group, University of Hawaii, 1833 Kalakaua Ave No 700, Honolulu, HA 96815.
Medical Missionary Association, 6 Canonbury Pl, London N12NJ, UK.
Mennonite Central Committee, 21 South 12th St, Akron, PA 17501.
Minnesota International Health Volunteers, 122 W Franklin Ave, Rm 5, Minneapolis, MN 55404.
National Council for International Health, 2100 Pennsylvania Ave NW No 740, Washington, DC 20037.
Operation California, 336 Foothill Rd No 1, Beverly Hills, CA 90210.
Operation Handicapp Internationale, 1 Impasse de l'Aigas, 69160 Tassin La Demi Lune, Lyon, France.
Overseas Development Council, West End Station, PO Box 57465, Washington, DC 20037.
OXFAM, 274 Banbury Road, Oxford OX2 7DZ, UK.
OXFAM America, 115 Broadway, Boston, MA 02116.
Oxford Polytechnic, Headington, Oxford, OX3 OBP, UK.
Oxford University Press, 200 Madison Ave, New York, NY 10016.
Pan American Health Organization, 525 23rd St NW, Washington, DC 20037.
Peace Corps, 806 Connecticut Ave NW, Washington, DC 20525.
POPLINE (Population Information Online), Population Information Program, The Johns Hopkins University, 624 N Broadway, Baltimore, MD 21205.
Primary Health Care Operations Research (PRICOR), 5530 Wisconsin Ave, Chevy Chase, MD 20815.
Public Health International of Oregon, PO Box 116, Roseburg, OR 97470.
Redd Barna, Lilletroget 1, Oslo 1, Norway.
Refugee International, 220 I St NE No 240, Washington, DC 20002.
Rescue Now, 870 Market St, San Francisco, CA 94102.
Ross Institute of Tropical Hygiene, London School of Hygiene and Tropical Medicine, Keppel St, London WC1 7HT, UK.
Save the Children Federation, 48 Wilton Rd, Westport, CT 06880.
Seventh-Day Adventist World Service, 6840 Eastern Ave NW, Washington, DC 20012.
Teaching Aids at Low Cost (TALC), 30 Guilford St, London WC1N 1EH, UK.
Tear Fund, 11 Station Rd, Teddington, Middlesex TW11 9AA, UK.
Tulane University School of Public Health, New Orleans, LA 70122.
United Nations Children's Fund (UNICEF), Palais des Nations, 1211 Geneva 10, Switzerland.
United Nations Disaster Relief Office (UNDRO), Palais des Nations, 1211 Geneva 10, Switzerland.
United Nations High Committee on Refugees (UNHCR), Palais des Nations, 1211 Geneva 10, Switzerland.
US Committee for Refugees, 20 W 40th St, New York, NY 10018.
US Department of State, 2201 C St NW, Washington, DC 20520.
Voluntary Service Overseas, 9 Belgrave Sq, London SWIX 8PW, UK.
Water and Sanitation for Health Project (WASH), 1611 N Kent St, Rm 1002, Arlington, VA 22209.
World Bank, 1818 H St NW, Washington, DC 20433.
World Concern, PO Box 33000, Seattle, WA 98133.
World Health Organization, 1211 Geneva 27, Switzerland.
World Vision International, 919 W Huntington Dr, Monrovia, CA 91016.
Worldwatch Institute, 1776 Massachusetts Ave, Washington, DC 20036.

APPENDIX C
Geographic Distribution of Communicable Diseases of Importance in Refugee Health Care

This appendix is designed to aid the health worker in the process of differential diagnosis by providing information on the regional distribution of common infectious diseases in the tropics and subtropics. The information included here must be supplemented by early assessment of disease distribution patterns in the area of refugee homeland and resettlement site. The Centers for Disease Control can also be contacted for up-to-date information on the prevalence of infectious diseases in a given region. As indicated in Chapter 22, this information will play a vital role in the differential diagnostic process, particularly in the absence of laboratory specific diagnostic facilities.

I. Communicable diseases in poor, crowded, migratory populations throughout the world:
  A. Viral and rickettsial diseases
    • Infectious hepatitis, some forms of typhus or spotted fever, some types of arthropod-borne virus, rabies.
  B. Bacterial diseases
    • Typhoid fever, shigellosis, leptospirosis, tuberculosis, brucellosis, meningococcus, anthrax, leprosy, diphtheria, trachoma.
  C. Fungi
    • Cutaneous mycoses.
  D. Protozoa
    • Amebiasis, malaria, giardiasis.
  E. Helminths
    • Ascariasis, strongyloidiasis, hookworm, hymenolepiasis, trichuriasis, enterobiasis.

II. Diseases of importance in specific geographic areas including Asia and Oceania, Central America, South America, Africa, Southern Europe, and Eastern Europe:
  A. Oceania (Pacific Islands)
    Viral and rickettsial diseases
    • Japanese B encephalitis, dengue fever, endemic and murine typhus, Q fever.
    Bacterial diseases
    • Leprosy
    Helminthic diseases
    • Paragonimiasis, eosinophilic meningitis, filariasis.
  B. East Asia
    Viral and rickettsial diseases
    • Japanese B encephalitis, dengue fever, hemorrhagic fever, scrub typhus.
    Bacterial diseases
    • Cholera, plague, tularemia.
    Fungal diseases
    • Histoplasmosis.
    Protozoal diseases
    • Visceral and cutaneous leishmaniasis.
    Helminthic diseases
    • Trichostrongyliasis, schistosomiasis japonicum, fasciolopsiasis, paragonimiasis, eosinophilic meningitis.
  C. Southeast Asia
    Viral and rickettsial diseases
    • Japanese B encephalitis, dengue fever, Sindbis, West Nile and chikungunya fever, scrub typhus.
    Bacterial diseases
    • Cholera, leprosy, plague.
    Fungal diseases

- Histoplasmosis.

Helminthic diseases
- Paragonimiasis, filariasis, eosinophilic meningitis, schistosomiasis japonicum.

D. Central Asia

Viral and rickettsial diseases
- Dengue fever, hemorrhagic fever, *Phlebotomus* fever, endemic typhus, scrub typhus, epidemic typhus.

Bacterial diseases
- Cholera, leprosy, borrelliosis, yaws, bejel.

Fungal diseases
- Maduromycosis.

Protozoal diseases
- Cutaneous and visceral leishmaniasis.

Helminthic diseases
- Dracunculiasis, filariasis, paragonimiasis.

E. West Asia

Viral and rickettsial diseases
- Phlebotomus, Sindbis and West Nile fever, scrub and murine typhus.

Bacterial diseases
- Cutaneous leishmaniasis.

Helminthic diseases
- Fascioliasis, echinococcosis, dracunculiasis, schistosomiasis.

F. Northern Africa

Viral and rickettsial diseases
- Phlebotomus fever, West Nile fever, epidemic typhus, boutonneuse fever.

Bacterial diseases
- Borrelliosis, leprosy.

Fungal diseases
- Histoplasmosis, maduromycosis.

Protozoal diseases
- Cutaneous and visceral leishmaniasis.

Helminthic diseases
- Schistosomiasis, filariasis.

G. East and West Central Africa

Viral and rickettsial diseases
- Yellow fever, chikungunya fever, dengue fever, Rift Valley fever, lassa fever, epidemic and murine typhus.

Bacterial diseases
- Borrelliosis, leprosy, yaws.

Protozoal diseases
- Cutaneous and visceral leishmaniasis, African trypanosomiasis.

Helminthic diseases
- Onchocerciasis, loiasis, filariasis, dracunculiasis, schistosomiasis, cysticercosis.

H. Central America and the Caribbean

Viral and rickettsial diseases
- Dengue fever, Venezuelan equine encephalitis, murine typhus.

Bacterial diseases
- Borrelliosis.

Fungal diseases
- Cutaneous leishmaniasis, Chagas' disease.

Helminthic diseases
- Onchocerciasis, filariasis, cysticercosis.

I. South America

Viral and rickettsial diseases
- Yellow fever, dengue fever, Venezuelan equine encephalitis, hemorrhagic fever, murine typhus, tick-borne spotted fever, epidemic typhus.

Bacterial diseases
- Borrelliosis, leprosy, plague, pinta, yaws.

Fungal diseases
- Coccidioidomycosis, paracoccidioidomycosis, histoplasmosis.

Protozoal diseases
- Chagas' disease, mucocutaneous and visceral leishmaniasis.

Helminthic diseases
- Schistosomiasis mansoni, paragonimiasis, filariasis, onchocerciasis, echinococcosis, cysticercosis.

J. Southern and Eastern Europe

Viral and rickettsial diseases

- West Nile fever, hemorrhagic fever, *Phlebotomus* fever, tick-borne encephalitis, Q fever, murine typhus.

Protozoal diseases

- Visceral and cutaneous leishmaniasis.

Helminthic diseases

- Fascioliasis, echinococcosis.

Index